EXTRANODAL LYMPHOMAS

EXTRANODAL LYMPHOMAS

Judith A. Ferry, MD

Associate Professor of Pathology

Massachusetts General Hospital

Boston, Massachusetts

1600 John F. Kennedy Blvd.
Ste 1800
Philadelphia, PA 19103-2899

Notice

Knowledge and best practice in this field are constantly changing. As new research and
experience broaden our understanding, changes in research methods, professional practices,
or medical treatment may become necessary.

Practitioners and researchers must always rely on their own experience and knowledge
in evaluating and using any information, methods, compounds, or experiments described
herein. In using such information or methods, they should be mindful of their own safety and
the safety of others, including parties for whom they have a professional responsibility.

With respect to any drug or pharmaceutical products identified, readers are advised to check
the most current information provided (i) on procedures featured or (ii) by the manufacturer
of each product to be administered, to verify the recommended dose or formula, the method
and duration of administration, and contraindications. It is the responsibility of practitioners, relying on their own experience and knowledge of their patients, to make diagnoses,
to determine dosages and the best treatment for each individual patient, and to take all
appropriate safety precautions.

To the fullest extent of the law, neither the Publisher nor the authors, contributors, or
editors assume any liability for any injury and/or damage to persons or property as a matter
of products liability, negligence or otherwise, or from any use or operation of any methods,
products, instructions, or ideas contained in the material herein.

International Standard Book Number   978-1-4160-4579-3

Executive Publisher: William R. Schmitt
Developmental Editor: Kathryn DeFrancesco
Publishing Services Manager: Anne Altepeter
Senior Project Manager: Cheryl A. Abbott
Design Direction: Ellen Zanolle

Printed in Canada

Last digit is the print number: 9 8 7 6 5 4 3 2 1

For my father, Dr. John F. Ferry,
and my daughters, Debbie and Cindy

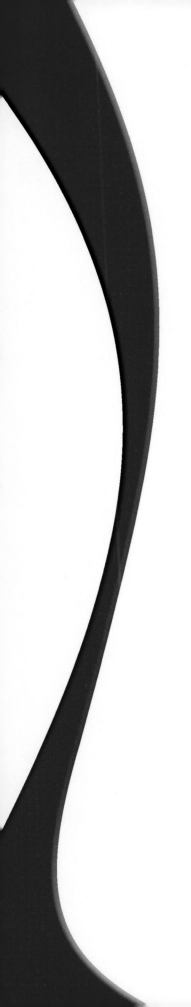

CONTRIBUTORS

Johanna L. Baran, MD
Dermatopathology Fellow
Department of Pathology
Massachusetts General Hospital
Boston, Massachusetts

Lyn M. Duncan, MD
Associate Professor of Pathology
Massachusetts General Hospital
Boston, Massachusetts

Judith A. Ferry, MD
Associate Professor of Pathology
Massachusetts General Hospital
Boston, Massachusetts

Robert P. Hasserjian, MD
Associate Professor of Pathology
Massachusetts General Hospital
Boston, Massachusetts

Aliyah Rahemtullah Sohani, MD
Assistant Professor of Pathology
Massachusetts General Hospital
Boston, Massachusetts

Lawrence R. Zukerberg, MD
Associate Professor of Pathology
Massachusetts General Hospital
Boston, Massachusetts

PREFACE

My interest in extranodal lymphomas dates back to my early years as a staff pathologist in the James Homer Wright Pathology Laboratories of the Massachusetts General Hospital, before our department was as subspecialized as it is today, and when I signed out general surgical pathology but had a focus on gynecologic pathology as well as hematopathology. Because of this unusual combination of special interests, I was often asked to review cases of female genital tract lymphomas and lymphoid infiltrates. An idiosyncrasy of our department was that testicular tumors were handled by the gynecologic pathology service, so I also had the opportunity to review many cases of testicular lymphoma. It soon became apparent that ovarian lymphomas have clinical and pathologic features that differ from those of lymphomas arising in the uterine cervix, that testicular lymphomas have their own set of distinctive features, and that the differential diagnosis of lymphoma differs greatly, depending on which of these sites is involved. This intriguing information gave rise to my interest in any and all extranodal lymphomas. Given the differences among lymphomas encountered in different sites, I decided to organize this book according to anatomic sites.

I would like to express my deep appreciation for the assistance and efforts of the many people who have made this book possible. During my years at the Massachusetts General Hospital, I have had the opportunity to receive teaching and guidance from masters in the field of pathology, most notably Drs. Nancy L. Harris, Robert E. Scully, and Robert H. Young. Without their help over the years, I doubt this book would have ever come into existence, and I thank them.

When I first thought of undertaking this project, Dr. Young encouraged me and found me a willing publisher. My goal was to have a book written exclusively by pathologists from the Massachusetts General Hospital, and so I am grateful to the members of the hematopathology and the dermatopathology units who have contributed chapters to this book. My staff and colleagues in the pathology department, our fellows, the residents rotating through hematopathology, and our clinical colleagues have also been a great source of interesting cases, intellectual stimulation, moral support, and camaraderie over the years.

I am indebted to our department's photographers, Michelle Lee and Stephen Conley, for their assistance with this book's images. I also appreciate the work of the technologists who have prepared our slides over the years. Special thanks go to Sharon Campbell, who prepared more of the immunohistochemical stains illustrated than anyone else. I also thank my assistant, Linda Arini, who patiently obtained and organized hundreds of the references.

Finally and most of all, I hope my daughters will forgive me if I devoted too much time to this book that I could have spent with them.

I have learned a huge amount during the preparation of this book, and I hope very much that the information given here will be helpful to other pathologists who confront definite or possible cases of extranodal lymphoma.

Judith A. Ferry, MD

CONTENTS

CHAPTER 1

Introduction to Extranodal Lymphomas

Judith A. Ferry

Lymphomas that arise in extranodal sites are intriguing. The types of lymphomas that occur differ from those encountered in lymph nodes and vary widely from one extranodal site to another. Almost all primary extranodal lymphomas are non-Hodgkin's lymphomas. Approximately one fourth of all non-Hodgkin's lymphomas arise in extranodal sites.[1] With the exception of the thymus (see Chapter 4), extranodal sites only rarely give rise to Hodgkin's lymphoma. Certain extranodal sites lack endogenous lymphoid tissue, which leaves incompletely resolved questions about the cell of origin of lymphomas that arise in these sites.

Many types of extranodal lymphomas have distinctive clinicopathologic features, which sometimes include association with an underlying immunodeficiency syndrome, autoimmune disease, infection, chronic inflammatory process or other immunologic disorder, or a predilection for patients of certain ethnic origins. In the gastrointestinal tract alone, for example, *Helicobacter pylori* infection, celiac disease, *Campylobacter jejuni* infection, a variety of immunodeficiency syndromes, and possibly inflammatory bowel disease predispose an individual to the development of different types of lymphoma; lymphomagenesis, therefore, appears to be related to chronic antigenic stimulation, inadequate immune regulation, or a combination of these factors (see Chapter 5).

The behavior of lymphomas of the same pathologic type sometimes differs, depending on the site of origin. For example, patients with gastric marginal zone lymphomas of mucosa-associated lymphoid tissue (MALT lymphomas; see Chapter 5) appear to have a higher disease-free survival rate than those with marginal zone lymphomas that arise in other sites. Marginal zone lymphomas may show different patterns of spread, depending on the site of origin.

Diffuse large B-cell lymphomas may show remarkably divergent behavior, depending on the site of origin. Primary diffuse large B-cell lymphoma of bone (see Chapter 12) has an excellent prognosis with optimal therapy; however, when it relapses, it has a tendency to spread to other bones. Diffuse large B-cell lymphoma that is primary in the central nervous system (see Primary Central Nervous System Lymphomas in Chapter 2) has a poor prognosis, even with aggressive therapy, but in most cases it remains confined to the central nervous system. Primary testicular diffuse large B-cell lymphoma (see Lymphomas of the Testis in Chapter 9) often behaves aggressively; it has a tendency to develop widespread disease, with preferential spread to the opposite testis and the central nervous system. Even when the histologic features are similar, differences may exist in the immunophenotype and in underlying genetic abnormalities; these differences may be responsible for site-specific differences in the prognosis.

The diagnosis of lymphoma in extranodal sites presents special challenges. Lymphoma is uncommon in certain extranodal sites; depending on the site, inflammatory conditions or other neoplasms may be much more common. Lymphoma, therefore, may not be considered a diagnostic possibility, which may lead to misdiagnosis. Flow cytometric analysis is useful for evaluating the possibility of lymphoma, but because lymphoma often is unexpected in extranodal sites, tissue may not be saved for flow cytometry. Familiarity with the types of lymphomas that may present in various extranodal sites is helpful for establishing a diagnosis. Subsequent chapters are thus organized by anatomic site; this chapter provides an overview of the lymphomas that may be encountered in extranodal sites.

Many different types of lymphoma of B-cell, T-cell, and natural killer (NK)-cell lineage can arise in extranodal sites or can involve extranodal sites. Marginal zone lymphoma of mucosa-associated lymphoid tissue (MALT lymphoma) can arise in any of a large number of anatomic sites (see Table 1-1). It is composed of marginal zone B cells with small numbers of large transformed cells; the proportion of plasma cells and the presence of plasmacytic differentiation of the neoplastic B cells vary from case to case. Evidence of underlying reactive lymphoid follicles almost always can be identified, either on routinely stained sections or through the use of antibodies to follicular dendritic cells. The underlying genetic changes in marginal zone lymphoma vary from case to case.

A particular set of chromosomal translocations is specific for or strongly associated with extranodal marginal zone lymphomas: t(11;18) *(API2-MALT1)*, t(14;18) *(IGH/MALT1)*, t(1;14) *(BCL10/IGH)*, and t(3;14) *(FOXP1/IGH)*. The first three of these translocations are believed to promote lymphomagenesis through activation of the NFκB pathway; the precise role of the fourth translocation is uncertain. The frequency of each of these translocations varies greatly, depending on the site of origin of the marginal zone lymphoma.[2-5] Immunoproliferative small intestinal disease (see Chapter 5) is a distinctive type of marginal zone lymphoma with marked plasmacytic differentiation and a possible pathogenetic association with *C. jejuni*.

Splenic marginal zone lymphoma (see Chapter 6) has a cellular composition similar to that of extranodal marginal zone lymphoma. However, it is biologically distinct from extranodal marginal zone lymphoma, showing a different anatomic distribution and clinical course, as well as some immunophenotypic and genetic differences. Hairy cell leukemia (see Chapter 6), in contrast to the predominant white pulp involvement of splenic marginal zone lymphoma, diffusely involves the red pulp, with loss of white pulp.

Follicular lymphoma (or, in the skin, primary cutaneous follicle center lymphoma) arises in extranodal sites in one of two main forms. One form is low-grade bcl2+ follicular lymphoma associated with a *BCL2* translocation [t(14;18)] as an underlying genetic event, similar to follicular lymphoma arising primarily in lymph nodes; this form of extranodal follicular lymphoma is encountered most often in the gastrointestinal tract (see Lymphomas of the

TABLE 1-1

Overview of Extranodal Lymphomas

Type of Lymphoma	Extranodal Anatomic Sites Involved	Cellular Composition	Usual Immunophenotype	Genetic Features	Associated Conditions
B-Cell Lymphomas					
Extranodal marginal zone lymphoma of mucosa-associated lymphoid tissue (MALT lymphoma)	GI tract, salivary glands, lung, thyroid, ocular adnexa, urinary tract, skin, dura mater	Marginal zone B cells, small lymphocytes, plasma cells, reactive follicles, lymphoepithelial lesions	Monotypic sIg+, cIg+/− (IgM > IgG or IgA), CD20+, CD5−, CD10−, bcl6−, bcl2+, CD43−/+, cyclin D1−	IGH clonal; t(11;18)(q21;q21) (API2-MALT1), t(14;18)(q32;q21) (IGH/MALT1), t(1;14)(p22;q32) (BCL10/IGH) or t(3;14)(p14.1;q32) (FOXP1/IGH) in some cases Trisomy 18 or trisomy 3 in some cases	Stomach: Helicobacter pylori gastritis Thyroid: Hashimoto's thyroiditis Parotid and thymus: Sjögren's syndrome Ocular adnexa: Chlamydia psittaci (some cases)
IPSID	Small intestine, long segments	Plasma cells, marginal zone B cells, reactive follicles, lymphoepithelial lesions	Alpha heavy chain+ without light chain	IGH clonal	Campylobacter jejuni, other factors (?)
Splenic marginal zone lymphoma	Spleen, abdominal lymph nodes, bone marrow +/− peripheral blood	Spleen: Expanded white pulp with small cells surrounded by marginal zone B cells +/− plasma cells; patchy red pulp involvement Blood: Villous lymphocytes	CD20+, CD5−, CD10−, CD23−, CD43−, cyclin D1−, IgM+, IgD+/−	IGH clonal Losses at 7q	Hepatitis C in some cases; no known risk factors in most cases
Hairy cell leukemia	Spleen, bone marrow, peripheral blood	Spleen: Diffuse infiltrate of cells with oval or bean-shaped nuclei, smooth chromatin, abundant clear cytoplasm Bone marrow: Interstitial or diffuse infiltrate of similar cells Blood and marrow aspirate: Hairy cells	CD20+, CD22+, CD11c+, CD25+, CD103+, DBA.44+, annexin A1+, cyclin D1+/−; rare CD10+ cases	IGH clonal	None known
Follicular lymphoma	GI tract, skin, testis, ocular adnexa, Waldeyer's ring	Mixture of centrocytes and centroblasts, follicular dendritic cells	Monotypic sIg+, CD20+, CD10+, bcl6+, CD5−, CD43, cyclin D1− Bcl2+ in most GI follicular lymphomas, variable or absent in other sites	IGH clonal; t(14;18) (IGH-BCL2) found in most GI follicular lymphomas; t(14;18) variable or absent in other sites	None known
Mantle cell lymphoma	GI tract, Waldeyer's ring, spleen, bone marrow	Small- to medium-sized, slightly irregular cells with scant cytoplasm	Monotypic sIg MD+, CD20+, CD5+, CD10−, CD43+, cyclin D1+	IGH clonal; t(11;14) (BCL1-IGH)	None known

Continued

TABLE 1-1

Overview of Extranodal Lymphomas—cont'd

Type of Lymphoma	Extranodal Anatomic Sites Involved	Cellular Composition	Usual Immunophenotype	Genetic Features	Associated Conditions
Diffuse large B-cell lymphoma, NOS	GI tract, CNS, Waldeyer's ring, paranasal sinuses, bone, heart, liver	Centroblasts, immunoblasts, and/or anaplastic large B-cells	Monotypic sIg+, CD20+, bcl6+/–, CD10–/+, bcl2+/–, MUM1/IRF4+/–, CD43+/–	*IGH* clonal, other changes variable	Some sporadic; some associated with immunodeficiency
Plasmablastic lymphoma	Oral cavity, GI tract, sinonasal tract	Plasmablasts, sometimes with more mature plasmacytoid cells, high mitotic rate	CD20–, MUM1/IRF4+, CD79a+/–, CD138+, cIg–/+, Ki67 high	EBV+ in most cases	HIV+ in most cases
Lymphomatoid granulomatosis	Lung; also skin, CNS, kidney, upper respiratory tract	Varying numbers of large atypical cells in a lymphohistiocytic background	*Large cells:* CD20+ B cells; *Small cells:* T cells (CD4 > CD8)	*B cells:* EBV+	Subtle or overt immunodeficiency
Primary effusion lymphoma	Pleural, peritoneal, or pericardial cavity; no discrete mass	Immunoblasts or large pleomorphic cells	HHV8+, CD45+, CD30+, CD20–, Ig–, MUM1/IRF4+, CD138+/–	EBV+ in most cases	HIV+ in most cases
Pyothorax-associated lymphoma	Pleura	Centroblasts, immunoblasts, some plasmacytoid	CD20+, MUM1/IRF4+, CD138+/–	EBV+	Many years status postiatrogenic pneumothorax to treat tuberculosis
Primary mediastinal (thymic) large B-cell lymphoma	Mediastinum (thymus)	Centroblasts, multilobated cells with clear cytoplasm, Reed-Sternberg–like cells in some cases; sclerosis	CD20+, CD45+, CD79a+, CD30+/–, CD15–, Oct2+, Bob1+, Ig–	*IGH* clonal, EBV–, activation of NFκB and JAK-STAT signaling pathways	None known
Intravascular large B-cell lymphoma	Vascular lumens in many extranodal sites	Centroblasts, immunoblasts	CD20+, subset CD5+	*IGH* clonal	None known
T-cell/histiocyte-rich large B-cell lymphoma	Spleen, liver, bone marrow	Scattered large cells (centroblasts, LP cell-like, or classical Reed-Sternberg cell-like) in background of many small lymphocytes and histiocytes; absence of eosinophils and plasma cells	*Large lymphoid cells:* B cells; CD20+, bcl6+, EMA+/–, CD15–, CD30–; *Small lymphocytes:* T cells; CD3+, CD5+; *Follicular dendritic meshworks (CD21+, CD23+):* Absent	EBV–	None known
EBV+ DLBCL of the elderly	Tonsil, skin, GI tract, lung	Polymorphous or monomorphous; large cells may include immunoblasts and/or Reed-Sternberg–like cells	CD20 and/or CD79a+, IRF4/MUM1+, CD30+/–, CD15–	EBV+	Advanced age
Cutaneous large B-cell lymphoma, leg type	Skin, especially lower extremities	Sheets of centroblasts and/or immunoblasts	CD20+, CD79a+, bcl2+, MUM1/IRF4+, CD10–, bcl6+/–	Variable	Preponderance of older women are affected

	Sites	Morphology	Immunophenotype	Genetics	Predisposing/Associated Factors
Burkitt's lymphoma	GI tract, Waldeyer's ring, bones of the jaw, ovaries, bone marrow	Medium-sized atypical lymphoid cells with round nuclei, basophilic cytoplasm, tingible-body macrophages	Monotypic sIgM+, CD20+, CD10+, bcl6+, bcl-2–, Ki67 ~ 100%	IGH clonal; t(8;14), t(2;8) or (8;22) (MYC); endemic cases and minority of sporadic cases EBV+	Some sporadic; some endemic; some associated with immunodeficiency, especially HIV
B-lymphoblastic lymphoma	Bone, skin	Small- to medium-sized blasts with scant cytoplasm	CD19+, CD20–, TdT+, CD10+, CD3–, MPO–	IGH clonal; other changes variable	None known
T-Cell and NK-Cell Lymphomas					
Extranodal NK/T-cell lymphoma, nasal type	Midline upper respiratory tract, especially nasal cavity; testis; GI tract; skin	Small-, medium-, and/or large-sized atypical lymphoid cells, necrosis, vascular damage	cCD3+, CD2+, CD5–, CD56+, granzyme B+, perforin+	NK-lineage cases: TCR germline; EBV+ T-lineage cases (minority): TCR clonal; EBV+	Asian, Native American ethnicity
Enteropathy-associated T-cell lymphoma	Small intestine, especially jejunum; multifocal	Type A: Medium-sized to large cells, sometimes bizarre; many admixed reactive cells Type B: Small- to medium-sized monomorphic cells; fewer admixed reactive cells	Type A: CD3+, CD4–/CD8– > CD8+, granzyme+, perforin+, CD56– Type B: CD3+, CD8+, CD56+	TCR clonal	Celiac disease
Hepatosplenic T-cell lymphoma	Liver, spleen, bone marrow	Medium-sized cells with clear cytoplasm in hepatic sinusoids, splenic red pulp, and bone marrow sinusoids	CD2+, CD3+, CD5–/+, CD4–, CD8–/+, TIA-1+	TCR clonal; isochromosome 7q and trisomy 8 common	Immune dysregulation or immunosuppression, some cases
Anaplastic large cell lymphoma, ALK+	Skin (with other sites of disease), bone, CNS	Large atypical cells with abundant cytoplasm, including hallmark cells	CD30+, ALK+, EMA+, variable expression of T-cell antigens	TCR clonal; t(2;5) (ALK/NPM)	None known
Primary cutaneous anaplastic large cell lymphoma	Skin (isolated)	Large cells with round or oval indented or pleomorphic nuclei and abundant cytoplasm	CD30+, ALK–, EMA–, most CD4+, variable expression of other T-cell antigens	TCR clonal	None known
T-lymphoblastic lymphoma	Mediastinum (thymus)	Small- to medium-sized blasts with round, irregular, or convoluted nuclei, finely dispersed to dark chromatin, variably prominent nucleoli, scant cytoplasm	CD3+, CD7+, TdT+, CD1a+, CD10+/–, often CD4+/CD8+ (double positive)	TCR clonal; IGH clonal in a minority of cases	None known
Hodgkin's Lymphoma					
Nodular lymphocyte-predominant Hodgkin's lymphoma	Spleen, bone marrow (very uncommon; isolated lymph node involvement is typical)	Large atypical LP cells in background of small lymphocytes and histiocytes	LP cells: CD45+, CD20+, bcl6+, CD30–, CD15–	EBV–	None known
Classical Hodgkin's lymphoma	Spleen, liver, thymus, lung, marrow, GI tract (less common than lymph node involvement)	Reed-Sternberg cells and variants in a reactive background	CD15+/–, CD30+, CD20–/+, Pax5+, MUM1/IRF4+, CD3–	EBV+ in approximately half of cases	In GI tract, some cases occur with inflammatory bowel disease

CNS, Central nervous system; DLBCL, diffuse large B-cell lymphoma; EBV, Epstein-Barr virus; GI, gastrointestinal; Ig, immunoglobulin; sIg, surface immunoglobulin; cIg, cytoplasmic immunoglobulin; HIV, human immunodeficiency virus; IGH, immunoglobulin heavy chain gene; IPSID, immunoproliferative small intestinal disease/Mediterranean lymphoma/alpha heavy chain disease. LP, lymphocyte predominant; MPO, myeloperoxidase; NK, natural killer; NOS, not otherwise specified; TCR, T-cell receptor genes.

Gastrointestinal Tract in Chapter 5). In other sites, such as the skin (see Chapter 11) and the testis (see Lymphomas of the Testis in Chapter 9), follicular lymphoma may test negative for bcl2 protein and may lack a *BCL2* translocation. These extranodal follicular lymphomas, particularly those that are bcl2−, may be associated with localized disease and a good prognosis.

Diffuse large B-cell lymphoma is the most common type of extranodal lymphoma overall, but the proportion of cases represented by this type of lymphoma varies widely from site to site. Nearly all primary central nervous system, testicular, and osseous lymphomas are the diffuse large B-cell type, whereas only a minority of lymphomas of the ocular adnexa, salivary glands, and lung are diffuse large B-cell lymphomas. A number of types and variants of diffuse large B-cell lymphoma that arise predominantly or exclusively in extranodal sites have been described, and each has its distinctive clinical and biologic features (see Table 1-1). These types of lymphoma include plasmablastic lymphoma (see Lymphomas of the Oral Cavity in Chapter 3), lymphomatoid granulomatosis (see Pulmonary Lymphomas in Chapter 4), primary effusion lymphoma and pyothorax-associated lymphoma (see Lymphomas of the Pleura and Pleural Cavity in Chapter 4), primary mediastinal large B-cell lymphoma (see Lymphomas of the Thymus in Chapter 4), intravascular large B-cell lymphoma (see Intravascular Lymphomas in Chapter 14), T-cell/histiocyte-rich large B-cell lymphoma (discussed primarily in Lymphomas of the Spleen in Chapter 6 and also in Hepatic Lymphomas in Chapter 5), Epstein-Barr virus (EBV)–positive diffuse large B-cell lymphoma of the elderly (discussed in Intestinal Diffuse Large B-Cell Lymphoma in Chapter 5 and in the Differential Diagnosis of Hodgkin's lymphoma of the Gastrointestinal Tract) and cutaneous large B-cell lymphoma, leg-type (see Cutaneous Lymphomas in Chapter 11).

Burkitt's lymphoma can involve a variety of extranodal sites as well as lymph nodes. In Western countries, in immunocompetent patients, Burkitt's lymphoma most often is seen in the ileocecal region of boys (Burkitt's lymphoma is discussed in detail in Burkitt's Lymphoma of the Gastrointestinal Tract in Chapter 5).

B-lymphoblastic neoplasms usually present as an acute leukemia (B-lymphoblastic leukemia). However, in a minority of cases, patients develop localized extranodal or nodal involvement by B-lymphoblastic lymphoma (see Lymphomas of Bone in Chapter 12). Most T-lymphoblastic neoplasms present with a mass lesion (T-lymphoblastic lymphoma) that most characteristically arises in the thymus, presenting as an anterior mediastinal mass (see Lymphomas of the Thymus in Chapter 4).

Extranodal NK/T-cell lymphoma, nasal type, is an EBV+ lymphoma that arises most often in the upper respiratory tract, most frequently in the nasal cavity (see Lymphomas of the Nasal Cavity and Paranasal Sinuses in Chapter 3). Enteropathy-associated T-cell lymphoma, an uncommon intestinal lymphoma with a poor prognosis, is strongly associated with celiac disease (see Enteropathy-Associated T-cell Lymphoma in Chapter 5). Hepatosplenic T-cell lymphoma, another T-cell lymphoma with a poor prognosis, presents with hepatosplenomegaly, sometimes in the setting of an immunologic abnormality (see Lymphomas of the Spleen in Chapter 6).

Anaplastic large cell lymphoma, both ALK+ and ALK−, may involve extranodal sites in the setting of widespread disease, but it also occasionally may present primarily with extranodal disease (see Anaplastic Large Cell Lymphoma in Chapter 2; Lymphomas of the Nervous System and the Meninges; and Lymphomas of Bone in Chapter 12). In contrast, primary cutaneous anaplastic large cell lymphoma characteristically is localized to the skin (primary cutaneous anaplastic large cell lymphoma and other cutaneous T-cell lymphomas are discussed in Chapter 11).

The key features of most lymphomas are outlined in Table 1-1 and discussed in the following chapters.

REFERENCES

1. Freeman C, Berg J, Cutler S: Occurrence and prognosis of extranodal lymphomas, *Cancer* 29:252-260, 1972.
2. Bertoni F, Zucca E: Delving deeper into MALT lymphoma biology [comment], *J Clin Invest* 116:22-26, 2006.
3. Farinha P, Gascoyne RD: Molecular pathogenesis of mucosa-associated lymphoid tissue lymphoma, *J Clin Oncol* 23: 6370-6378, 2005.
4. Hu S, Du M-Q, Park S-M et al: cIAP2 is a ubiquitin protein ligase for *BCL10* and is dysregulated in mucosa-associated lymphoid tissue lymphomas, *J Clin Invest* 116:174-181, 2006.
5. Isaacson PG, Du MQ: Gastrointestinal lymphoma: where morphology meets molecular biology, *J Pathol* 205:255-274, 2005.

CHAPTER 2

Lymphomas of the Nervous System and the Meninges

Judith A. Ferry

■ PRIMARY CENTRAL NERVOUS SYSTEM LYMPHOMAS

Introduction

Primary central nervous system lymphoma (PCNSL) is defined as lymphoma that arises in the brain, spinal cord, eyes, or leptomeninges without evidence of previous or concurrent lymphoma outside the central nervous system.[1] (Intraocular lymphoma is discussed separately later in the chapter.) PCNSL has a worse prognosis than nearly all other primary extranodal lymphomas. Diffuse large B-cell lymphoma that arises in the central nervous system has a worse prognosis than diffuse large B-cell lymphoma arising in any other site, although recent advances in therapy offer some hope for patients with this disease.

Epidemiology

PCNSL develops in two distinct clinical settings: in immunocompetent patients and in immunosuppressed patients. Among immunocompetent patients, PCNSL is uncommon, currently accounting for approximately 4% to 5% of all neoplasms primary in the central nervous system and for approximately 1% to 2% of all non-Hodgkin's lymphomas.[2-5] Immunocompetent patients are predominantly older adults (median age of 55 to 65 in different series), and a slight male preponderance is seen.[4-14] Only rarely are patients under age 21.[13,15,16]

Most immunodeficient patients who develop PCNSL have human immunodeficiency virus (HIV) infection, a status that poses a risk estimated to be 1000 times that of immunocompetent individuals.[17] Overall, patients with HIV are younger, and the male preponderance is more striking.[6,18] The increased risk of PCNSL is seen with HIV infection of various transmission types.[18,19] The disease is found mainly in patients with advanced immunodeficiency, with CD4 counts lower than 50 cells/mm³.[6,18,20] In contrast to PCNSL in immunocompetent individuals, HIV-associated PCNSL can occur in children as young as 2 years of age.[12,19] Patients with congenital immunodeficiency, iatrogenically immunosuppressed transplant recipients, and patients with autoimmune disease also are at increased risk of developing PCNSL.[6,12]

A sharp increase in PCNSL has occurred in recent decades. This is partly because of the acquired immunodeficiency syndrome (AIDS) epidemic; however, an unexplained increase also has been seen among immunocompetent patients in the United States and several other countries since the 1970s.[16,21-23] The incidence of PCNSL among HIV-positive patients appears to have peaked in the 1990s.[12] Since then, the introduction of highly active antiretroviral therapy (HAART) for HIV-positive patients has been associated with a substantial decrease in the occurrence of PCNSL in these patients,[18,24] correlating with the improved CD4 counts that result from HAART.[20]

Immunologic abnormalities, therefore, are important in the pathogenesis of a major subset of PCNSL. The etiology is unknown for cases that occur sporadically.

Clinical Features

Signs and Symptoms

Patients present with symptoms that usually are of short duration. Signs and symptoms depend on the site of the lesion; constitutional symptoms are uncommon.[4] In one large series of immunocompetent patients, 70% had focal neurologic deficits (e.g., aphasia, hemiparesis, or ataxia); 43% had neuropsychiatric symptoms (e.g., apathy, depression, or confusion); 33% had manifestations of elevated intracranial pressure (e.g., headache, papilledema, nausea, or vomiting); 14% had seizures; and 4% had ocular symptoms.[15]

Focal deficits are the result of discrete intracerebral lesions. Neuropsychiatric changes are likely related to infiltration of white matter tracts. Leptomeningeal involvement may lead to cranial nerve palsies, headache, and neck stiffness. Spinal cord involvement is rare and may result in sensory or motor deficits of the extremities or bowel or bladder dysfunction. A higher proportion of HIV-positive patients, compared with immunocompetent patients, present with mental status changes or seizures.[6]

Anatomic Distribution of Disease

PCNSL can present as one or more intracranial lesions, leptomeningeal disease, or spinal cord disease. In immunocompetent patients, intracranial lesions are more often solitary than multiple. Multiple lesions are found in approximately one third of cases.[4,14] They are much more often supratentorial than infratentorial. Also, they often are in contact with meningeal or ventricular surfaces; this may lead to disease spread through seeding of the cerebrospinal fluid. Involvement of the basal ganglia, thalamus, and corpus callosum is common. Frontal and parietal lobe involvement is slightly more common than temporal lobe disease. Disease is uncommon in the occipital lobe, cerebellum, and brainstem.[4,6,12,15,16] Primary leptomeningeal lymphoma (limited to leptomeninges and cerebrospinal fluid) is rare. Secondary leptomeningeal lymphoma is common in patients with PCNSL and may be asymptomatic. Spinal cord involvement is seen in only 1% of patients with PCNSL; primary spinal cord involvement is extremely rare.[2,12] Rare cases of PCNSL arising in the pituitary[25] and the hypothalamus[26] have been described; these cases have been associated with diabetes insipidus and panhypopituitarism, respectively.

Radiographic Features

At one time, angiography and brain scans were used to detect intracranial lesions. Computed tomography (CT) and magnetic resonance imaging (MRI) now

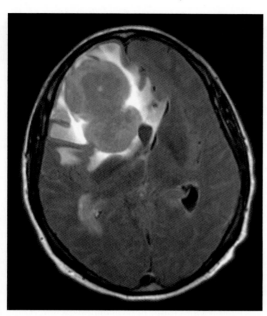

Figure 2-1 Magnetic resonance imaging (MRI) shows a large bilobed frontal lobe lesion that is dark in this image; the lesion is associated with prominent peritumoral edema, which is bright in this image.

are both widely used. Gadolinium-enhanced MRI is an especially powerful tool for imaging lymphoma. PCNSLs in immunocompetent patients typically have one or more homogeneously enhancing lesions in a periventricular distribution or in contact with meningeal surfaces. Nearly all are 1 to 6 cm. Lesions are single in 60% to 70% of cases and multiple in 30% to 40% of cases. Most appear well demarcated (Figure 2-1). The most common sites are the cerebral hemispheres, basal ganglia, thalamus, and corpus callosum. Linear enhancement tracking along the Virchow-Robin perivascular spaces is strongly associated with lymphoma. Evidence of hemorrhage, calcification, or necrosis may be present, but these findings are uncommon before therapy.[6,12,15]

HIV-associated PCNSLs usually are supratentorial and more often are multiple rather than single.[6,12,18] Compared with PCNSL in immunocompetent patients, the lesions are more often ring enhancing or heterogeneously enhancing[6,12,18]; the appearance can mimic that of *Toxoplasma* encephalitis. Posttransplantation PCNSL shares many features with HIV-associated PCNSL. Both tend to be multifocal and to involve the cerebral cortex, white matter, and basal ganglia (Table 2-1).[27]

Diagnostic Techniques

The possibility of lymphoma often is suspected, based on radiographic characteristics (see previous section), before pathologic evaluation. The diagnosis may then be established by biopsy of the tumor. Cytologic examination of cerebrospinal fluid (CSF) occasionally can be diagnostic, particularly if serial lumbar punctures are performed. However, the technique is relatively insensitive[6]; in one large series

of cases with both brain and ocular involvement by lymphoma, CSF cytology was positive in 23% of cases.[28] The sensitivity of diagnosis by CSF evaluation may be augmented by flow cytometry and/or polymerase chain reaction (PCR) procedures to investigate for a clonal B-cell population.

When a biopsy is performed, stereotactic biopsy is preferred, because the lesions are often deep and involve vital structures. If fresh material is available, touch preps or smears, in addition to routine sections, can be helpful in establishing a diagnosis.[29] At the Massachusetts General Hospital, tissue from stereotactic biopsies typically is submitted for intraoperative diagnosis in cases of suspected PCNSL and other intracranial lesions. A "squash prep," in addition to a frozen section, is prepared to increase diagnostic accuracy.

For immunosuppressed patients in whom PCNSLs almost always test positive for the Epstein-Barr virus (EBV), EBV deoxyribonucleic acid (DNA) (detected by PCR) in the cerebrospinal fluid of patients with intracranial mass lesions is reported to be a relatively sensitive and specific technique for diagnosing PCNSL. This test could be used as an alternative to routine diagnostic methods in selected cases, such as when the lesion is inaccessible to biopsy.[4,12,30,31] Some investigators have identified EBV DNA in the cerebrospinal fluid of HIV-positive patients with a variety of disorders other than PCNSL, and these researchers have advised caution in using this test alone to establish a diagnosis. However, they also found that the absence of EBV DNA provided strong evidence against a diagnosis of PCNSL.[32]

Pathologic Features: Overview

Nearly 95% of PCNSLs in Western countries are diffuse large B-cell lymphomas (Figures 2-2 to 2-5). (Virtually all HIV-associated PCNSLs are diffuse large B-cell lymphomas [see Table 2-1]).[18,33] The remaining 5% are T-cell lymphomas, low-grade B-cell lymphomas,[34] and Burkitt's lymphomas (rare).[19] We have seen a case of B-lymphoblastic lymphoma primary in the central nervous system (CNS) (Figure 2-6). T-cell lymphoma is more common in Asian series than in Western series (Table 2-2).[35]

Diffuse Large B-Cell Lymphoma

Gross examination (usually based on examination at autopsy and, in rare cases, on a surgical resection specimen) typically reveals one or more well-circumscribed or ill-defined, infiltrative mass lesions, with replacement or displacement of normal structures. The lesions usually are relatively large (greater than 2 cm). They may be homogeneous and pale; when ill defined, they may be difficult to distinguish from normal brain.[36] The lesions often show areas of necrosis or hemorrhage. Some patients have diffuse meningeal involvement resembling meningitis or, in rare cases, diffuse subependymal periventricular involvement by tumor.[16]

TABLE 2-1

Primary Central Nervous System Lymphomas: Principal Features of Diffuse Large B-Cell Lymphoma in Immunocompetent and Immunodeficient Patients

Feature	Immunocompetent Patients	Immunodeficient Patients
Patients affected	• Mainly older adults • Males slightly more often than females	• Most HIV positive • Younger; higher male to female ratio than in immunocompetent patients • CD4 usually <50 cells/mm^3 • Decreased risk of lymphoma for HIV-positive patients on HAART
Symptoms	Neurologic defects, neuropsychiatric symptoms, headache, papilledema; less often seizures, ocular symptoms	Mental status changes, seizures more common than in immunocompetent patients
Anatomic distribution	• Supratentorial more often than infratentorial • Solitary more often than multiple • Often in contact with meningeal or ventricular surfaces • Secondary leptomeningeal involvement (common) • Primary leptomeningeal lymphoma (rare) • Spinal cord involvement (rare)	Similar to distribution in immunocompetent patients, but multiple lesions more common than single lesions
Radiographic features	Homogeneously enhancing lesions	More often heterogeneously enhancing or ring enhancing
Histology	Diffuse and perivascular proliferation of large lymphoid cells, often centroblasts	Similar to histology seen in immunocompetent patients, except tumor cells more often are immunoblasts
Immunophenotype	CD45+, CD20+, CD10−/+, bcl6+/−, MUM1/IRF4+, SHP1+, CD138−	CD45+, CD20+
Genetic features	• EBER negative • *IGH, IGL:* Clonally rearranged • *IGV*: High load of somatic mutations, intraclonal diversity • *IGVH:* Preferential use of certain gene families • Aberrant somatic hypermutation of non-Ig genes, including *PIM1, Pax5, RhoH/TTF, MYC* • Gene expression analysis: High expression of regulators of UPR signaling pathway (e.g., XBP-1); high expression of c-MYC • Abnormalities of tumor suppressor genes p14 and p16 (common)	• EBER positive • *IGH, IGL:* Clonally rearranged • Most but not all cases show somatic hypermutation, no ongoing somatic hypermutation • Preferential use of *IGLV6-57*
Cytogenetic features	Gains of chromosomes 12, 18q, and X and loss of 6q (common)	
Outcome	Median survival of 30-60 mo in optimally treated patients	Less favorable than for immunocompetent patients
Differential diagnosis based on clinical and radiographic features	• Glioma • Metastasis • Chronic infarct • Demyelinating lesion	• Toxoplasmosis • Progressive multifocal leukoencephalopathy
Differential diagnosis based on pathologic features	• Other tumors: Oligodendroglioma, small cell astrocytoma, primitive neuroectodermal tumor, undifferentiated carcinoma, melanoma • Reactive process (if biopsy is not representative or is taken status post steroids) • Astrocytoma (if biopsy contains surrounding glial reaction) • Germinoma (for lymphomas at base of brain) • Arteritis (because of prominent perivascular tumor growth)	Similar to that for immunocompetent patients

EBER, Epstein-Barr virus–encoded RNA; *HAART,* highly active antiretroviral therapy; *HIV,* human immunodeficiency virus; *IGH,* immunoglobulin heavy chain gene; *IGL,* immunoglobulin light chain gene; *IGV,* variable regions of immunoglobulin genes; *IGVH,* variable region of the immunoglobulin heavy chain gene; *UPR,* unfolded protein response; *XBP-1,* X-box binding protein-1.

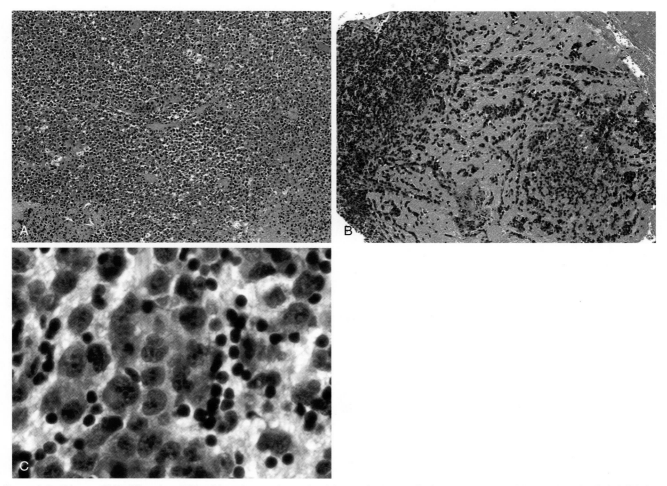

Figure 2-2 Primary CNS diffuse large B-cell lymphoma. In contrast to most primary CNS lymphomas, which are supratentorial, this lymphoma arose in the cerebellum. **A,** In this area the lymphoma is composed of densely packed, atypical lymphoid cells. **B,** In other areas, the lymphoma cells are present in clusters as they infiltrate the parenchyma of the brain. **C,** This lymphoma is composed of large atypical cells with irregular, multilobated nuclei that were CD20+ B cells, whereas the scattered small, round, nonneoplastic lymphocytes proved to be T cells (not shown).

The characteristic microscopic appearance is a diffuse proliferation of atypical cells with areas of perivascular growth that are especially conspicuous at the periphery of the lesion (see Figures 2-2 to 2-4). Perivascular tumor cells commonly are found at a substantial distance from the main tumor mass (see Figure 2-4). In areas with prominent perivascular growth, tumor cells also may be found scattered singly and in small clusters within brain parenchyma between small blood vessels (see Figure 2-2, *B*). Necrosis is common; when it is extensive, viable tumor cells often are found around blood vessels.[3,16,36] The neoplastic cells are discohesive, large, atypical lymphoid cells with oval or irregular nuclei, prominent nucleoli, and usually scant cytoplasm. A minority have multilobated nuclei (see Figure 2-2).

Most of these tumors can be subclassified as diffuse large B-cell lymphomas of the centroblastic type. A component of immunoblasts with large, oval nuclei, vesicular chromatin, and large, centrally placed nucleoli may be present. In immunocompetent patients, diffuse large B-cell lymphomas occasionally are composed almost entirely of immunoblasts (see Figure 2-3, *B*)[13,37-39]; among immunosuppressed patients, immunoblastic or immunoblastic plasmacytoid morphology is more common.[*] Examination of a well-prepared squash prep reveals large, atypical, discohesive cells that are readily identifiable as centroblasts or immunoblasts (see Figure 2-3, *C*). A case of plasmablastic lymphoma primary in the CNS in an HIV-positive man has been described (see Lymphomas of the Oral Cavity in Chapter 3 for additional discussion of plasmablastic lymphoma).[42]

In contrast to post-transplantation lymphoproliferative disorders (PTLDs) that arise in sites other than the CNS, which show a range of morphology from polymorphic to monomorphic lymphoid proliferations, PTLDs that arise in the CNS are nearly all monomorphic B-cell tumors with the pathologic features of diffuse large B-cell lymphoma (Figure 2-5). Necrosis is common in these PTLDs.[27,36]

Lymphomatosis cerebri is a very rare type of PCNSL characterized by a diffusely infiltrative process without formation of a discrete mass. Most of

---

[*]References 3, 7, 9, 16, 29, 33, 40, and 41.

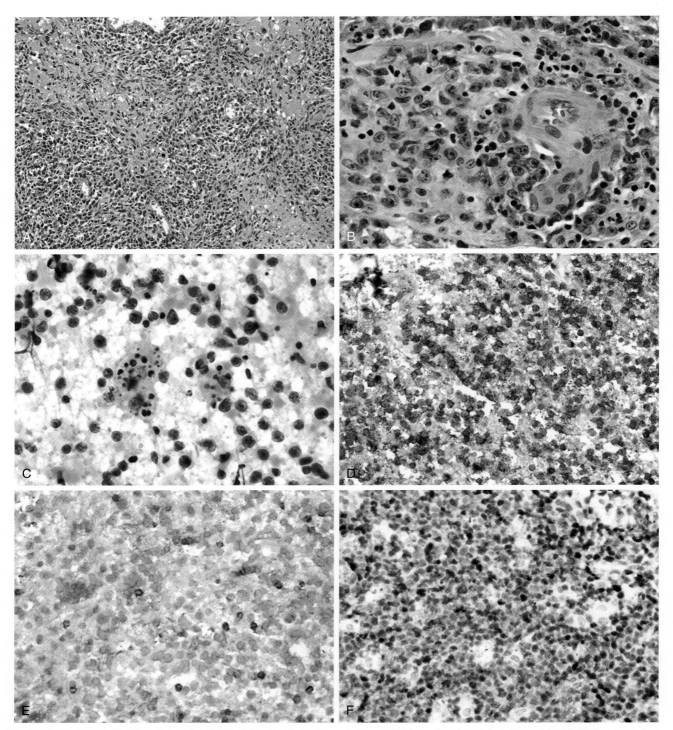

Figure 2-3 Primary CNS diffuse large B-cell lymphoma. **A,** Lymphoma is present in broad perivascular aggregates. **B,** High power shows a dense infiltrate of large lymphoid cells. Many have the appearance of immunoblasts, with oval, vesicular nuclei and prominent central nucleoli. **C,** "Squash prep" from another case shows numerous, discohesive, large lymphoid cells with relatively coarse chromatin and scant cytoplasm. Scattered tingible-body macrophages with abundant cytoplasm containing cellular debris are present. **D,** The neoplastic cells are CD20+. **E,** Few scattered small T cells (CD3+) are present. **F,** The large B cells are MUM1/IRF4+. (*D, E,* and *F,* Immunoperoxidase technique on frozen (*D* and *E*) and paraffin (*F*) sections.)

these patients are HIV negative. Large atypical B cells are scattered diffusely, and often sparsely, with some perivascular growth, with admixed small lymphocytes, macrophages, and reactive glial cells.[36,43] Variably dense tumor cell infiltrates may be found throughout the brain and in the spinal cord, mainly affecting white matter. Both clinically and pathologically, lymphomatosis cerebri can mimic a variety of nonneoplastic inflammatory, infectious, and neurodegenerative disorders. One percent to 2% of

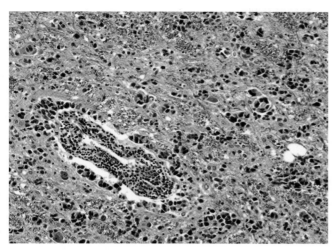

Figure 2-4 Primary CNS diffuse large B-cell lymphoma. This lymphoma, initially diagnosed at autopsy, shows conspicuous spread in a perivascular distribution. (Luxol fast blue/hematoxylin and eosin.)

PCNSLs are intravascular large B-cell lymphomas[3,16] (this distinctive type of lymphoma is discussed in Chapter 14).

If steroids are administered before biopsy, neoplastic cells may undergo a remarkable degree of apoptosis, and the tumor may temporarily shrink or even disappear, making diagnosis difficult or impossible; this has been referred to as the "vanishing tumor" phenomenon.[1] However, a recent study found that only in a small number of cases was the loss of tumor cells after steroid therapy so striking as to require a second biopsy for diagnosis.[14] These investigators also noted that shrinkage or disappearance of a lesion may be seen with other neoplasms and with some nonneoplastic disorders; a response to steroids, therefore, is not sufficient for a diagnosis of PCNSL. In any case, areas previously involved by lymphoma may contain many macrophages and show reactive gliosis.

In both immunocompetent and immunodeficient patients, diffuse large B-cell lymphomas typically

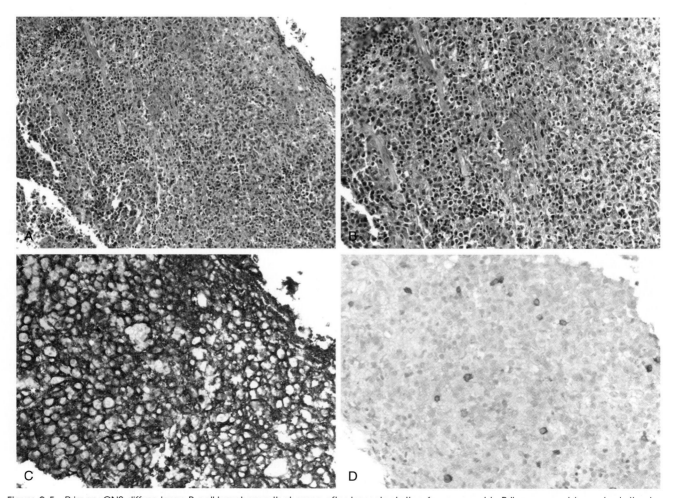

Figure 2-5 Primary CNS diffuse large B-cell lymphoma that arose after transplantation (monomorphic B-lineage post-transplantation lymphoproliferative disorder). **A,** Normal tissue is replaced by a dense lymphoid infiltrate. **B,** Higher power shows large atypical lymphoid cells. **C,** Lymphoid cells are CD20+. **D,** Immunostain for CD3 highlights a few reactive T cells sections. (*C* and *D,* Immunoperoxidase technique on paraffin sections.)

Continued

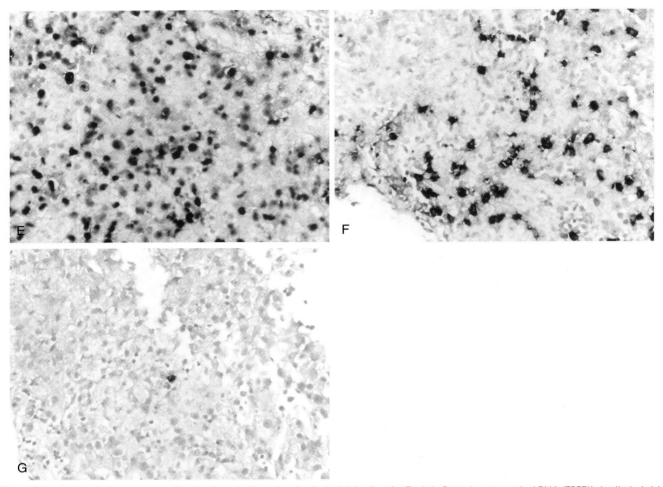

Figure 2-5, cont'd E, B cells are positive for Epstein-Barr virus (in situ hybridization for Epstein-Barr virus–encoded RNA (EBER)). In situ hybridization for kappa (F) and lambda (G) immunoglobulin light chain shows strong monotypic staining of many cells for kappa, indicating plasmacytic differentiation.

express the leukocyte common antigen (CD45); pan–B cell antigens (e.g., CD20; see Figure 2-3, D); and monotypic immunoglobulin.[3,18,27,39,41] Almost all PCNSLs are IgM+; they fail to undergo the immunoglobulin heavy chain class switch.[44]

Virtually all diffuse large B-cell lymphomas in immunosuppressed patients (including patients who are HIV positive, iatrogenically immunosuppressed, or congenitally immunodeficient) are pathogenetically linked to EBV and have neoplastic cells that are infected by EBV (see Figure 2-5). This is best demonstrated using in situ hybridization for Epstein-Barr virus–encoded RNA (EBER). A subset of cases is EBV latent membrane protein (EBV-LMP) positive and/or EBV nuclear antigen (EBNA) positive.[16,18,27,30] PCNSL in immunocompetent patients is negative for EBV (see Table 2-1).[5,7,17]

A number of studies have focused on more detailed immunophenotypic and genetic analysis to better define the immunophenotype of PCNSL and to investigate the stage of differentiation of the neoplastic cells. Most of these studies have included only immunocompetent patients. Results have

varied somewhat from one series to another, but in general, a minority (less than 20%) are CD10+,[13,37-39] and a majority (50% to 80%) are bcl6+.[13,35,37-39] Nearly all cases (75% to 97%) are positive for MUM1/IRF4 (see Figure 2-3, F), a marker of the late germinal center/post-germinal center stage of differentiation[13,37,38]; MUM1/IRF4 expression is more common in PCNSL than in nodal diffuse large B-cell lymphoma.[13] PCNSLs are negative for the plasma cell marker CD138.[37-39] Nearly all cases are positive for SHP1, a non-germinal center marker.[39] In summary, a minority of cases have a germinal center B-cell type immunophenotype (CD10+, bcl6+ or CD10−, bcl6+, MUM1−),[45] but in most cases, the expression of MUM1/IRF4 and SHP1 is consistent with a post-germinal center immunophenotype. A germinal center B-cell immunophenotype is seen less often in PCNSL than in nodal diffuse large B-cell lymphoma.[13]

The cytokine interleukin 4 (IL-4) is an important regulator of B-cell activation, proliferation, aggregation, and survival. It regulates expression of X-box binding protein-1 (XBP-1) and angiogenesis.

Immunohistochemical analysis has shown IL-4 expression by endothelial cells and by tumor cells near blood vessels in PCNSL. IL-4 staining is reduced or absent in nodal diffuse large B-cell lymphoma, in endothelium in brain away from lymphoma, and in other types of tumors in the CNS (glioblastomas and carcinomas metastatic to the brain). IL-4 may well be important in the pathogenesis of PCNSL. Signal transducer and activator of transcription 6 (STAT6) mediates IL-4–dependent gene expression. As is IL-4, the activated, phosphorylated form of STAT6 (P-STAT6) is expressed in PCNSL in both tumor cells and endothelium; however, it is only rarely found in nodal diffuse large B-cell lymphomas.[46]

Expression of the chemokine stroma-derived factor 1 (SDF-1 also known as CXCL-12), a key regulator of B- and T-cell lymphopoiesis, lymphocyte trafficking, and lymphocyte maturation, has been demonstrated in normal elements of the brain, as well as by tumor cells in most cases of PCNSL. The SDF-1 receptor, CXCR4, is expressed by PCNSL. This pattern of chemokine and chemokine-receptor expression may play a role in attracting neoplastic lymphoid cells to the central nervous system. Targeting of this signaling pathway may play a role in the treatment of PCNSL.[47]

Molecular genetic analysis shows monoclonal rearrangement of immunoglobulin genes.[11,17,39] PCNSL is characterized by an unusually high load of somatic mutations in the variable regions of the immunoglobulin heavy chain gene (*IGH*) and light chain genes (*IGL*), which suggests prolonged participation of tumor cells or their precursors in the germinal center reaction,[11,41,48] with evidence of ongoing somatic hypermutation accompanied by intraclonal diversity.[11,41] Translocations of *BCL6* to *IGH* or to a nonimmunoglobulin partner gene are relatively common.[5,48]

The characteristic cell surface IgM expression seen in PCNSL is reflected at the messenger ribonucleic acid (mRNA) level, because PCNSLs show a strong tendency for exclusive IgM or IgD transcription. This could be due to internal switch mu region deletion,[44,48] but it also could be due to a different cytokine milieu or derivation from a distinct subset of B cells not destined to undergo class switch, such as IgM+ memory B cells. In contrast to the tendency of PCNSLs to maintain expression of IgM, many other lymphoid cells typically switch their Ig class isotype (most often to IgG) during the process of somatic hypermutation in the germinal center.[44]

Strong evidence suggests preferential use of certain immunoglobulin heavy chain variable region (*IGHV*) families, especially the *IGHV4* family and in particular *IGHV4-34*.[11,17,41,44,49] The combination of extensive somatic hypermutation, which sometimes is ongoing, and skewed *IGHV* family use suggests that the neoplastic cells are derived from antigen-selected B cells of the germinal center.

Aberrant somatic hypermutation (i.e., involving genes other than those encoding immunoglobulin)

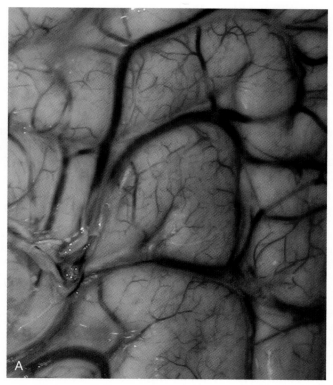

Figure 2-6 B-lymphoblastic lymphoma/leukemia, confined to the central nervous system, with involvement of the brain and the cerebrospinal fluid. Systemic involvement was not demonstrated at any time during the course of the disease or at postmortem examination. **A,** Gross photograph of the cerebral cortex shows opaque white meninges; this change is most conspicuous over sulci (photograph available through the courtesy of Dr. Michael Lawlor).

Continued

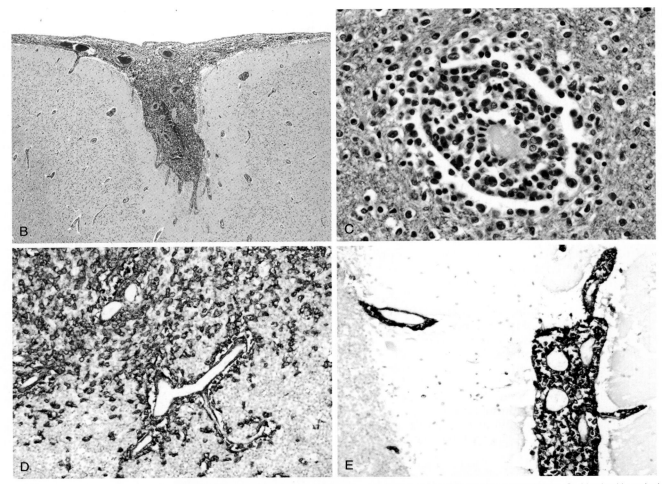

Figure 2-6, cont'd **B,** Microscopic examination reveals a layer of monotonous lymphoid cells in the leptomeninges. **C,** Atypical lymphoid cells also occupy Virchow-Robin spaces. (*C,* Luxol fast blue/hematoxylin and eosin.) **D,** Immunostain for CD20 highlights lymphoblasts in a perivascular and also diffuse distribution. **E,** Lymphoblasts were bright CD10+ cells. (*D* and *E,* immunoperoxidase technique on paraffin sections.) Neoplastic cells were CD19+, CD20dim+, CD10+, CD34+/−, TdT+, surface immunoglobulin light chain–negative B lymphoblasts, as demonstrated on a biopsy of the brain and in cerebrospinal fluid during the patient's life using flow cytometry and immunohistochemistry.

TABLE 2-2

Primary Central Nervous System Lymphomas: Principal Features of Rare Types				
Feature	**Low-Grade B-Cell Lymphomas**	**Peripheral T-Cell Lymphoma, Unspecified**	**Anaplastic Large Cell Lymphoma, ALK+**	**Anaplastic Large Cell Lymphoma, ALK−**
Clinical features	Similar to diffuse large B-cell lymphoma	Similar to diffuse large B-cell lymphoma	Affects children, adolescents, and young adults	Affects adults
Pathologic features	Most composed of small lymphocytes with or without plasmacytic differentiation	Variable	Usually supratentorial, single or multifocal Involvement of overlying meninges (common) Histologically similar to ALCL in other sites	Usually supratentorial, single or multifocal
Prognosis	Better than for primary CNS diffuse large B-cell lymphoma	Better for cases with low-grade histology	Probably worse than for ALCL/ALK+ in other sites	Worse than for ALCL/ALK+
Differential diagnosis	Reactive processes	Reactive processes	• Infection • Metastasis • Other high-grade primary CNS neoplasms	As for ALCL/ALK+

ALCL, Anaplastic large cell lymphoma; *CNS,* central nervous system.

occurs relatively often in a number of genes that play an important role in B-cell development and the regulation of proliferation and apoptosis, including *PIM1, PAX5, RhoH/TTF,* and *MYC*.[50] These genetic changes may play a role in the pathogenesis of PCNSL. The same mechanism that gives rise to the frequency of somatic hypermutation in immunoglobulin genes may be responsible for the aberrant hypermutation.

Using gene expression analysis, diffuse large B-cell lymphomas have been divided into three groups: germinal center B-cell (GCB)–like lymphomas, activated B-cell (ABC)–like lymphomas, and type 3 lymphomas.[51] Similar analysis of primary central nervous system diffuse large B-cell lymphomas has shown that all cases could be assigned to one of these three categories. However, some ABC-type PCNSLs did show upregulated expression of certain GCB genes, such as *BCL6*, suggesting an overlapping state of differentiation.[46] PCNSL is distinct from primary nodal diffuse large B-cell lymphoma (DLBCL) in that PCNSL shows high expression of regulators of the unfolded protein response (UPR) signaling pathway (e.g., XBP-1), high expression of certain oncogenes (e.g. *MYC*), and expression of distinct regulators of apoptosis.[46] XBP-1 and UPR are important for tumor growth under conditions of hypoxia and hypoglycemia. Pharmacologic blockade of UPR may be an effective therapeutic option in selected cases.[46]

In the *CDKN2A* or *INK4a/ARF* locus on 9p21 are two tumor suppressor genes coding for p14 and p16; abnormalities related to these genes may play an important role in the pathogenesis of PCNSL. p16 protein inactivates cyclin-dependent kinases 4 and 6, resulting in activation of retinoblastoma (Rb) protein, which suppresses cell growth. p14 protein inactivates *MDM2*, stabilizing p53, which also suppresses cell growth. In one study of PCNSL, material from the gene coding for p14 was homozygously or hemizygously deleted in 90% of cases.[52] In contrast, p14 abnormalities were uncommon in systemic diffuse large B-cell lymphomas.[52] In another study, the gene coding for p16 showed homozygous or hemizygous deletion in more than 60% of cases. Those with homozygous deletion had no p16 expression by immunohistochemistry, confirming the deletion of genetic material at the protein level.[38] Hypermethylation of CpG islands in the promoter regions of tumor suppressor genes plays a role in the pathogenesis of various neoplasms; epigenetic silencing of tumor suppressor genes by this mechanism may be important in the pathogenesis of PCNSL. The genes most commonly affected include *DAPK, p16^INK4a, p14^ARF,* and *MGMT*.[53]

Comparative genomic hybridization (CGH) studies have shown an average of nearly seven chromosomal alterations per case. The most common abnormalities are gains of chromosomes 12, 18q, and X, and loss of 6q.[54] Gains of chromosome 12 could lead to amplification of the proto-oncogene *MDM2*. Additional material from chromosome 18 could involve alterations in the *BCL2* gene. The frequent deletion of 6q in PCNSL, which has been demonstrated by fluorescence in situ hybridization (FISH) as well as by CGH,[5] is more common in PCNSL than in systemic diffuse large B-cell lymphomas. However, it has been found in testicular lymphoma and is common in aggressive lymphoma in general. The significance of loss of chromosomal material from 6q may be related to loss of one or more tumor suppressor genes.[5,54]

The genetic features of HIV-associated PCNSLs have not been studied as extensively as PCNSL in immunocompetent patients; however, some distinctive features have been noted. In virtually all cases, analysis of immunoglobulin heavy and light chain genes suggests a functional rearrangement that would lead to expression of immunoglobulin. Most cases show evidence of somatic hypermutation of *IGHV*, although a subset shows no evidence of somatic hypermutation, suggesting origin from naïve B cells that have not participated in the germinal center reaction.[33] In contrast to PCNSL in immunocompetent patients, HIV-associated PCNSLs do not show evidence of ongoing somatic hypermutation.[33] In addition, analysis of immunoglobulin heavy and light chain gene family use shows no preferential use of *IGHV4-34*, a feature of PCNSL in immunocompetent patients. In a disproportionate number of HIV-positive cases, *IGLV6-57* is used (see Table 2-1).[33]

Staging, Treatment, and Outcome

Staging procedures should be performed to exclude systemic lymphoma with secondary involvement of the central nervous system. Ophthalmic evaluation, including a slit lamp examination, also is important because of the frequency of concurrent ocular involvement. A lumbar puncture and examination of the CSF also should be performed. PCNSL is an aggressive neoplasm that requires prompt diagnosis and treatment. Without therapy, survival is only a few months.

Treatment has evolved considerably over time. Surgical removal of the lesion is not associated with prolonged survival and may result in severe, irreversible neurologic complications; therefore that approach currently is rarely used.[55] Traditional therapy for PCNSL in years past was whole brain radiation therapy combined with steroids. This resulted in complete remission in 90% of cases; however, the lymphoma usually relapsed within 1 year, with a median survival of 12 to 18 months and a 5-year survival rate of only 3% to 4%.[9,29,55]

Adriamycin-doxorubicin based chemotherapy (e.g., cyclophosphamide, doxorubicin, vincristine, and prednisone [CHOP]) combined with radiation did not improve survival compared to radiation alone, probably because of poor penetration into the CNS.[55] The addition of high-dose methotrexate, an agent able to penetrate the blood-brain barrier, to radiation has improved survival, with a median survival of 30 to 60 months. Unfortunately, long-term survivors, particularly older patients who receive radiation either alone or in combination with chemotherapy, are at high risk for developing a leukoencephalopathy, manifested by severe, progressive dementia, ataxia, and urinary incontinence.[29,56] Patients with this severe neurotoxicity are reported to have cortical atrophy, ventricular enlargement, and diffuse leukoencephalopathy, characterized by axonal loss, myelin loss, gliosis, and spongiosis, as well as vascular damage.[57] In an effort to prevent this devastating complication, regimens without radiation have been tested.

Relatively good outcomes with a lower risk of cognitive loss may be achieved using methotrexate-based regimens.[2,55] However, methotrexate-based chemotherapy is very aggressive, and some patients are unable to complete the planned course.[56] Methotrexate-based regimens can be used to treat elderly patients with PCNSL, and good responses have been achieved in these patients. However, careful monitoring for toxicity and evaluation of the effect of underlying medical problems are required.[58,59] The optimal therapy for PCNSL has yet to be determined.

When patients relapse, the central nervous system is involved in most cases. In fewer cases, lymphoma spreads outside the central nervous system; the sites of spread, which usually are extranodal, include the testes, paranasal sinuses, bone, kidneys, epidural space, breasts, gastrointestinal tract, lungs, adrenals, liver, and others.[8,10,38,60] Relapses also may involve lymph nodes.

The prognosis is better for younger patients (the most commonly used cutoff age is 60 years).[9,10,13,37] A favorable performance status usually is associated with a better outcome.[2,15] Immunodeficient patients have a worse prognosis, although this may be due at least in part to other medical problems rather than the biology of the lymphoma itself.[6,18] Other factors associated with a worse prognosis in some series include involvement of deep structures, such as the basal ganglia, corpus callosum, cerebellum, and brainstem; multiple lesions; elevated protein levels in the cerebrospinal fluid; and an elevated serum lactate dehydrogenase (LDH).[15,61] In some studies, better survival is described for patients with bcl6+ primary CNS diffuse large B-cell lymphomas compared to those without bcl6 expression,[13,38] although this result has not been uniform.[37,39] High expression of the activated form of STAT6 (P-STAT6) in PCNSL has been associated with a worse outcome.[46] Del6q22 and *BCL6* rearrangements have been associated with an inferior overall survival.[5]

Survival after relapse is very poor, usually only a few months. Systemic relapses have been associated with a better outcome than relapses in the central nervous system.[60] Although survival has improved over time in clinical trials, this is not reflected in large population-based studies; therefore, recent improvements in therapy have not clearly translated into widespread improvement in patient survival.[55,56]

Cell of Origin

Normally, lymphoid cells are extremely sparse to absent in the central nervous system, and it is unclear whether neoplastic transformation of lymphoid cells takes place in the CNS or before entry into the CNS. The origin of PCNSL, therefore, is uncertain. Several possibilities exist: PCNSLs could derive from circulating neoplastic B cells that randomly seed multiple sites but are able to form tumors only in the immunologically privileged site of the CNS; they could arise through neoplastic transformation of lymphoid cells already in the central nervous system as part of a chronic inflammatory process; or they could derive from circulating neoplastic B cells expressing adhesion molecules that confer an affinity for localization in the CNS.[2,6,36]

The specific type of B cell that gives rise to diffuse large B-cell lymphoma of the CNS is also uncertain. The immunophenotype and the gene expression profile of the lymphomas suggest that only a minority correspond to a germinal center stage of differentiation, and the majority correspond to a post-germinal center stage of differentiation, or by gene expression signature, to ABC-type lymphomas (see previous discussion). However, the extent of somatic hypermutation suggests prolonged exposure to the germinal center environment, which may be ongoing in cases with intraclonal diversity. A stage of differentiation corresponding to overlapping late germinal center/early post-germinal center B cells has been suggested.[37]

Although identifying the precise stage of differentiation that corresponds to B cells in PCNSL is difficult, the important role of the germinal center in at least some stage of the development of B cells destined to give rise to PCNSL tends to suggest an origin outside the CNS,[38] because the CNS normally is devoid of lymphoid follicles. It is intriguing that in some cases, small numbers of B cells clonally related to the PCNSL can be identified in peripheral blood or bone marrow (or both); these peripherally located B cells may show ongoing mutation of the immunoglobulin variable region genes, yielding clones distinct from those in the CNS.[49,62] This indicates that at least low-level trafficking of abnormal B cells from the CNS to the periphery may occur in patients with PCNSL; however, whether the clone that gave rise to the PCNSL initially arose systemically or in the CNS remains unclear, as does the reason the abnormal B cells present systemically so infrequently lead to clinically significant disease outside the CNS.

Low-Grade B-Cell Lymphomas

Histologically low-grade lymphomas account for only about 3% of PCNSLs. Among low-grade PCNSLs, 80% are B-cell lymphomas and 20% are T-cell lymphomas.[34,63] Low-grade PCNSLs are even less common among HIV-positive patients than among immunocompetent individuals. The clinical manifestations of these lymphomas overlap with those of the more common diffuse large B-cell lymphoma, although the low-grade lymphomas are more likely to present with seizures.[34] The B-cell lymphomas have been classified most often as lymphoplasmacytic lymphoma or small lymphocytic lymphoma. Very rare cases of extranodal marginal zone lymphoma of mucosa-associated lymphoid tissue (MALT lymphoma) have been reported; these apparently arose within the brain, including one that arose in the basal ganglia.[64] Follicular lymphoma has been described. A number of cases have not been subclassified.

Microscopic examination reveals a perivascular and/or diffuse infiltrate of small lymphoid cells. The immunophenotypic and genetic features of the low-grade B-cell lymphomas have not been studied in detail.[34] Treatment has not been uniform, but it often has been less aggressive than considered appropriate for diffuse large B-cell lymphoma. Despite this, the prognosis appears significantly better than for diffuse large B-cell lymphoma.[16,34] Age is an important prognostic factor for patients with low-grade lymphomas, as is seen with diffuse large B-cell lymphoma (see Table 2-2).[34]

T-Cell and Natural Killer (NK)–Cell Lymphomas

Peripheral T-Cell Lymphoma, Not Otherwise Specified (NOS)

Three percent to 4% of PCNSLs in Western series[15] and up to 17% of PCNSL in Asian series[35] are peripheral T-cell lymphomas. Although some authors suggest that T-cell lymphomas are more likely than B-cell lymphomas to arise in the posterior fossa or the leptomeninges,[65] other investigators have observed that, like B-cell lymphomas, T-cell lymphomas are mostly supratentorial.[35,66] Compared with B-cell lymphomas, a higher proportion of T-cell lymphomas are histologically low-grade. T-cell lymphomas include cases classified as small lymphocytic lymphoma and angiocentric lymphoma.[34] Some tumors are composed of small or (occasionally) medium-sized cells; a minority of cases are composed of pleomorphic cells, or medium to large atypical cells.[35,66,67] Some cases are described as showing loosely scattered cells without formation of a discrete mass; a perivascular pattern of growth is common.[34,35] Immunohistochemistry reveals a normal or an aberrant T-cell immunophenotype.[67]

Some cases have been CD8+[35]; T-cell lymphomas that have been CD4/CD8 double positive and double negative have been described.[34,35,67] Some cases show admixed reactive B cells and T cells.[67] The cases studied have shown clonal rearrangement of T-cell receptor genes.[35,66] Documenting clonality is important for distinguishing histologically low-grade T-cell lymphoma from reactive lymphoid infiltrates, such as encephalitis caused by infection or autoimmune disease.[35,67] No significant difference in outcome overall is seen for patients with T-cell lymphoma compared with those with B-cell lymphoma.

T-cell lymphomas with low-grade histologic features may have a more favorable outcome than high-grade lymphomas.[34]

Anaplastic Large Cell Lymphoma

Anaplastic large cell lymphoma (ALCL) that is primary in the central nervous system is a rare type of peripheral T-cell lymphoma. Both ALK+ and ALK– types have been described (see Table 2-2).

Anaplastic Large Cell Lymphoma, ALK+

ALCL/ALK+ that is primary in the CNS has distinctive clinical and pathologic features (Figure 2-7). Males and females are both affected, from early childhood to young adulthood, with an approximate median age of 15 years.[68-71] Underlying immunologic abnormalities do not appear to be a risk factor.[68] Most patients present with supratentorial disease, sometimes accompanied by infratentorial involvement. Lesions may be single or multiple. In most cases, involvement of the leptomeninges or dura (or both) is seen, and some lymphomas are adherent to the dura.[68,69] In one case, ALCL invaded the bone of the overlying skull.[70] ALCL/ALK+ that is primary in the leptomeninges has been reported.[71] The tendency to affect young people and to invade the leptomeninges or dura are features that may help distinguish ALCL from other PCNSLs.

Based on clinical and radiographic features, ALCL sometimes is mistaken for infection or metastasis. The histologic and immunohistologic features are similar to those of ALCL in other sites[68,70,71]: a diffuse proliferation of large atypical cells with abundant cytoplasm, with a component of "hallmark cells" with horseshoe-shaped or bean-shaped nuclei, often with an eosinophilic paranuclear area. Rare examples of the lymphohistiocytic variant and the small cell variant have been described.[69] Neoplastic cells in the cerebrospinal fluid may have the appearance of atypical large granular lymphocytes.[71] Tumor cells are CD30+, ALK+, and EMA+; they lack B-cell antigens and usually express some T-cell antigens.

Based on the small number of reported cases, the prognosis for ALCL/ALK+ that arises in the CNS appears worse than for ALCL/ALK+ that arises in other sites. At least some failures are systemic.[68-71]

Anaplastic Large Cell Lymphoma, ALK–

ALCL/ALK– is a disease of adults, and both males and females are affected. As in ALCL/ALK+, single or multiple lesions, usually supratentorial, are seen, with pathologic features similar to those of ALCL/ALK+ but without expression of the ALK protein. The prognosis for ALCL/ALK– that is primary in the CNS appears to be worse than for primary CNS ALCL/ALK+.[68]

Extranodal NK/T-Cell Lymphoma

Rare cases of extranodal NK/T-cell lymphoma, nasal type, that are primary in the brain have been reported (see Lymphomas of the Nasal Cavity and Paranasal Sinuses, Chapter 3, for a detailed discussion of this

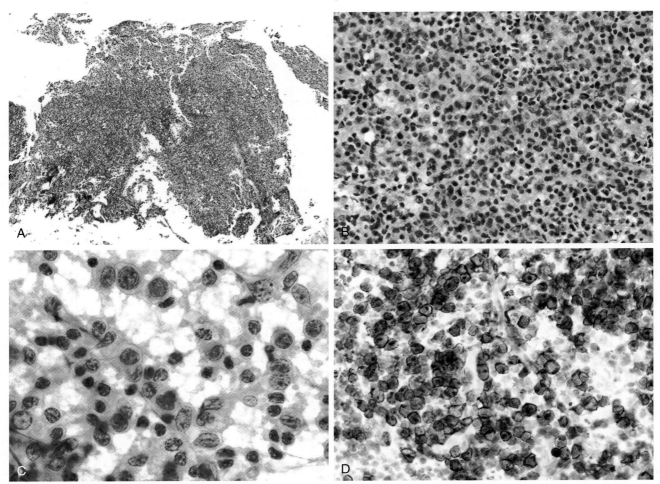

Figure 2-7   Anaplastic large cell lymphoma, ALK+. **A,** Low power shows fragments of brain replaced by lymphoma. **B,** Higher power shows a dense infiltrate of medium-sized to large atypical lymphoid cells. **C,** Squash prep reveals large lymphoid cells with moderately abundant pink cytoplasm. The neoplastic cells appear loosely cohesive in this field. **D,** Tumor cells are CD30+ *(D)*. **E,** Cytoplasmic ALK+.

type of lymphoma). In one case, a young man who had received a renal allograft developed a highly unusual post-transplantation lymphoproliferative disorder in the form of an EBV+ nasal-type NK/T-cell lymphoma; he became well after whole brain irradiation and a decrease in immunosuppressive therapy.[72] More often, this type of lymphoma behaves aggressively. A patient in another case, a Korean man, did not respond well to therapy and succumbed to the NK/T-cell lymphoma.[73]

Hodgkin's Lymphoma

Classical Hodgkin's lymphoma rarely involves the brain or meninges; when such involvement does occur, it usually is in the setting of widespread disease or at the time of relapse.[74,75] CNS involvement at the time of initial presentation with Hodgkin's lymphoma also has been reported.[74,76,77] Classical Hodgkin's lymphoma that arises within and is confined to the brain is even more unusual but has been described.[74,78] Parenchymal disease may be unifocal or multifocal. The lymphomas usually have been of nodular sclerosis or mixed cellularity type; some cases have not been subclassified. The histologic

and immunohistologic features are similar to those of classical Hodgkin's lymphoma in other sites. The prognosis is not favorable, but some patients have achieved long-term, disease-free survival.[74]

Differential Diagnosis

1. **PCNSL versus inflammatory disorders.** For cases of diffuse large B-cell lymphoma, sampling artifact or previous steroid therapy could result in a biopsy showing a predominance of small reactive T cells, mimicking a chronic inflammatory process.[3] Arteritis can mimic areas of lymphoma with perivascular growth.[16] In any case of suspected PCNSL, avoiding steroids before biopsy and obtaining intraoperative frozen sections to make sure tissue is representative are helpful for establishing a diagnosis. For low-grade B-cell and T-cell lymphomas, excluding a reactive process can be challenging; thorough immunophenotyping and evaluation of clonality can help establish a diagnosis.[67]

2. **PCNSL versus other neoplasms.** PCNSLs may be associated with a surrounding glial reaction that may mimic astrocytoma. Other neoplasms,

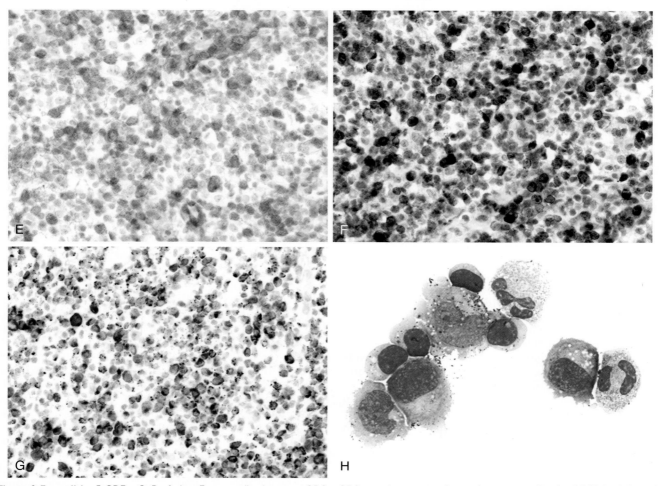

Figure 2-7, cont'd   F, CD7+. **G,** Perforin+. Tumor cells also were CD2+, CD3+, and granzyme B+ and were negative for CD20 (not shown). **H,** Cerebrospinal fluid shows several large neoplastic cells with oval or indented nuclei and abundant cytoplasm, sometimes with azurophilic granules. Scattered nonneoplastic small lymphocytes and neutrophils also are present. (Wright-Giemsa stain.)

including primitive neuroectodermal tumors, undifferentiated carcinoma, melanoma, anaplastic oligodendroglioma, and small cell astrocytoma, can grow in sheets and mimic lymphoma.[16] The neoplastic cells of germinomas have oval nuclei and prominent nucleoli and thus may mimic immunoblasts. As with lymphomas, many admixed small lymphocytes may be seen. In contrast to lymphoid cells, the neoplastic cells of a germinoma have abundant clear, glycogen-rich cytoplasm, and they express placental alkaline phosphatase (PLAP) and Oct4. Also, germinomas arise in the midline, in the area of the pineal gland; therefore, their anatomic localization should give a clue to the diagnosis.

■ SECONDARY INVOLVEMENT OF THE CENTRAL NERVOUS SYSTEM BY LYMPHOMA

Secondary involvement of the CNS by lymphoma is much more common than PCNSL. Approximately 5% of patients with aggressive non-Hodgkin's lymphomas (most of which are diffuse large B-cell lymphomas) who do not receive CNS prophylaxis develop relapse of their lymphomas in the CNS. The risk is even higher for those with Burkitt's lymphoma and lymphoblastic lymphoma/leukemia, and lower for low-grade lymphomas.[79,80] In contrast to other aggressive lymphomas, ALCL only rarely involves the CNS secondarily.[68] Hodgkin's lymphoma rarely involves the CNS; when it does, it almost always is in the setting of relapsed Hodgkin's lymphoma and usually is associated with widespread, concurrent disease outside the CNS.[75,78]

Other factors associated with a higher risk of spread to the CNS have varied from one study to another; they include involvement of certain anatomic sites (e.g., bone marrow, testes, and paranasal sinuses); involvement of more than one extranodal site; advanced-stage disease; a high serum LDH; B symptoms (e.g., fever, night sweats, weight loss); and others.[80,81] Patients present with neurologic deficits, mental status changes, cranial neuropathy, radicular pain, seizures, headache, or visual impairment.[3,29,81] In some patients, relapse is confined to the CNS, whereas in others, concurrent systemic relapse occurs[79,81];

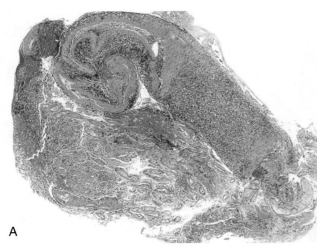
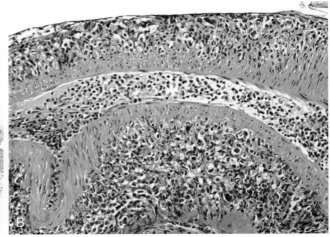

Figure 2-8 Meningeal involvement by primary mediastinal large B-cell lymphoma. **A**, Large leptomeningeal deposit of lymphoma. **B**, Large atypical lymphoid cells surround and invade a large blood vessel.

patients also may have symptoms related to systemic sites of involvement. In contrast to PCNSL, lymphomas with secondary involvement more often involve the meninges than the brain itself (Figure 2-8).[3,29,80] An exception is testicular lymphoma; when it spreads to the CNS, parenchymal lesions are more common than meningeal involvement.[82,83]

The prognosis for lymphoma that relapses in the CNS is poor; survival usually is only a few months.[3,29] Therefore, patients considered at high risk for spread to the CNS often receive CNS prophylaxis (e.g., intrathecal methotrexate and/or high-dose intravenous methotrexate) as part of their initial therapy. Some patients with CNS relapse are successfully salvaged.[79]

Studies on a small number of cases of diffuse large B-cell lymphomas arising systemically and secondarily involving the CNS show high levels of genes such as *MYC* and *XBP-1*, similar to PCNSL, and in contrast to diffuse large B-cell lymphoma in lymph nodes.[46] This could be due to some effect of the CNS microenvironment, or it could be that the genetic features of lymphomas capable of spreading to the CNS overlap with those of PCNSL.

■ INTRAOCULAR LYMPHOMAS

Primary Intraocular Lymphoma

Intraocular lymphoma, or ocular lymphoma (lymphoma involving the eye itself), is nearly always the diffuse large B-cell type[84-87]; other types of lymphoma are rare.

Diffuse Large B-Cell Lymphoma

Clinical Features

Intraocular lymphoma is uncommon, but its frequency has increased in recent years.[23,84-86] Intraocular lymphoma is a subset of PCNSL; it may occur in isolation or in association with lymphoma in the brain. Ten percent to 25% of all patients with PCNSL have ocular involvement.[12,38,88] Intraocular lymphoma predominantly affects older adults[28,84,86,89,90]; most series show a median age in the 60s,[28,87,88,91,92] although occasionally young adults,[91,93] and in rare cases children,[84,94] are affected. In contrast to PCNSL overall, intraocular lymphoma shows a female preponderance.[*] Most patients have no known predisposing conditions, but a number of cases have been described in HIV-positive patients[85,96] and iatrogenically immunosuppressed allograft recipients.[94]

Patients typically complain of floaters, blurred vision, or loss of vision.[84,86-88] Although symptoms often are more severe in one eye, ophthalmologic examination reveals involvement of both eyes in about 80% of cases.[23,87,88] Neoplastic cells are found between Bruch's membrane and the retinal pigment epithelium, especially early in the course of the disease. Tumor usually involves the retina and the vitreous and may involve the head of the optic nerve.[36,96-98] Slit lamp examination reveals a variable number of cells with a translucent gray appearance suspended in the vitreous in sheets and clumps. Whitish, yellow-white, or gray-white infiltrates, plaquelike lesions, or large masses may be seen beneath the retinal pigment epithelium or invading the optic nerve, sometimes with edema, hemorrhage, necrosis, or retinal detachment. Other manifestations include increased intraocular pressure, keratic precipitates (deposits of cells on the posterior surface of the cornea), and anterior chamber cells and flare (i.e., the presence of increased protein, which causes the normally clear fluid of the anterior chamber to become cloudy [flare] with tiny particles [cells] suspended in the fluid).[†]

A variety of techniques may be used to establish a diagnosis, including vitreous aspiration, vitrectomy, biopsy or, in patients with a blind, painful eye, ocular enucleation. The method most commonly used is

---

[*]References 23, 28, 84, 86, 88, 91, 92, and 95.
[†]References 23, 84, 86, 89, 96, 99, and 100.

microscopic examination of the vitreous, but the sensitivity of this procedure may be limited by admixed inflammatory cells or by previous steroid therapy, which may eliminate many of the tumor cells.[28,84,86] Diagnostic yield may be improved by combining routine light microscopy with flow cytometry and molecular genetic analysis.[91,95]

Determining the IL-10 and IL-6 levels in the vitreous also can be a useful adjunct for evaluating the possibility of lymphoma. An elevated IL-10 level in the vitreous is strongly associated with ocular lymphoma and could prompt rebiopsy if the initial specimen is nondiagnostic.[23,92,96] IL-10 is a growth and differentiation factor for B cells, as well as an immunosuppressive cytokine that inhibits cell-mediated immunity. IL-10 probably promotes proliferation of neoplastic B cells and protects them from the immune system. In ocular lymphoma, IL-10 is released by neoplastic B cells. IL-6 may be released by a variety of cell types but presumably is released by the reactive population in cases of ocular lymphoma. An IL-10 to IL-6 ratio greater than 1 suggests lymphoma rather than inflammation,[96] although in the early stages of lymphoma, the IL-10 to IL-6 ratio may not be elevated, because few tumor cells are present. Uveitis usually has a ratio less than 1.[96]

Pathologic Features

The pathologic features of ocular lymphoma are similar to those of diffuse large B-cell lymphoma presenting in the brain. Microscopic examination of a biopsy or enucleation specimen reveals a retina or an optic nerve with a diffuse or perivascular infiltrate of large atypical lymphoid cells.[36,96] Cytologic evaluation of vitreous specimens shows large pleomorphic cells with round, oval, or lobated nuclei, scant cytoplasm, prominent nucleoli (usually in small numbers) in a background of reactive T cells, necrotic cells, fibrin, and debris (Figure 2-9).[92,96] The choroid may contain reactive lymphocytes.[36]

Among immunocompetent patients, the usual immunophenotype is CD20+, bcl2+, bcl6+, MUM1+/RF4, and monotypic IgM+, with CD10 expression in a minority of cases and without EBV.[98] As with other B-cell lymphomas, clonal rearrangement of the immunoglobulin heavy chain gene is seen.[91,92,96,98] Sequencing of *IGH* reveals preferential use of certain variable region families; in one study, eight sequenced cases showed four using VH4-34, two using VH3-23, and one each using VH3-7 and VH3-30. The lymphomas also showed a high load of somatic mutations of *IGH*. In some cases of both ocular and cerebral involvement, the same clone has been demonstrated in both sites.[98]

The immunophenotypic and genetic features of intraocular lymphoma in immunocompetent patients appear to correspond to a late germinal center/early post-germinal center stage of differentiation, analogous to PCNSL in the brain. Intraocular lymphoma in immunocompromised patients typically is composed of large atypical B cells latently infected by EBV.[96,101]

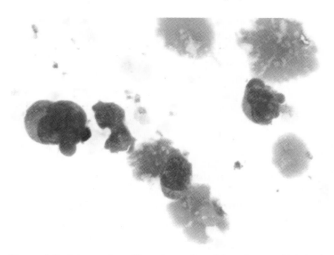

Figure 2-9 Intraocular diffuse large B-cell lymphoma. Cytologic preparation of a vitreous aspirate reveals large atypical lymphoid cells with oval to lobated nuclei and deep blue cytoplasm. (Wright stain.)

Pathogenesis

As with PCNSLs in the brain, the pathogenesis of ocular lymphoma is uncertain. Possibilities include attraction of reactive lymphoid cells to the eye, with subsequent neoplastic transformation in a subset of individuals, and homing to the eye of cells that have already undergone neoplastic transformation. In support of the latter hypothesis, tumor cells have been found to stain for chemokine receptors CXCR4 and CXCR5, whereas retinal pigment epithelium has been shown to stain for their respective chemokines BLC (also known as CXCL-13) and SDF-1 (stromal-derived factor-1, also known as *CXCL-12*). B-cell chemokines, therefore, may be involved in the pathogenesis of primary intraocular lymphoma by attracting neoplastic cells from the choroidal circulation.[97]

Staging, Treatment, and Outcome

Most cases of intraocular lymphoma are associated with lymphoma involving the brain either at presentation or, without treatment, on follow-up; a minority of cases are associated with systemic lymphoma or remain confined to the eye. Aggressive treatment of isolated intraocular lymphoma can reduce the risk of progression.*

Untreated intraocular lymphoma often results in blindness.[89] Intraocular lymphoma frequently responds well to radiation therapy,[87,89] but restoration of sight is not guaranteed, because the retina may already be irreversibly damaged and because radiation may be associated with dry eyes, optic neuropathy, retinopathy, and cataracts. The best treatment remains to be determined.

Patients treated with ocular radiation alone often develop local recurrence or progress to involvement of the brain or, less often, systemic involvement.[23,28,99] Testicular relapse has been described.[87]

---

*References 23, 84, 86, 89, 98, and 102.

Because radiation alone does not yield optimal results, other types of therapy have been suggested, including combined chemotherapy and radiation, chemotherapy alone, intensive chemotherapy with autologous stem cell transplantation, and intravitreal methotrexate.[23,87,95,99] Addition of methotrexate may inhibit progression to involvement of the brain. Most patients eventually die of lymphoma.[28,88,98]

Differential Diagnosis

1. **Intraocular large B-cell lymphoma versus non-neoplastic disorders.** Intraocular lymphoma can mimic a variety of nonneoplastic conditions, including chronic idiopathic uveitis, acute retinal necrosis, retinal vasculitis,[86,88] optic neuritis, amyloidosis, and sarcoidosis; it also can mimic infections, including herpes simplex viral infection, toxoplasmosis, syphilis, tuberculosis, Whipple's disease and cytomegalovirus infection.[23,91] The possibility of lymphoma may be raised if a poor response to steroids or antimicrobial therapy is seen, or with the onset of neurologic symptoms as a result of CNS involvement.[23,86] Because signs and symptoms are somewhat nonspecific and because obtaining a diagnostic specimen can be difficult, the interval from onset of symptoms to diagnosis may be prolonged; some series have reported a median interval as long as 1 to 2 years.[87,92]

T-Cell Lymphomas

Rare cases of peripheral T-cell lymphoma presenting with intraocular involvement have been described.[87,92,93,103] A case recently seen in our department was diagnosed on chorioretinal biopsy (Figure 2-10).

Primary Uveal Tract Lymphoma

Primary uveal tract lymphoma, an unusual subtype of ocular lymphoma, is also referred to as *primary choroidal lymphoma* or *uveal lymphoid neoplasia.* It typically is a low-grade B-cell lymphoma. Because of uncertainty about the nature of this condition, the older literature refers to it as "reactive lymphoid hyperplasia of the uvea" and "uveal lymphoid infiltration."[101,104-107] The clinical and pathologic features indicate that these are likely extranodal marginal zone lymphomas of mucosa-associated lymphoid tissue.

Clinical Features

Patients with primary uveal tract lymphoma are mostly middle aged or older adults, ranging in age from 30 to 94 years (the mean age is approximately 60 years).[106] Involvement is usually unilateral, but occasionally both eyes are involved.[104] Patients often present with visual disturbances that may progress to blindness. Some patients develop glaucoma. Examination of the fundus reveals single or multiple creamy, white, or yellow lesions at the level of the choroid or diffuse thickening of the choroid; this may result in retinal detachment.[104,106,107] In cases with anterior involvement, pink discoloration of the eyeball is visible on physical examination. Because the infiltrate may extend to involve extraocular tissue, sometimes in a retrobulbar location, patients may have proptosis. In some cases the overlying conjunctiva is involved, resulting in salmon-pink conjunctival lesions that are fixed to the sclera and not mobile.[106,107] Changes evolve slowly; the disease process is indolent.[104,107]

Pathologic Features

Enucleation of the eye occasionally has been performed because of a clinical impression of uveal melanoma or other types of aggressive malignant neoplasms or because the eyes may become blind and painful.[104] Examination of enucleation specimens typically discloses extensive infiltration of the uveal tract by tumor, sometimes accompanied by retrobulbar or epibulbar involvement.[104] Currently, a diagnosis typically is established on biopsy of the lesions (when possible, of foci of extraocular or conjunctival extension). Microscopic examination typically shows a diffuse infiltrate of small lymphocytes and plasma cells (sometimes with Dutcher bodies or Russell bodies) with interspersed reactive germinal centers and scattered polykaryocytes.[104-107] Immunophenotypic features have not been extensively studied, but light chain restriction has been documented.[105,106]

Staging, Treatment, and Outcome

The disease almost always is confined to the eye and surrounding tissue. Patients have been treated with steroids, radiation or, in older series, enucleation. Survival has been excellent, with only a small minority developing recurrences in lymph nodes or extranodal sites.[104,106,107]

Differential Diagnosis

1. **Primary uveal tract lymphoma versus other neoplasms and inflammatory conditions.** The clinical differential includes choroidal melanoma, metastatic carcinoma, and a variety of inflammatory conditions. Conjunctival lymphoma is more common than uveal lymphoma, but they may have a similar appearance on physical examination. In contrast to uveal lymphoma with involvement of the overlying conjunctiva, conjunctival lymphomas are freely mobile over the surface of the eye. The pathologic differential diagnosis includes a reactive, chronic inflammatory process and secondary involvement of the eye by systemic lymphoma. Clinical correlation and immunophenotyping can help establish a diagnosis.[105-107]

Secondary Intraocular Involvement by Lymphoma

The eyes can be secondarily involved by spread from PCNSL or from systemic lymphoma arising in nodal or extranodal primary sites.[23,108,109] When systemic lymphomas (and other tumors) spread to the eye, they

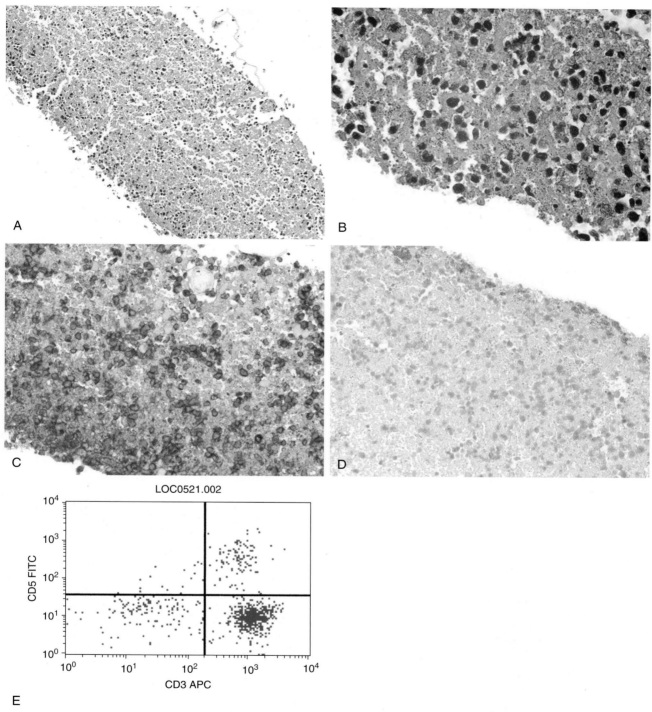

Figure 2-10 Intraocular peripheral T-cell lymphoma, not otherwise specified (NOS). **A,** Chorioretinal biopsy shows scattered lymphoid cells in a background of extensive necrosis. Normal tissue is not recognizable. **B,** Higher power shows medium-sized to large atypical lymphoid cells with dark chromatin and scant cytoplasm in a background of cellular debris. Pigment derived from the retinal pigment epithelium is interspersed. **C** and **D,** Atypical cells are CD3+ *(C)* and negative for CD5 *(D)*. Atypical T cells also were positive for CD2 and negative for CD8, CD30, TdT, B-cell markers, and Epstein-Barr virus using in situ hybridization for EBER (not shown). (Immunoperoxidase technique on paraffin sections.) **E,** Flow cytometry on vitreous fluid confirmed an aberrant CD3+, CD2+, CD5–, CD7–, CD4+, CD8–, CD56–, TCR alpha/beta+ T-cell immunophenotype. This scattergram shows abnormal CD3+, CD5– T cells in the right lower quadrant; a small population of immunophenotypically normal CD3+, CD5+ T cells is present in the right upper quadrant. A clonal T-cell receptor gamma chain gene rearrangement was identified in tissue from a concurrent brain lesion that, in conjunction with histologic and immunophenotypic features confirmed the diagnosis of peripheral T-cell lymphoma. (**E,** Image courtesy Dr. Fred Preffer, Massachusetts General Hospital, Boston.)

tend to metastasize through the blood to the uvea, especially the choroid.[36] When PCNSL involves the eye, the anatomic distribution is like that of primary intraocular lymphoma. The most common lymphoma to secondarily involve the eye is diffuse large B-cell lymphoma, but rare cases of peripheral T-cell lymphoma, NOS; extranodal NK/T-cell lymphoma[110]; mycosis fungoídes[100]; and disseminated adult T-cell lymphoma/leukemia[111] have been reported. The eye has also been the site of large cell transformation (Richter's syndrome) in rare cases of chronic lymphocytic leukemia.[112]

■ LYMPHOMAS OF THE PERIPHERAL NERVOUS SYSTEM

Introduction

Lymphoma can affect the peripheral nervous system in a variety of ways.[113] A peripheral neuropathy may be seen in association with lymphoproliferative disorders that have a monoclonal serum protein, such as Waldenström's macroglobulinemia or polyneuropathy, organomegaly, endocrinopathy, M-component, and skin changes (POEMS) syndrome; it also may be seen with immunologically mediated neural damage in conditions such as Guillain-Barré syndrome or chronic inflammatory demyelinating polyneuropathy (CIDP). In lymphomas associated with cryoglobulinemia, vasculitis may result in neuropathy. Compression of nerves or direct extension into nerves by lymphoma in adjacent tissues may be seen (Figure 2-11). Certain agents used to treat lymphoma can cause peripheral neuropathy.

Preferential infiltration of the nerves themselves is uncommon. In such cases, the patient may present with symptoms related to neural involvement, but staging usually reveals more widespread disease that involves sites outside the nervous system or, less often, within the CNS (brain parenchyma or leptomeninges with CSF involvement).[114-116] Involvement of peripheral or cranial nerves, with or without involvement of spinal nerve roots or dorsal root ganglia, is referred to as *neurolymphomatosis*.[115,117,118] Also, lymphoma that arises in other sites can relapse in peripheral nerves.[113,114,117]

Clinical Features

Patients with peripheral nerve lymphoma usually are middle-aged or older adults; males and females are equally affected. They typically present with a subacute onset of neuritic pain and/or sensory and motor deficits. Four categories of clinical presentation have been described: (1) painful involvement of nerves or nerve roots; (2) cranial neuropathy, with or without pain; (3) painless involvement of peripheral nerves; and (4) painful or painless involvement of a single peripheral nerve.[114] Involvement of a single peripheral nerve is the least common pattern.[114,117] When a single nerve is involved, it is most often the sciatic nerve.[117,119] Gross examination or MRI reveals a tumor expanding nerves, sometimes imparting a fusiform contour.[116,117]

A few patients will have a long history of neuropathy before the development of neurolymphomatosis. It is suggested that in those cases, the patients had an inflammatory process involving nerves and that B lymphocytes involved in the inflammation eventually underwent neoplastic transformation to produce a lymphoma. Some patients have a history of an autoimmune disease or other chronic inflammatory process. It can be speculated that immunologic mechanisms play a role in the development of lymphoma of the peripheral nerve. However, an increased risk for lymphoma of the peripheral nerve in patients with such disorders has not been confirmed in epidemiologic studies.[114]

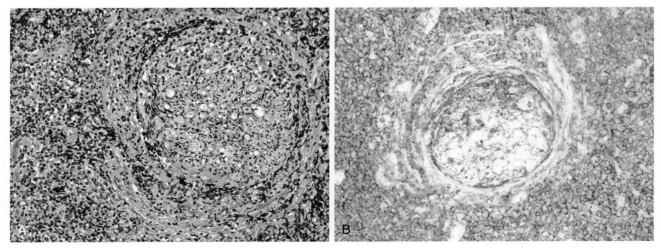

Figure 2-11 Diffuse large B-cell lymphoma involving a peripheral nerve. This patient had a past history of diffuse large B-cell lymphoma. **A,** Lymphoma surrounds and invades a peripheral nerve. **B,** B-lineage is demonstrated with an immunostain for CD20. (Immunoperoxidase technique on a paraffin section.)

Pathologic Features

Establishing a diagnosis may be challenging. Because of the rarity of lymphoma in the peripheral nervous system, the possibility of neurolymphomatosis often is not an initial consideration. Delay in diagnosis is common; in many cases, the diagnosis is not established until autopsy.[114] Once enlarged nerves have been identified, neural biopsy can establish a diagnosis. Lymphoma infiltrates the nerve, resulting in segmental demyelination and axonal degeneration.[115,118] Diffuse large B-cell lymphoma is the most common type, but low-grade B-cell lymphomas and T-cell lymphomas have been described.[113,114,117,119] Because of the difficulty associated with performing a biopsy on certain nerves, some authorities accept a diagnosis of neurolymphomatosis if there is radiographic evidence of nerve enlargement or enhancement in a patient already known to have lymphoma.

Treatment and Outcome

Patients may respond to chemotherapy, which sometimes has included methotrexate[113] or rituxan,[119] with or without radiation.[113,114,117] However, most develop relapses in other nerves, the CNS, or a variety of extranodal sites, and most succumb to the lymphoma.[117] In a study of four patients with primary peripheral nerve lymphoma, two patients who died of the disease had deletion of the *CDKN2A/p16* gene (one case tested) and loss of p16 expression (both cases). Two patients were alive at last follow-up, and both had normal *CDKN2A/p16* genes and intact p16 expression, which suggests that loss of p16 is associated with more aggressive behavior.[117]

Differential Diagnosis

The differential diagnosis on clinical grounds can include a paraneoplastic syndrome, Guillain-Barré syndrome, schwannoma, chronic inflammatory demyelinating polyneuropathy unrelated to underlying lymphoma, and other entities.[117,118] Histologically, early involvement by low-grade lymphoma could be difficult to distinguish from an inflammatory process.

■ LYMPHOMAS OF THE DURA MATER

Clinical Features

Lymphoma that arises in the dura mater is much less common than lymphoma that arises in the brain.[120] Patients with primary lymphoma of the dura are mostly middle-aged adults, but adults over a broad age range are affected. A striking female preponderance is seen.[120-122] No established risk factors have been identified, but one patient with marginal zone lymphoma had a long previous history of multiple sclerosis.[121] Patients present with seizures, headache, visual changes, focal neurologic deficits, cranial nerve abnormalities, radicular pain, syncope, or a combination of these findings.[4,120,121,123-127]

Radiologic evaluation usually reveals a localized, expansile mass or plaquelike thickening of the dura overlying the brain,[4,120,121,125] which most often is thought to be a meningioma and less often is thought to be a nerve sheath tumor or subdural hematoma preoperatively.[124,125]

Pathologic Features

Dural lymphomas are almost all extranodal marginal zone lymphomas of mucosa-associated lymphoid tissue (MALT lymphomas).[125,127] The marginal zone lymphomas have histologic and immunohistologic features similar to those seen in other sites. They are composed of small lymphocytes and marginal zone cells, usually with plasmacytic differentiation, sometimes with remnants of reactive follicles and follicular colonization.* Occasionally, associated amyloid deposition is seen,[121,127] and entrapped meningothelial cells may be present.[124,125,127] Dural marginal zone lymphomas may arise in association with meningothelium, just as marginal zone lymphomas usually arise in association with epithelium in other sites.[124,125]

The immunophenotype is similar to that of marginal zone lymphoma in other sites (Figure 2-12). Clonal rearrangement of the immunoglobulin heavy chain gene has been detected by PCR in some cases.[124,125,128] Trisomy 3 is common.[121] A translocation involving the *MALT1* and *IGH* genes, consistent with *IGH/MALT1* fusion [t(14;18)(q32;q21)], has been documented using FISH in one case.[128]

Rare cases of diffuse large B-cell lymphoma have been described.[122] In rare cases, classical Hodgkin's lymphoma arises in the meninges, and the radiographic appearance can mimic that of meningioma.[129]

Staging, Treatment, and Outcome

The lymphomas typically are localized to the dura,[120,121,124,125,127] although some marginal zone lymphomas produce multiple lesions in the dura.[120] Invasion into underlying brain, infiltration of the optic nerve, positive CSF cytology, bony erosion, and hyperostosis of the overlying skull have been described.[120,122,128] Therapy has varied from case to case, but almost all patients attain complete remission and remain in remission,[120,121,124,125,127] although systemic relapse has been described in a few patients.[120] Only a few cases of other types of lymphoma have been reported in recent years, but the prognosis for these patients appears relatively good.

---

*References 120, 121, 124, 125, 127, and 128.

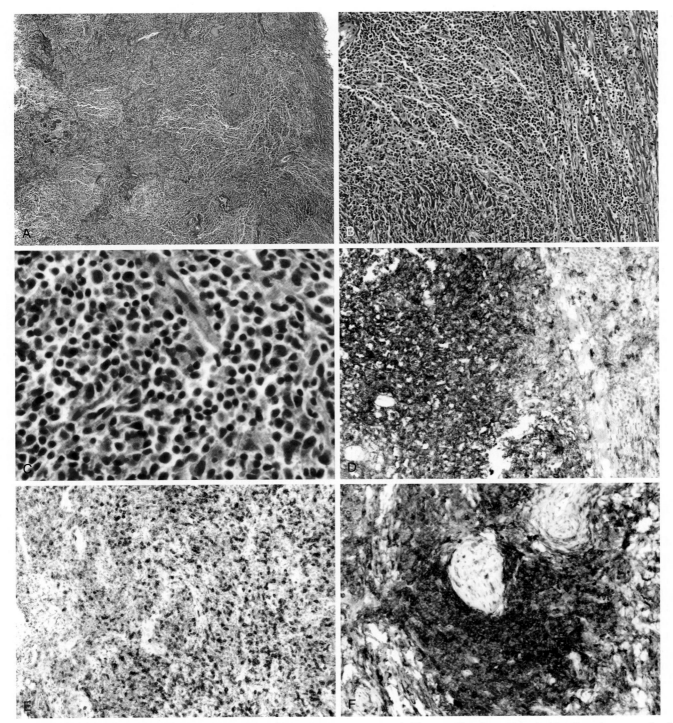

Figure 2-12 Marginal zone lymphoma arising in the dura. **A,** Vaguely nodular and diffuse proliferation of lymphoid cells replaces much of the specimen. **B,** Lymphoid cells infiltrate coarse dural collagen. **C,** High power shows small, dark lymphoid cells with smooth chromatin and many scattered plasma cells with eccentrically placed nuclei and abundant pink cytoplasm. **D to F,** Most of the cells are CD20+ B cells (*D*) with scattered CD3+ T cells (*E*). CD43+ cells are present in substantial excess of CD3+ cells, consistent with co-expression of CD43 by B cells.

Differential Diagnosis

1. **Marginal zone lymphoma versus other low-grade B-cell lymphomas.** Histologic features of other low-grade B-cell lymphomas (e.g., lympho-plasmacytic lymphoma and chronic lymphocytic

leukemia) can mimic those of marginal zone lymphoma, but marginal zone lymphomas usually are localized, in contrast to many other low-grade lymphomas; immunophenotyping is helpful.

2. **Marginal zone lymphoma versus plasmacytoma.** Some cases previously interpreted as dural

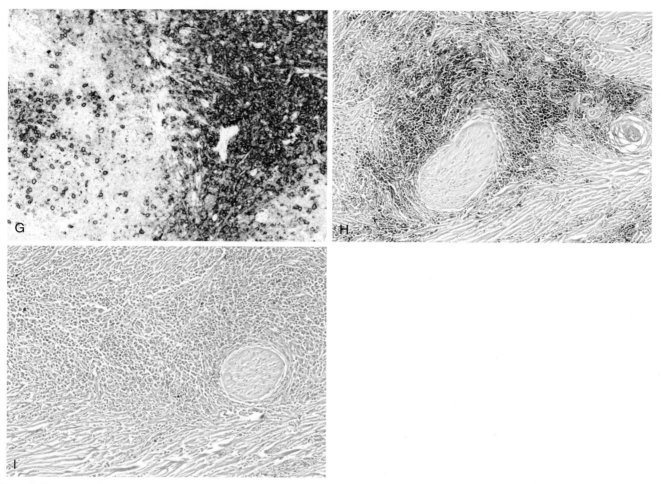

Figure 2-12, cont'd G to I, Broad bands of CD138+ plasma cells are present **(G)**. Plasma cells express monotypic kappa immunoglobulin light chain **(H)**, with only rare lambda-positive cells **(I)**. (*D* to *G*, Immunoperoxidase technique on paraffin sections; *H* and *I*, in situ hybridization on paraffin sections.)

plasmacytoma may actually represent marginal zone lymphoma with marked plasmacytic differentiation.[124,125] As in other sites, the presence of a component of B cells with the appearance of marginal zone cells should raise the question of lymphoma.

3. **Marginal zone lymphoma versus inflammatory processes.** Chronic inflammatory processes (e.g., chronic pachymeningitis) are important in the differential diagnosis of marginal zone lymphoma and other low-grade lymphomas that may involve the dura. Immunophenotyping and/or genotyping can help establish a diagnosis. Rosai-Dorfman disease can involve the dura and is associated with a prominent lymphoplasmacytic infiltrate. Rosai-Dorfman disease can be diagnosed upon recognition of the characteristic large S100+ histiocytes showing emperipolesis. A case of IgG4-related sclerosing pachymeningitis has been described.[130] The dense lymphoplasmacytic infiltrate found in this case and in cases of IgG4-related sclerosing disease in other sites could raise the question of lymphoma. Demonstration of polytypic immunoglobulin light chain expression by the plasma cells and of IgG4 by most of the plasma cells supports a diagnosis of IgG4-related sclerosing disease rather than lymphoma.

4. **Marginal zone lymphoma versus lymphoplasmacyte-rich meningioma.** Rare meningiomas are associated with a prominent lymphoplasmacytic infiltrate that may obscure the neoplastic meningothelial cells. Careful evaluation of routine sections to identify foci recognizable as meningioma is required to establish a diagnosis. The lymphoplasmacytic infiltrate is reactive and does not fulfill the criteria for lymphoma.

■ EPIDURAL LYMPHOMAS

Introduction

A minority of cases of non-Hodgkin's lymphoma (less than 5%) are associated with spinal epidural involvement. Epidural involvement can occur in the setting of widespread disease[131,132] or through direct extension from lymphoma in a vertebral body or the retroperitoneum.[133] Epidural involvement can occur at the time of initial diagnosis or at relapse of lymphoma.[131] Even more uncommon is primary spinal epidural lymphoma, defined as lymphoma primarily occurring in the epidural space in the absence of previously detected foci of lymphoma.[133-135] Fewer than 10% of all lymphomas with epidural involvement are primary in this site.[133] Lymphoma accounts for 10% of primary epidural neoplasms.[134]

Clinical Features

Primary epidural lymphoma affects males roughly twice as often as females.[133,134] Almost all patients are adults, and 80% or more are over age 40.[133,134] No specific risk factors for lymphoma in this site have been identified. Patients present with symptoms related to extrinsic compression of the spinal cord or cauda equina; the manifestations depend on the anatomic level of involvement. The most common symptoms are back pain, weakness of extremities, paraplegia, sensory deficits, and bowel or bladder dysfunction.[133-135] Patients with secondary lymphomatous involvement of the epidural space may present with similar symptoms,[131,132] but occasionally, asymptomatic epidural disease is detected during staging.[131] Primary epidural lymphoma most often affects the thoracic area, followed by the lumbar and cervical regions.[133-135] In a few cases, lymphoma has involved the lumbosacral, cervicothoracic, or thoracolumbar areas.[134]

Pathologic Features

The pathologic features of epidural lymphoma have not been described in detail in many cases, but most of these lymphomas are B-cell lymphomas. Diffuse large B-cell lymphoma is the most common type of primary epidural lymphoma. A few B-cell lymphomas of other types and a few T-cell lymphomas have been described.[135]

Staging, Treatment, and Outcome

When a patient presents with symptoms related to epidural lymphoma, staging should be performed, because many such patients are found to have widespread disease.[131,132] Patients often are treated with a combination of decompressive laminectomy with subtotal resection of tumor, and radiation, often with the addition of chemotherapy.[133-135] Primary epidural lymphoma usually responds fairly well to therapy. In one large multiinstitution series, the 5-year overall survival rate was 69%; the 5-year disease-free survival rate was 57%; and local control at 5 years was 88%.[134] Even when treatment effectively eliminates disease in the epidural space, neurologic recovery may not be complete.[133,134]

REFERENCES

1. Kluin P, Deckert M, Ferry J: Primary diffuse large B-cell lymphoma of the CNS. In Swerdlow S, Campo E, Harris N et al, editors: *WHO classification: tumours of haematopoietic and lymphoid tissues,* pp 240-241, Lyon, 2008, IARC.
2. Iwamoto FM, DeAngelis LM: An update on primary central nervous system lymphoma, *Hematol Oncol Clin North Am* 20:1267-1285, 2006.
3. van der Valk P: Central nervous system lymphomas, *Curr Diagn Pathol* 3:45-52, 1996.
4. Rubenstein J, Ferreri AJ, Pittaluga S: Primary lymphoma of the central nervous system: epidemiology, pathology and current approaches to diagnosis, prognosis and treatment, *Leuk Lymphoma* 49(suppl 1):43-51, 2008.
5. Cady FM, O'Neill BP, Law ME et al: Del(6)(q22) and BCL6 rearrangements in primary CNS lymphoma are indicators of an aggressive clinical course, *J Clin Oncol* 26:4814-4819, 2008.
6. Fine H, Mayer R: Primary central nervous system lymphoma, *Ann Intern Med* 119:1093-1104, 1993.
7. Camilleri-Broet S, Martin A, Moreau A et al: Primary central nervous system lymphomas in 72 immunocompetent patients: pathologic findings and clinical correlations, *Am J Clin Pathol* 110:607-612, 1998.
8. Herrlinger U, Schabet M, Clemens M et al: Clinical presentation and therapeutic outcome in 26 patients with primary CNS lymphoma, *Acta Neurol Scand* 97:257-264, 1998.
9. Herrlinger U, Schabet M, Brugger W et al: Primary central nervous system lymphoma, 1991-1997: outcome and late adverse effects after combined modality treatment, *Cancer* 91:130-135, 2001.
10. McAllister LD, Doolittle ND, Guastadisegni PE et al: Cognitive outcomes and long-term follow-up results after enhanced chemotherapy delivery for primary central nervous system lymphoma, *Neurosurgery* 46:51-61, 2000.
11. Sekita T, Tamaru J, Kaito K et al: Primary central nervous system lymphomas express Vh genes with intermediate to high somatic mutations, *Leuk Lymphoma* 41:377-385, 2001.
12. Eichler AF, Batchelor TT: Primary central nervous system lymphoma: presentation, diagnosis and staging, *Neurosurg Focus* 21:E15, 2006.
13. Lin CH, Kuo KT, Chuang SS et al : Comparison of the expression and prognostic significance of differentiation markers between diffuse large B-cell lymphoma of central nervous system origin and peripheral nodal origin, *Clin Cancer Res* 12:1152-1156, 2006.
14. Porter AB, Giannini C, Kaufmann T et al : Primary central nervous system lymphoma can be histologically diagnosed after previous corticosteroid use: a pilot study to determine whether corticosteroids prevent the diagnosis of primary central nervous system lymphoma, *Ann Neurol* 63:662-667, 2008.
15. Bataille B, Delwail V, Menet E et al: Primary intracerebral malignant lymphoma: report of 248 cases, *J Neurosurg* 92:261-266, 2000.
16. Miller D, Hochberg F, Harris N et al: Pathology with clinical correlations of primary central nervous system non-Hodgkin's lymphoma: the Massachusetts General Hospital experience, 1958-1989, *Cancer* 74:1383-1397, 1994.
17. Larocca L, Capello D, Rinelli A et al: The molecular and phenotypic profile of primary central nervous system lymphoma identifies distinct categories of the disease and is consistent with histogenetic derivation from germinal center related B cells, *Blood* 92:1011-1019, 1998.
18. Haldorsen IS, Krakenes J, Goplen AK et al: AIDS-related primary central nervous system lymphoma: a Norwegian national survey, 1989-2003, *BMC Cancer* 8:225, 2008.
19. Epstein L, DiCarlo F, Joshi V et al: Primary lymphoma of the central nervous system in children with acquired immunodeficiency syndrome, *Pediatrics* 82:355-363, 1988.
20. Bower M, Powles T, Nelson M et al: Highly active antiretroviral therapy and human immunodeficiency virus–associated primary cerebral lymphoma, *J Natl Cancer Inst* 98:1088-1091, 2006.
21. Olson JE, Janney CA, Rao RD et al : The continuing increase in the incidence of primary central nervous system non-Hodgkin lymphoma: a surveillance, epidemiology, and end results analysis, *Cancer* 95:1504-1510, 2002.
22. Makino K, Nakamura H, Kino T et al: Rising incidence of primary central nervous system lymphoma in Kumamoto, Japan, *Surg Neurol* 66:503-506, 2006.

23. Cassoux N, Merle-Beral H, Leblond V et al: Ocular and central nervous system lymphoma: clinical features and diagnosis, *Ocul Immunol Inflamm* 8:243-250, 2000.

24. Kirk O, Pedersen C, Cozz-Lepri A et al: Non-Hodgkin's lymphoma in HIV-infected patients in the era of highly active antiretroviral therapy, *Blood* 98:3406-3412, 2001.

25. Gottfredsson M, Oury T, Bernstein C et al: Lymphoma of the pituitary gland: an unusual presentation of central nervous system lymphoma in AIDS, *Am J Med* 101:563-564, 1996.

26. Lee MT, Lee TI, Won JG et al: Primary hypothalamic lymphoma with panhypopituitarism presenting as stiff-man syndrome, *Am J Med Sci* 328:124-128, 2004.

27. Castellano-Sanchez AA, Li S, Qian J et al: Primary central nervous system posttransplant lymphoproliferative disorders, *Am J Clin Pathol* 121:246-253, 2004.

28. Grimm SA, McCannel CA, Omuro AM et al: Primary CNS lymphoma with intraocular involvement: International PCNSL Collaborative Group Report, *Neurology* 71:1355-1360, 2008.

29. DeAngelis L: Primary central nervous system lymphoma, *J Neurol Neurosurg Psychiatry* 66:699-701, 1999.

30. Antinori A, Larocca L, Fassone L et al: HHV-8/KSHV is not associated with AIDS-related primary central nervous system lymphoma, *Brain Pathol* 9:199-208, 1999.

31. DeLuca A, Antinori A, Cingolani A et al: Evaluation of cerebrospinal fluid EBV-DNA and IL-10 as markers for in vivo diagnosis of AIDS-related primary central nervous system lymphoma, *Br J Haematol* 90:844-849, 1995.

32. Corcoran C, Rebe K, van der Plas H et al: The predictive value of cerebrospinal fluid Epstein-Barr viral load as a marker of primary central nervous system lymphoma in HIV-infected persons, *J Clin Virol* 42:433-436, 2008.

33. Capello D, Martini M, Gloghini A et al: Molecular analysis of immunoglobulin variable genes in human immunodeficiency virus–related non-Hodgkin's lymphoma reveals implications for disease pathogenesis and histogenesis, *Haematologica* 93:1178-1185, 2008.

34. Jahnke K, Korfel A, O'Neill BP et al: International study on low-grade primary central nervous system lymphoma, *Ann Neurol* 59:755-762, 2006.

35. Choi JS, Nam DH, Ko YH et al: Primary central nervous system lymphoma in Korea: comparison of B- and T-cell lymphomas, *Am J Surg Pathol* 27:919-928, 2003.

36. Commins DL: Pathology of primary central nervous system lymphoma, *Neurosurg Focus* 21:E2, 2006.

37. Camilleri-Broet S, Criniere E, Broet P et al: A uniform activated B-cell–like immunophenotype might explain the poor prognosis of primary central nervous system lymphomas: analysis of 83 cases, *Blood* 107:190-196, 2006.

38. Braaten KM, Betensky RA, de Leval L et al: BCL-6 expression predicts improved survival in patients with primary central nervous system lymphoma, *Clin Cancer Res* 9:1063-1069, 2003.

39. Sugita Y, Tokunaga O, Nakashima A, Shigemori M: SHP-1 expression in primary central nervous system B-cell lymphomas in immunocompetent patients reflects maturation stage of normal B-cell counterparts, *Pathol Int* 54:659-666, 2004.

40. Nuckols J, Liu K, Burchette J et al: Primary central nervous system lymphomas: a 30-year experience at a single institution, *Mod Pathol* 12:1167-1173, 1999.

41. Thompsett A, Ellison D, Stevenson F, Zhu D: VH gene sequences from primary central nervous system lymphomas indicate derivation from highly mutated germinal center B cells with ongoing mutational activity, *Blood* 94:1738-1746, 1999.

42. Shuangshoti S, Assanasen T, Lerdlum S et al: Primary central nervous system plasmablastic lymphoma in AIDS, *Neuropathol Appl Neurobiol* 34:245-247, 2008.

43. Rollins KE, Kleinschmidt-DeMasters BK, Corboy JR et al: Lymphomatosis cerebri as a cause of white matter dementia, *Hum Pathol* 36:282-290, 2005.

44. Montesinos-Rongen M, Schmitz R, Courts C et al: Absence of immunoglobulin class switch in primary lymphomas of the central nervous system, *Am J Pathol* 166:1773-1779, 2005.

45. Hans CP, Weisenburger DD, Greiner TC et al: Confirmation of the molecular classification of diffuse large B-cell lymphoma by immunohistochemistry using a tissue microarray, *Blood* 103:275-282, 2004.

46. Rubenstein JL, Fridlyand J, Shen A et al: Gene expression and angiotropism in primary CNS lymphoma, *Blood* 107:3716-3723, 2006.

47. Smith JR, Falkenhagen KM, Coupland SE et al: Malignant B cells from patients with primary central nervous system lymphoma express stromal cell–derived factor-1, *Am J Clin Pathol* 127:633-641, 2007.

48. Schwindt H, Akasaka T, Zuhlke-Jenisch R et al: Chromosomal translocations fusing the BCL6 gene to different partner loci are recurrent in primary central nervous system lymphoma and may be associated with aberrant somatic hypermutation or defective class switch recombination, *J Neuropathol Exp Neurol* 65:776-772, 2006.

49. McCann KJ, Ashton-Key M, Smith K et al: Primary central nervous system lymphoma: tumor-related clones exist in the blood and bone marrow with evidence for separate development, *Blood* 113:4677-4680, 2009.

50. Montesinos-Rongen M, Van Roost D, Schaller C et al: Primary diffuse large B-cell lymphomas of the central nervous system are targeted by aberrant somatic hypermutation, *Blood* 103:1869-1875, 2004.

51. Rosenwald A, Wright G, Chan W et al: The use of molecular profiling to predict survival after chemotherapy for diffuse large B-cell lymphoma, *N Engl J Med* 346:1937-1947, 2002.

52. Zhang SJ, Endo S, Saito T et al : Primary malignant lymphoma of the brain: frequent abnormalities and inactivation of p14 tumor suppressor gene, *Cancer Sci* 96:38-41, 2005.

53. Chu LC, Eberhart CG, Grossman SA et al: Epigenetic silencing of multiple genes in primary CNS lymphoma, *Int J Cancer* 119:2487-2491, 2006.

54. Harada K, Nishizaki T, Kubota H et al: Distinct primary central nervous system lymphoma defined by comparative genomic hybridization and laser scanning cytometry, *Cancer Genet Cytogenet* 125:147-150, 2001.

55. Panageas KS, Elkin EB, DeAngelis LM et al: Trends in survival from primary central nervous system lymphoma, 1975-1999: a population-based analysis, *Cancer* 104:2466-2472, 2005.

56. Shenkier TN, Voss N, Chhanabhai M et al: The treatment of primary central nervous system lymphoma in 122 immunocompetent patients: a population-based study of successively treated cohorts from the British Columbia Cancer Agency, *Cancer* 103:1008-1017, 2005.

57. Lai R, Abrey LE, Rosenblum MK, DeAngelis LM: Treatment-induced leukoencephalopathy in primary CNS lymphoma: a clinical and autopsy study, *Neurology* 62:451-456, 2004.

58. Illerhaus G, Marks R, Muller F et al: High-dose methotrexate combined with procarbazine and CCNU for primary CNS lymphoma in the elderly: results of a prospective pilot and phase II study, *Ann Oncol* 20:319-325, 2009.

59. Zhu JJ, Gerstner ER, Engler DA et al : High-dose methotrexate for elderly patients with primary CNS lymphoma, *Neuro Oncol* 11:211-215, 2009.

60. Jahnke K, Thiel E, Martus P et al: Relapse of primary central nervous system lymphoma: clinical features, outcome and prognostic factors, *J Neurooncol* 80:159-165, 2006.

61. Ferreri AJ, Reni M: Prognostic factors in primary central nervous system lymphomas, *Hematol Oncol Clin North Am* 19:629-649, vi, 2005.

62. DeAngelis LM: Primary central nervous system lymphoma: coming or going? *Blood* 113:4483-4484, 2009.

63. Jahnke K, Thiel E, Schilling A et al: Low-grade primary central nervous system lymphoma in immunocompetent patients, *Br J Haematol* 128:616-624, 2005.

64. Park I, Huh J, Kim JH et al: Primary central nervous system marginal zone B-cell lymphoma of the basal ganglia mimicking low-grade glioma: a case report and review of the literature, *Clin Lymphoma Myeloma* 8:305-308, 2008.

65. Villegas E, Villa S, Lopez-Guillermo A et al: Primary central nervous system lymphoma of T-cell origin: description of two cases and review of the literature, *J Neurooncol* 34:157-161, 1997.

66. Shenkier TN, Blay JY, O'Neill BP et al: Primary CNS lymphoma of T-cell origin: a descriptive analysis from the international primary CNS lymphoma collaborative group, *J Clin Oncol* 23:2233-2239, 2005.

67. Dulai MS, Park CY, Howell WD et al: CNS T-cell lymphoma: an under-recognized entity? *Acta Neuropathol* 115:345-356, 2008.

68. George DH, Scheithauer BW, Aker FV et al: Primary anaplastic large cell lymphoma of the central nervous system: prognostic effect of ALK-1 expression, *Am J Surg Pathol* 27:487-493, 2003.

69. Ponzoni M, Terreni MR, Ciceri F et al: Primary brain CD30+ ALK1+ anaplastic large cell lymphoma ("ALKoma"): the first case with a combination of 'not common' variants, *Ann Oncol* 13:1827-1832, 2002.

70. Rupani A, Modi C, Desai S, Rege J: Primary anaplastic large cell lymphoma of central nervous system: a case report, *J Postgrad Med* 51:326-327, 2005.

71. Merlin E, Chabrier S, Verkarre V et al: Primary leptomeningeal ALK+ lymphoma in a 13-year-old child, *J Pediatr Hematol Oncol* 30:963-967, 2008.

72. Omori N, Narai H, Tanaka T et al : Epstein-Barr virus–associated T/NK cell type central nervous system lymphoma which manifested as a post-transplantation lymphoproliferative disorder in a renal transplant recipient, *J Neurooncol* 87:189-191, 2008.

73. Kaluza V, Rao DS, Said JW, de Vos S: Primary extranodal nasal-type natural killer/T-cell lymphoma of the brain: a case report, *Hum Pathol* 37:769-772, 2006.

74. Gerstner ER, Abrey LE, Schiff D et al: CNS Hodgkin lymphoma, *Blood* 112:1658-1661, 2008.

75. Sapoznik M, Kaplan H: Intracranial Hodgkin's disease: a report of 12 cases and review of the literature, *Cancer* 52:1301-1307, 1983.

76. Hirmiz K, Foyle A, Wilke D et al: Intracranial presentation of systemic Hodgkin's disease, *Leuk Lymphoma* 45:1667-1671, 2004.

77. Re D, Fucjs M, Schober T et al: CNS involvement in Hodgkin's lymphoma, *J Clin Oncol* 25:3182, 2007.

78. Klein R, Mullges W, Bendszus M et al: Primary intracerebral Hodgkin's disease: report of a case with Epstein-Barr virus association and review of the literature, *Am J Surg Pathol* 23:477-481, 1999.

79. Haioun C, Besson C, Lepage E et al: Incidence and risk factors of central nervous system relapse in histologically aggressive non-Hodgkin's lymphoma uniformly treated and receiving intrathecal central nervous system prophylaxis: a GELA study on 974 patients, Groupe d'Etudes des Lymphomes de l'Adulte, *Ann Oncol* 11:685-690, 2000.

80. Hollender A, Kvaloy S, Nome O et al: Central nervous system involvement following diagnosis of non-Hodgkin's lymphoma: a risk model, *Ann Oncol* 13:1099-1107, 2002.

81. Boehme V, Zeynalova S, Kloess M et al: Incidence and risk factors of central nervous system recurrence in aggressive lymphoma: a survey of 1693 patients treated in protocols of the German High-Grade Non-Hodgkin's Lymphoma Study Group (DSHNHL), *Ann Oncol* 18:149-157, 2007.

82. Hasselblom S, Ridell B, Wedel H et al: Testicular lymphoma: a retrospective, population-based, clinical and immunohistochemical study, *Acta Oncol* 43:758-765, 2004.

83. Zucca E, Conconi A, Mughal TI et al: Patterns of outcome and prognostic factors in primary large-cell lymphoma of the testis in a survey by the International Extranodal Lymphoma Study Group, *J Clin Oncol* 21:20-27, 2003.

84. Peterson K, Gordon K, Heinemann M-H, DeAngelis L: The clinical spectrum of ocular lymphoma, *Cancer* 72:843-849, 1993.

85. Rivero M, Kuppermann B, Wiley C et al: Acquired immunodeficiency syndrome–related intraocular B-cell lymphoma, *Arch Ophthalmol* 117:616-622, 1999.

86. Whitcup S, de Smet M, Rubin B et al: Intraocular lymphoma: clinical and histopathologic diagnosis, *Ophthalmology* 100:1399-1406, 1993.

87. Isobe K, Ejima Y, Tokumaru S et al: Treatment of primary intraocular lymphoma with radiation therapy: a multi-institutional survey in Japan, *Leuk Lymphoma* 47:1800-1805, 2006.

88. Karma A, von Willebrand EO, Tommila PV et al: Primary intraocular lymphoma: improving the diagnostic procedure, *Ophthalmology* 114:1372-1377, 2007.

89. Freeman L, Schachat A, Knox D et al: Clinical features, laboratory investigations, and survival in ocular reticulum cell sarcoma, *Ophthalmology* 94:1631-1639, 1987.

90. Wilson D, Braziel R, Rosenbaum J: Intraocular lymphoma: immunopathologic analysis of vitreous biopsy specimens, *Arch Ophthalmol* 110:1455-1458, 1992.

91. Baehring JM, Androudi S, Longtine JJ et al: Analysis of clonal immunoglobulin heavy chain rearrangements in ocular lymphoma, *Cancer* 104:591-597, 2005.

92. Merle-Beral H, Davi F, Cassoux N et al: Biological diagnosis of primary intraocular lymphoma, *Br J Haematol* 124:469-473, 2004.

93. Brown S, Jampol L, Cantrill H: Intraocular lymphoma presenting as retinal vasculitis, *Surv Ophthalmol* 39:133-140, 1994.

94. Clark W, Scott I, Murray T et al: Primary intraocular post-transplantation lymphoproliferative disorder, *Arch Ophthalmol* 116:1667-1669, 1998.

95. Frenkel S, Hendler K, Siegal T et al: Intravitreal methotrexate for treating vitreoretinal lymphoma: 10 years of experience, *Br J Ophthalmol* 92:383-388, 2008.

96. Chan CC: Molecular pathology of primary intraocular lymphoma, *Trans Am Ophthalmol Soc* 101:275-292, 2003.

97. Chan CC, Shen D, Hackett JJ et al: Expression of chemokine receptors, CXCR4 and CXCR5, and chemokines, BLC and SDF-1, in the eyes of patients with primary intraocular lymphoma, *Ophthalmology* 110:421-426, 2003.

98. Coupland SE, Hummel M, Muller HH, Stein H: Molecular analysis of immunoglobulin genes in primary intraocular lymphoma, *Invest Ophthalmol Vis Sci* 46:3507-3514, 2005.

99. Buggage R, Chan C, Nussenblatt R: Ocular manifestations of central nervous system, *Curr Opin Oncol* 13:137-142, 2001.

100. Keltner J, Fritsch E, Cykiert R, Albert D: Mycosis fungoides: intraocular and central nervous system involvement, *Arch Ophthalmol* 95:645-650, 1977.

101. Gunduz K, Pulido JS, McCannel CA, O'Neill BP: Ocular manifestations and treatment of central nervous system lymphomas, *Neurosurg Focus* 21:E9, 2006.

102. Hormigo A, Abrey L, Heinemann MH, DeAngelis LM: Ocular presentation of primary central nervous system lymphoma: diagnosis and treatment, *Br J Haematol* 126:202-208, 2004.

103. Kohno T, Uchida H, Inomata H et al: Ocular manifestations of adult T-cell leukemia/lymphoma: a clinicopathologic study, *Ophthalmology* 100:1794-1799, 1993.

104. Ryan S, Zimmerman L, King F: Reactive lymphoid hyperplasia: an unusual form of intraocular pseudotumor, *Trans Am Acad Ophthalmol Otolaryngol* 76:652-671, 1972.

105. Ciulla TA, Bains RA, Jakobiec FA et al: Uveal lymphoid neoplasia: a clinical-pathologic correlation and review of the early form, *Surv Ophthalmol* 41:467-476, 1997.

106. Grossniklaus HE, Martin DF, Avery R et al: Uveal lymphoid infiltration: report of four cases and clinicopathologic review, *Ophthalmology* 105:1265-1273, 1998.

107. Jakobiec FA, Sacks E, Kronish JW et al: Multifocal static creamy choroidal infiltrates: an early sign of lymphoid neoplasia, *Ophthalmology* 94:397-406, 1987.

108. Hochberg F, Miller D: Primary central nervous system lymphoma (review), *J Neurosurg* 68:835-853, 1988.

109. Ridley M, McDonald H, Sternberg P Jr et al: Retinal manifestations of ocular lymphoma (reticulum cell sarcoma), *Ophthalmology* 99:1153-1161, 1992.

110. Coupland S, Foss H, Assaf C et al: T-cell and T/natural killer cell lymphomas involving ocular and ocular adnexal tissues, *Ophthalmology* 106:2109-2120, 1999.

111. Kumar S, Gill P, Wagner D et al: Human T-cell lymphotropic virus type I–associated retinal lymphoma: a clinicopathologic report, *Arch Ophthalmol* 112:954-959, 1994.

112. Fernandez-Suntay J, Gragoudas E, Ferry J et al: High grade uveal B-cell lymphoma as the initial feature in Richter syndrome, *Arch Ophthalmol* 120:1383-1385, 2002.

113. Ghobrial IM, Buadi F, Spinner RJ et al: High-dose intravenous methotrexate followed by autologous stem cell transplantation as a potentially effective therapy for neurolymphomatosis, *Cancer* 100:2403-2407, 2004.

114. Baehring JM, Damek D, Martin EC et al: Neurolymphomatosis, *Neuro Oncol* 5:104-115, 2003.

115. Abad S, Zagdanski A, Sabine B et al: Neurolymphomatosis in Waldenstrom's macroglobulinaemia, *Br J Haematol* 106:100-103, 1999.

116. Quinones-Hinojosa A, Friedlander R, Boyer P et al: Solitary sciatic nerve lymphoma as an initial manifestation of diffuse neurolymphomatosis, *J Neurosurg* 92:165-169, 2000.

117. Misdraji J, Ino Y, Louis D et al: Primary lymphoma of peripheral nerve, *Am J Surg Pathol* 24:1257-1265, 2000.

118. Diaz-Arrastia R, Younger D, Hair L et al: Neurolymphomatosis: a clinicopathologic syndrome re-emerges, *Neurology* 42:1136-1141, 1992.

119. Descamps MJ, Barrett L, Groves M et al: Primary sciatic nerve lymphoma: a case report and review of the literature, *J Neurol Neurosurg Psychiatry* 77:1087-1089, 2006.

120. Iwamoto FM, DeAngelis LM, Abrey LE: Primary dural lymphomas: a clinicopathologic study of treatment and outcome in eight patients, *Neurology* 66:1763-1765, 2006.

121. Tu PH, Giannini C, Judkins AR et al: Clinicopathologic and genetic profile of intracranial marginal zone lymphoma: a primary low-grade CNS lymphoma that mimics meningioma, *J Clin Oncol* 23:5718-5727, 2005.

122. Yamada SM, Ikawa N, Toyonaga S et al: Primary malignant B-cell–type dural lymphoma: case report, *Surg Neurol* 66:539-43; discussion, 543; 2006.

123. Altundag M, Ozisik Y, Yalcin S et al: Primary low grade B-cell lymphoma of the dura in an immunocompetent patient, *J Exp Clin Cancer Res* 19:249-251, 2000.

124. Kambham N, Chang Y, Matsushima A: Primary low-grade B-cell lymphoma of mucosa-associated lymphoma tissue (MALT) arising in dura, *Clin Neuropathol* 17:311-317, 1998.

125. Kumar S, Kumar D, Kaldjian E et al: Primary low-grade B-cell lymphoma of the dura: a mucosa associated lymphoid tissue–type lymphoma, *Am J Surg Pathol* 21:81-87, 1997.

126. Freudenstein D, Bornemann A, Ernemann U et al: Intracranial malignant B-cell lymphoma of the dura, *Clin Neuropathol* 19:34-37, 2000.

127. Lehman N, Horoupian D, Warnke R et al: Dural marginal zone lymphoma with massive amyloid deposition: rare low-grade primary central nervous system B-cell lymphoma, *J Neurosurg* 96:368-372, 2002.

128. Bhagavathi S, Greiner T, Kazmi S et al: Extranodal marginal zone lymphoma of the dura mater with IgH/MALT1 translocation and review of the literature, *J Hematopathol* 1:131-137, 2008.

129. Ashby MA, Barber PC, Holmes AE et al: Primary intracranial Hodgkin's disease: a case report and discussion, *Am J Surg Pathol* 12:294-299, 1988.

130. Chan SK, Cheuk W, Chan KT, Chan JK: IgG4-related sclerosing pachymeningitis: a previously unrecognized form of central nervous system involvement in IgG4-related sclerosing disease, *Am J Surg Pathol* 33:1249-1252, 2009.

131. Wong ET, Portlock CS, O'Brien JP, DeAngelis LM: Chemosensitive epidural spinal cord disease in non-Hodgkin's lymphoma, *Neurology* 46:1543-1547, 1996.

132. Simiele Narvarte A, Gomez Rodriguez N, Novoa Sanjurjo F: [Spinal epidural involvement as presentation form of non-Hodgkin's lymphoma: report of 6 cases], *An Med Interna* 20:466-469, 2003.

133. Lyons MK, O'Neill BP, Kurtin PJ, Marsh WR: Diagnosis and management of primary spinal epidural non-Hodgkin's lymphoma, *Mayo Clin Proc* 71:453-457, 1996.

134. Monnard V, Sun A, Epelbaum R et al: Primary spinal epidural lymphoma: patients' profile, outcome, and prognostic factors: a multicenter Rare Cancer Network study, *Int J Radiat Oncol Biol Phys* 65:817-823, 2006.

135. Schwechheimer K, Hashemian A, Ott G, Muller-Hermelink: Primary spinal epidural manifestation of malignant lymphoma, *Histopathology* 29:265-269, 1996.

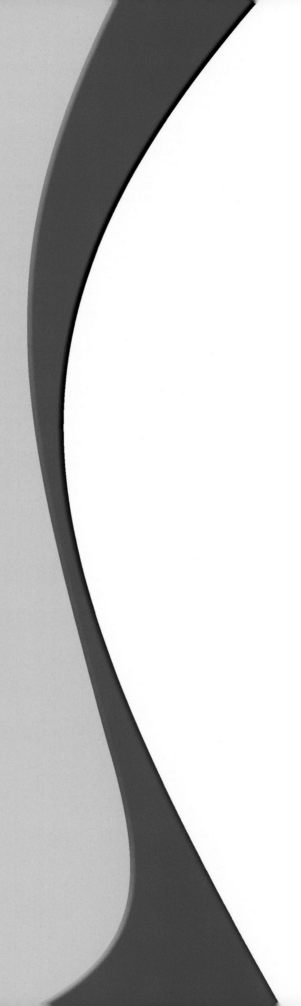

CHAPTER 3

Lymphomas of the Head and Neck

Judith A. Ferry

■ OCULAR ADNEXAL LYMPHOMAS

Primary Ocular Adnexal Lymphomas

Clinical Features

Primary ocular adnexal lymphoma is defined as lymphoma that arises in the tissues and structures surrounding the eye, including the orbital soft tissue, lacrimal gland, lacrimal sac, conjunctiva, and eyelids. One percent to 2% of all lymphomas[1] and approximately 8% of all extranodal lymphomas[2] arise in the ocular adnexa. Lymphoid tumors comprise 10% of orbital mass lesions, and lymphoma is the most common orbital malignancy.[1] Lymphomas in this site predominantly affect older women (the male to female ratio is 3:4) with a median age in the 60s.[3-5] Children are only rarely affected.[3] Occasionally, patients have a history of an autoimmune disorder,[3] another malignancy,[6] human immunodeficiency virus (HIV) infection,[7] or contact lens wear.[8] Some patients have a history of hepatitis C infection,[9,10] which could play a role in lymphomagenesis.

Some ocular adnexal marginal zone lymphomas have been associated with *Chlamydia psittaci* infection; in a subset of patients harboring *C. psittaci*, the lymphoma responded to antibiotic therapy.[11] However, marked geographic variation is seen in the proportion of cases associated with *C. psittaci*,[12] and some studies have found no association with the bacterium.[13-15] Therefore, most cases of ocular adnexal marginal zone lymphoma cannot be attributed to infection with this microorganism.

Recently, several cases of lymphoma have been described that have arisen in association with IgG4+ chronic sclerosing dacryoadenitis (sclerosing inflammatory pseudotumor); the lymphomas included marginal zone lymphoma (one case with large cell transformation) and follicular lymphoma.[16] However, in most series, most patients with ocular adnexal lymphoma have no recognizable predisposing conditions for the development of lymphoma.[3]

Patients present with symptoms related to the presence of a mass; these symptoms vary, depending on the location of the lesion. The patient may have a palpable or visible mass, exophthalmos, ptosis, diplopia, swelling or fullness, nasolacrimal duct obstruction, tearing, or discomfort.[3,5,17,18] Systemic symptoms are rare. The orbital soft tissue most often is involved, followed by the conjunctiva (bulbar or palpebral) and lacrimal gland. Lacrimal sac involvement is uncommon.[3,19] Conjunctival lymphoma usually produces a salmon-colored plaque ("salmon patch") that is mobile over the surface of the eye (Figure 3-1). Bilateral involvement is seen in approximately 13% of cases.[3]

Pathologic Features

Almost all ocular adnexal lymphomas are non-Hodgkin's lymphomas of B-lineage.[3] Extranodal marginal zone lymphoma is the most common type,

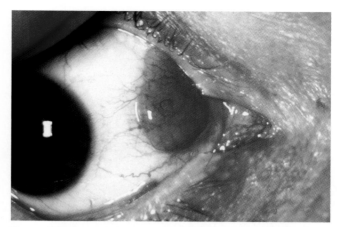

Figure 3-1 Conjunctival marginal zone lymphoma (MALT lymphoma). The lymphoma takes the form of a "salmon patch" medial to the pupil on the bulbar conjunctiva. (From Ferry JA, Harris NL: *Atlas of lymphoid hyperplasia and lymphoma,* Philadelphia, 1997, Saunders.)

accounting for roughly 60% to 75% of cases.[4,5,7,17] Most of the remainder (up to about 20% of cases) are follicular lymphomas, followed by diffuse large B-cell lymphomas, which account for fewer than 10% of cases. Occasional cases of chronic lymphocytic leukemia and mantle cell lymphoma, and rare cases of B-lymphoblastic lymphoma, present with ocular adnexal involvement.[3] Rare cases of marginal zone lymphoma with concurrent[18] or subsequent[4] diffuse large B-cell lymphoma have been described, consistent with large cell transformation.

The histologic, immunophenotypic, and genetic features of the various lymphomas overall are similar to those of the same types of lymphomas that arise in other anatomic sites, although some distinctive features have been noted (those features are discussed in this chapter).

Extranodal Marginal Zone Lymphoma of Mucosa-Associated Lymphoid Tissue (MALT Lymphoma)

The marginal zone lymphomas typically are composed of small, round to slightly irregular, lymphoid cells with a scant to moderate amount of pale cytoplasm (Figure 3-2). Monocytoid B cells with abundant, clear cytoplasm, which typically are seen in marginal zone lymphomas of the parotid gland, are uncommon. Lymphoepithelial lesions also are uncommon, even when only the subset of marginal zone lymphomas involving the lacrimal gland is considered. In most cases, residual reactive follicles can be found. In about one third of cases, plasma cells are abundant and form aggregates. In the remainder of cases, plasma cells are less numerous. Dutcher bodies can be found in more than one fourth of cases and are more common in cases with abundant plasma cells.

Multinucleated polykaryocytes are scattered among neoplastic cells in nearly half of cases

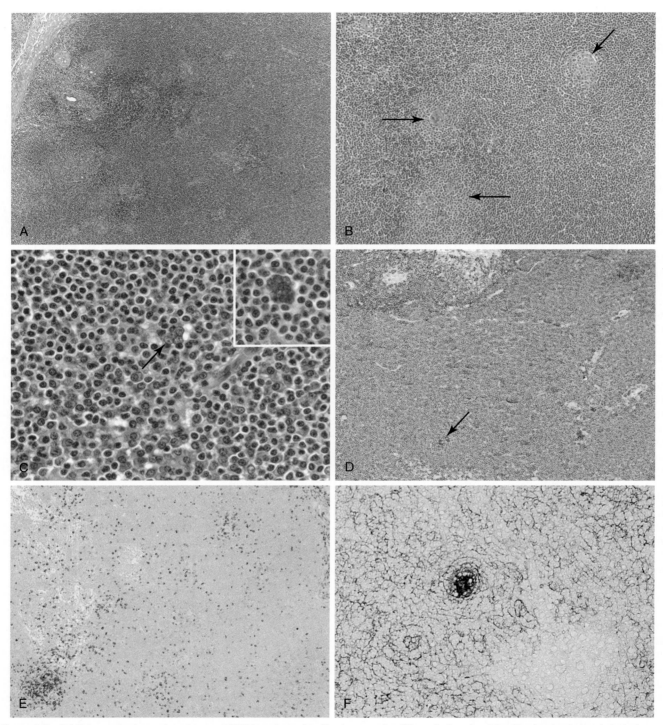

Figure 3-2   Orbital marginal zone lymphoma (MALT lymphoma), with plasmacytic differentiation, involving the lacrimal gland. **A,** A dense, diffuse lymphoid infiltrate obliterates nearly all normal tissue. A small amount of lacrimal gland epithelium remains in the left middle and left lower area of the image. **B,** Slightly higher power shows a small lymphoid follicle *(arrow, upper right)* overrun by lymphoma. Small aggregates of small neoplastic lymphoid cells with slightly more abundant, pale cytoplasm *(arrows)* surround atrophic epithelial structures in a background of numerous small lymphocytes with scant cytoplasm. **C,** High power shows small lymphoid cells and plasma cells in aggregates; plasma cells are most numerous in the left lower corner of the image. Also present is a polykaryocyte *(arrow).* An inset shows one additional polykaryocyte. Polykaryocytes are common in marginal zone lymphomas but are a nonspecific finding. **D,** An immunostain for CD20 highlights sheets of B cells; the remnant of a reactive follicle has slightly more coarse staining in a dendritic pattern *(arrow).* **E,** A small number of the cells present are small T lymphocytes (CD2+). **F,** An immunostain for CD21 densely stains a lymphoid follicle and also highlights a markedly expanded follicular dendritic meshwork infiltrated by the lymphoma.

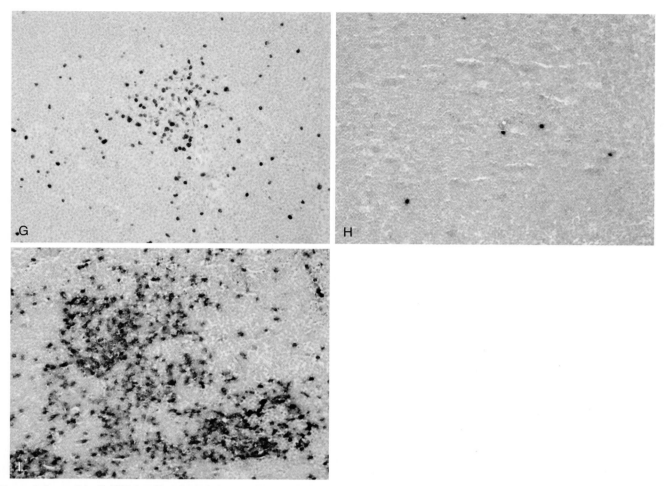

Figure 3-2, cont'd *G,* Ki67 (proliferation) stains a higher proportion of cells in the area of a follicle, likely as a result of residual reactive follicle center cells. Away from the follicle, the proliferation index is quite low. (*D* to *G,* Immunoperoxidase technique on paraffin sections.) **H** and **I,** In situ hybridization for kappa and lambda light chains shows only rare kappa-positive plasma cells **(H)** and numerous lambda-positive plasma cells **(I),** consistent with plasmacytic differentiation of the marginal zone lymphoma. (In situ hybridization on paraffin sections.)

(see Figure 3-2, *C*). The marginal zone lymphomas may show perivascular hyalinization, but interstitial sclerosis is uncommon. Rare cases are associated with amyloid deposition.[3] The marginal zone lymphomas are CD20+, CD5−, and CD10−; rare marginal zone lymphomas have been reported to express CD5 (see Figure 3-2, *D*). Approximately 25% of cases are CD43+.

Monotypic surface immunoglobulin expression almost always can be detected when fresh or frozen tissue is available for flow cytometry or immunostaining. IgM most often is expressed, followed by IgG; only rare cases are IgA+ or IgD+. Monotypic kappa and lambda are expressed in roughly equal numbers of cases. Cases with many plasma cells usually show monotypic cytoplasmic immunoglobulin expression (see Figure 3-2, *H* and *I*). Nearly all cases have CD21+ or CD23+ follicular dendritic meshworks, consistent with remnants of reactive follicles (see Figure 3-2, *F*).[3]

Ocular adnexal marginal zone lymphomas show a tendency for site-specific genetic changes. Approximately one fourth of ocular adnexal marginal zone lymphomas harbor t(14;18), a translocation involving the immunoglobulin heavy chain gene (*IGH*) and the *MALT1* gene. This translocation also has been found in marginal zone lymphomas arising in the liver, skin, and salivary glands, but it is vanishingly rare in marginal zone lymphomas in other sites. Conversely, t(11;18), a translocation involving *API2* and *MALT1* that is common in gastric marginal zone lymphoma, is not frequently encountered in the ocular adnexa.[20] A subset of ocular adnexal marginal zone lymphomas shows a loss of genetic material in the area of the NFκB inhibitor *A20* (also known as TNF α-induced protein 3, or *TNFAIP3*) and at 6q23, and a gain of genetic material in the area of the tumor necrosis factor (TNF) A/B/C locus at 6p21.[21] In some cases, *A20* promoter methylation can be demonstrated; this appears to

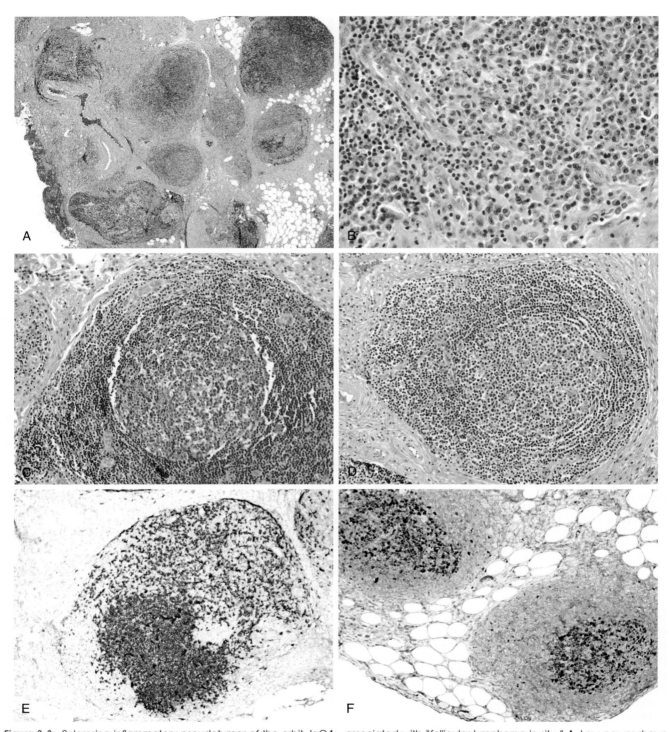

Figure 3-3 Sclerosing inflammatory pseudotumor of the orbit, IgG4+, associated with "follicular lymphoma in situ." **A,** Low power shows lymphoid follicles scattered in a sclerotic background. **B,** Many plasma cells and scattered eosinophils are present around the follicles. **C,** Some follicles have discrete, active, hyperplastic-appearing follicle centers. **D,** Other follicles have follicle centers with a more monotonous cellular composition that are less well delineated from their mantle. **E,** CD20+ B cells occupy follicles and are also scattered outside follicles. **F,** Follicles centers are bcl6+.

be most common in cases with heterozygous deletion of *A20*, leading functionally to homozygous deletion of *A20*.[22] These changes could promote lymphomagenesis through activation of the NFκB pathway, analogous to several of the chromosomal translocations that have been associated with marginal zone lymphomas (see Table 1-1). Cases with *A20* deletion have a shorter relapse-free survival.[21]

In patients with bilateral ocular adnexal lymphoma, the morphologic, immunophenotypic, and

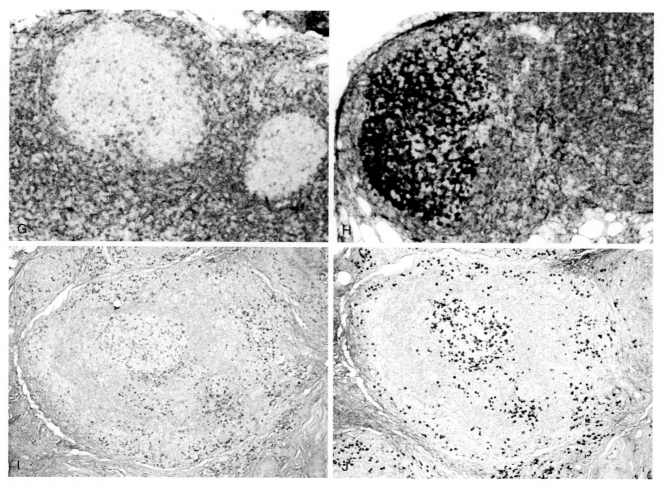

Figure 3-3, cont'd   G, Reactive-appearing follicles have bcl2– follicle centers. **H,** The monotonous follicles show bright overexpression of bcl2 without distortion of the underlying architecture of the lymphoid tissue, a pattern referred to as *follicular lymphoma in situ*. **I,** Many IgG+ plasma cells surround follicles and also are scattered within follicles. **J,** IgG4+ plasma cells are present in numbers and distribution similar to those of IgG, consistent with this pseudotumor representing an IgG4-associated sclerosing lesion. (*E* to *J,* Immunoperoxidase technique on paraffin sections.)

molecular genetic features are reported to be identical, consistent with a single neoplastic clone involving both sites rather than two distinct, unrelated primary tumors.[7,8,23]

Follicular Lymphoma

Most follicular lymphomas have a predominantly follicular pattern, and most are low-grade (grade 1 or 2 of 3). Half of follicular lymphomas are associated with sclerosis.[3] The neoplastic follicles are CD20+, CD10+, bcl6+, and CD43–; although most are bcl2+, a subset of the follicular lymphomas does not express the bcl2 protein.[3] One example of pediatric-type follicular lymphoma that arose in the conjunctiva has been described; this lymphoma was grade 3 of 3, and the neoplastic cells in this case were CD43+, in contrast to other ocular adnexal follicular lymphomas.[3] We have seen a case of IgG4-associated sclerosing inflammatory pseudotumor in which were several follicles with bright expression

of the bcl2 protein, so-called follicular lymphoma in situ (Figure 3-3).

Diffuse Large B-Cell Lymphoma

The diffuse large B-cell lymphomas usually are composed of centroblasts with round or oval, vesicular nuclei; however, multilobated large lymphoid cells or immunoblasts occasionally predominate.[3]

Peripheral T-Cell Lymphoma

Rare cases of T-cell lymphoma[24,25] have manifested ocular adnexal lymphoma at presentation.

Extranodal Natural Killer (NK)/T-Cell Lymphoma, Nasal Type

Extranodal NK/T-cell lymphoma, nasal type, is an EBV+ lymphoma that rarely involves the ocular adnexa.[3] Males are affected more often than females. Patients, on average, are younger than other patients with ocular adnexal lymphoma; in one recent series, the mean age was 45 years.[26] In a few patients with NK/T-cell lymphoma, the lymphoma is confined to the ocular adnexa at presentation[3,26]; most patients, however, have ocular adnexal involvement with concurrent sinonasal lymphoma or even more widespread involvement by lymphoma.[26] The pathologic features are similar to those of NK/T-cell lymphoma in the nasal cavity (see Lymphomas of the Nasal Cavity and Paranasal Sinuses, later in the chapter). The prognosis is poor; most patients succumb to the lymphoma less than 1 year after diagnosis.[26]

Staging, Treatment, and Outcome

Overall, in approximately 80% to 90% of patients with marginal zone lymphoma, the disease is confined to the ocular adnexa unilaterally or bilaterally.[13,27] Other types of primary ocular adnexal lymphoma also usually present as a localized disease, although in some studies, marginal zone lymphomas have been more likely to present as stage I disease than other types of lymphoma.[28,29]

Localized low-grade lymphomas usually are treated with radiation. Intermediate or high-grade lymphoma, whether localized or widespread, usually is treated with a combination of ocular adnexal radiation and chemotherapy. Chemotherapy usually is added to radiation for disseminated low-grade lymphoma.[29-31] Radiation therapy achieves excellent local control of the disease; absence of local recurrence is close to 100%.[5,28,30,32] In a large series from our hospital, the 5- and 10-year relapse-free survival rates for patients with marginal zone lymphoma were 65% and 35%, respectively; the 5- and 10-year overall survival rates were 93% and 88%, respectively.[27] Of the few patients with marginal zone lymphoma who died, one had developed large cell transformation. The relapse-free and overall survival rates for follicular lymphoma were similar to those for marginal zone lymphoma. Patients with diffuse large B-cell lymphoma had excellent relapse-free and overall survival rates.

Thus, patients with low-grade (marginal zone or follicular lymphoma) had frequent relapses but a very good overall survival rate. Patients with diffuse large B-cell lymphoma usually attained complete remission and remained in remission. Relapses of marginal zone lymphoma often were extranodal; the skin and soft tissue and the same or opposite ocular adnexa were the most common extranodal sites of relapse.[27]

Prognostically important features vary from one series to another. Patients who present with disease localized to the ocular adnexa have a much better prognosis than those with more widespread disease.[4,7,29,33] Ironically, considering how strongly the stage affects the prognosis, isolated bilateral ocular adnexal disease does not have a worse prognosis than unilateral disease.[30,34] The histologic type of lymphoma also is important in defining the outcome. In most reports, patients with high-grade lymphoma had a worse outcome.[4,17,18,29] Bony erosion also has been associated with a worse prognosis,[29] but most lymphomas with bony erosion are large cell lymphomas.[6] A high proportion of mib-1 or p53+ cells (or both) correlates with an unfavorable outcome,[7] but these markers also correlate with more aggressive histologic types. Of the marginal zone lymphomas studied at the Massachusetts General Hospital, those involving the lacrimal gland showed a trend for worse relapse-free survival rates than did those involving the orbital soft tissue or conjunctiva; however, no difference in survival was noted with respect to age, gender, stage, or unilateral versus bilateral disease.[27]

Differential Diagnosis

1. **Lymphoma versus reactive lymphoid infiltrates.** Because most ocular adnexal lymphomas are low-grade lymphomas, the main entity in the differential diagnosis is a reactive process, including sclerosing inflammatory pseudotumor and reactive lymphoid hyperplasia. Inflammatory pseudotumor is a lesion with a variably cellular, polymorphous infiltrate of small lymphocytes, plasma cells, immunoblasts, and histiocytes, sometimes with hyperplastic follicles, eosinophils and/or neutrophils, in a stroma with areas that are hyalinized, edematous, or both. Immunohistochemical studies in such cases show a mixture of T cells, B cells, and polytypic plasma cells. In some cases inflammatory pseudotumors are part of the spectrum of IgG4+ sclerosing disease, and numerous IgG4+ plasma cells are seen in these cases. Reactive lymphoid hyperplasia usually consists of follicular hyperplasia without a prominent diffuse lymphoid proliferation and without cytologic atypia. A dense, diffuse infiltrate composed predominantly of B cells favors marginal zone lymphoma. Lymphomas typically express monotypic surface immunoglobulin on frozen section immunostains or by flow cytometry. A subset of cases shows plasmacytic differentiation, with monotypic cytoplasmic immunoglobulin demonstrable with immunohistochemistry on paraffin sections. Follicular lymphomas usually are composed of atypical, crowded follicles occupied by a monotonous population of centrocytes with small numbers of centroblasts. Neoplastic cells usually express monotypic immunoglobulin and usually co-express bcl2, in contrast to reactive follicles.[3] Bilateral lesions and bony erosion are more common in lymphoma than in reactive lesions.[35]

Secondary Ocular Adnexal Lymphoma

The ocular adnexa may be secondarily involved by lymphomas that arise in other sites. An estimated 5% of patients with non-Hodgkin's lymphoma develop ocular adnexal involvement during the course of the disease. Patients with secondary ocular adnexal lymphoma usually are adults and, on average, are slightly younger or about the same age as patients with primary ocular adnexal lymphoma.[1,3,6] A variety of types of non-Hodgkin's lymphoma can be found in this setting. The most common is follicular lymphoma, followed by marginal zone lymphoma.[3,4] Diffuse large B-cell lymphoma, mantle cell lymphoma and, rarely, splenic marginal zone lymphoma,[3] hairy cell leukemia,[7] and T-cell or extranodal NK/T-cell lymphomas also may secondarily involve the ocular adnexa.[3,7,24] In the rare cases in which NK/T-cell lymphoma, nasal type, affects the ocular adnexa, the primary site may be sinonasal.[26] In rare cases, Hodgkin's lymphoma can relapse in the ocular adnexa.[3]

Secondary ocular adnexal marginal zone and follicular lymphomas have worse failure-free survival rates than do primary lymphomas of the same types, although their disease-specific survival rates are similar. Secondary ocular adnexal involvement by diffuse large B-cell lymphoma has a moderately poor prognosis.[27] Patients are more likely to have disseminated disease at presentation.[36] Although the ocular adnexal lymphoma usually can be eradicated, the extraorbital disease frequently persists or progresses.[1,6]

■ LYMPHOMAS OF WALDEYER'S RING

Introduction

Waldeyer's ring includes the palatine tonsils, the nasopharynx, and the base of the tongue. The ring of organized lymphoid tissue in these sites guards the entrance to the alimentary and respiratory tracts. Waldeyer's ring is the most common primary site for lymphomas that arise in the upper aerodigestive tract,[37] giving rise to 5% to 10% of all non-Hodgkin's lymphomas. More than half of all non-Hodgkin's lymphomas that are primary in the head and neck arise in Waldeyer's ring.[38] The incidence of Waldeyer's ring lymphoma appears to be somewhat higher in Asia than in the United States.[39]

Primary Non-Hodgkin's Lymphomas of Waldeyer's Ring

Clinical Features

Most patients with primary non-Hodgkin's lymphomas of Waldeyer's ring are adults (median age in the 50s), and the male to female ratio is 1:1 to 1:1.5.[38,40,41] Children also may develop lymphoma in this site.[42,43] Among patients with diffuse large B-cell lymphoma, the male preponderance is slightly more pronounced in some series,[43] whereas patients with extranodal marginal zone lymphoma (MALT lymphoma) are more likely to be female.[40,44] A few patients are HIV positive[45] or iatrogenically immunosuppressed. Patients with marginal zone lymphoma typically do not have an identifiable predisposing condition, such as an autoimmune disease, in contrast to those with marginal zone lymphoma arising in some other sites.[40,44] Patients present with dyspnea caused by airway obstruction, a sore throat, or a neck mass caused by

cervical lymphadenopathy. A minority of patients have systemic symptoms.[37,42,43,45]

The tonsil is the most frequently involved site (accounting for more than half of Waldeyer's ring lymphomas), followed by the nasopharynx and the base of the tongue.[19,37,38,41] In some cases, more than one component of Waldeyer's ring is involved.[40] Physical examination reveals a mass that is unilateral and exophytic in most cases; it may be polypoid, fungating, or ulcerated, with invasion of adjacent tissues. The lymphoma is localized (stage I or stage II) in more than 75% of cases; however, as a result of cervical lymph node involvement, stage II disease is more common than stage I disease in most series.[41,43]

Pathologic Features

Diffuse large B-cell lymphoma is by far the most common type of lymphoma in Waldeyer's ring, accounting for 60% to 84% of cases (Figure 3-4). Other, less common types include follicular lymphoma (Figure 3-5), Burkitt's lymphoma, mantle cell lymphoma, extranodal marginal zone lymphoma (MALT lymphoma [see Figure 3-6]), and peripheral T-cell lymphoma.[19,37,38,41] Extranodal NK/T-cell lymphoma, nasal type, also may arise in Waldeyer's ring; this is more often encountered in Asia than in Western countries.[46] Mantle cell lymphoma can present with involvement of Waldeyer's ring, but in contrast to diffuse large B-cell lymphoma, mantle cell lymphoma usually is widespread at the time of diagnosis. Burkitt's lymphoma is much more common in children with Waldeyer's ring lymphoma than it is in adults with lymphoma in this site[42]; children also may develop diffuse large B-cell lymphoma.[40,43]

Diffuse Large B-Cell Lymphoma

Diffuse large B-cell lymphomas are composed of a diffuse proliferation of large lymphoid cells, including centroblasts, immunoblasts, and large, atypical cells with irregular nuclei, with distortion or obliteration of the normal architecture. Neoplastic cells are CD20+, usually bcl6+, and CD10+ in nearly half of cases. EBV is found in a minority of cases.[40] In one study, 51% of cases showed diffuse, uniform expression of bcl6 similar to that seen in germinal centers, usually accompanied by CD10 expression; these cases were considered to be of germinal center B-cell origin. Other cases either had nonuniform bcl6 expression or failed to express bcl6; these cases usually did not co-express CD10 and were considered to be of non-germinal center derivation.[39] This potentially is an important distinction, because deoxyribonucleic acid (DNA) microarray studies indicate that patients with germinal center B-cell–like diffuse large B-cell lymphoma have a better prognosis than patients with other activated B-cell or type 3 diffuse large B-cell lymphomas.[47,48] In addition, diffuse large B-cell lymphoma that arises as a histologic progression of marginal zone lymphoma (see Extranodal Marginal Zone Lymphoma, later in

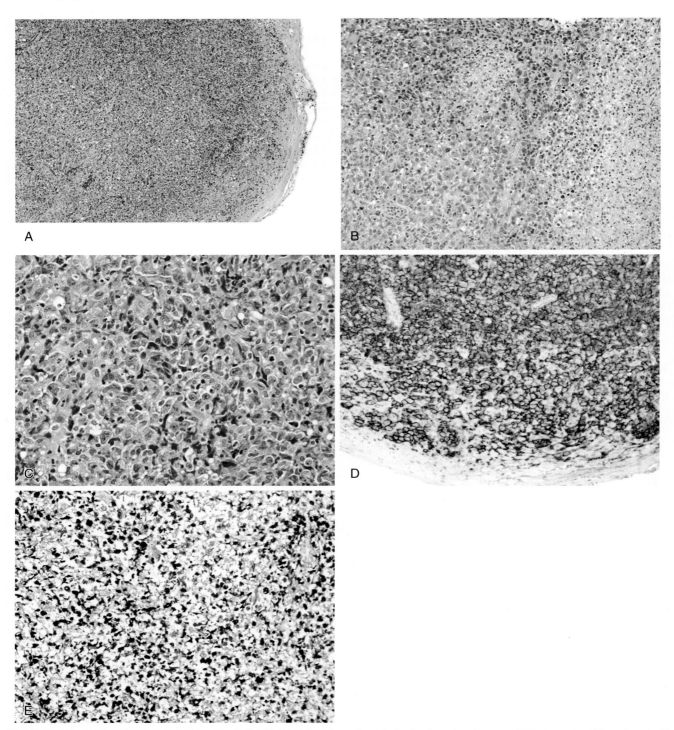

Figure 3-4 EBV+ diffuse large B-cell lymphoma of the elderly involving the tonsil of a 74-year-old woman. **A,** A dense, diffuse lymphoid infiltrate lies beneath and also invades the overlying squamous epithelium. **B,** In these areas, the epithelium is ulcerated and the surface of the tissue consists of necrotic debris *(right)*. **C,** High power shows sheets of large atypical cells with oval or irregular nuclei, vesicular chromatin, and prominent nucleoli. In this example, the lymphoma has a monomorphous composition. **D,** Diffuse, strong CD20 expression by the neoplastic B cells. (Immunoperoxidase technique on a paraffin section.) **E,** In situ hybridization demonstrates the presence of Epstein-Barr virus (EBV) in the tumor cells. (In situ hybridization for Epstein-Barr virus–encoded RNA (EBER) on a paraffin section.)

the chapter) would be expected not to show the uniform pattern of bcl6 expression.[39]

EBV+ diffuse large B-cell lymphoma of the elderly is a subtype of diffuse large B-cell lymphoma that affects individuals over age 50 who do not have any specific underlying immunodeficiency. The presence of EBV suggests that the lymphoma arose because of the decreased immunosurveillance that may occur with advancing age. Extranodal involvement is common, and the tonsil is among the more common

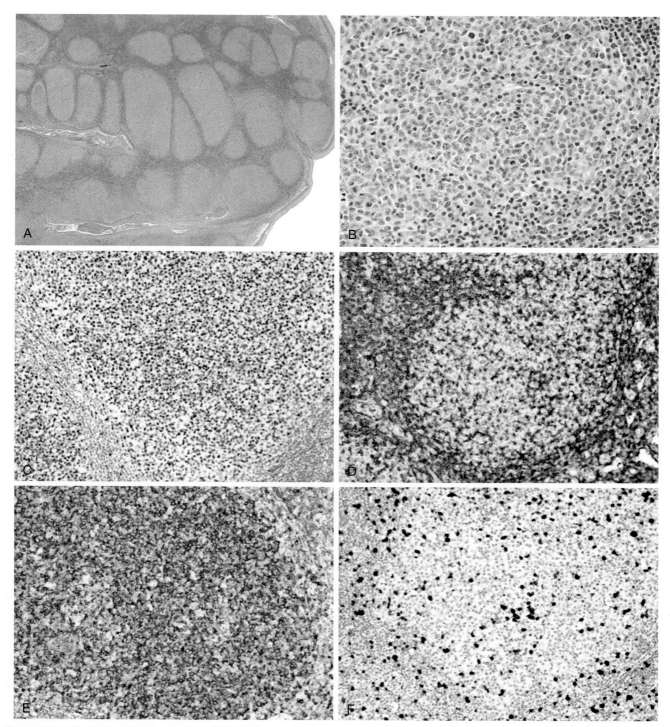

Figure 3-5 Follicular lymphoma, grade 2 of 3, involving the tonsil. **A,** Low power shows that although several intact crypts remain, the rest of the tissue has been replaced by crowded follicles lacking mantles. **B,** High power shows a follicle occupied by centrocytes and occasional centroblasts. **C,** Follicles are composed mainly of B cells (Pax5+). **D,** T cells (CD2+) are scattered within follicles and are present in larger numbers in the interfollicular area. **E** and **F,** B cells co-express bcl2 **(E)** and have a low proliferation index using Ki67 **(F)**; the histologic and immunohistologic features together support a diagnosis of follicular lymphoma over follicular hyperplasia. (*C* to *F,* Immunoperoxidase technique on paraffin sections.)

sites of involvement. The lymphoma can be monomorphous or polymorphous. Neoplastic cells typically are CD20+, CD79a+, or both. They usually lack markers of the germinal center stage of differentiation (CD10, bcl6), and they do express MUM1/IRF4,

a later stage differentiation marker and, often, CD30. EBV is present, by definition (see Figure 3-4).[49]

Patients with diffuse large B-cell lymphoma respond well to therapy, and a high proportion achieve complete remission. However, distant relapse frequently occurs, particularly in patients treated with radiation alone.[38, 41] Relapses may occur in the lymph nodes and a variety of extranodal sites,[38] but some observers have reported a predilection for spread to the gastrointestinal tract.[41]

A better prognosis has been reported for patients with tonsillar primaries compared to those with lymphoma that arises elsewhere in Waldeyer's ring.[38] In a recent study of tonsillar diffuse large B-cell lymphoma, the 10-year disease-free survival rate was 66%, and the overall survival rate was 82%. The prognosis was worse with higher stage disease, a bulky primary tumor (greater than 7 cm), the presence of B symptoms, and a performance score of 2 or higher.[43] Patients treated with combined modality therapy (e.g., chemotherapy, either cyclophosphamide, doxorubicin, vincristine, and prednisone [CHOP] or a CHOP-like regimen, and radiation) had a better outcome than those treated with chemotherapy alone.[43]

Extranodal Marginal Zone Lymphoma of Mucosa-Associated Lymphoid Tissue (MALT Lymphoma)

The marginal zone lymphomas are characterized by a parafollicular, interfollicular, or diffuse proliferation of marginal zone cells with slightly irregular nuclei and a moderate amount of clear cytoplasm (Figure 3-6). Monocytoid B cells with abundant, clear cytoplasm, plasmacytoid differentiation, and follicular colonization may be present. Neoplastic cells routinely invade crypt epithelium to form lymphoepithelial lesions,[40,44] although this histologic feature also is characteristic of nonneoplastic lymphoid tissue in this site. In some cases increased numbers of large B cells are seen, consistent with progression to diffuse large B-cell lymphoma.[40] Some have suggested that the frequency of marginal zone lymphoma in Waldeyer's ring has been underestimated, because it may be difficult to render a diagnosis of marginal zone lymphoma from small biopsy samples. Similarly, a small biopsy sample may disclose diffuse large B-cell lymphoma but fail to reveal an underlying marginal zone lymphoma.[40]

The neoplastic cells typically are CD20+, CD5−, CD10−, CD43+/−, bcl2+, bcl6−, IRF4/MUM1+/−, cyclin D1−, IgM+, and cytoplasmic light chain+/− (Figure 3-6, F to K); residual reactive follicle centers, if present, are CD20+, CD10+, bcl6+, and bcl2−. Immunostains for follicular dendritic cells such as CD21 and CD23 demonstrate disrupted follicular dendritic meshworks.[40,44] Neoplastic cells are negative for EBV. Genetic features have not been studied in detail, but a clonal rearrangement of the immunoglobulin heavy chain gene has been seen, and one case was negative for trisomy 3 and for t(11;18) (q21;q21) involving the *API2* and *MALT1* genes.[44]

Patients with extranodal marginal zone lymphoma have an excellent prognosis,[40,44] although some with progression to diffuse large B-cell lymphoma may have a more aggressive course and succumb to the lymphoma.[40]

Extranodal NK/T-Cell Lymphoma, Nasal Type

Extranodal NK/T-cell lymphomas of the type most often encountered in the nasal cavity may occur in a variety of other anatomic sites (see Extranodal NK/T-Cell Lymphoma, Nasal Type, later in the chapter). The most common of these nonnasal sites is the upper aerodigestive tract, and the most common site in the aerodigestive tract is Waldeyer's ring.[46] Within Waldeyer's ring, the nasopharynx is the most common primary site, followed by the tonsil. The base of the tongue and the oropharynx only rarely serve as the primary site. As is true of this type of lymphoma in the nasal cavity, when it arises in Waldeyer's ring, the patients mostly are male and, on average, younger than patients with most other types of Waldeyer's ring lymphoma (in one recent series, the median age was 37).[46]

Lymph node involvement (and therefore a higher proportion of cases with Ann Arbor stage II disease) appears to be more common with Waldeyer's ring nasal-type NK/T-cell lymphoma than for nasal primaries. The lymphomas are sensitive to radiation therapy, and the addition of combination chemotherapy appears to reduce the chance of systemic failure. The 5-year overall survival rate is estimated to be 65%. Older age, a higher stage, and the presence of B symptoms are reported to be associated with a worse survival outcome.[46]

Secondary Non-Hodgkin's Lymphoma of Waldeyer's Ring

Patients with a variety of types of lymphoma may show spread to Waldeyer's ring. This situation seems to be less common than lymphoma with primary involvement of Waldeyer's ring.[41]

Hodgkin's Lymphoma of Waldeyer's Ring

Hodgkin's lymphoma, almost always the classical type, rarely presents with involvement of Waldeyer's ring. These cases account for as few as 1% of all Waldeyer's ring lymphomas.[50] In rare cases, relapse in Waldeyer's ring may occur in patients with Hodgkin's lymphoma that arises in another site. These lymphomas affect the nasopharynx and tonsils, but involvement of the base of the tongue is rare.[50-52] Patients presenting with involvement of Waldeyer's ring are affected over a broad age range, but almost all are adults (median age in the 40s), and a slight male preponderance is seen.[52] Rare patients have had previous or have concurrent non-Hodgkin's lymphoma, including follicular lymphoma and chronic lymphocytic leukemia.[52] Rare patients have been HIV positive.[52] Patients present with symptoms similar to those of patients with non-Hodgkin's lymphomas. In fewer than one-half of cases, the disease is localized to Waldeyer's ring. Often the disease also involves the cervical lymph nodes and occasionally more distant sites as well.[51,52]

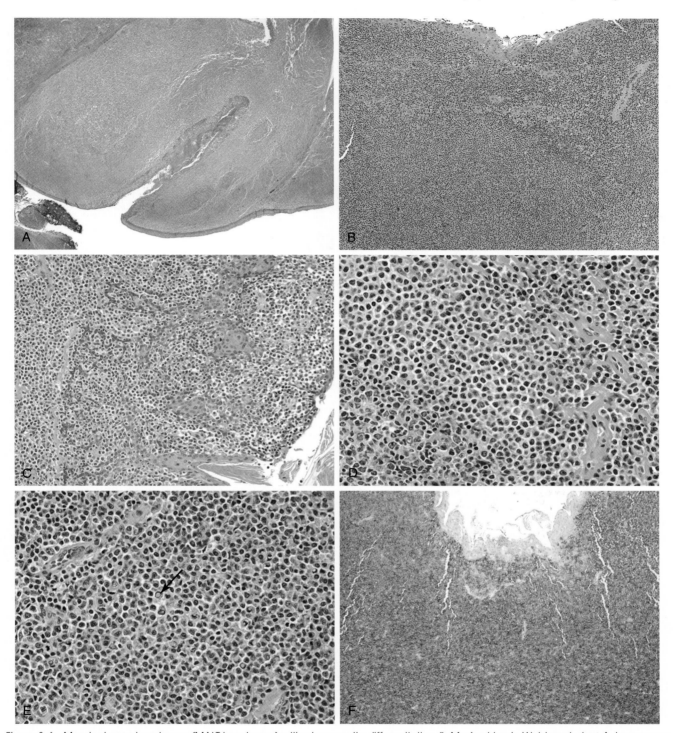

Figure 3-6 Marginal zone lymphoma (MALT lymphoma) with plasmacytic differentiation (IgMκ+) arising in Waldeyer's ring. **A,** Low power shows distortion of the normal architecture. **B,** Slightly higher power shows that most cells present are small lymphoid cells; reactive follicles are much less conspicuous than usual. **C,** Numerous monocytoid B cells with clear cytoplasm and also many plasma cells infiltrate crypt epithelium; this is seen in normal tonsils and is not a finding specific for lymphoma in this site. **D,** High power shows a portion of a reactive follicle with a polymorphous population of small and large cells *(lower left);* the remainder of the image is occupied by small lymphoid cells and plasma cells. **E,** Plasma cells are numerous in areas; many of the plasma cells in this image contain Dutcher bodies, which are intranuclear protrusions of cytoplasm containing immunoglobulin (the *arrow* points to a Dutcher body). **F,** Sheets of CD20+ B cells are present.

Continued

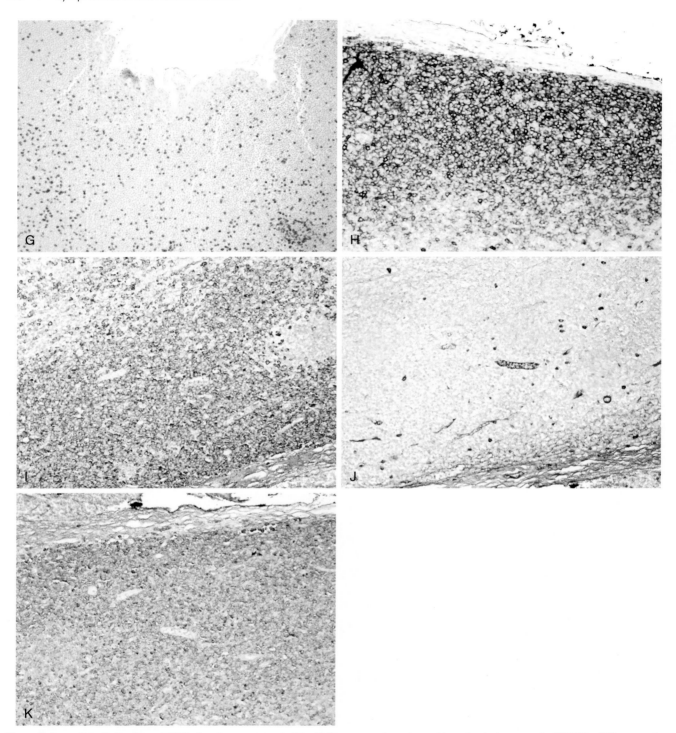

Figure 3-6, cont'd   G, Scattered CD3+ T cells are present. **H** to **K,** Also present are broad bands of plasma cells (CD138+ **(H)**) expressing monotypic kappa light chain **(I)**; only a few lambda light chain–positive plasma cells are present **(J)**. Plasma cells co-express mu heavy chain **(K)**, consistent with a marginal zone lymphoma with plasmacytic differentiation expressing monotypic IgMκ. (*F* to *K,* Immunoperoxidase technique on paraffin sections.)

The most common types of Hodgkin's lymphoma in Waldeyer's ring are nodular sclerosis, mixed cellularity, and lymphocyte-rich classical Hodgkin's lymphoma; only rare cases of nodular lymphocyte–predominant and lymphocyte-depleted types are described.[50,52] In one study, among the cases confined to Waldeyer's ring, lymphocyte-rich classical Hodgkin's lymphoma was the most common type.[52] In several cases of Hodgkin's lymphoma of the nodular sclerosis type, lacunar cell variants and a nodular pattern of growth were seen but without fibrous bands, consistent with the cellular phase of nodular sclerosis.[50] Several cases have had a predominantly interfollicular pattern of growth and therefore were not subclassified.[50]

The immunophenotype of the neoplastic cells (CD15+, CD30+, and CD20–/+) is similar to that found in other sites.[50,52] Tumor cells in most cases contain EBV (67% in two large series).[50,52] The Epstein-Barr virus may be more prevalent in Hodgkin's lymphoma in this anatomic site than in Hodgkin's lymphoma arising elsewhere, possibly because Waldeyer's ring is a reservoir for EBV.[50,52]

Differential Diagnosis

1. **Reactive lymphoid hyperplasia versus lymphoma.** Reactive lymphoid hyperplasia often causes enlargement of one or more of the components of Waldeyer's ring, sometimes forming mass lesions that mimic a neoplasm. Preservation of reactive follicles and crypts favors a reactive process.

   a. *Infectious mononucleosis versus diffuse large B-cell lymphoma.* Infectious mononucleosis, in particular, can mimic a diffuse large B-cell lymphoma. However, some architectural preservation, a polymorphous composition, positive in situ hybridization for EBER (Figure 3-7), and clinical features can be helpful for making the differential diagnosis. In addition, the immunophenotype of the immunoblasts in infectious mononucleosis is distinctive and may help exclude lymphoma. The immunoblasts typically are CD20+, CD10–, bcl6–, bcl2+/–, and MUM1/IRF4+, with polytypic immunoglobulin light chain expression (see Figure 3-7, *E* to *L*).[53] This immunophenotype corresponds to a post-germinal center stage of differentiation. Most diffuse large B-cell lymphomas are bcl6+, and some are CD10+; therefore lack of CD10 and bcl6 may raise the question of an alternative diagnosis. Polytypic light chain expression in the large, atypical EBV+ immunoblasts strongly supports a reactive process. In addition, CD8+ T cells typically outnumber CD4+ T cells in infectious mononucleosis,[53] whereas in most B-cell lymphomas in immunocompetent patients, the opposite is true. Therefore, careful examination of the histologic features, combined with focused immunophenotypic evaluation, can help prevent misdiagnosis.

   b. *Infectious mononucleosis versus Hodgkin's lymphoma.* Infectious mononucleosis is characterized by a proliferation of EBV-infected immunoblasts, some of which may be large, atypical, and/or binucleated, potentially mimicking Reed-Sternberg cells (see Figure 3-7, *D*). Infectious mononucleosis is associated with distortion of the architecture of the lymphoid tissue, showing interfollicular expansion but without architectural obliteration. Hodgkin's lymphoma is more likely to obliterate the normal architecture. Although some of the large cells in infectious mononucleosis may closely resemble Reed-Sternberg cells, most have the morphology of immunoblasts. The background reactive population contains lymphoid cells in a range of sizes, in contrast to Hodgkin's lymphoma, in which nonneoplastic lymphocytes typically are uniform small cells. Granulocytes, especially eosinophils, are much more common in Hodgkin's lymphoma. The EBV-infected large cells typically are CD20+, CD30+/–, and CD15– (see Figure 3-7, *E* and *G*), in contrast to Hodgkin's lymphoma. Also, as noted previously, the reactive T cells in infectious mononucleosis typically have an inverted CD4:CD8 ratio,[53] whereas T cells in Hodgkin's lymphoma typically have a normal or elevated CD4:CD8 ratio.

   c. *Reactive lymphoid hyperplasia versus extranodal marginal zone lymphoma.* The reactive lymphoid tissue present in Waldeyer's ring is characterized by reactive follicles and prominent bands of marginal zone B cells along crypts. Infiltration of crypt epithelium by lymphoid cells is normal and alone does not indicate marginal zone lymphoma. A diagnosis of marginal zone lymphoma may be considered when substantial distortion of the normal architecture by a parafollicular and diffuse proliferation of B cells with the morphology and immunophenotype of marginal zone cells is seen. Demonstration of monotypic immunoglobulin light chain by flow cytometry or immunohistochemistry is very helpful for confirming lymphoma.

   Atypical marginal zone hyperplasia of mucosa-associated lymphoid tissue is an uncommon condition that has been described in the tonsils and appendices of children.[54] It is characterized by expansion of the marginal zone with an admixture of large cells and colonization of reactive follicles. The expanded marginal zones are composed of B cells that are CD20+ and CD43+, as well as monotypic lambda light chain positive, with expression of both mu and delta heavy chains. The atypical histologic findings, together with co-expression of CD43 and the monotypic lambda light chain, make these proliferations highly suspicious for marginal zone lymphoma. However, these cases have not shown clonal immunoglobulin gene rearrangement, and patients have been alive and well with no evidence of lymphoma, although follow-up has not been long. The authors describing these cases suggest that they represent preferential expansion of immunoglobulin light chain lambda–expressing B cells, the etiology of which is uncertain.[54] This entity is somewhat controversial, however, because others have described similar cases involving Waldeyer's ring in children and have interpreted them as marginal zone lymphoma.[55]

   d. *Reactive lymphoid hyperplasia related to HIV infection versus lymphoma.* Lymphoid hyperplasia due to HIV infection can result in prominent enlargement of the components of Waldeyer's ring. Patients may present with

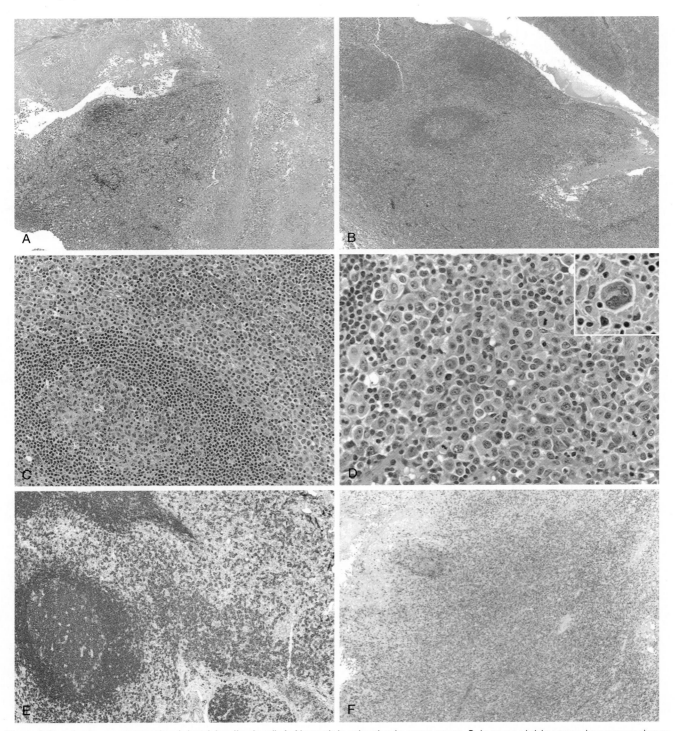

Figure 3-7 Infectious mononucleosis involving the tonsil. **A,** Necrosis is extensive in some areas. **B,** In more viable areas, low power shows expansion of the interfollicular area, although follicles remain and crypts are intact. **C,** Adjacent to this reactive follicle are many large lymphoid cells; many small lymphoid cells and plasma cells also are present. **D,** In some foci, large lymphoid cells are numerous, forming aggregates. Rare Reed-Sternberg-like cells are present *(inset)*. **E** to **H,** Most cells in follicles, as well as the interfollicular large cells, are CD20+ B cells **(E)**; many admixed CD3+ T cells also are present **(F)**.

airway obstruction and a sore throat or fever, sometimes accompanied by cervical lymphade-nopathy[56]; this constellation of findings may raise the question of lymphoma. The histologic changes are similar to those seen in lymph nodes in HIV-positive individuals. The early stages of HIV infection are marked by florid follicular hyperplasia with follicle lysis and attenuation or loss of follicular mantles (Figure 3-8). Multinucleated giant cells also are often present, especially adjacent to surface epithe-lium or epithelium lining crypts; these giant

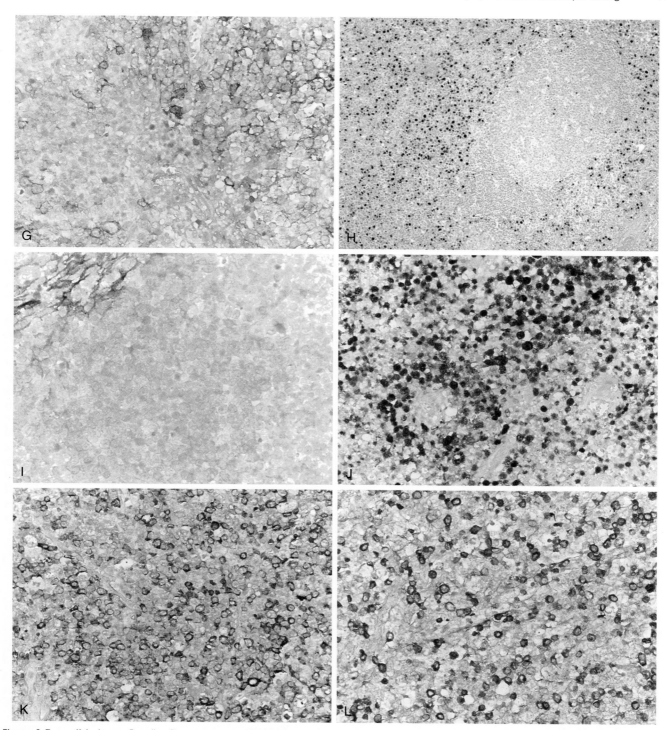

Figure 3-7, cont'd Large B cells often co-express CD30 **(G)**; the presence of EBV is documented in the interfollicular B cells using in situ hybridization **(H)**; note the sparing of the reactive follicle by the EBV+ B-cell proliferation. I to L, EBV-infected cells are negative for CD10 **(I)**, negative for BCl6, weakly positive for BCl2 (not shown), and strongly express nuclear MUM1/IRF4 **(J)**. Large cells and some smaller plasmacytoid cells stain in a polytypic pattern for kappa **(K)** and lambda **(L)**. (*E* to *G* and *I* to *L*, Immunoperoxidase technique on paraffin sections; *H*, in situ hybridization for EBER on a paraffin section.)

cells are reported to be CD68+, S100+, HIV p24 core protein+ and HIV ribonucleic acid (RNA)+.[56] In the late stages of HIV infection, the lymphoid tissue shows involuted or absent follicles and lymphoid depletion with small lymphocytes, plasma cells, and immunoblasts scattered in the tissue, along with increased vascularity and stroma.

The mantle zone attenuation of floridly hyperplastic follicles in early HIV infection may lead to failure to recognize them as follicles and to misinterpretation of them as a diffuse

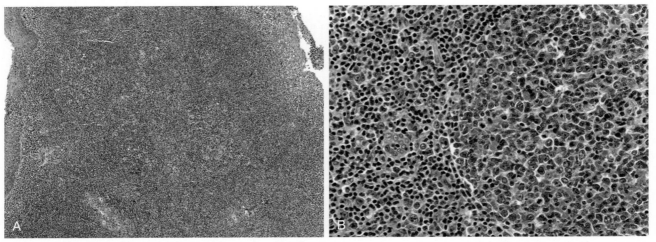

Figure 3-8　Adenoids from an HIV-positive patient. **A,** Follicles are present but ill-defined on low power examination. **B,** Higher power shows a reactive follicle occupied mainly by large cells. Because the follicle mantle is absent, the follicle is poorly delineated from the interfollicular area.

proliferation of B cells (see Figure 3-7). Familiarity with these changes, accompanied by a basic panel of immunostains for B and T cells and for follicular dendritic cells, confirms preservation of architecture and helps exclude lymphoma. Clinical correlation is helpful. If the patient is not known to be HIV positive, the pathologist may suggest testing for HIV infection if histologic changes of the type associated with HIV infection are encountered.

2. **Undifferentiated nasopharyngeal carcinoma versus diffuse large B-cell lymphoma.** Undifferentiated nasopharyngeal carcinoma and diffuse large B-cell lymphoma may be difficult to distinguish on routine sections, because undifferentiated carcinoma often is composed of cells with large, oval nuclei with vesicular chromatin, prominent nucleoli, and scant cytoplasm with indistinct cell borders; this closely resembles the appearance of large lymphoid cells, especially immunoblasts, but immunophenotyping readily establishes a diagnosis.

3. **Follicular lymphoma versus mantle cell lymphoma.** Mantle cell lymphoma typically is characterized by a vaguely nodular and diffuse, monotonous proliferation of small to slightly enlarged lymphoid cells with dark, slightly irregular nuclei and scant cytoplasm. Follicular lymphoma is characterized by a proliferation of neoplastic follicles composed of centrocytes with a variable admixture of centroblasts, with or without diffuse areas. Some overlap may be seen in the histologic features of these two lymphomas, particularly for follicular lymphoma, grade 1, in which few centroblasts are present. However, some histologic clues are useful: the follicles of follicular lymphoma usually are better defined than the nodules of mantle cell lymphoma; large cells, such as centroblasts, are virtually absent in mantle cell lymphoma unless they represent remnants of a reactive follicle; single epithelioid

histiocytes sometimes are scattered among neoplastic mantle cells, but this is very uncommon in follicular lymphoma. Immunophenotyping is very helpful. Both lymphomas are almost always CD20+ and bcl2+, but follicular lymphoma usually is CD10+, bcl6+, and cyclin D1–, whereas mantle cell lymphoma is CD10–, bcl6–, and cyclin D1+.

4. **Diffuse large B-cell lymphoma versus mantle cell lymphoma, blastoid variant.** In some cases of mantle cell lymphoma, the neoplastic cells are relatively large and mitoses are common; the appearance can mimic that of diffuse large B-cell lymphoma. Areas of vague nodularity and areas with a range of cell sizes with some smaller cells may raise the possibility of mantle cell lymphoma. An immunostain for cyclin D1 can exclude or confirm a diagnosis of mantle cell lymphoma.

■ LYMPHOMAS OF THE NASAL CAVITY AND PARANASAL SINUSES

Among malignancies that arise in the sinonasal area, lymphoma is second in frequency only to squamous cell carcinoma.[57] Sinonasal lymphoma accounts for 0.2% to 2% of all lymphomas[58] and for fewer than 5% of extranodal lymphomas.[19] Two main types of lymphoma are found in the sinonasal tract: diffuse large B-cell lymphoma and extranodal NK/T-cell lymphoma, nasal type. Lymphomas that arise in the paranasal sinuses are almost always the diffuse large B-cell type,[59,60] whereas most of the lymphomas arising in the nasal cavity are extranodal NK/T-cell lymphomas, followed by diffuse large B-cell lymphomas.[59,61-63] Other types of lymphoma are uncommon or rare in the sinonasal tract. In many cases lymphomas involve both the paranasal sinuses and the nasal cavity[59] and assigning a primary site is difficult. Therefore, lymphomas of the nasal cavity and paranasal sinuses are discussed together.

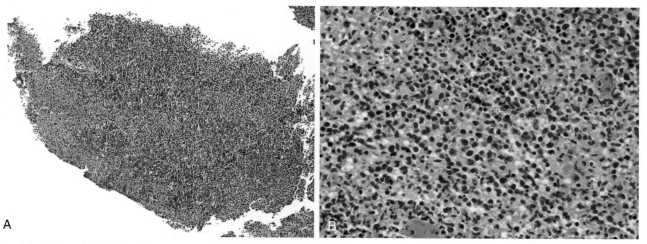

Figure 3-9 Extranodal NK/T-cell lymphoma, nasal type, involving the nasal septum of an Asian male who presented with septal perforation. **A,** Low power shows a fragment of tissue with necrosis along one surface. Other fragments of tissue were entirely necrotic. **B,** High power shows medium and large atypical lymphoid cells in a background of apoptotic debris and fibrin.

Extranodal NK/T-Cell Lymphoma, Nasal Type

Introduction

Extranodal NK/T-cell lymphoma is a rare malignancy in the United States and Europe; it is more common among Asians and individuals of native American descent in Mexico, Central America, and South America. In years past it was a poorly understood disorder; many cases were designated as polymorphic reticulosis or lethal midline granuloma. Now it is recognized as a distinctive type of lymphoma that in most cases is of NK-cell lineage but in a few cases is composed of cytotoxic T cells.[64] The pathogenesis of this type of lymphoma is strongly linked to the Epstein-Barr virus.

Clinical Features

Extranodal NK/T-cell lymphoma affects adults over a broad age range (the median age is about 40 years); children occasionally are affected. The male to female ratio is at least 2:1.[65-69] In rare cases, patients are iatrogenically immunosuppressed transplant recipients.[70,71] Patients present with nasal obstruction, bleeding, pain, or local swelling.[59,65] This type of lymphoma produces ulcerative, destructive lesions in extranodal sites. The nasal cavity is the typical site of origin, but this lymphoma may present with involvement of other midline structures in the upper aerodigestive tract, including the palate and the nasopharynx. The lymphoma may involve the paranasal sinuses along with the nasal cavity or (uncommonly) principally involve the paranasal sinuses.[59,60] Lymphoma in the nasal cavity or paranasal sinuses may invade locally to involve the facial skin, orbit, nasopharynx, or tonsil.[65] In rare cases extranodal NK/T-cell lymphoma, nasal type, arises in other extranodal sites, including the skin,[72] testis,[73] gastrointestinal tract, and soft tissue. Primary lymph nodal involvement is extremely uncommon.[64]

Pathologic Features

Extranodal NK/T-cell lymphoma usually is composed of a diffuse proliferation of small and large, atypical lymphoid cells, with a variable admixture of small lymphocytes, plasma cells, histiocytes, and sometimes eosinophils, often with ulceration and zonal necrosis. The appearance of the neoplastic population varies from case to case. In some, obviously malignant, large lymphoid cells with dark, irregular, or convoluted nuclei predominate (Figure 3-9), whereas in others, small to medium-sized cells with subtle atypia are the predominant type (Figures 3-10 and 3-11). The neoplastic cells may have distinct rims of clear cytoplasm. Angioinvasion and angiodestruction with fibrinoid change of vascular walls are common, although angiodestruction, necrosis, and vascular thrombosis may be absent, especially with a predominance of small neoplastic cells (Figure 3-10).[74] Necrosis of both tumor cells and normal tissue usually is seen and ranges from focal to extensive. Karyorrhectic debris may be abundant. Residual epithelium may show squamous metaplasia, sometimes with prominent pseudoepitheliomatous hyperplasia. Cytoplasmic azurophilic granules corresponding to cytotoxic granules often are seen in neoplastic cells when Wright-Giemsa–stained touch preps are examined.[64]

Most cases show an NK-cell immunophenotype: cCD3+, sCD3–, CD2+, CD5–, CD4–, CD8–, CD45RO+, CD43+, CD56+, CD20–, TCRαβ–, and TCRγδ– (see Figure 3-10). Surface CD3 (sCD3, as would be assessed by flow cytometry or by frozen section immunohistochemistry) usually is absent, but cytoplasmic CD3 (cCD3) usually is detected on paraffin sections. Although the entire CD3 complex is not expressed by NK cells, the CD3 epsilon chain, which is recognized by paraffin section antibodies to CD3, may be found in NK cells. The neoplastic cells express cytotoxic molecules (TIA-1, granzyme B, and perforin); this may contribute to the extensive necrosis characteristic of this type of lymphoma.

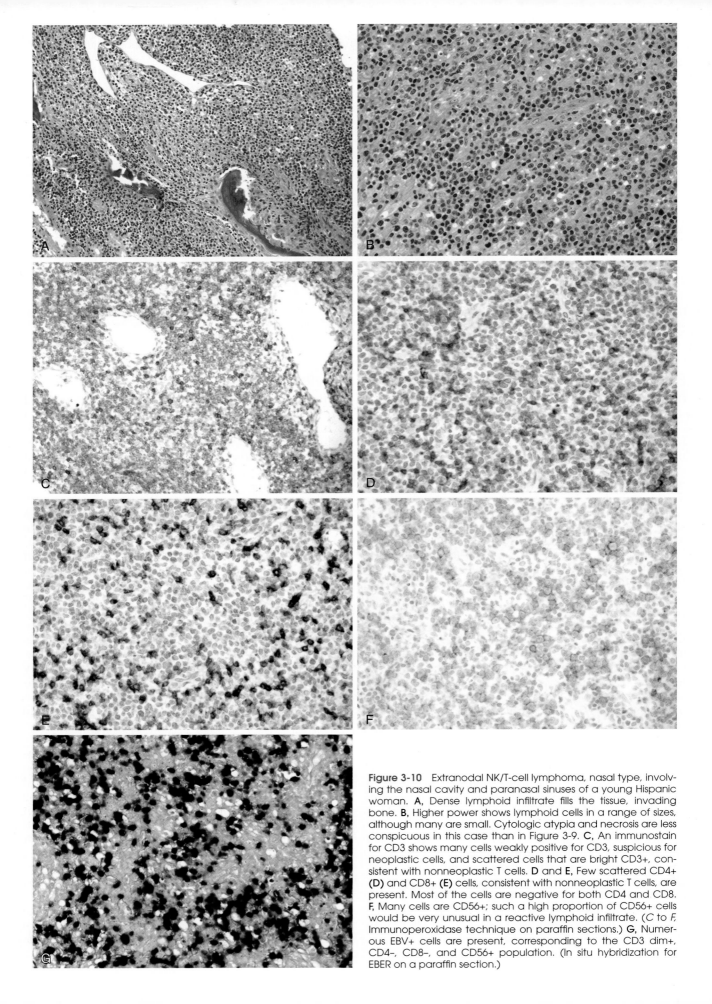

Figure 3-10 Extranodal NK/T-cell lymphoma, nasal type, involving the nasal cavity and paranasal sinuses of a young Hispanic woman. **A,** Dense lymphoid infiltrate fills the tissue, invading bone. **B,** Higher power shows lymphoid cells in a range of sizes, although many are small. Cytologic atypia and necrosis are less conspicuous in this case than in Figure 3-9. **C,** An immunostain for CD3 shows many cells weakly positive for CD3, suspicious for neoplastic cells, and scattered cells that are bright CD3+, consistent with nonneoplastic T cells. **D** and **E,** Few scattered CD4+ **(D)** and CD8+ **(E)** cells, consistent with nonneoplastic T cells, are present. Most of the cells are negative for both CD4 and CD8. **F,** Many cells are CD56+; such a high proportion of CD56+ cells would be very unusual in a reactive lymphoid infiltrate. (*C* to *F,* Immunoperoxidase technique on paraffin sections.) **G,** Numerous EBV+ cells are present, corresponding to the CD3 dim+, CD4–, CD8–, and CD56+ population. (In situ hybridization for EBER on a paraffin section.)

A few cases are CD8+.[59,64,65] Some cases are CD30+. T-cell receptor (TCR) and immunoglobulin (Ig) genes usually are germline (NK lineage); T-lineage cases have clonally rearranged TCR genes and may express sCD3 (Figure 3-11). EBV can be detected in most neoplastic cells in virtually all cases with in situ hybridization for Epstein-Barr virus–encoded RNA (EBER). The EBV genomes are clonal. Some cases express EBV latent membrane protein (LMP); however, in this type of lymphoma, LMP expression is much less sensitive than EBER in detecting EBV.[59,64,75,76]

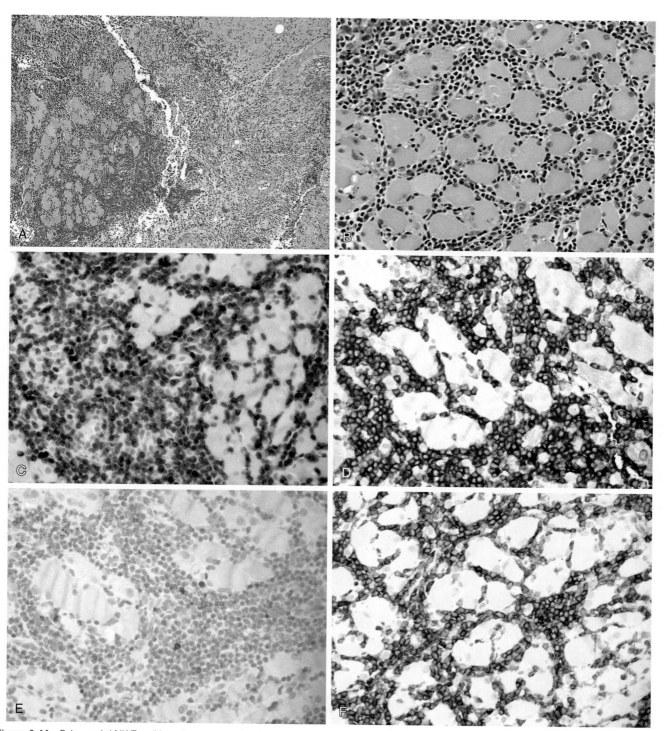

Figure 3-11   Extranodal NK/T-cell lymphoma, nasal type, T lineage, involving the buccal mucosa and underlying soft tissue. **A,** Dense lymphoid infiltrate invades skeletal muscle in an interstitial pattern, with foci of hemorrhage and necrosis. **B,** Lymphoid cells are small to slightly enlarged and irregular; cytologic atypia is subtle. **C** to **I,** Lymphoid infiltrate is CD3+ **(C),** CD5+ **(D),** CD4– **(E),** CD8+ **(F),** CD7–**(G),**

Continued

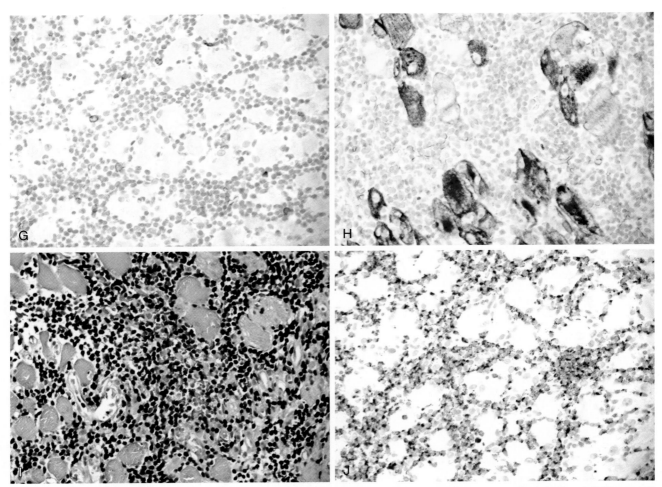

Figure 3-11, cont'd   CD56− **(H)**, EBV+ **(I)**, and granzyme B+ **(J)**. The expression of CD5 and CD8 and the lack of CD7 and CD56 would be unusual in extranodal NK/T-cell lymphoma of NK lineage and suggested T lineage. Polymerase chain reaction (PCR) confirmed the presence of a clonal T-cell population (not shown). (*C* to *H* and *J*, Immunoperoxidase technique on paraffin sections; *I*, in situ hybridization for EBER on a paraffin section.)

Mutations of *p53* have been identified in approximately half of cases. Beta-catenin mutations have been found in about 20% of cases, and smaller numbers of cases show mutations of *c-kit* or *K-ras*. This suggests that *p53* may play a role in the pathogenesis of nasal NK/T-cell lymphoma, and mutations of the other genes studied probably are less important.[77] The cell of origin is believed to be an activated cytotoxic T or NK cell infected by EBV.

Staging, Treatment, and Outcome

Most patients present with localized disease (Ann Arbor stage I).[59,65,66,78] Higher stage disease will have spread to local or distant lymph nodes, the testis, skin, subcutis, or other sites.[65] Bone marrow involvement at presentation is uncommon.[66]

The clinical course usually is aggressive, and in many series, NK/T-cell lymphoma has been associated with a high mortality. The 5-year overall survival rate is approximately 50%.[67,78,79] Variation in cytologic features does not appear to have a significant impact on the stage, response to therapy, or outcome.[65]

Factors that affect the prognosis have varied among series, but a worse outcome has been associated with extensive local invasion (e.g., to skin or into bone),[67] B symptoms,[78,79] a high lactate dehydrogenase (LDH) level,[69,79] a higher stage,[59,79] regional lymphadenopathy,[79] and an Eastern Cooperative Oncology Group (ECOG) performance score of 2 or higher.[69] A better prognosis has been associated with a low proliferation fraction (Ki67 less than 65%),[68] lower EBV viral load in tumor tissue,[66] and lower serum levels of EBV DNA.[78] Serum EBV DNA also may be useful for monitoring disease status.[78] Most extranodal NK/T-cell lymphomas are Skp2+/p27−. Cases that are Skp2+/p27−, Skp+/p27+, and Skp2−/p27− are reported to have a worse prognosis than those that are Skp2−/p27+. p27 is a major negative regulator at the G1/S transition. Skp2 mediates p27 degradation. Some have suggested that upregulation of Skp2, perhaps by EBV-encoded proteins may promote tumor cell proliferation and tumor progression, at least in some cases.[80]

Extranodal NK/T-cell lymphomas seem to be relatively resistant to CHOP chemotherapy.[67] Radiation therapy appears to be very important for optimal survival.[65,67] Patients with localized disease who receive radiation therapy up front or alone have shown fairly good survival rates in some series.[59, 67] High-dose chemotherapy with bone marrow transplantation may have a role in the treatment of recurrences, but additional studies are needed.[69]

The main cause of death is progressive disease. Relapses may be local or distant; distant sites include the skin, liver, bone marrow, testis, and lung.[67] Hemophagocytic syndromes may develop and are responsible for some of the fatalities in patients with extranodal NK/T-cell lymphoma.[59,67]

Diffuse Large B-Cell Lymphoma

Clinical Features

Sinonasal diffuse large B-cell lymphoma affects men more often than women (male to female ratio of 1.5 to 2:1). It predominantly affects middle-aged or older adults[58-60,81] and occasionally affects children.[59] A few patients have been HIV positive[59,82] or iatrogenically immunosuppressed.[59,83] Symptoms include nasal obstruction or discharge, facial pain or swelling, numbness, epistaxis, sinus pressure, toothache, or headache. The lymphoma may invade adjacent structures, such as the orbit, base of the skull, central nervous system (CNS), pterygopalatine fossa, nasopharynx, and palate.[60,82,84] In these cases, the patient may present with neurologic abnormalities, proptosis, diplopia, decreased visual acuity, and even blindness.[58,59,82,85-88] Patients occasionally have fever and night sweats.[59,82] Among the paranasal sinuses, the maxillary sinus is the most common site of involvement, followed by the ethmoid sinus, sphenoid sinus, and frontal sinus. Frequently, multiple sinuses are involved concurrently.[58,59,82,89] The lymphomas often are associated with destruction of adjacent bone.

Pathologic Features

The pathologic features of sinonasal diffuse large B-cell lymphomas are similar to those found in other sites; a subset of cases is composed predominantly of immunoblasts (immunoblastic lymphoma).[60] Rare large B-cell lymphomas of the lymphomatoid granulomatosis type have presented with involvement of the paranasal sinuses.[59] Occasional cases of plasmablastic lymphoma in the sinonasal area have been described in both HIV-positive[91] and HIV-negative patients.[92] (See Lymphomas of the Oral Cavity, later in the chapter, for a more detailed discussion of plasmablastic lymphoma.)

The immunophenotypic features are similar to those seen in other sites. Some authors have described the presence of EBV in up to 40% of sinonasal B-cell lymphomas.[61,87,93] However, in a study at the Massachusetts General Hospital, EBV was found in B-cell lymphomas only in immunodeficient patients.[59]

Staging, Treatment, and Outcome

Approximately 75% of cases are localized at presentation (Ann Arbor stage I or II).[59,81] Patients with stage IV disease may have involvement of the CNS, lung, bone, kidney, or gastrointestinal tract.[81,82] In earlier times patients usually were treated with radiation alone; however, that approach was associated with a high proportion of treatment failures.[94] Currently, most patients receive radiation and chemotherapy. Some authorities recommend prophylactic treatment of the CNS to improve long-term, disease-free survival.[60,81]

When paranasal sinus lymphomas relapse or progress, they frequently involve lymph nodes and may also involve a variety of extranodal sites, including the CNS, lung, bone, ovary, testis, marrow, liver, spleen and skin.* Local failures are uncommon when optimal radiation is included in the therapeutic regimen.[95] The results of follow-up have varied widely, with 5-year survival rates ranging from 29%[87] to 80%[89] in different series of patients with paranasal sinus lymphoma treated with combined modality therapy. In one large series of patients, most of whom received chemotherapy, radiation, and prophylactic intrathecal chemotherapy, the 5-year overall survival rate was 54%, and the 5-year disease-specific survival rate was 67%.[60]

Miscellaneous Lymphomas

Paranasal sinus involvement has been described for Burkitt's lymphoma, follicular lymphoma,[82,85,87,89] marginal zone lymphoma,[59] peripheral T-cell lymphoma not otherwise specified (NOS),[60] and adult T-cell leukemia/lymphoma (human T-lymphocyte virus-1 [HTLV-1] positive) (Figure 3-12).[59,88] Among children, diffuse large B-cell lymphoma is less common than Burkitt's lymphoma.[59,96]

Differential Diagnosis of Sinonasal Lymphoma

1. **Reactive/infectious process with extensive necrosis versus extranodal NK/T-cell lymphoma.** A difficulty in making a diagnosis of NK/T-cell lymphoma is obtaining adequate viable tissue. When lymphoma is a consideration, the surgeon must biopsy until diagnostic tissue has been obtained. In our laboratory, we encourage surgeons to submit tissue for frozen section to ensure that viable tissue is available for evaluation.
2. **Chronic inflammation versus extranodal NK/T-cell lymphoma.** Cases of extranodal NK/T-cell lymphoma in which the neoplastic cells are relatively small may be difficult to distinguish from an inflammatory process. When CD3+ cells in the infiltrate have nuclear atypia, rims of clear cytoplasm, mitotic activity, and demonstrable EBV, a diagnosis of lymphoma is favored. Also, because

---

*References 58, 60, 63, 81, 84, and 87.

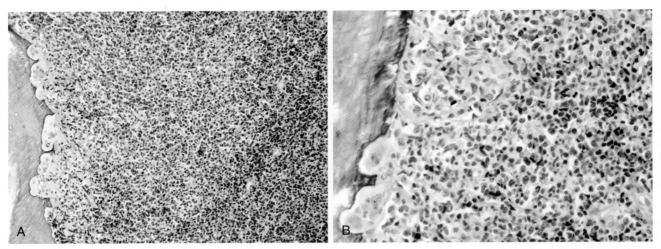

Figure 3-12 Adult T-cell leukemia/lymphoma involving the paranasal sinuses. **A,** Low power shows a dense lymphoid infiltrate eroding into bone. **B,** Higher power shows a population of medium-sized to large atypical lymphoid cells with irregular nuclei. Osteoclasts are present at the interface with the bone, with scalloping and bony resorption. Additional studies demonstrated that the neoplastic cells were T lineage and that the patient was seropositive for human T-lymphocyte virus-1 (HTLV-1) (results not shown).

CD56+ lymphocytes typically are found in very small numbers in reactive lymphoid infiltrates, the presence of many CD56+ cells supports a diagnosis of lymphoma.

3. **Diffuse large B-cell lymphoma versus extranodal NK/T-cell lymphoma.** Diffuse large B-cell lymphoma and extranodal NK/T-cell lymphoma may be difficult to differentiate on routine sections. Angioinvasion and angiocentric localization, prominent necrosis, epitheliotropism, and pseudoepitheliomatous hyperplasia favor extranodal NK/T-cell lymphoma. B-cell lymphomas more commonly arise in the paranasal sinuses, whereas nasal localization and midfacial destructive disease favor NK/T-cell lymphoma. Most sinonasal B cell lymphomas are composed of a diffuse proliferation of large cells; therefore, any other cellular composition with a diffuse pattern, especially a mixture of small and large cells or of medium-sized cells, should raise the question of NK/T-cell lymphoma. B-cell and NK/T-cell lymphomas can be distinguished easily with immunophenotyping. B-cell lymphoma is nearly always CD20+. NK/T-cell lymphoma is usually CD2+, cCD3+, CD56+, CD5−, CD4−, and CD8−. Extranodal NK/T-cell lymphomas are EBV+; therefore, absence of EBV provides strong evidence against NK/T-cell lymphoma.

4. **Peripheral T-cell lymphoma versus extranodal NK/T-cell lymphoma.** Rare lymphomas expressing T-cell antigens but without CD56 or EBV present with nasal involvement. They should be diagnosed as peripheral T-cell lymphomas and further subclassified, if possible, but they should not be classified as extranodal NK/T-cell lymphoma.

5. **Wegener's granulomatosis versus extranodal NK/T-cell lymphoma.** Like extranodal NK/T-cell lymphoma, Wegener's granulomatosis may cause midfacial destructive disease, with biopsies showing a mixed cellular infiltrate, vascular damage, and necrosis. Unlike extranodal NK/T-cell lymphoma, Wegener's granulomatosis lacks a component of abnormal, EBV+ lymphoid cells and may be associated with granulomas. Patients with Wegener's granulomatosis often have evidence of systemic disease, with pulmonary and renal involvement, and the test for antineutrophil cytoplasmic antibodies often is positive; these findings are unlikely in extranodal NK/T-cell lymphoma.

6. **Squamous cell carcinoma versus extranodal NK/T-cell lymphoma.** Extranodal NK/T-cell lymphoma can be associated with marked hyperplasia of the overlying epithelium, which may mimic squamous cell carcinoma. The atypia of the lymphoid infiltrate and lack of significant atypia of the epithelial cells favor lymphoma.

■ LYMPHOMAS AND OTHER LYMPHOPROLIFERATIVE DISORDERS OF THE SALIVARY GLANDS

Reactive and Neoplastic Lymphoproliferative Disorders Primary in the Salivary Glands

Introduction

The salivary glands provide the setting for a variety of lymphoproliferative disorders, a number of which are intimately associated with the epithelium. These lymphoproliferative disorders range from reactive processes to indolent and aggressive lymphomas.

Simple Lymphoepithelial Cyst

Lymphoepithelial cysts occur predominantly as solitary lesions in the area of the parotid gland. Patients of any age may be affected, but most are middle-aged or older adults, and a slight female preponderance is seen. The lesions arise unassociated with immunodeficiency, Sjögren's syndrome, IgG4-related sclerosing disease, or any other autoimmune disorder.[97,98] They most likely arise within the parotid gland,[98] although some alternatives have been proposed, including an origin from dilatation of ducts in the intraparotid lymph nodes or from branchial cleft remnants. The typical histologic picture is that of a unilocular cyst lined by simple or stratified squamous epithelium or columnar epithelium, or a mixture of epithelia, surrounded by reactive lymphoid tissue.[97]

In one large series, the authors described three types of lymphoepithelial cysts, which they proposed represented three stages in the development of the lesion: (1) cystic dilatation of ducts in the parotid glands, surrounded by lymphoid cells; (2) partially demarcated cystic lesions with lymphoid stroma; and (3) well-encapsulated cystic lesions with lymphoid stroma with conspicuous lymphoid follicles.[98] Columnar lining epithelium was most likely to be encountered in early stage (type 1) lymphoepithelial cysts, whereas most later stage cysts were lined by squamous epithelium.[98]

"Myoepithelial islands" (see Lymphoepithelial Sialadenitis, later in the chapter) may be present in the walls of the cyst, but diffuse changes of lymphoepithelial sialadenitis are not seen.[98]

Cystic Lymphoid Hyperplasia

Cystic lymphoid hyperplasia mainly involves the parotid gland rather than other salivary glands; however, whether the lesion primarily involves periparotid or intraparotid lymph nodes or the salivary gland parenchyma is the subject of debate.[99] The process often is bilateral and typically consists of multiple dilated ducts surrounded by floridly hyperplastic follicles with attenuated mantles. Lymphoepithelial lesions are not usually conspicuous, although large numbers of lymphoid cells may be found in the epithelium of dilated ducts. Small numbers of monocytoid B cells may be present.

Most patients with cystic lymphoid hyperplasia are HIV positive. Most are adults,[99,100] but children may also be affected.[101] The process may occur in patients who also have HIV-associated persistent generalized lymphadenopathy.[101] The cysts most likely form when the expanded lymphoid tissue causes ductal obstruction and dilatation behind the obstruction. Some morphologic overlap with lymphoepithelial sialadenitis is seen. Involvement of one or more lymph nodes with sparing of the salivary gland parenchyma, prominent ductal dilatation, few or absent monocytoid B cells, a decreased CD4:CD8 ratio, and a history of HIV seropositivity favor cystic lymphoid hyperplasia over lymphoepithelial sialadenitis.

Chronic Sclerosing Sialadenitis

Chronic sclerosing sialadenitis, or Küttner's tumor, is a fairly common type of chronic sialadenitis. It occurs in adults, and males are affected more often than females in some series. The submandibular gland is by far the salivary gland most often involved, but in rare cases Küttner's tumor involves the parotid gland. It produces a hard mass that may be unilateral or bilateral.[102-104] Some cases classified as Küttner's tumor are thought to be due to sialolithiasis, but currently Küttner's tumor is thought to be in the spectrum of IgG4-associated sclerosing disease.[102,103]

Microscopic examination reveals fibrosis and a variably prominent lymphoid infiltrate. Sclerosis typically begins in a periductal location and over time progresses to involve lobules, with resultant parenchymal atrophy but preserved lobular architecture. Ducts are dilated and filled with inspissated material; they often display acute and chronic sialodochitis. An infiltrate of small lymphocytes and plasma cells is present; reactive lymphoid follicles commonly are found.[103] Lymphoepithelial lesions are not typically found but have been described.[104] Cases related to IgG4-associated sclerosing disease show florid lymphoid hyperplasia with reactive lymphoid follicles and numerous plasma cells, sometimes accompanied by obliterative phlebitis.

Immunophenotyping reveals a high proportion of IgG4+ plasma cells (Figure 3-13).[102] Some patients with Küttner's tumor have manifestations of IgG4-associated sclerosing disease at sites distant from the salivary glands.[102]

Lymphoepithelial Sialadenitis

The history of the process that has come to be known as lymphoepithelial sialadenitis began in 1892, when Mikulicz reported a patient with symmetric enlargement of the salivary glands and lacrimal glands; the disorder appeared to be benign, but the etiology was unknown. Subsequently, a variety of disorders producing lacrimal or salivary gland enlargement came to be labeled as "Mikulicz's disease" or "Mikulicz's syndrome." In 1952 Godwin reported 10 cases of lymphoid proliferations of the salivary glands associated with epithelial alterations. He suggested the term "benign lymphoepithelial lesion" to describe his cases, which he believed represented what had come to be called Mikulicz's disease. In a study from the Massachusetts General Hospital, Morgan and Castleman described additional cases and suggested that the altered ducts be called "epimyoepithelial islands," also known as "myoepithelial islands." They also made the important observation of an association with Sjögren's syndrome and suggested that the pathologic changes in their cases represented one aspect of this systemic disease (reviewed by Harris).[100] The term "myoepithelial sialadenitis" (MESA) later came into wide use, although this term has proven to be inaccurate, because the altered ductal structures consist of lymphoid cells and epithelial cells but not myoepithelial cells. Currently, the term *lymphoepithelial sialadenitis (LESA)* is the preferred designation for the disease, and *lymphoepithelial lesion* is used to refer to individual ductal structures infiltrated by lymphoid cells.

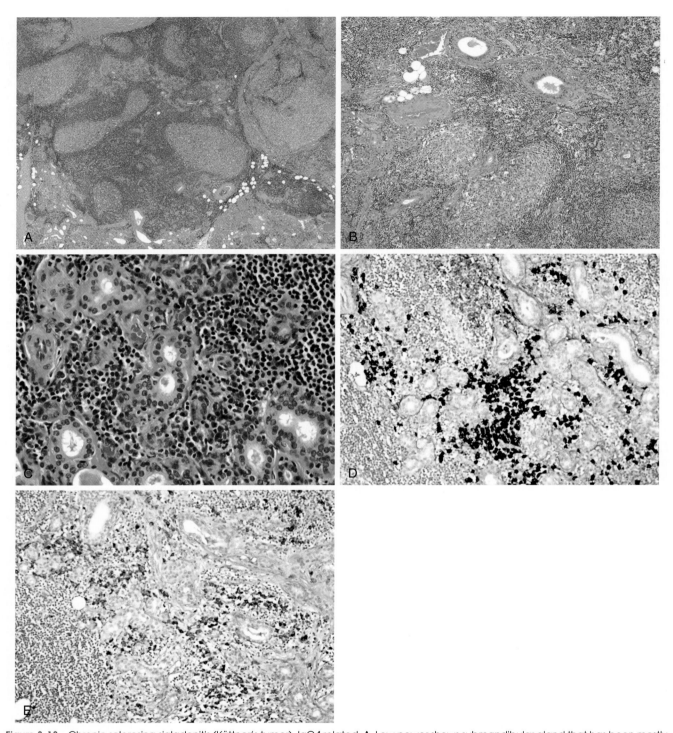

Figure 3-13 Chronic sclerosing sialadenitis (Küttner's tumor), IgG4 related. **A,** Low power shows submandibular gland that has been mostly replaced by a proliferation of reactive lymphoid follicles with foci of fibrosis. **B,** Higher power shows reactive follicles with polarization of follicle centers adjacent to acini and ductules. **C,** Small lymphocytes and plasma cells are present in large numbers among acini. **D** and **E,** IgG4+ plasma cells **(D)** are almost as numerous as IgG+ plasma cells **(E).** (*D* and *E*, Immunoperoxidase technique on paraffin sections.)

Clinical Features

LESA affects patients over a broad age range; the median age is in the 50s. A female predominance is seen (male to female ratio of about 1:4). Nearly all patients with Sjögren's syndrome have LESA, but only about half of individuals with LESA have Sjögren's syndrome. The remainder may be otherwise well or may have other types of autoimmune disease, especially rheumatoid arthritis.[100] The changes seen with LESA are most prominent in the

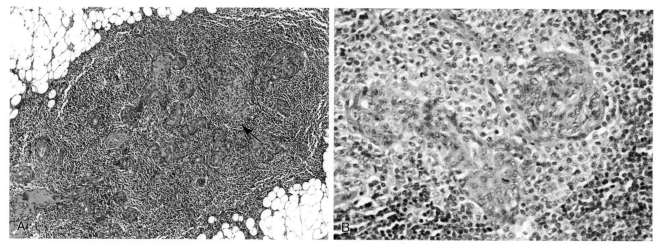

Figure 3-14   Lymphoepithelial sialadenitis (LESA). **A,** An aggregate of lymphoid cells is present in a background of salivary gland with areas of fatty replacement. Lymphocytes surround and invade epithelial structures, with epithelial proliferation and loss of lumens, to produce lymphoepithelial lesions. A reactive follicle *(arrow)* is present among the lymphoepithelial lesions. Monocytoid B cells are not conspicuous. **B,** This lymphoepithelial lesion is surrounded by a halo of monocytoid B cells with oval or bean-shaped nuclei and abundant, clear cytoplasm.

parotid gland, but other salivary glands, including minor salivary glands, also may be involved.

Pathologic Features

LESA is marked by salivary gland parenchyma with a multifocal or diffuse lymphoid proliferation, characterized by the formation of lymphoepithelial lesions in ductal structures, surrounded by reactive lymphoid follicles, small lymphocytes, plasma cells, and occasional immunoblasts. Lymphoepithelial lesions show infiltration of ducts by lymphoid cells, which is associated with proliferation and disorganization of the epithelial cells. The ductal lumen often is lost; infrequently, the ducts may become dilated. The lymphoid cells in the lymphoepithelial lesions are monocytoid B cells; this type of B cell has a small to medium-sized oval or indented nucleus without conspicuous nucleoli and with abundant, pale to clear cytoplasm. The monocytoid B cells are confined to the lymphoepithelial lesion or form a narrow halo around the lesion (Figure 3-14); more extensive monocytoid B-cell proliferation should prompt consideration of extranodal marginal zone lymphoma. Lymphoepithelial lesions are most conspicuous in the parotid gland; they may not be found in other salivary glands.

Immunophenotyping shows that the monocytoid B cells express pan–B-cell markers, such as CD20, and are negative for CD5 and CD10. Plasma cells are polytypic.

In clonality studies, most cases of LESA can be shown to harbor clonal B-cell populations. Over time, the same clone may persist or may regress and new clones may appear. Demonstration of clonality does not necessarily predict clinical or morphologic evidence of lymphoma; therefore, results must be evaluated with caution.[100,105,106]

Primary Salivary Gland Lymphomas

Introduction

Lymphoma accounts for 2% to 5% of salivary gland malignancies.[97,107] Approximately 5% of extranodal lymphomas are primary in the salivary glands.[2] In one study, 10.9% of all nodal and extranodal non-Hodgkin's lymphomas in the head and neck arose from the major salivary glands.[108] The lymphomas arise in the parotid gland in at least 70% of cases, in the submaxillary gland in 15% to 25% of cases, and in the sublingual and minor salivary glands in fewer than 10% of cases. Patients present with an enlarging mass that usually is painless, although occasionally it is accompanied by facial nerve paralysis or cervical lymphadenopathy.[97,107-110] Roughly one fourth of the lymphomas affect the parotid and submandibular glands bilaterally.[110] B symptoms are very unusual.[109] Extranodal marginal zone lymphoma of mucosa-associated lymphoid tissue (MALT lymphoma), follicular lymphoma, and diffuse large B-cell lymphoma together account for nearly all salivary gland lymphomas.

Risk Factors for Salivary Gland Lymphoma

Sjögren's Syndrome and Lymphomagenesis

An association between Sjögren's syndrome and lymphoma was first noted in the 1960s by Talal and colleagues[111] at the National Institutes of Health. In two series published in 1964 and 1967, they described a total of 12 patients with Sjögren's syndrome and *extrasalivary* lymphoid proliferations (four reticulum cell sarcomas, two macroglobulinemias, five pseudolymphomas, and one atypical lymphoid infiltrate). Some of their patients may have had salivary gland lymphoma, but because most salivary gland lymphomas are marginal zone lymphomas and because this type of lymphoma had not yet been described, any salivary marginal lymphomas may have been mistaken for the lesion that later came to be known as LESA. Another study from the same institution, published in 1978, estimated the risk of lymphoma to be 43.8 times that expected for patients with Sjögren's syndrome.[112] Subsequent studies have confirmed that Sjögren's syndrome is indeed associated with an increased risk of lymphoma,[113,114] and this risk is most pronounced for lymphoma arising in the salivary gland. In one large study, Sjögren's syndrome was associated with a 250-fold increase in risk for salivary gland lymphoma and a 1000-fold increase in risk for salivary gland marginal zone lymphoma.[113]

Patients with Sjögren's syndrome also develop marginal zone lymphoma in other extranodal sites, such as the stomach, thymus, and lung; they less often develop lymph nodal lymphoma.[115] Among patients with Sjögren's syndrome, the presence of parotid enlargement, lymphadenopathy, splenomegaly, cryoglobulinemia, decreased complement, and cutaneous vasculitis with palpable purpura have been associated with an increased likelihood of lymphoma.[111,112,116]

Sjögren's Syndrome, Hepatitis C, and Lymphomagenesis

Some investigators contend that the hepatitis C virus (HCV) is involved in the pathogenesis of a subset of cases of LESA and the lymphomas that subsequently arise. The topic is controversial, but it is suggested that HCV is characterized by sialotropism and the ability to replicate in salivary glands, as well as by lymphotropism. These features could contribute to the development of Sjögren's syndrome or a Sjögren's syndrome–like illness accompanied by LESA, as well as mixed cryoglobulinemia.[117,118] As with other patients with Sjögren's syndrome, those who also have HCV are mostly older females; the parotid is among the most frequent locations for the development of lymphoma. Other sites include the liver and stomach.[118]

Most salivary gland lymphomas are extranodal marginal zone lymphomas and have a good prognosis, although large cell transformation may occur.[118] It should be noted that patients with HCV who do not have a Sjögren's syndrome-like illness do not have an increased risk of lymphoma in the salivary glands. However, most series studying salivary gland lymphoma[109,110] or lymphomas associated with Sjögren's syndrome[115] include few or no HCV-positive patients. The overall importance of HCV in the pathogenesis of lymphomas arising in the setting of Sjögren's syndrome remains uncertain.

Extranodal Marginal Zone Lymphoma of Mucosa-Associated Lymphoid Tissue (MALT Lymphoma)

Clinical Features

Marginal zone lymphoma is the most common type of lymphoma that arises in the salivary gland parenchyma. The salivary glands are one of the more common primary sites for marginal zone lymphoma,[110,119] giving rise to approximately 4% of such cases.[119] Up to approximately one fourth of nongastric marginal zone lymphomas arise in the salivary glands.[120] As noted previously, patients with salivary gland marginal zone lymphoma often have underlying Sjögren's syndrome, and less often they have other associated diseases, including rheumatoid arthritis, hypothyroidism, systemic lupus erythematosus, membranoproliferative glomerulonephritis, or cryoglobulinemia.[110,121] Salivary gland lymphomas in patients with Sjögren's syndrome are almost always the marginal zone type. Patients are mostly middle-aged or older adults with a mean and median age of about 60 years. Women are affected approximately twice as often as men, reflecting the high ratio of women to men in Sjögren's syndrome.[109,121]

One case of marginal zone lymphoma arising in association with Küttner's tumor has been reported.[104] The authors suggested that chronic inflammatory processes other than Sjögren's syndrome occasionally may predispose an individual to the development of marginal zone lymphoma.[104] In the reported case, the lesion was not tested for IgG4+ plasma cells, but the patient had no evidence of systemic disease.[104]

Pathologic Features

Marginal zone lymphoma in the parotid gland usually arises in a background of LESA (Figure 3-15).[110,121] In contrast to LESA without lymphoma, when lymphoma is present, it takes the form of large haloes; broad, intersecting strands; and sheets of monocytoid B cells that surround the lymphoepithelial lesions and distort and obliterate the salivary gland parenchyma. The monocytoid B-cell proliferation may link several or multiple lymphoepithelial lesions (Figure 3-15, *A*). Also present are scattered reactive lymphoid follicles and plasma cells; the latter sometimes form large aggregates, often correlating with plasmacytic differentiation of the lymphoma. Cases with numerous plasma cells may have Dutcher bodies, PAS+ intranuclear protrusions of cytoplasm containing immunoglobulin; the presence of Dutcher bodies is highly suspicious for lymphoma with plasmacytic differentiation. Rare cases are associated with amyloid deposition.[100,109] Ductal structures occasionally are dilated.

In salivary glands other than the parotid, lymphoepithelial lesions may be less conspicuous, but the histologic features are otherwise similar. Compared to marginal zone lymphomas in other sites, the salivary glands typically have a more prominent component of monocytoid B cells, which are slightly larger and have more abundant cytoplasm than marginal zone B cells. In a small number of cases, areas of histologic progression to diffuse large B-cell lymphoma are seen (see Diffuse Large B-Cell Lymphoma, later in the chapter).

The immunophenotype is similar to that of marginal zone lymphomas in other sites: CD20+, CD79a+, CD5−, CD10−, CD43+/−, bcl2+, bcl6−, and

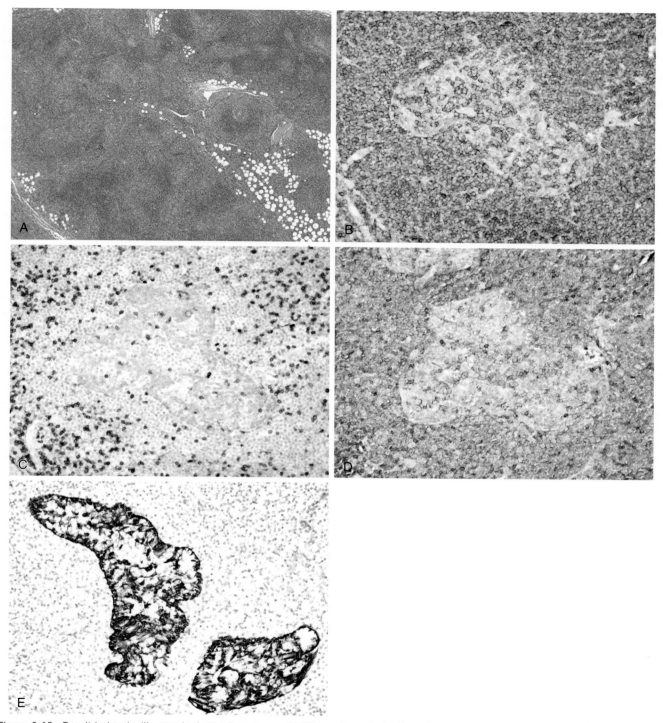

Figure 3-15 Parotid gland with marginal zone lymphoma (MALT lymphoma). **A,** Along the upper edge of the image, changes of LESA can be seen, with lymphoepithelial lesions with absent or narrow haloes of monocytoid B cells. Most of the image shows broad strands of monocytoid B cells linking adjacent lymphoepithelial lesions, consistent with marginal zone lymphoma. **B** to **E,** Higher power image of a lymphoepithelial lesion within the lymphoma shows a preponderance of CD20+ B cells **(B)** in and around the lymphoepithelial lesion. CD3+ T cells are scattered among B cells **(C)**. B cells co-express CD43 **(D)**. An immunostain for cytokeratin highlights the epithelial cells **(E)**. (*B* to *E,* Immunoperoxidase technique on paraffin sections)

cyclin D1− (see Figure 3-15, *B* to *E*).[109,121,122] Clonal rearrangement of the *IGH* often can be demonstrated.[121] Of the four chromosomal translocations strongly associated with marginal zone B-cell lymphoma [t(11;18) involving *API* and *MALT1*, t(14;18) involving *IGH* and *MALT1*, t(1;14) involving *BCL10* and *IGH*, and t(3;14) involving *FOXP1* and *IGH*], only the t(14;18) translocation is encountered with any frequency, ranging from 0% to 18% in different studies.[20,121,123,124] Trisomy 3 and trisomy 18 both are fairly common in salivary gland marginal zone lymphomas.[20,123]

Staging, Treatment, and Outcome

Most patients with marginal zone lymphoma of the salivary gland present with localized disease (Ann Arbor stage I or II). Lymph nodes, when involved, are usually local or regional.[109,110] In occasional cases, staging reveals involvement of other MALT sites. Relapses are not uncommon and may involve the primary site, lymph nodes (especially cervical nodes), and other extranodal sites; however, relapses usually can be treated successfully.[110] The overall survival rate is excellent.[109,110]

In a few cases, the lymphoma undergoes large cell transformation[97,107,110]; these diffuse large B-cell lymphomas sometimes have resulted in the death of the patient.[109,110,118]

Follicular Lymphoma

Clinical Features

Follicular lymphoma of the salivary gland is a somewhat controversial entity. The proportion of cases arising in the area of the salivary glands varies widely from one series to another, ranging from fewer than 5%[110] to 30%.[125] Many investigators have proposed that most of these follicular lymphomas involve intraparotid or periparotid lymph nodes rather than the salivary glands themselves; they note that even when the salivary gland parenchyma is involved, it usually is in the setting of concurrent lymph node involvement.[100] Others maintain that a subset of salivary gland lymphomas is truly extranodal follicular lymphoma.[109,125] The mean or median age of patients with follicular lymphoma ranges from 10 years[109] to 15 years[121] younger than that of patients with marginal zone lymphoma. No association with autoimmune disease is seen.[109,121]

Pathologic Features

Whether nodal or extranodal, the histologic features overall are similar to those of follicular lymphoma in other sites, with a proliferation of crowded, poorly delineated follicles with ill-defined or absent mantles. Most are low grade (grade 1 or 2 of 3)[109,121]; rare cases are grade 3.[109] In some cases, distinguishing lymphoma in an intraparotid lymph node from lymphoma involving a salivary gland itself can be difficult; however, a well-circumscribed lesion surrounded by a discrete, fibrous capsule is more likely nodal. In a few cases, follicular lymphoma is associated with lymphoepithelial lesions,[100,125] but ductal structures are not usually conspicuous and are not usually infiltrated by lymphocytes.[100] The follicular lymphomas typically are CD20+, CD10+, and bcl6+. Most express the bcl2 protein, and clonal *IGH* and *IGH/BCL2* fusion often can be demonstrated; however, a minority of these lymphomas are bcl2 protein negative and do not have detectable *IGH/BCL2* fusion.[121,125]

A number of cases of Warthin's tumor, in which the lymphoid stroma of the tumor is composed of follicular lymphoma, have been described.[126] Warthin's tumor is believed to arise from salivary gland ducts in lymph nodes; therefore, the follicular lymphoma in these cases would be node based. It is not known whether the follicular lymphoma and the Warthin's tumor represent collision tumors, or whether the Warthin's tumor could be a source of chronic antigenic stimulation that promotes lymphomagenesis.[126]

Staging and Outcome

For the most part, the follicular lymphomas behave in a manner similar to that of nodal follicular lymphoma arising elsewhere. Staging typically reveals widespread disease, particularly if the lymphoma clearly involves lymph nodes rather than salivary gland parenchyma; relapses are common.[100,108] Similarly, the follicular lymphomas associated with Warthin's tumor occasionally are localized at presentation, but staging often reveals widespread disease.[126] Those that appear to be truly extranodal may present with localized disease; in such cases, relapse is infrequent, and the prognosis is excellent.[125] The clinical and pathologic features of these extranodal follicular lymphomas are reminiscent of those of primary cutaneous follicle center lymphoma: a primary extranodal location, lack of bcl2 protein and of *IGH/BCL2* fusion in some cases, localized disease, and a favorable outcome.[125]

Diffuse Large B-Cell Lymphoma

Clinical Features

Approximately 10% of salivary gland lymphomas are diffuse large B-cell lymphomas without an identifiable low-grade lymphoma. A slightly smaller number are diffuse large B-cell lymphomas with a component of marginal zone lymphoma.[109,110,118,121] At least some diffuse large B-cell lymphomas in which no low-grade lymphoma is identified probably represent large cell transformation of an underlying marginal zone lymphoma. It is also possible that some are transformed follicular lymphomas, but this is not well documented.[97,100,107,109,110]

Patients with diffuse large B-cell lymphoma (with or without an associated marginal zone lymphoma) are similar in age or slightly older than patients presenting with marginal zone lymphoma. Some have a history of Sjögren's syndrome,[109,110,121] and rare patients have a history of both Sjögren's syndrome and HCV infection.[118] The parotid gland is by far the salivary gland most often involved. Most patients present with localized disease; however, the clinical behavior of diffuse large B-cell lymphoma is more aggressive than that of either marginal zone lymphoma or follicular lymphoma. Some patients, including those with and without an associated marginal zone lymphoma, succumb to the diffuse large B-cell lymphoma.[109,121]

Pathologic Features

Microscopic examination reveals sheets of large transformed cells, as are seen in diffuse large B-cell lymphomas in other sites. For cases with a component of marginal zone lymphoma, the presence in addition of solid aggregates or sheets of large cells or of areas in which large cells make up 50% of the population has been suggested to establish a diagnosis of large cell transformation.[109] The immunophenotype, which has been reported in only a small number of cases, has been CD20+, CD5−, and CD10−.[109]

Miscellaneous Lymphomas

Rare cases of Burkitt's lymphoma,[107] peripheral T-cell lymphoma not otherwise specified (NOS), anaplastic large cell lymphoma, and NK/T-cell lymphoma also have been reported.[127] Chronic lymphocytic leukemia and mantle cell lymphoma can involve the salivary glands, although they usually involve adjacent lymph nodes rather than salivary gland parenchyma.[108] We have seen a case of peripheral T-cell lymphoma NOS with morphology that mimicked that of marginal zone lymphoma in a young Asian woman. This lymphoma had an abnormal T-cell immunophenotype by both flow cytometry and immunohistochemistry (CD2+, CD3+, and CD5+; CD4−, CD8−, CD7−, CD1a−, CD10−, CD56−, and CD34−); it also showed clonal rearrangement of TCR genes but had the unusual feature of dim CD20 co-expression by the neoplastic T cells, which may rarely be observed in T-cell lymphomas (Figure 3-16).[128]

Differential Diagnosis

A morphologic continuum is seen between LESA, with increasingly prominent monocytoid B-cell proliferation, and marginal zone lymphoma; therefore, distinguishing between the two can be difficult. The presence of broad strands of monocytoid B cells between lymphoepithelial lesions or monotypic immunoglobulin expression by lymphoid cells or plasma cells is closely related to the risk of developing extrasalivary lymphoma; these features, therefore, have been proposed as establishing a diagnosis of marginal zone lymphoma.[97] Monocytoid B cells confined to lymphoepithelial lesions and even discrete haloes around lymphoepithelial lesions can be seen in lymphoepithelial sialadenitis; however, broad, intersecting bands of monocytoid B cells support a diagnosis of lymphoma. Molecular genetic studies are not usually definitive, because B-cell clones are found in more than 50% of cases of lymphoepithelial sialadenitis.[105,106]

Secondary Salivary Gland Lymphoma

Secondary involvement of the salivary glands by lymphoma is less common than primary salivary gland lymphoma.[107] Relapse of marginal zone lymphomas arising in other MALT sites accounts for some cases.

■ LYMPHOMAS OF THE ORAL CAVITY

Primary Lymphoma of the Oral Cavity

Introduction

Oral cavity lymphomas are rare. They include lymphomas of the palate, gingiva, tongue, buccal mucosa, floor of the mouth, and lips, as well as lymphomas that arise in the bones of the jaw and protrude into the oral cavity. Only about 2% of all extranodal lymphomas arise in the oral cavity.[2,129] A heterogeneous assortment of lymphomas arises in the oral cavity. For the most part, the various lymphomas of the oral cavity do not emerge as distinct entities. This is not surprising, because lymphomas that present primarily in the oral cavity arise from the diverse tissues and structures surrounding the oral cavity. An exception to this is plasmablastic lymphoma,[130] a rare, aggressive lymphoma usually associated with immunodeficiency that was first recognized in this site.[131]

Clinical Features

Lymphoma that arises in the oral cavity can affect individuals of any age, but most patients are middle-aged or older adults with a median age in the sixth or seventh decade. Men and women are affected roughly equally, although the male to female ratio varies quite a bit among series.[129,132-137] Most patients are immunocompetent. However, in recent years, the number of cases of lymphoma of the oral cavity has increased, because patients with HIV tend to develop lymphoma in this site.[136-139] HIV+ oral cavity lymphoma patients are almost all males who overall are younger, with an approximate median age of 40 years.[131,136,139] Oral lymphoma also has been reported in rare cases in transplant recipients.[137]

Patients present with soft tissue swelling, a discrete mass, pain, mucosal ulceration or discoloration, gingival thickening, paresthesias, anesthesia, and loosening of teeth.[37,134,137,139-144] The sites most often affected, in both HIV-positive and HIV-negative patients, are the palate (bone or soft tissue), maxilla, and gingiva; the tongue, buccal mucosa, floor of the mouth, and lips are less often affected.* Physical examination reveals an exophytic mass that may be smooth surfaced and polypoid or fungating and ulcerated. In other cases, the lymphoma is an infiltrative, ill-defined lesion.[129,142,143]

Pathologic Features

Plasmablastic Lymphoma

Plasmablastic lymphoma is a distinctive variant of diffuse large B-cell lymphoma that was first described in the oral cavity by Delecluse and colleagues in 1997.[131] According to the WHO

---

*References 129, 131, 132, 134, 136, 139, and 142.

classification, it is defined as a diffuse proliferation of large neoplastic cells, most with the morphology of immunoblasts but with the immunophenotype of plasma cells.[130] Since its initial description, plasmablastic lymphoma has been found in other extranodal sites, including other sites in the head and neck, gastrointestinal tract, bone, skin, and soft tissue and less often in lymph nodes.[92,145,146] Almost all patients with this type of lymphoma are HIV positive, although a few cases have been described in iatrogenically immunosuppressed patients. A few cases also have occurred

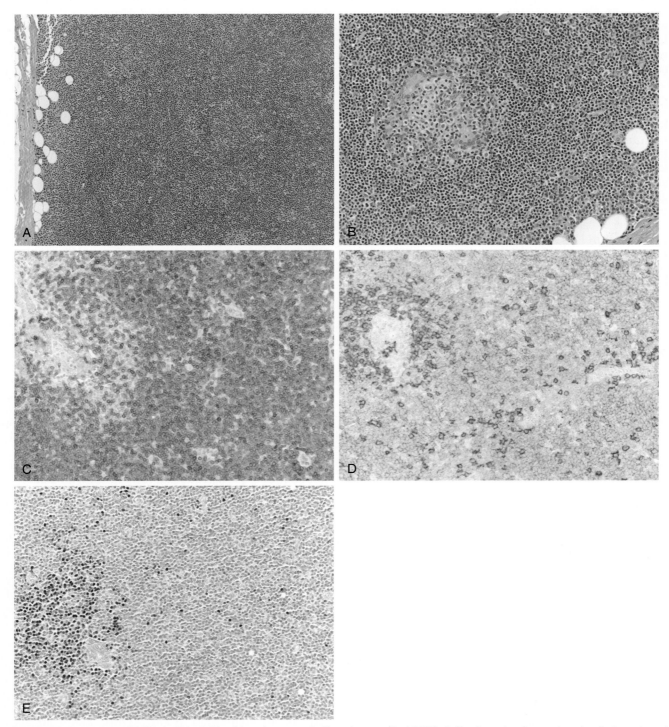

Figure 3-16 Parotid with CD20+ peripheral T-cell lymphoma, not otherwise specified (NOS). **A,** The tissue has been almost entirely replaced by a diffuse infiltrate of lymphoid cells. **B,** Higher power shows a small aggregate of pale cells with the appearance of monocytoid B cells infiltrating residual epithelial elements; most of the cells are small and round or slightly irregular with scant, pale cytoplasm. **C to E,** Immunostains show that most cells are CD3+ T cells **(C)**. The monocytoid B cells are CD20bright+, whereas the T cells are CD20dim+ **(D)**. B cells, but not T cells, express Pax5 **(E)** and CD79a (not shown).

in HIV-negative, immunocompetent individuals, mostly older adults. The disease is rare in children.[92,143] The development of plasmablastic lymphoma after extraction of a tooth, in the extraction site, has been described.[143]

In some cases the lymphoma is composed of a monotonous population of large cells with the appearance of immunoblasts, plasmacytoid immunoblasts, or plasmablasts, with vesicular nuclei and prominent nucleoli (Figure 3-17). In other cases plasmacytic differentiation is seen, with a subset of cells showing maturation toward plasma cells. These neoplasms have a high mitotic rate, frequent single cell or zonal necrosis, and scattered tingible body macrophages (Figure 3-17, B). The immunophenotype is distinctive: neoplastic cells often lack the leukocyte common antigen (CD45), typically lack CD20 and Pax5,[92,131,143] and almost always lack bcl6, a marker associated with the germinal center stage of B-cell differentiation. Some have reported CD10 expression to be rare or absent,[92,138,146] and others occasionally have observed CD10 expression.[147] A subset of cases is CD79a+. These cases typically express

markers associated with post-germinal center stage of differentiation or with plasma cells, including MUM1/IRF4 and CD138 (Figure 3-17, D to F). More than half express monotypic cytoplasmic immunoglobulin (kappa more often than lambda).[92,131,143,146] A high proliferation fraction (typically 60% to 90%) is seen among the neoplastic cells.[92,130,142]

In approximately 75% of cases,[143,146] tumor cells are infected by the Epstein-Barr virus (see Figure 3-17, G). Detection of EBV using in situ hybridization with a probe for EBER is much more sensitive than immunohistochemical staining for EBV-LMP, because the latter often is negative.[138,142,143] Molecular genetic analysis demonstrates clonal immunoglobulin heavy chain (IGH) gene rearrangement.[92,131] Human herpes virus type 8 (HHV8, the Kaposi's sarcoma–associated herpes virus) is absent.[130,142,145] A translocation between *MYC* and *IGH* [t(8;14)] has been reported in plasmablastic lymphoma, but the prevalence of this finding is uncertain.[148] Mutational analysis has shown that a subset of plasmablastic lymphoma has somatically hypermutated immunoglobulin heavy chain variable region genes

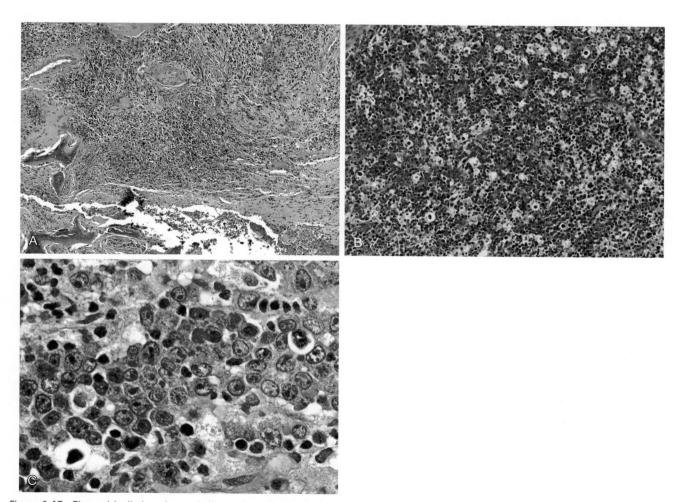

Figure 3-17 Plasmablastic lymphoma in the oral cavity (gingiva) of an HIV-positive male. The clinical differential diagnosis included periodontal disease. **A,** Low power shows a dense lymphoid infiltrate invading underlying bone. **B,** In many areas the lymphoma has a starry sky pattern, with many tingible body macrophages. **C,** High power shows large lymphoid cells, many of which have the appearance of immunoblasts, with large oval nuclei, vesicular chromatin, and prominent central nucleoli.

Continued

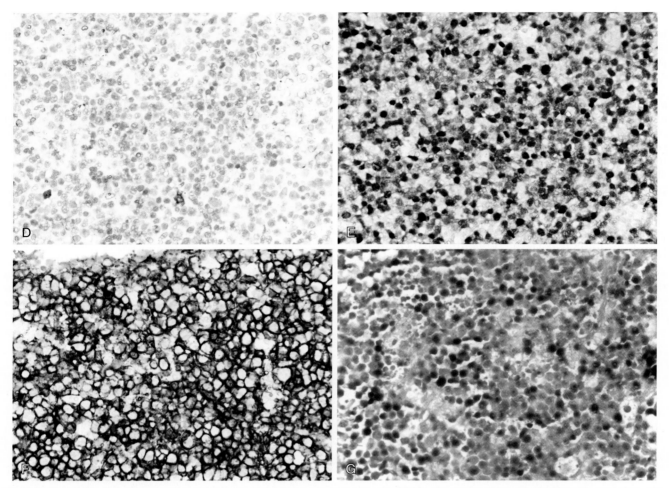

Figure 3-17, cont'd   D to G, Immunostains show that the large atypical cells are CD20– **(D)**, MUM1/IRF4+ **(E)**, CD138+ **(F)**, and EBV+ **(G)**. (*D* to *F,* Immunoperoxidase technique on paraffin sections; *G,* in situ hybridization for EBER on a paraffin section.)

(*IGHV*), presumably acquired during transit through the germinal center, indicating a derivation from post-germinal center B cells; in other cases, *IGHV* is germline, consistent with an origin from naïve B cells. Therefore, although the histologic and immunohistologic features are fairly uniform from case to case, analysis of genetic features indicates that plasmablastic lymphomas are genetically diverse.[138]

Other Oral Cavity Lymphomas Associated with HIV Infection

Other types of oral lymphomas in patients with HIV are almost all diffuse high-grade lymphomas. Most are diffuse large B-cell lymphomas, with occasional peripheral T-cell lymphoma NOS, and a few cases of Burkitt's lymphoma and anaplastic large cell lymphoma of T-lineage.[97,136,137,139]

Most HIV-associated oral lymphomas, both the B-cell and T-cell types, contain EBV. When in situ hybridization for EBER is used, approximately 80% of cases test positive.[131,136,137,139] In contrast, only a minority (9% to 19%) of oral lymphomas in nonimmunosuppressed patients test positive for EBER; most of these are diffuse large B-cell lymphomas.[133,136,137] EBV may play a role in the pathogenesis of most HIV-associated

lymphomas, but it is not a major factor in the pathogenesis of oral lymphoma in the general population.

Oral Cavity Lymphomas in Immunocompetent Patients

Oral cavity lymphomas in immunocompetent patients show a wider variety of high- and low-grade types than in immunodeficient patients. However, almost all are B-cell lymphomas, and at least half are diffuse large B-cell lymphomas. The next most common type is follicular lymphoma, followed by marginal zone lymphoma.[132-136] The follicular lymphomas have shown a predilection for involving the palate.[137] The marginal zone lymphomas may arise in minor salivary glands[149] and may show formation of lymphoepithelial lesions with minor salivary gland epithelium. Association with amyloid deposition has been described.[149] A few cases of various other types of lymphoma have been described, including mantle cell lymphoma; small lymphocytic lymphoma/chronic lymphocytic leukemia; peripheral T-cell lymphoma NOS; extranodal NK/T-cell lymphoma, nasal type; Burkitt's lymphoma; anaplastic large cell lymphoma; and B lymphoblastic lymphoma.[37,132,134-136]

Peripheral T-cell lymphoma that arose in the oral cavity in the form of painful ulcers has been described in an adult with celiac disease, probably representing an unusual manifestation of enteropathy-associated T-cell lymphoma.[144] A case of adult T-cell lymphoma (HTLV-1+) that presented as a painful ulcer on the hard palate has been reported; staging revealed widespread disease involving bones and other sites.[150] Mycosis fungoí des rarely involves the oral cavity. Most cases are found with long-standing, advanced disease, but in exceptional cases, mycosis fungoí des first manifests in the oral cavity.[151-153] Rare cases of Hodgkin's lymphoma primary in the oral cavity have been described.[154]

Staging, Treatment, and Outcome

Staging reveals localized disease in approximately 70% of cases.[131,134] The proportion of patients with localized and disseminated disease is similar in HIV-positive and HIV-negative patients. The outcome depends on the stage, the type of lymphoma, and the patient's HIV status; patients with localized, histologically low-grade lymphomas have an excellent outcome, whereas patients with high-grade lymphoma or disseminated disease have a significantly worse survival rate.[97,134,140] Patients with acquired immunodeficiency syndrome (AIDS), including those with plasmablastic lymphoma, have a poor prognosis. Most have died of lymphoma, although other HIV-associated illnesses sometimes contributed to the patients' deaths.[*]

Differential Diagnosis

1. **Lymphoma versus inflammatory processes.** An important pitfall in diagnosis is failure to consider lymphoma on physical examination. Oral lymphoma can mimic dental conditions such as periodontal disease, acute necrotizing gingivitis, and dental infections.[139,141,144] The appearance on physical examination may suggest carcinoma. In HIV-positive patients, Kaposi's sarcoma, deep fungal infections, and HIV-associated periodontal disease also enter the clinical differential diagnosis.[139] Once a biopsy sample has been obtained, assuming that the tissue is well preserved and representative of the tumor, the differential diagnosis is similar to that for the same type of lymphoma in other sites. Because inflammatory conditions are so much more common than lymphoma in this site, reactive processes must be considered carefully before a diagnosis of lymphoma is rendered. A distinctive, incompletely understood oral disease known as *traumatic eosinophilic granuloma* or *traumatic ulcerative granuloma with stromal eosinophilia* has been described. The tongue is the most common site of this disorder. It is characterized by a polymorphic infiltrate of T lymphocytes, B lymphocytes, histiocytes, eosinophils,

and large atypical cells that often prove to be CD30+ T cells.[156,157] The large cells usually are mononuclear but may be binucleated, occasionally resembling Reed-Sternberg cells. Occasionally, molecular studies have documented a clonal T-cell population.[156] The ulcerated lesions may persist for weeks to months or even a year before healing. Despite the suspicious clinical appearance and the atypical cells, follow-up usually has been uneventful. Some investigators suggest that traumatic eosinophilic granuloma represents the oral equivalent of the cutaneous CD30+ lymphoproliferative disorders.[156] The histologic features of such lesions may raise the question of Hodgkin's lymphoma, underscoring the importance of adhering to strict criteria for the diagnosis of lymphoma in this site.

2. **Plasmablastic lymphoma versus other neoplasms.** Plasmablastic lymphoma is associated with special problems in differential diagnosis. Because the neoplastic cells may grow in sheets and appear cohesive, undifferentiated carcinoma may be included in the differential on routine sections. Lack of CD45 and CD20 expression may lead to failure to consider the possibility of lymphoma. Familiarity with the entity, augmented by additional post-germinal center B-cell markers (e.g., MUM1/IRF4 and CD138), immunostains or in situ hybridization for immunoglobulin light chains, and in situ hybridization for EBV, help exclude carcinoma. Surprisingly, a case of plasmablastic lymphoma expressing cytokeratin has been described[92]; this emphasizes the need for careful interpretation of a panel of immunostains in conjunction with other clinical and pathologic features.

   The differential diagnosis of plasmablastic lymphoma also includes a variety of lymphomas with histologic and/or immunophenotypic evidence of plasmacytic or plasmablastic differentiation, such as extramedullary plasmacytoma, plasma cell myeloma with plasmablastic morphology,[147] Burkitt's lymphoma with plasmacytic differentiation, ALK+ large B-cell lymphoma, and extracavitary primary effusion lymphoma. Cases of EBV+ diffuse large B-cell lymphoma of the elderly can have a monomorphous, or large cell lymphoma, morphology, as well as a polymorphous morphology. Cases with monomorphous morphology may be considered in the differential of plasmablastic lymphoma. The various lymphoid and plasmacytic neoplasms in the differential diagnosis of plasmablastic lymphoma all have some morphologic and immunophenotypic features that overlap with those of plasmablastic lymphoma; some occur in the setting of immunodeficiency, and some are also EBV+; therefore, classifying them correctly requires careful correlation of clinical and pathologic features and thorough immunophenotypic analysis. Although the appearance of neoplastic cells in some cases of diffuse large B-cell lymphoma

---

*References 90, 131, 138, 143, 145, 146, 148, and 155.

NOS can overlap with that of neoplastic cells in plasmablastic lymphoma, the former type of lymphoma can be distinguished from the latter by its diffuse, strong expression of CD20 and other pan—B-cell markers. Diffuse large B-cell lymphoma NOS usually occurs in immunocompetent patients and usually is negative for EBV. In the differential diagnosis with an extramedullary plasmacytoma and plasma cell myeloma, factors favoring plasmablastic lymphoma include a history of immunodeficiency, especially HIV infection; involvement of extranodal sites, especially the oral cavity; a high proliferation fraction; and the presence of EBV.[130,147] In some cases plasma cell myeloma with plasmablastic morphology has a high proliferation fraction[147]; therefore this characteristic should not be used by itself to make a distinction. Plasma cell myeloma is more likely to show prominent bone marrow involvement, lytic bone lesions, and a serum M component.

EBV+ diffuse large B-cell lymphoma of the elderly affects older adults without a specific underlying immunodeficiency. Neoplastic cells typically express CD20 and/or CD79a,[49] in contrast to plasmablastic lymphoma. A minority of cases of Burkitt's lymphoma shows histologic and immunophenotypic evidence of plasmacytic differentiation. Burkitt's lymphoma with plasmacytic differentiation tends to occur in immunodeficient patients and, as does plasmablastic lymphoma, has a high mitotic rate. The neoplastic cells in these cases of Burkitt's lymphoma may have single central nucleoli, heightening the resemblance to plasmablastic lymphoma. Like Burkitt's lymphoma, plasmablastic lymphoma may have an *IGH-MYC* translocation.[148] In contrast to plasmablastic lymphoma, Burkitt's lymphoma has diffuse, strong expression of CD10 and bcl6; virtually every neoplastic cells is Ki67+; and except for endemic Burkitt's lymphoma, only a minority of Burkitt's lymphomas are EBV+. ALK+ large B-cell lymphoma is another large B-cell lymphoma that typically lacks CD20 expression and is composed of neoplastic cells with morphology that overlaps with that of plasmablastic lymphoma. In contrast to plasmablastic lymphoma, ALK+ diffuse large B-cell lymphoma has no particular association with immunodeficiency; principally involves lymph nodes (with a preferential sinusoidal distribution); usually expresses cytoplasmic IgA; does not harbor EBV; and by definition expresses the ALK protein.[158,159]

HHV8+ lymphomas that have pathologic features similar to those of primary effusion lymphoma but that produce mass lesions in lymph nodes or in extranodal sites may enter the differential diagnosis of plasmablastic lymphoma. These extracavitary primary effusion lymphomas have clinical, histologic, and immunophenotypic features that overlap with those of plasmablastic lymphoma. However, by definition, they are HHV8+, whereas plasmablastic lymphoma, by definition, lacks HHV8.[160-162] (HHV8+ lymphomas are discussed in Lymphomas of the Pleura and Pleural Cavity, in Chapter 4.) The clinical and pathologic features of plasmablastic lymphoma and neoplasms in its differential diagnosis are shown in Table 3-1.

■ THYROID LYMPHOMAS

Primary Lymphomas of the Thyroid

Introduction

Primary lymphoma of the thyroid is uncommon but has characteristic clinical and pathologic features. It accounts for 1% to 5% of thyroid malignancies and for 1% to 2.5% of all lymphomas.[163]

Extranodal Marginal Zone Lymphoma of Mucosa-Associated Lymphoid Tissue (MALT Lymphoma) and Diffuse Large B-Cell Lymphoma

Clinical Features

Marginal zone lymphoma of the thyroid and diffuse large B-cell lymphoma of the thyroid are discussed together because they share many clinical features; this is not surprising, because a subset of the diffuse large B-cell lymphomas represents large cell transformation of marginal zone lymphomas. Together they account for nearly all lymphomas arising in the thyroid. These lymphomas affect patients over a wide age range, but most are older adults with a median age of 60 to 70 years. A striking female preponderance is seen; females are affected more than three times as often as males.[163-169] Almost all patients with marginal zone lymphoma and a subset of patients with diffuse large B-cell lymphoma have evidence of chronic lymphocytic thyroiditis/Hashimoto's thyroiditis.[164,167,170] Patients with chronic lymphocytic thyroiditis have an estimated 67-fold increase in risk for thyroid lymphoma compared with patients without this disorder.[171] Rare lymphomas, including both marginal zone lymphoma and diffuse large B-cell lymphoma, have developed in patients with Graves' disease.[172]

The most common complaint is the presence of a mass or swelling,[164,166] sometimes described as rapidly enlarging. Patients also may have dysphagia, cough, dyspnea, hoarseness, stridor, dysphonia, or pain. The symptoms reflect the presence of the lesion, sometimes complicated by compression or obstruction of adjacent structures. Symptoms may be more severe and evolve more rapidly in patients with diffuse large B-cell lymphoma than in those with marginal zone lymphoma. A neck mass almost always is identified on physical examination.[163-165,167-169]

Pathologic Features

On gross examination, the lymphomas range from 0.5 to 19 cm (mean, 7 cm) and form multinodular or diffuse, firm or soft masses with smooth, pale tan,

TABLE 3-1

Differential Diagnosis of Plasmablastic Lymphoma

	DLBCL, NOS	Plasmablastic Lymphoma	Plasma Cell Myeloma and Plasmacytoma	EBV+ DLBCL of the Elderly	Burkitt's Lymphoma with Plasmacytoid Differentiation	Large B-Cell Lymphoma (ALK+)	Extracavitary Primary Effusion Lymphoma (HHV8+)
Clinical features	Mostly adults, occasionally children	Most patients are HIV positive, young to middle-aged; males are affected much more often than females	Adults, no underlying immunodeficiency; serum M component common with myeloma	Age >50 yr; no previous lymphoma, no underlying immunodeficiency	Often immunodeficient adults, some children	Any age but mostly adults; males are affected more often than females	Most are HIV positive, young to middle-aged; males are affected more often than females; minority are HIV negative and elderly
Common anatomic sites	Lymph nodes, many extranodal sites	Oral cavity; other sites include GI tract, sinonasal, skin, bone, lymph nodes	Bone marrow, bones, head and neck sites	Skin, upper and lower respiratory tract, stomach, lymph nodes	Many extranodal sites, with or without lymph nodes	Lymph nodes are affected much more often than extranodal sites	GI tract, skin, soft tissue, lung, spleen, lymph nodes
Histology	Diffuse proliferation of centroblasts, immunoblasts, and/or multilobated cells	Diffuse proliferation of immunoblasts and plasmacytoid immunoblasts; overt plasmacytic differentiation in some cases	Diffuse proliferation of mature or slightly to markedly atypical plasma cells or plasmablasts	*Monomorphous subtype:* Large lymphoid cells, including immunoblasts, plasmacytoid immunoblasts, and/or Reed-Sternberg–like cells, in diffuse pattern	As for other Burkitt's lymphomas but with eccentric cytoplasm and often a single central nucleolus	Plasmacytoid immunoblasts with sinusoidal growth in lymph nodes; Reed-Sternberg–like cells may be present	Large immunoblast-like or pleomorphic bizarre cells
Usual immunophenotype	CD20+, CD45+; CD10, bcl6, bcl2, MUM1/IRF4 variable; CD138–	CD20–, Pax5–/+, CD45–/+, CD79a–/+, bcl6–, MUM1/IRF4+, CD138+, CD56–/+, CD30+/–, EMA+/–, Ki67 ~60% to 90%, monotypic cIg +/– (kappa or lambda), usually IgG	CD20–, CD138+, MUM1/IRF4+, cyclin D1–/+, CD56+/–, monotypic cIg+, usually IgG or IgA	CD20+ and/or CD79a+, CD10–, bcl6–, MUM1/IRF4+, CD30+/–, CD15–	CD20+, CD10+, bcl6+, bcl2–, Ki67: 100% (as for other Burkitt's lymphomas); monotypic cIg+	Cytoplasmic ALK+, rarely nuclear ALK+; CD45dim+/–, CD20–, bcl6–, CD30–, CD138+, EMA+, monotypic cIg+;IgA is expressed much more often than IgG	CD20–/+, MUM1/IRF4+, CD138+/–, Ig–/+ (lambda is expressed much more often than kappa)
EBV	Usually negative	Most cases positive	Negative	Positive	Minority of cases positive	Negative	Majority of cases positive
HHV8	Negative	Negative	Negative	Negative	Negative	Negative	Positive
Genetic and cytogenetic features	IGH clonal; other abnormalities variable	IGH clonal; IGH/MYC has been described	IGH clonal, other abnormalities variable	IGH clonal	IGH clonal; IGH/MYC or IGL/MYC, as for other Burkitt's lymphomas	IGH clonal; t(2;17)(p23;q23) [CLTG-ALK] is characteristic	IGH clonal; no translocations of BCL1, BCL2, BCL6, or MYC

cIg, Cytoplasmic immunoglobulin; DLBCL, diffuse large B-cell lymphoma; EBV, Epstein-Barr virus; GI, gastrointestinal; HHV8, human herpes virus type 8; HIV, human immuno-deficiency virus; LBCL, large B-cell lymphoma; NOS, not otherwise specified.

or white-gray surfaces on sectioning.[167] Diffuse large B-cell lymphoma is the most common type of lymphoma in most series, accounting for the majority of cases. Extranodal marginal zone lymphoma is the next most common. However, up to half of the diffuse large B-cell lymphomas have a marginal zone lymphoma component, consistent with large cell transformation of the low-grade lymphoma[163,167-169]; for this reason, these lymphomas are discussed together.

The histologic features of these lymphomas are similar to those seen in other sites, although thyroid marginal zone lymphoma has some distinctive characteristics (Figure 3-18). It often has a characteristic type of lymphoepithelial lesion, which shows round aggregates of marginal zone cells filling and expanding the lumens of thyroid follicles, known as *"MALT ball" lymphoepithelial lesions* (Figure 3-18, *D*).[167] Follicular colonization tends to be prominent, in some cases resulting in a follicular architecture so striking that it mimics follicular lymphoma (Figure 3-18, *B*). Large cell transformation of neoplastic cells within colonized follicles is more common in the thyroid than elsewhere.[173] The histologic changes of Hashimoto's thyroiditis often are seen adjacent to the lymphoma.[167]

Marginal zone lymphoma of the thyroid has an immunophenotype similar to that found in other sites (CD20+, CD5−, CD10−, bcl6−, and cIg+/−; see Figure 3-18, *E*). The lymphomas have clonally rearranged *IGH*.[174] Recently three of six marginal zone lymphomas of the thyroid were found to have a previously undescribed translocation involving *FOXP1* and *IGH* [t(3;14)(p14.1;q32)] that resulted in upregulation of *FOXP1;* this translocation could play a role in the pathogenesis of marginal zone lymphoma.[175]

Diffuse large B-cell lymphomas are almost always CD20+ and CD5−. Most are bcl6+. Bcl2 is variably expressed. CD10 and MUM1/IRF4 are each expressed in a minority of cases. Diffuse large B-cell lymphomas with a component of marginal zone lymphoma have been CD10−, but some have expressed bcl6 or MUM1/IRF4.[170] Most diffuse large B-cell lymphomas have a germinal center–like immunophenotype.[170] Cytogenetic analysis by routine karyotyping or fluorescence in situ hybridization (FISH) has revealed occasional cases with a t(8;14) involving *MYC* and *IGH* and some with a translocation involving the *BCL6* locus at chromosome 3q27. No *IGH/BCL2* or *IGH/MALT1* translocations have been identified among the relatively small number of cases studied.[170]

Staging, Treatment, and Outcome

Extranodal marginal zone lymphomas are almost always localized (stage I or II). Patients with diffuse large B-cell lymphoma also usually have localized disease.[163,165,167,169,172] A minority of patients, usually those with diffuse large B-cell lymphoma, have widespread nodal and/or extranodal involvement. Extranodal sites that may be involved include the bone marrow, gastrointestinal tract, lungs, liver, and bladder.[165,167-169]

Treatment has not been uniform, but in general, marginal zone lymphoma usually can be treated successfully with local therapy (surgery or radiation or a combination of these techniques). Most authorities consider radiation alone to be inadequate therapy for diffuse large B-cell lymphoma. Chemotherapy or combined modality therapy (chemotherapy and radiation) is a more effective treatment for diffuse large B-cell lymphoma.[170,176] Patients with marginal zone lymphoma have an excellent prognosis.[163,164,166,167,169] Patients with localized diffuse large B-cell lymphoma usually can be treated successfully. When disease recurs, it often involves lymph nodes, but it also may involve a variety of extranodal sites (CNS, liver, stomach, and others). Local recurrence can occur but is uncommon.[166] In one series of patients with stage I or II diffuse large B-cell lymphoma of the thyroid who were treated with chemotherapy or combined modality therapy, 90% achieved complete remission. The 5-year progression-free survival rate was 84%, and the 5-year overall survival rate was 90%.[170]

The outcome is less favorable for those with diffuse large B-cell lymphoma who have higher stage disease or are treated with radiation only.[163,165,167,169] Among diffuse large B-cell lymphomas of the thyroid, the germinal-center–like B-cell immunophenotype has been associated with a better progression-free survival and overall survival, and bcl6 expression with better progression-free survival.[170] Patients with diffuse large B-cell lymphoma with a component of marginal zone lymphoma do not have an obvious survival benefit compared with those without a component of low-grade lymphoma.[170]

Follicular Lymphoma of the Thyroid

Follicular lymphoma rarely presents with thyroid involvement; 5% or fewer of primary lymphomas of the thyroid are follicular lymphomas.[167-169,177] The histologic features are similar to those of follicular lymphoma in other sites, although surprisingly, in the thyroid, follicular lymphoma may be associated with lymphoepithelial lesions.[177] In most cases, concurrent chronic lymphocytic thyroiditis is seen. In one study, follicular lymphoma of the thyroid could be divided into two groups based on clinical and pathologic features: In the first group, the follicular lymphomas were low grade (grade 1 or 2 of 3), usually expressed CD10 and expressed bcl2 and/or displayed a t(14;18)/*IGH/BCL2* translocation. These patients usually had spread of disease beyond the thyroid gland, typically involving lymph nodes and sometimes the bone marrow. The second group was characterized by grade 3 of 3 histology, frequent lack of CD10, lack of bcl2 and lack of *IGH/BCL2* translocation. In these patients, the lymphoma typically was confined to the thyroid.[177] Cases in the first group, therefore, share many features with lymph node follicular lymphomas, whereas those in the second group share some features with follicular lymphomas arising in certain extranodal sites, such as the testis (see Chapter 9) and the skin (see Chapter 11).

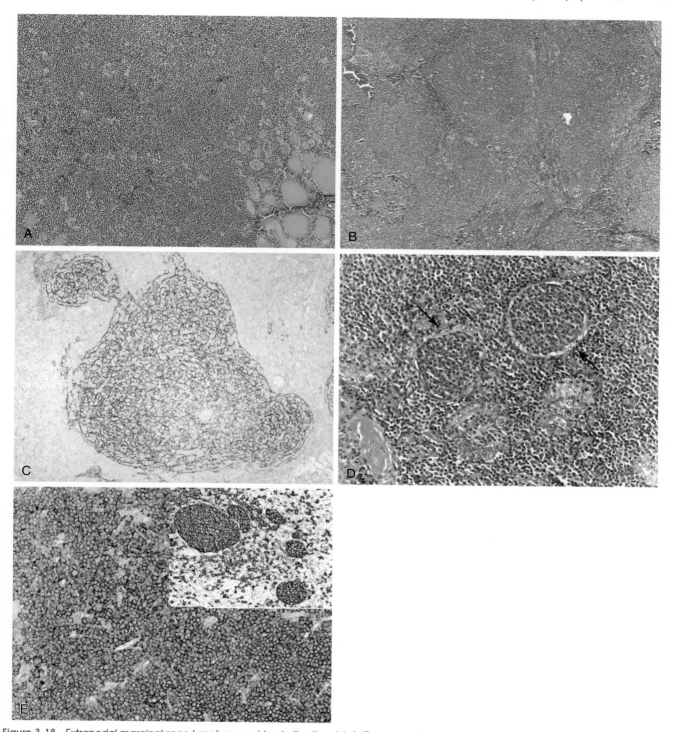

Figure 3-18 Extranodal marginal zone lymphoma arising in the thyroid. **A,** The normal parenchyma of the thyroid has been almost completely obliterated by lymphoma, which has a diffuse pattern in this field. **B,** In other areas, the lymphoma has a vaguely nodular pattern. **C,** Nodular areas correspond to large follicular dendritic meshworks, consistent with follicular colonization by neoplastic marginal zone cells. (Immunostain for CD21 on a paraffin section.) **D,** "MALT ball" lymphoepithelial lesions *(arrows)* are present within the lymphoma. **E,** Neoplastic cells are CD20+, as are nearly all cells in the MALT balls *(inset).* (Immunoperoxidase technique on a paraffin section.)

Patients presenting with localized disease usually appear to remain free of lymphoma after treatment. Those presenting with more widespread disease may achieve a complete remission, although some have progressive disease, sometimes with histologic transformation to diffuse large B-cell lymphoma, and are alive with lymphoma or succumb to their lymphoma.[177]

The main differential is with marginal zone lymphoma, which often can have a follicular pattern as a result of conspicuous follicular colonization, as noted previously. Other features strongly associated with marginal zone lymphoma, such as lymphoepithelial lesions and chronic lymphocytic thyroiditis, may also be found in follicular lymphoma; therefore, these features cannot be used to differentiate the two. Careful study of the cytologic features, augmented by immunohistochemistry, helps establish a diagnosis.

Miscellaneous Lymphomas of the Thyroid

Other types of lymphoma are uncommon; among those reported are Burkitt's lymphoma and rare peripheral T-cell lymphomas, including anaplastic large cell lymphoma.[163,168,169] A few peripheral T-cell lymphomas NOS considered to be primary in the thyroid have been reported. These have mainly affected older adults, and women are affected more often than men.[178] Some patients have a history of thyroiditis, and some are reported to have hypothyroidism or antithyroid antibodies or both. These lymphomas have been composed of small cells, medium-sized or large cells, or cells in a range of sizes. The formation of lymphoepithelial lesions has been described. Often, extensive immunophenotyping has not been performed, but most cases tested have been CD3+ and CD4+. Four have been TCRαβ+; one case was TCRγδ+. The outcome is variable.[178]

We have seen a case of mantle cell lymphoma presenting with involvement of the thyroid (Figure 3-19). The patient had a thyroidectomy and excision of a cervical lymph node after a diagnosis of papillary carcinoma was made on a fine needle aspiration biopsy specimen. In this difficult and unusual case, the lymphoma suggested extranodal marginal zone lymphoma in the thyroid (Figure 3-19, *A* to *C*) and low-grade follicular lymphoma in the lymph node (Figure 3-19, *D*). Establishment of a diagnosis was complicated by the lack of CD5 expression by the neoplastic B cells (Figure 3-19, *J*). However, lymphoma in both the lymph node and the thyroid clearly expressed cyclin D1 (Figure 3-19, *H* and *I*), and staging revealed more widespread disease.

Differential Diagnosis of Non-Hodgkin's Lymphomas of the Thyroid

1. **Hashimoto's thyroiditis versus marginal zone lymphoma.** Hashimoto's thyroiditis is characterized by a lymphoid infiltrate extensively involving the thyroid. The infiltrate is composed of well-delineated, reactive lymphoid follicles and an interfollicular infiltrate of small lymphocytes and plasma cells, sometimes with fibrosis. Thyroid follicles are present in the lymphoid infiltrate and show oxyphil metaplasia. Lymphoepithelial lesions, when present, are small and inconspicuous. Often, marginal zone lymphoma also has reactive follicles and a lymphoplasmacytic infiltrate; however, factors favoring marginal zone lymphoma include obliteration of thyroid parenchyma by the lymphoid infiltrate; interfollicular

cells with the morphology and immunophenotype of marginal zone B cells; large, prominent lymphoepithelial lesions; lymphoid follicles with follicular colonization; and, on paraffin sections, plasma cells expressing monotypic immunoglobulin. If fresh tissue is available for flow cytometry, a monotypic B-cell population can be identified. Lymphoepithelial lesions in Hashimoto's thyroiditis are more often composed of T cells, whereas in marginal zone lymphoma they contain mainly B cells.[174]

In a subset of cases of Hashimoto's thyroiditis, molecular studies using polymerase chain reaction (PCR) to search for clonal rearrangement of *IGH* reveal the presence of clonal bands, typically in a background smear. The same clonal population may not be found in different areas of the tissue, in contrast to lymphoma, which typically shows strong reproducible bands. Follow-up suggests that patients with Hashimoto's thyroiditis with clonal B cells by PCR do not have any obvious increased risk for lymphoma.[174] Therefore, in the setting of typical histologic features of Hashimoto's thyroiditis, a diagnosis of marginal zone lymphoma should not be made, even if a clonal B-cell population is identified by PCR.

2. **Marginal zone lymphoma versus follicular lymphoma.** Marginal zone lymphoma of the thyroid often shows prominent follicular colonization, imparting a follicular pattern that may raise the question of follicular lymphoma. Marginal zone lymphoma is much more common than follicular lymphoma in this site; therefore, the possibility of marginal zone lymphoma with follicular colonization should always be considered for a thyroid lymphoma with a follicular pattern. Factors favoring marginal zone lymphoma are atypical cells with the morphology of marginal zone B cells (typically less irregular and angulated than the centrocytes of follicular lymphoma), lack of CD10 and bcl6 expression by atypical cells, coexpression of CD43 by atypical cells, and plasmacytic differentiation, in the form of a plasma cell population expressing monotypic cytoplasmic immunoglobulin light chain.

3. **Plasmacytoma versus marginal zone lymphoma.** A number of cases of extramedullary plasmacytoma arising in the thyroid have been described; at least some of these may represent marginal zone lymphomas with marked plasmacytic differentiation. Reactive follicles; an extrafollicular component of B cells, particularly if they have the morphology of marginal zone cells; and lymphoepithelial lesions make plasmacytoma unlikely.[167,169]

4. **Hashimoto's thyroiditis versus follicular lymphoma.** The floridly hyperplastic follicles of Hashimoto's thyroiditis are not usually difficult to distinguish from follicular lymphoma. However, flow cytometry sometimes shows an unusually high kappa to lambda ratio (as high as 14.4 in one series) among CD10+ B cells in cases of otherwise

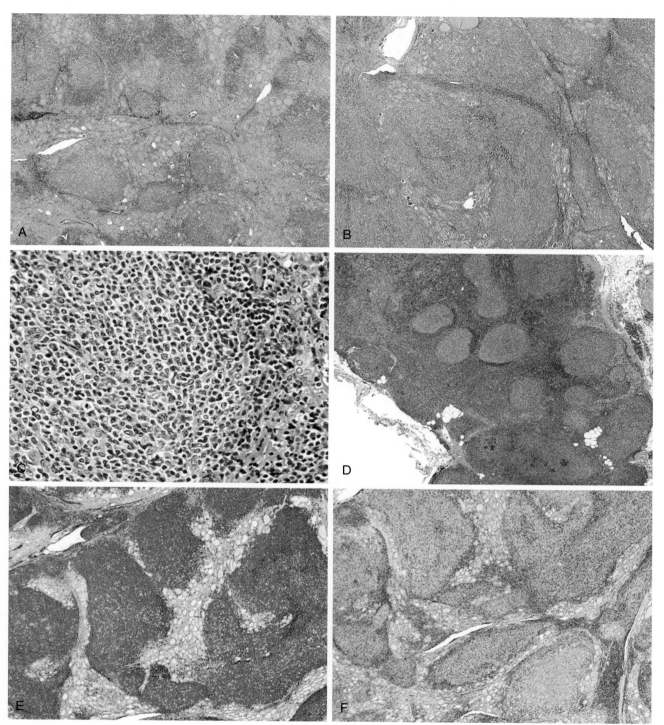

Figure 3-19 Mantle cell lymphoma, CD5–, presenting with involvement of the thyroid. The patient, who had a history of chronic lympho-cytic thyroiditis, underwent thyroidectomy and excision of a cervical lymph node after a diagnosis of papillary carcinoma was made on a fine needle aspiration biopsy. **A,** In some areas, multiple lymphoid follicles suggesting chronic lymphocytic thyroiditis can be seen. The thyroid parenchyma overall is preserved. **B,** In other areas, the lymphoid follicles are enlarged, crowded, and poorly delineated, and normal thyroid tissue has been obliterated. **C,** Some of the enlarged follicles had remnants of reactive follicle centers; however, most of the cells present, as seen in this image, are small, oval, or slightly irregular lymphoid cells with scant cytoplasm. The histologic findings suggested early involvement by marginal zone lymphoma. Papillary carcinoma also was present (not illustrated). **D,** The lymph node contains multiple follicles occupied by a monotonous population of small lymphoid cells; the appearance of the lymph node would be unusual for marginal zone lymphoma. **E to H,** Immunostains on the thyroid show that the follicles are composed mostly of CD20+ B cells **(E),** with fewer CD3+ T cells **(F).** Most lymphoid cells are bcl2+, although a few small clusters of bcl2– residual reactive follicle center cells are present **(G).**

Continued

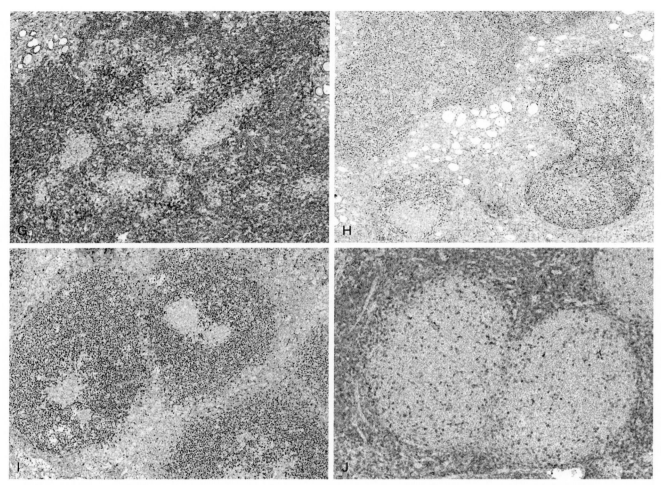

Figure 3-19, cont'd   The monotonous small cells were CD43dim+ and were negative for CD10 and bcl6 (not shown). The monotonous cells are cyclin D1+ **(H)**, which confirms a diagnosis of mantle cell lymphoma. **I** and **J**, The mantle cell lymphoma in this case was unusual in that it lacked expression of CD5; immunostains on the lymph node showed cyclin D1+ lymphoid cells **(I)** that were negative for CD5 **(J)**. (*E* to *J*, Immunoperoxidase technique on paraffin sections.)

typical Hashimoto's thyroiditis.[179] In such cases, no clonal B-cell population and no *BCL2/IGH* fusion is found by PCR, and these patients do not appear to have an increased risk for progression to lymphoma.[179]

5. **Poorly differentiated carcinoma versus diffuse large B-cell lymphoma.** Undifferentiated carcinoma may be difficult to distinguish from diffuse large B-cell lymphoma on routine sections, but a diagnosis can be established using immunohistochemical studies.

Hodgkin's Lymphoma of the Thyroid

Introduction

Fewer than two dozen cases of Hodgkin's lymphoma presenting with thyroid involvement have been described; however, when this occurs, characteristic clinical and pathologic features are seen, which suggests that Hodgkin's lymphoma of the thyroid is a distinct entity.

Clinical Features

Patients range in age from 18 to 64 years, and the median age is in the early 40s. The male to female ratio is approximately 1:3.[180] A history of Hashimoto's thyroiditis, lymphocytic thyroiditis, or hypothyroidism is common. As do other types of lymphoma of the thyroid, Hodgkin's lymphoma shows a female preponderance and often occurs in the setting of thyroiditis; it tends to affect patients who are overall slightly younger than those with other types of thyroid lymphoma. Patients often have evidence of tracheal or esophageal obstruction at presentation. They have hoarseness, stridor, dysphagia, or a painless mass that may be rapidly enlarging. Physical examination reveals unilateral or bilateral lesions that often are quite hard. Some patients have concurrent lymphadenopathy or a mediastinal mass. Occasionally, the thyroid disease may be in continuity with a mediastinal mass, which suggests that some of these cases may represent secondary involvement of the thyroid. The prognosis is favorable.[180]

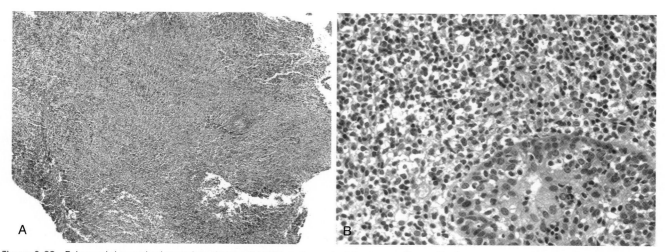

Figure 3-20 Extranodal marginal zone lymphoma (MALT lymphoma) of the larynx. The patient was a young woman who presented with a lesion of the vocal cord. **A,** Low power shows a lesion composed of a diffuse infiltrate of lymphoid cells. **B,** High power shows small, oval, lymphoid cells with clear cytoplasm invading a submucosal gland to form a lymphoepithelial lesion. As is typical of marginal zone lymphoma in other sites, the lymphoid cells in this case were CD20+, CD5–, CD10–, and cyclin D1–, with scattered disrupted follicular dendritic meshworks. Molecular studies using PCR revealed the presence of a clonal B-cell population; in conjunction with the other pathologic features, this result confirmed a diagnosis of marginal zone lymphoma.

Pathologic Features

All published cases have been classical Hodgkin's lymphoma, and nearly all have been the nodular sclerosis type. One case of mixed cellularity classical Hodgkin's lymphoma has been described.[180] The predominance of nodular sclerosis–type cases may be related to the sites involved, because many cases are associated with cervical or mediastinal involvement, and when Hodgkin's lymphoma involves those sites, it usually is the nodular sclerosis type. The pathologic features are similar to those of classical Hodgkin's lymphoma in other sites, except that sclerosis may be unusually extensive and sometimes is more prominent than in involved lymph nodes.

Differential Diagnosis of Hodgkin's Lymphoma of the Thyroid

The prominent sclerosis may suggest the possibility of the fibrosclerosing variant of Hashimoto's thyroiditis, or Riedel's thyroiditis.[180] Careful examination in cases of Hodgkin's lymphoma reveals large, atypical Reed-Sternberg cells and variants. Information about lymphadenopathy also may alert the pathologist that a case is less likely to represent an uncomplicated inflammatory disorder of the thyroid.

■ LARYNGEAL LYMPHOMAS

Primary Laryngeal Lymphomas

Clinical Features

Primary laryngeal lymphoma is rare, accounting for fewer than 1% of laryngeal neoplasms.[181] Patients are mostly middle-aged or older adults, although a few young adults and children also have been affected.

A slight male preponderance is seen.[97,181-185] Several patients have had concurrent laryngeal squamous cell carcinoma or other malignancies.[184,185] Individual case reports have described patients with Sjögren's syndrome,[186] rheumatoid arthritis,[187] or chronic laryngitis secondary to extraesophageal reflux with *Helicobacter pylori* gastritis.[188] In rare cases patients are HIV positive[97,183] or have another underlying immunodeficiency.[189]

Patients present with hoarseness, dyspnea, progressive or acute airway obstruction, sore throat, foreign body sensation, or dysphagia.[37,97,181,184,185] The tumors usually are smooth surfaced, submucosal, raised, often polypoid lesions.[183,184,188,190] Circumferential involvement of the larynx is also described.[186] Pedunculated tumors may prolapse into the airway.[183,185] Laryngeal lymphomas may arise from the lymphoid tissue that can be found in the larynx, mainly in the epiglottis and supraglottic larynx, which correlates with the distribution of lymphomas of this site.[190] Lymphomas are only rarely subglottic.[186]

Pathologic Features

Diffuse large B-cell lymphoma and extranodal marginal zone lymphoma of mucosa-associated lymphoid tissue (MALT lymphoma) together account for nearly all cases of laryngeal lymphoma. Their histologic and immunophenotypic features are similar to those found in other sites (Figure 3-20).[37,181,182,184-188,190] Marginal zone lymphomas may form lymphoepithelial lesions in submucosal glands (Figure 3-20, *B*).[188] Rare cases of follicular lymphoma[181] and peripheral T-cell lymphoma,[184,191] several cases of extranodal NK/T-cell lymphoma,[183,191,192] and an EBV+ B-cell lymphoma in a boy with Wiskott-Aldrich syndrome[189] have been described.

Staging, Treatment, and Outcome

Most patients present with localized (Ann Arbor stage I) disease.[97,181,183-185,188,192] In a few cases of marginal zone lymphoma, the larynx has been involved simultaneously with other extranodal sites in the head and neck.[97,193] Laryngeal lymphoma may cause sudden death as a result of acute airway obstruction,[190] but most patients with marginal zone lymphoma and diffuse large B-cell lymphoma can be treated successfully by surgery, radiation, chemotherapy, or a combination of these techniques.[97,186-188,194] In marginal zone lymphoma, relapses tend to be isolated, extranodal tumors in the upper respiratory tract, stomach, orbit, and skin, and even when relapses occur, the patient may have long, disease-free intervals. This behavior is similar to that of marginal zone lymphoma in other sites.[97,184]

Secondary Laryngeal Involvement by Lymphoma

The larynx occasionally is involved by lymphomas of a variety of types that arise in other sites. The larynx may be the only site of relapse, or it may be involved as a result of disseminated disease.[192,195] A case of oral cavity marginal zone lymphoma with multiple relapses confined to the upper aerodigestive tract, including the larynx, has been described.[149]

Differential Diagnosis

Because of the rarity of laryngeal lymphoma, it may not be suspected before biopsy. The clinical impression may be that of another type of neoplasm or, particularly if the lesion results in stenosis rather than an exophytic mass, an inflammatory process.[186] On pathologic evaluation, the differential diagnosis of laryngeal lymphoma is similar to that of the same types of lymphoma in other extranodal sites. The larynx is a common site for tumor-forming amyloidosis; it should be noted that amyloid deposition in the larynx (and in other extranodal sites) may be due to marginal zone lymphoma. Any lymphoplasmacytic infiltrate associated with the amyloid should be carefully evaluated to determine whether it represents lymphoma.[149]

REFERENCES

1. Bairey O, Kremer I, Rakowsky E et al: Orbital and adnexal involvement in systemic non-Hodgkin's lymphoma, *Cancer* 73:2395-2399, 1994.
2. Freeman C, Berg J, Cutler S: Occurrence and prognosis of extranodal lymphomas, *Cancer* 29:252-260, 1972.
3. Ferry J, Fung C, Zukerberg L et al: Lymphoma of the ocular adnexa: a study of 353 cases, *Am J Surg Pathol* 31:170-184, 2007.
4. Auw-Haedrich C, Coupland S, Kapp A et al: Long term outcome of ocular adnexal lymphoma subtyped according to the REAL classification, *Br J Ophthalmol* 85:63-69, 2001.
5. Baldini L, Blini M, Guffanti A et al: Treatment and prognosis in a series of primary extranodal lymphomas of the ocular adnexa, *Ann Oncol* 9:779-781, 1998.
6. White WL, Ferry JA, Harris NL, Grove AS: Ocular adnexal lymphoma: a clinicopathologic study with identification of lymphomas of mucosa-associated lymphoid tissue (MALT) type, *Ophthalmology* 102:1994-2006. 1995.
7. Coupland S, Krause L, Delecluse H-J et al: Lymphoproliferative lesions of the ocular adnexa: analysis of 112 cases, *Ophthalmology* 105:1430-1441, 1998.
8. Wotherspoon A, Diss T, Pan L et al: Primary low-grade B-cell lymphoma of the conjunctiva: a mucosa-associated lymphoid tissue type lymphoma, *Histopathology* 23:417-424, 1993.
9. Arcaini L, Burcheri S, Rossi A et al: Prevalence of HCV infection in nongastric marginal zone B-cell lymphoma of MALT, *Ann Oncol* 18:346-350, 2007.
10. Ferreri AJ, Viale E, Guidoboni M et al: Clinical implications of hepatitis C virus infection in MALT-type lymphoma of the ocular adnexa, *Ann Oncol* 17:769-772, 2006.
11. Ferreri AJ, Guidoboni M, Ponzoni M et al: Evidence for an association between *Chlamydia psittaci* and ocular adnexal lymphomas, *J Natl Cancer Inst* 96:586-594, 2004.
12. Chanudet E, Zhou Y, Bacon CM et al: *Chlamydia psittaci* is variably associated with ocular adnexal MALT lymphoma in different geographical regions, *J Pathol* 209:344-351, 2006.
13. Stefanovic A, Lossos IS: Extranodal marginal zone lymphoma of the ocular adnexa, *Blood* 114:501-510, 2009.
14. Rosado M, Byrne G, Ding F et al: Ocular adnexal lymphoma: a clinicopathologic study of a large cohort of patients with no evidence for an association with *Chlamydia psittaci*, *Blood* 107:467-472, 2006.
15. Zhang GS, Winter JN, Variakojis D et al: Lack of an association between *Chlamydia psittaci* and ocular adnexal lymphoma, *Leuk Lymphoma* 48:577-583, 2007.
16. Cheuk W, Yuen HK, Chan AC et al: Ocular adnexal lymphoma associated with IgG4+ chronic sclerosing dacryoadenitis: a previously undescribed complication of IgG4-related sclerosing disease, *Am J Surg Pathol* 32:1159-1167, 2008.
17. Jenkins C, Rose G, Bunce C et al: Histological features of ocular adnexal lymphoma (REAL classification) and their association with patient morbidity and survival, *Br J Ophthalmol* 84:907-913, 2000.
18. Mannami T, Yoshimo T, Oshima K et al: Clinical histopathological and immunogenetic analysis of ocular adnexal lymphoproliferative disorders: characterization of MALT lymphoma and reactive lymphoid hyperplasia, *Mod Pathol* 14:641-649, 2001.
19. Vega F, Lin P, Medeiros L: Extranodal lymphomas of the head and neck, *Ann Diagn Pathol* 9:340-350, 2005.
20. Streubel B, Simonitsch-Klupp I, Mullauer L et al: Variable frequencies of MALT lymphoma–associated genetic aberrations in MALT lymphomas of different sites, *Leukemia* 18:1722-1726, 2004.
21. Chanudet E, Ye H, Ferry J et al: A20 deletion is associated with copy number gain at the TNFA/B/C locus and occurs preferentially in translocation-negative MALT lymphoma of the ocular adnexa and salivary glands, *J Pathol* 217:420-430, 2009.
22. Chanudet E, Ichimura K, Hamoudi R et al: A20 is targeted by deletion and promotermethylation in MALT lymphoma, *Leukemia* 24:483-487, 2010.
23. McNally L, Jakobiec F, Knowles D: Clinical, morphologic, immunophenotypic, and molecular genetic analysis of bilateral ocular adnexal lymphoid neoplasms in 17 patients, *Am J Ophthalmol* 103:555-568, 1987.
24. Coupland S, Foss H, Assaf C et al: T-cell and T/natural killer cell lymphomas involving ocular and ocular adnexal tissues, *Ophthalmology* 106:2109-2120, 1999.
25. Sherman M, Van Dalen J, Conrad K: Bilateral orbital infiltration as the initial sign of a peripheral T-cell lymphoma presenting in a leukemic phase, *Ann Ophthalmol* 22:93-95, 1990.
26. Woog JJ, Kim YD, Yeatts RP et al: Natural killer/T-cell lymphoma with ocular and adnexal involvement, *Ophthalmology* 113:140-147, 2006.
27. Ferry J, Fung C, Hasserjian R et al: Ocular adnexal lymphomas: outcome in 181 patients, *Mod Pathol* 21(suppl 1):253A, 2008.

28. Fung C, Ferry J, Linggood R et al: Extranodal marginal zone (MALT type) lymphoma of the ocular adnexa: a localized tumor with favorable outcome after radiation therapy. Proceedings of ASTRO Thirty-Seventh Annual Meeting, *Int J Radiat Oncol Phys* 36:199, 1996.

29. Bennett C, Putterman A, Bitran J et al: Staging and therapy of orbital lymphomas, *Cancer* 57:1204-1208, 1986.

30. Smitt M, Donaldson S: Radiotherapy is successful treatment for orbital lymphoma, *Int J Radiat Oncol Biol Phys* 26:59-66, 1993.

31. Platanias L, Putterman A, Vijayakumar S et al: Treatment and prognosis of orbital non-Hodgkin's lymphomas, *Am J Clin Oncol* 15:79-83, 1992.

32. Eulau S, Hildebrand R, Warnke R et al: Primary radiotherapy is curative for CS 1E orbital MALT lymphoma, *Int J Radiat Oncol Biol Phys* 39:176, 1997.

33. Knowles D, Jakobiec F, McNally L, Burke J: Lymphoid hyperplasia and malignant lymphoma occurring in the ocular adnexa (orbit, conjunctiva, and eyelids): a prospective multiparametric analysis of 108 cases during 1977 to 1987, *Hum Pathol* 21:959-973, 1990.

34. Medeiros L, Harmon D, Linggood R, Harris N: Immunohistologic features predict clinical behavior of orbital and conjunctival lymphoid infiltrates, *Blood* 74:2121-2129, 1989.

35. Knowles D, Jakobiec F: Ocular adnexal lymphoid neoplasms: clinical, histopathologic, electron microscopic, and immunologic characteristics, *Hum Pathol* 13:148-162, 1982.

36. Medeiros L, Harris N: Lymphoid infiltrates of the orbit and conjunctiva: a morphologic and immunophenotypic study of 99 cases, *Am J Surg Pathol* 13:459-471, 1989.

37. Assanasen T, Wannakrairot P, Keelawat S et al: Extranodal malignant lymphoma of the upper aerodigestive tract in King Chulalongkorn Memorial Hospital according to WHO classification, *J Med Assoc Thai* 87(suppl 2):S249-S254, 2004.

38. Ezzat AA, Ibrahim EM, El Weshi AN et al: Localized non-Hodgkin's lymphoma of Waldeyer's ring: clinical features, management, and prognosis of 130 adult patients, *Head Neck* 23:547-558, 2001.

39. Ree HJ, Ohsima K, Aozasa K et al: Detection of germinal center B-cell lymphoma in archival specimens: critical evaluation of Bcl-6 protein expression in diffuse large B-cell lymphoma of the tonsil, *Hum Pathol* 34:610-616, 2003.

40. Kojima M, Nakamura N, Shimizu K et al: Marginal zone B-cell lymphoma among primary B-cell lymphoma of Waldeyer's ring: histopathologic and immunohistochemical study of 16 tonsillectomy specimens, *Int J Surg Pathol* 16:164-170, 2008.

41. Krol AD, Le Cessie S, Snijder S et al: Waldeyer's ring lymphomas: a clinical study from the Comprehensive Cancer Center West population-based NHL registry, *Leuk Lymphoma* 42:1005-1013, 2001.

42. Tewfik T, Bond M, al-Ghamdi K, Bernard C: Burkitt's lymphoma of the tonsil in children, *J Otolaryngol* 25:205-238, 1996.

43. Laskar S, Bahl G, Muckaden MA et al: Primary diffuse large B-cell lymphoma of the tonsil: is a higher radiotherapy dose required? *Cancer* 110:816-823, 2007.

44. Sakabe H, Bamba M, Nomura K et al: MALT lymphoma at the base of the tongue developing without any background of immunodeficiency or autoimmune disease, *Leuk Lymphoma* 44:875-878, 2003.

45. Sobol S, Kost KM: Nasopharyngeal Burkitt's lymphoma causing acute airway obstruction, *Otolaryngol Head Neck Surg* 124:334-335, 2001.

46. Li YX, Fang H, Liu QF et al: Clinical features and treatment outcome of nasal-type NK/T-cell lymphoma of Waldeyer ring, *Blood* 112:3057-3064, 2008.

47. Alizadeh A, Eisen M, Davis R et al: Distinct types of diffuse large B-cell lymphoma identified by gene expression profiling, *Nature* 403:503-511, 2000.

48. Rosenwald A, Wright G, Chan W et al: The use of molecular profiling to predict survival after chemotherapy for diffuse large B-cell lymphoma, *N Engl J Med* 346:1937-1947, 2002.

49. Nakamura S, Jaffe E, Swerdlow S: EBV positive diffuse large B-cell lymphoma of the elderly. In Swerdlow S, Campo E, Harris N et al, editors: *WHO classification tumours of haematopoietic and lymphoid tissues*, pp 243-244, Lyon, 2008 IARC.

50. Kapadia SB, Roman LN, Kingma DW et al: Hodgkin's disease of Waldeyer's ring: clinical and histoimmunophenotypic findings and association with Epstein-Barr virus in 16 cases, *Am J Surg Pathol* 19:1431-1439, 1995.

51. Treaba DO, Eklund JW, Wayne J et al: Classical Hodgkin's lymphoma presenting with tongue involvement: a case report and review of the literature, *Clin Lymphoma Myeloma* 6:410-413, 2006.

52. Quinones-Avila MdP, Gonzalez-Longoria AA, Admirand JH, Medeiros LJ: Hodgkin lymphoma involving Waldeyer ring: a clinicopathologic study of 22 cases, *Am J Clin Pathol* 123:651-656, 2005.

53. Louissaint A, Soupir C, Ganguly A et al: Infectious mononucleosis: morphology and immunophenotype in cervical lymph nodes and Waldeyer's ring, *Mod Pathol* 21(suppl 1): 263A, 2008.

54. Attygalle AD, Liu H, Shirali S et al: Atypical marginal zone hyperplasia of mucosa-associated lymphoid tissue: a reactive condition of childhood showing immunoglobulin lambda light chain restriction, *Blood* 104:3343-3348, 2004.

55. Taddesse-Heath L, Pittaluga S, Sorbara L et al: Marginal zone B-cell lymphoma in children and young adults, *Am J Surg Pathol* 27:522-531, 2003.

56. Wenig BM, Thompson LDR, Frankel SS et al: Lymphoid changes of the nasopharyngeal and palatine tonsils that are indicative of human immunodeficiency virus infection: a clinicopathologic study of 12 cases, *Am J Surg Pathol* 20:572-587, 1996.

57. Harbo G, Grau C, Bundgaard T et al: Cancer of the nasal cavity and paranasal sinuses: a clinico-pathological study of 277 patients, *Acta Oncol* 36:45-50, 1997.

58. Quraishi M, Bessell E, Clark D et al: Non-Hodgkin's lymphoma of the sinonasal tract, *Laryngoscope* 110:1489-1492, 2000.

59. Cuadra-Garcia I, Proulx G, Wu C et al: Sinonasal lymphoma: a clinicopathologic analysis of 58 cases from the Massachusetts General Hospital, *Am J Surg Pathol* 23:1356-1369, 1999.

60. Laskin JJ, Savage KJ, Voss N et al: Primary paranasal sinus lymphoma: natural history and improved outcome with central nervous system chemoprophylaxis, *Leuk Lymphoma* 46:1721-1727, 2005.

61. Tomita Y, Ohsawa M, Mishiro Y et al: The presence and subtype of Epstein-Barr virus in B and T cell lymphomas of the sino-nasal region from the Osaka and Okinawa districts of Japan, *Lab Invest* 73:190-196, 1995.

62. Tomita Y, Ohsawa M, Qiu K et al: Epstein-Barr virus in lymphoproliferative diseases in the sino-nasal region: close association with CD56+ immunophenotype and polymorphic-reticulosis morphology, *Int J Cancer* 70:9-13, 1997.

63. Kim GE, Koom WS, Yang WI et al: Clinical relevance of three subtypes of primary sinonasal lymphoma characterized by immunophenotypic analysis, *Head Neck* 26:584-593, 2004.

64. Chan J, Quintanilla-Martinez L, Ferry J, Peh S-C: Extranodal NK/T-cell lymphoma, nasal type. In Swerdlow S, Campo E, Harris N et al, editors: *WHO classification tumours of haematopoietic and lymphoid tissues*, pp 285-288, Lyon 2008, IARC.

65. Barrionuevo C, Zaharia M, Martinez MT et al: Extranodal NK/T-cell lymphoma, nasal type: study of clinicopathologic and prognosis factors in a series of 78 cases from Peru, *Appl Immunohistochem Mol Morphol* 15:38-44, 2007.

66. Hsieh PP, Tung CL, Chan AB et al: EBV viral load in tumor tissue is an important prognostic indicator for nasal NK/T-cell lymphoma, *Am J Clin Pathol* 128:579-584, 2007.

67. Huang MJ, Jiang Y, Liu WP et al: Early or up-front radiotherapy improved survival of localized extranodal NK/T-cell lymphoma, nasal-type, in the upper aerodigestive tract, *Int J Radiat Oncol Biol Phys* 70:166-174, 2008.

68. Kim SJ, Kim BS, Choi CW et al: Ki-67 expression is predictive of prognosis in patients with stage I/II extranodal NK/T-cell lymphoma, nasal type, *Ann Oncol* 18:1382-1387, 2007.

69. Wang B, Lu JJ, Ma X et al: Combined chemotherapy and external beam radiation for stage IE and IIE natural killer T-cell lymphoma of nasal cavity, *Leuk Lymphoma* 48:396-402, 2007.

70. Hoshida Y, Li T, Dong Z et al: Lymphoproliferative disorders in renal transplant patients in Japan, *Int J Cancer* 91:869-875, 2001.

71. Momose A, Mizuno H, Kajihara S et al: EBV-associated nasal-type NK/T-cell lymphoma of the nasal cavity/paranasal sinus in a renal allograft recipient, *Nephrol Dial Transplant* 21:1413-1416, 2006.

72. Kohler S, Iwatsuki K, Jaffe E, Chan J: Extranodal NK/T-cell lymphoma, nasal-type. In LeBoit P, Burg G, Weedon D, Sarasin A, editors: *Pathology and genetics: skin tumours*, pp 191-192 Lyon, 2006, IARC.

73. Kim Y, Chang S, Yang W-I et al: Primary NK/T cell lymphoma of the testis, *Acta Haematol* 109:95-100, 2003.

74. Kuo TT, Shih LY, Tsang NM: Nasal NK/T cell lymphoma in Taiwan: a clinicopathologic study of 22 cases, with analysis of histologic subtypes, Epstein-Barr virus LMP-1 gene association, and treatment modalities, *Int J Surg Pathol* 12:375-387, 2004.

75. Chan J, Sin V, Wong K et al: Nonnasal lymphoma expressing the natural killer cell marker CD56: a clinicopathologic study of 49 cases of an uncommon aggressive neoplasm, *Blood* 89:4501-4513, 1997.

76. Chan JKC, Tsang WYW, Lau W-H et al: Aggressive T/natural killer cell lymphoma presenting as testicular tumor, *Cancer* 77:1198-1205, 1996.

77. Hongyo T, Hoshida Y, Nakatsuka S et al: p53, K-ras, c-kit and beta-catenin gene mutations in sinonasal NK/T-cell lymphoma in Korea and Japan, *Oncol Rep* 13:265-271, 2005.

78. Ishii H, Ogino T, Berger C et al: Clinical usefulness of serum EBV DNA levels of BamHI W and LMP1 for Nasal NK/T-cell lymphoma, *J Med Virol* 79:562-572, 2007.

79. Lee J, Suh C, Park YH et al: Extranodal natural killer T-cell lymphoma, nasal type: a prognostic model from a retrospective multicenter study, *J Clin Oncol* 24:612-618, 2006.

80. Xiang-Lan M, Zu-Lan S, Dan H et al: Skp2/p27 expression profile is correlated with Epstein-Barr virus status in extranodal nasal-type natural killer cell lymphoma, *Transl Res* 151:303-308, 2008.

81. Oprea C, Cainap C, Azoulay R et al: Primary diffuse large B-cell non-Hodgkin lymphoma of the paranasal sinuses: a report of 14 cases, *Br J Haematol* 131:468-471, 2005.

82. Pomilla P, Morris A, Jaworek A: Sinonasal non-Hodgkin's lymphoma in patients infected with human immunodeficiency virus: report of three cases and review, *Clin Infect Dis* 21:137-149, 1995.

83. Shiong YS, Lian JD, Lin CY: Epstein-Barr virus associated T-cell lymphoma of the maxillary sinus in a renal transplant recipient, *Transplant Proc* 24:1929-1931, 1992.

84. Tran L, Mark R, Fu Y et al: Primary non-Hodgkin's lymphomas of the paranasal sinuses and nasal cavity: a report of 18 cases with stage IE disease, *Am J Clin Oncol (CCT)* 15:222-225, 1992.

85. Abbondanzo S, Wenig B: Non-Hodgkin's lymphoma of the sinonasal tract: a clinicopathologic and immunophenotypic study of 120 cases, *Cancer* 75:1281-1291, 1995.

86. Frierson H Jr, Innes D Jr, Mills S, Wick M: Immunophenotypic analysis of sinonasal non-Hodgkin's lymphomas, *Hum Pathol* 20:636-642, 1989.

87. Hausdorff J, Davis E, Long G et al: Non-Hodgkin's lymphoma of the paranasal sinuses: clinical and pathological features, and response to combined-modality therapy, *Cancer J Sci Am* 3:303-311, 1997.

88. Inaki S, Okamura H, Chikamori Y: Adult T-cell leukemia/lymphoma originating in the paranasal sinus, *Arch Otolaryngol Head Neck* 114:1471-1473, 1988.

89. Nakamura K, Uehara S, Omagari J et al: Primary non-Hodgkin lymphoma of the sinonasal cavities: correlation of CT evaluation with clinical outcome, *Radiology* 204:431-435, 1997.

90. Chetty R, Hlatswayo N, Muc R et al: Plasmablastic lymphoma in HIV+ patients: an expanding spectrum, *Histopathology* 42:605-609, 2003.

91. Schichman S, McClure R, Schaefer R, Mehta P: HIV and plasmablastic lymphoma manifesting in sinus, testicles and bones: a further expansion of the disease spectrum, *Am J Hematol* 77:291-295, 2004.

92. Kim JE, Kim YA, Kim WY et al: Human immunodeficiency virus–negative plasmablastic lymphoma in Korea, *Leuk Lymphoma* 50:582-587, 2009.

93. Weiss L, Gaffey M, Chen Y-Y, Frierson H: Frequency of Epstein-Barr viral DNA in "western" sinonasal and Waldeyer's ring non-Hodgkin's lymphomas, *Am J Surg Pathol* 16:156-162, 1992.

94. Duncavage J, Campbell B, Hanson G et al: Diagnosis of malignant lymphomas of the nasal cavity, paranasal sinuses and nasopharynx, *Laryngoscope* 93:1276-1280, 1983.

95. Jacobs C, Hoppe R: Non-Hodgkin's lymphomas of head and neck extranodal sites, *Int J Radiat Oncol Biol Phys* 11:357-364, 1985.

96. Lewis WB, Perlman P, Lasi J: Pediatric American Burkitt's lymphoma of the sphenoid sinus, *Otolaryngol Head Neck Surg* 123:642-644, 2000.

97. Ferry J, Harris N: Lymphoma and lymphoid hyperplasia in head and neck sites. In Pilch B, editor: *Head and neck surgical pathology,* Philadelphia, 2001, Lippincott, Williams & Wilkins.

98. Wu L, Cheng J, Maruyama S et al: Lymphoepithelial cyst of the parotid gland: its possible histopathogenesis based on clinicopathologic analysis of 64 cases, *Hum Pathol* 40:683-692, 2009.

99. Ihrler S, Zietz C, Riederer A et al: HIV-related parotid lymphoepithelial cysts: immunohistochemistry and 3-D reconstruction of surgical and autopsy material with special reference to formal pathogenesis, *Virchows Arch* 429:139-147, 1996.

100. Harris N: Lymphoid proliferations of the salivary glands, *Am J Clin Pathol* 111:S94-S103, 1999.

101. Dave SP, Pernas FG, Roy S: The benign lymphoepithelial cyst and a classification system for lymphocytic parotid gland enlargement in the pediatric HIV population, *Laryngoscope* 117:106-113, 2007.

102. Geyer J, Ferry J, Harris NL et al: Chronic sclerosing sialadenitis is an IgG4-associated disease, *Am J Surg Pathol* 34:202-210, 2010.

103. Kitagawa S, Zen Y, Harada K et al: Abundant IgG4-positive plasma cell infiltration characterizes chronic sclerosing sialadenitis (Küttner's tumor), *Am J Surg Pathol* 29:783-791, 2005.

104. Ochoa ER, Harris NL, Pilch BZ: Marginal zone B-cell lymphoma of the salivary gland arising in chronic sclerosing sialadenitis (Küttner tumor), *Am J Surg Pathol* 25:1546-1550, 2001.

105. Hsi ED, Siddiqui J, Schnitzer B et al: Analysis of immunoglobulin heavy chain gene rearrangement in myoepithelial sialadenitis by polymerase chain reaction, *Am J Clin Pathol* 106:498-503, 1996.

106. Carbone A, Gloghini A, Ferlito A: Pathological features of lymphoid proliferations of the salivary glands: lymphoepithelial sialadenitis versus low-grade B-cell lymphoma of the MALT type, *Ann Otol Rhinol Laryngol* 109:1170-1175, 2000.

107. Barnes L, Myers E, Prokopakis E: Primary malignant lymphoma of the parotid gland, *Arch Otolaryngol Head Neck Surg* 124:573-577, 1998.

108. Jaehne M, Ussmuller J, Jakel KT, Zschaber R: The clinical presentation of non-Hodgkin lymphomas of the major salivary glands, *Acta Otolaryngol* 121:647-651, 2001.

109. Kojima M, Shimizu K, Nishikawa M et al: Primary salivary gland lymphoma among Japanese: a clinicopathological study of 30 cases, *Leuk Lymphoma* 48:1793-1798, 2007.

110. Dunn P, Kuo TT, Shih LY et al: Primary salivary gland lymphoma: a clinicopathologic study of 23 cases in Taiwan, *Acta Haematol* 112:203-208, 2004.

111. Talal N, Sokoloff L, Bargh W: Extrasalivary lymphoid abnormalities in Sjögren's syndrome (reticulum cell sarcoma, "pseudolymphoma," macroglobulinemia), *Am J Med* 43:50-65, 1967.

112. Kassan S, Thomas T, Moutsopoulos H et al: Increased risk of lymphoma in sicca syndrome, *Ann Intern Med* 89:888-892, 1979.

113. Ekstrom Smedby K, Vajdic CM, Falster M et al: Autoimmune disorders and risk of non-Hodgkin lymphoma subtypes: a pooled analysis within the InterLymph Consortium, *Blood* 111:4029-4038, 2008.

114. Engels EA, Cerhan JR, Linet MS et al: Immune-related conditions and immune-modulating medications as risk factors for non-Hodgkin's lymphoma: a case-control study, *Am J Epidemiol* 162:1153-1161, 2005.

115. Royer B, Cazals-Hatem D, Sibilia J et al: Lymphomas in patients with Sjögren's syndrome are marginal zone B-cell neoplasms, arise in diverse extranodal and nodal sites, and are not associated with viruses, *Blood* 90:766-775, 1997.

116. Voulgarelis M, Skopouli FN: Clinical, immunologic, and molecular factors predicting lymphoma development in Sjögren's syndrome patients, *Clin Rev Allergy Immunol* 32:265-274, 2007.

117. Carrozzo M: Oral diseases associated with hepatitis C virus infection. Part 1. Sialadenitis and salivary gland lymphoma, *Oral Dis* 14:123-130, 2008.

118. Ramos-Casals M, la Civita L, de Vita S et al: Characterization of B cell lymphoma in patients with Sjögren's syndrome and hepatitis C virus infection, *Arthritis Rheum* 57:161-170, 2007.

119. Papaxoinis G, Fountzilas G, Rontogianni D et al: Low-grade mucosa-associated lymphoid tissue lymphoma: a retrospective analysis of 97 patients by the Hellenic Cooperative Oncology Group (HeCOG), *Ann Oncol* 19:780-786, 2008.

120. Zucca E, Conconi A, Pedrinis E et al: Nongastric marginal zone B-cell lymphoma of mucosa-associated lymphoid tissue, *Blood* 101:2489-2495, 2003.

121. Nakamura S, Ichimura K, Sato Y et al: Follicular lymphoma frequently originates in the salivary gland, *Pathol Int* 56:576-583, 2006.

122. Lai R, Arber DA, Chang KL et al: Frequency of bcl-2 expression in non-Hodgkin's lymphoma: a study of 778 cases with comparison of marginal zone lymphoma and monocytoid B-cell hyperplasia, *Mod Pathol* 11:864-869, 1998.

123. Remstein ED, Dogan A, Einerson RR et al: The incidence and anatomic site specificity of chromosomal translocations in primary extranodal marginal zone B-cell lymphoma of mucosa-associated lymphoid tissue (MALT lymphoma) in North America, *Am J Surg Pathol* 30:1546-1553, 2006.

124. Streubel B, Lamprecht A, Dierlamm J et al: t(14;18)(q32;q21) involving IgH and MALT1 is a frequent chromosomal aberration in MALT lymphoma, *Blood* 101:2335-2339, 2003.

125. Kojima M, Nakamura S, Ichimura K et al: Follicular lymphoma of the salivary gland: a clinicopathological and molecular study of six cases, *Int J Surg Pathol* 9:287-293, 2001.

126. Park CK, Manning JT Jr, Battifora H, Medeiros LJ: Follicle center lymphoma and Warthin tumor involving the same anatomic site: report of two cases and review of the literature, *Am J Clin Pathol* 113:113-119, 2000.

127. Hew W, Carey F, Kernohan N et al: Primary T cell lymphoma of salivary gland: a report of a case and review of the literature, *J Clin Pathol* 55:61-63, 2002.

128. Rahemtullah A, Longtine JA, Harris NL et al: CD20+ T-cell lymphoma: clinicopathologic analysis of 9 cases and a review of the literature, *Am J Surg Pathol* 32:1593-1607, 2008.

129. Takahashi H, Fujita S, Okabe H et al: Immunophenotypic analysis of extranodal non-Hodgkin's lymphomas in the oral cavity, *Pathol Res Pract* 189:300-311, 1993.

130. Stein H, Harris N, Campo E: Plasmablastic lymphoma. In Swerdlow S, Campo E, Harris N et al, editors: *WHO classification tumours of haematopoietic and lymphoid tissues*, Lyon, 2008, IARC.

131. Delecluse H, Anagnostopoulos I, Dallenbach F et al: Plasmablastic lymphomas of the oral cavity: a new entity associated with the human immunodeficiency virus infection, *Blood* 89:1413-1420, 1997.

132. Kemp S, Gallagher G, Kabani S et al: Oral non-Hodgkin's lymphoma: review of the literature and World Health Organization classification with reference to 40 cases, *Oral Surg Oral Med Oral Pathol Oral Radiol Endod* 105:194-201, 2008.

133. Solomides CC, Miller AS, Christman RA et al: Lymphomas of the oral cavity: histology, immunologic type, and incidence of Epstein-Barr virus infection, *Hum Pathol* 33:153-157, 2002.

134. van der Waal RI, Huijgens PC, van der Valk P, van der Waal I: Characteristics of 40 primary extranodal non-Hodgkin lymphomas of the oral cavity in perspective of the new WHO classification and the International Prognostic Index, *Int J Oral Maxillofac Surg* 34:391-395, 2005.

135. Takahashi H, Kawazoe K, Fujita S et al: Expression of bcl-2 oncogene product in primary non-Hodgkin's malignant lymphoma of the oral cavity, *Pathol Res Pract* 192:44-53, 1996.

136. Gulley M, Sargeant K, Grider D et al: Lymphomas of the oral soft tissues are not preferentially associated with latent or replicative Epstein-Barr virus, *Oral Surg Oral Med Oral Pathol Oral Radiol Endod* 80:425-431, 1995.

137. Leong I, Fernandes B, Mock D: Epstein-Barr virus detection in non-Hodgkin's lymphoma of the oral cavity: an immunocytochemical and in situ hybridization study, *Oral Surg Oral Med Oral Pathol Oral Radiol Endod* 92:184-193, 2001.

138. Gaidano G, Cerri M, Capello D et al: Molecular histogenesis of plasmablastic lymphoma of the oral cavity, *Br J Haematol* 119:622-628, 2002.

139. Lozada-Nur F, de Sanz S, Silverman S Jr et al: Intraoral non-Hodgkin's lymphoma in seven patients with acquired immunodeficiency syndrome, *Oral Surg Oral Med Oral Pathol Oral Radiol Endod* 82:173-178, 1996.

140. Shindoh M, Takami T, Arisue M et al: Comparison between submucosal (extra-nodal) and nodal non-Hodgkin's lymphoma (NHL) in the oral and maxillofacial region, *J Oral Pathol Med* 26:283-289, 1997.

141. Rosenburg A, Biesma D, Sie-Go D, Slootweg P: Primary extranodal CD30-positive T-cell non-Hodgkin's lymphoma of the oral mucosa: report of two cases, *Int J Oral Maxillofac Surg* 25:57-59, 1996.

142. Folk GS, Abbondanzo SL, Childers EL, Foss RD: Plasmablastic lymphoma: a clinicopathologic correlation, *Ann Diagn Pathol* 10:8-12, 2006.

143. Scheper MA, Nikitakis NG, Fernandes R et al: Oral plasmablastic lymphoma in an HIV-negative patient: a case report and review of the literature, *Oral Surg Oral Med Oral Pathol Oral Radiol Endod* 100:198-206, 2005.

144. Shiboski C, Greenspan D, Dodd C, Daniels T: Oral T-cell lymphoma associated with celiac sprue: a case report, *Oral Surg Oral Med Oral Pathol* 76:54-58, 1993.

145. Dong HY, Scadden DT, de Leval L et al: Plasmablastic lymphoma in HIV-positive patients: an aggressive Epstein-Barr virus–associated extramedullary plasmacytic neoplasm, *Am J Surg Pathol* 29:1633-1641, 2005.

146. Castillo J, Pantanowitz L, Dezube BJ: HIV-associated plasmablastic lymphoma: lessons learned from 112 published cases, *Am J Hematol* 83:804-809, 2008.

147. Vega F, Chang CC, Medeiros LJ et al: Plasmablastic lymphomas and plasmablastic plasma cell myelomas have nearly identical immunophenotypic profiles, *Mod Pathol* 18:806-815, 2005.

148. Dawson MA, Schwarer AP, McLean C et al: AIDS-related plasmablastic lymphoma of the oral cavity associated with an IGH/MYC translocation: treatment with autologous stem-cell transplantation in a patient with severe haemophilia A, *Haematologica* 92:e11-e12, 2007.

149. Kojima M, Sugihara S, Iijima M et al: Marginal zone B-cell lymphoma of minor salivary gland representing tumor-forming amyloidosis of the oral cavity: a case report, *J Oral Pathol Med* 35:314-316, 2006.

150. Albuquerque M, Migliari D, Sugaya N et al: Adult T-cell leukemia/lymphoma with predominant bone involvement initially diagnosed by its oral manifestation: a case report, *Oral Surg Oral Med Oral Pathol Oral Radiol Endod* 100:315-320, 2000.

151. Quarterman M, Lesher J Jr, Davis L et al: Rapidly progressive CD8-positive cutaneous T-cell lymphoma with tongue involvement, *Am J Dermatol* 17:287-291, 1995.

152. Sirois D, Miller A, Harwick R, Vonderheid E: Oral manifestations of cutaneous T-cell lymphoma: a report of eight cases, *Oral Surg Oral Med Oral Pathol* 75:700-705, 1993.

153. May SA, Jones D, Medeiros LJ et al: Oral-cutaneous CD4-positive T-cell lymphoma: a study of two patients, *Am J Dermatopathol* 29:62-67, 2007.

154. Whitt JC, Dunlap CL, Martin KF: Oral Hodgkin lymphoma: a wolf in wolf's clothing, *Oral Surg Oral Med Oral Pathol Oral Radiol Endod* 104:e45-e51, 2007.

155. Colomo L, Loong F, Rives S et al: Diffuse large B-cell lymphomas with plasmablastic differentiation represent a heterogeneous group of disease entities, *Am J Surg Pathol* 28:736-747, 2004.

156. Agarwal M, Shenjere P, Blewitt RW et al: CD30-positive T-cell lymphoproliferative disorder of the oral mucosa—an indolent lesion: report of 4 cases, *Int J Surg Pathol* 16:286-290, 2008.

157. Hirshberg A, Amariglio N, Akrish S et al: Traumatic ulcerative granuloma with stromal eosinophilia: a reactive lesion of the oral mucosa, *Am J Clin Pathol* 126:522-529, 2006.

158. Laurent C, Do C, Gascoyne RD et al: Anaplastic lymphoma kinase–positive diffuse large B-cell lymphoma: a rare clinicopathologic entity with poor prognosis, *J Clin Oncol* 27:4211-4216, 2009.

159. Delsol G, Campo E, Gascoyne RD: ALK positive DLBCL. In Swerdlow S, Campo E, Harris N et al, editors: *WHO classification tumours of haematopoietic and lymphoid tissues,* Lyon, 2008, IARC.

160. Carbone A, Gloghini A, Vaccher E et al: KSHV/HHV-8 associated lymph node based lymphomas in HIV seronegative subjects: report of two cases with anaplastic large cell morphology and plasmablastic immunophenotype, *J Clin Pathol* 58:1039-1045, 2005.

161. Chadburn A, Hyjek E, Mathew S et al: KSHV-positive solid lymphomas represent an extra-cavitary variant of primary effusion lymphoma, *Am J Surg Pathol* 28:1401-1416, 2004.

162. Carbone A, Gloghini A, Vaccher E et al: Kaposi's sarcoma–associated herpesvirus/human herpesvirus type 8-positive solid lymphomas: a tissue-based variant of primary effusion lymphoma, *J Mol Diagn* 7:17-27, 2005.

163. Thieblemont C, Mayer A, Dumontet C et al: Primary thyroid lymphoma is a heterogeneous disease, *J Clin Endocrinol Metab* 87:105-111, 2002.

164. Cho JH, Park YH, Kim WS et al: High incidence of mucosa-associated lymphoid tissue in primary thyroid lymphoma: a clinicopathologic study of 18 cases in the Korean population, *Leuk Lymphoma* 47:2128-2131, 2006.

165. Harrington KJ, Michalaki VJ, Vini L et al: Management of non-Hodgkin's lymphoma of the thyroid: the Royal Marsden Hospital experience, *Br J Radiol* 78:405-410, 2005.

166. Laing RW, Hoskin P, Hudson BV et al: The significance of MALT histology in thyroid lymphoma: a review of patients from the BNLI and Royal Marsden Hospital, *Clin Oncol (R Coll Radiol)* 6:300-304, 1994.

167. Derringer G, Thompson L, Frommelt R et al: Malignant lymphoma of the thyroid gland, *Am J Surg Pathol* 24:623-639, 2000.

168. Pederson R, Pederson N: Primary non-Hodgkin's lymphoma of the thyroid gland: a population based study, *Histopathology* 28:25-32, 1996.

169. Skacel M, Ross C, Hsi E: A reassessment of primary thyroid lymphoma: high-grade MALT-type lymphoma as a distinct subtype of diffuse large B-cell lymphoma, *Histopathology* 37:10-18, 2000.

170. Niitsu N, Okamoto M, Nakamura N et al: Clinicopathologic correlations of stage IE/IIE primary thyroid diffuse large B-cell lymphoma, *Ann Oncol* 18:1203-1208, 2007.

171. Holm L, Blomgren H, Lowhagen T: Cancer risks in patients with chronic lymphocytic thyroiditis, *N Engl J Med* 312:601-604, 1985.

172. Doi Y, Goto A, Murakami T et al: Primary thyroid lymphoma associated with Graves' disease, *Thyroid* 14:772-776, 2004.

173. Isaacson P, Androulakis-Papachristou A: Follicular colonization in thyroid lymphoma, *Am J Pathol* 141:43-52, 1992.

174. Saxena A, Alport EC, Moshynska O et al: Clonal B cell populations in a minority of patients with Hashimoto's thyroiditis, *J Clin Pathol* 57:1258-1263, 2004.

175. Streubel B, Vinatzer U, Lamprecht A et al: T(3;14)(p14.1;q32) involving IGH and FOXP1 is a novel recurrent chromosomal aberration in MALT lymphoma, *Leukemia* 19:652-658, 20005.

176. Mack LA, Pasieka JL: An evidence-based approach to the treatment of thyroid lymphoma, *World J Surg* 31:978-986, 2007.

177. Bacon CM, Diss TC, Ye H et al: Follicular lymphoma of the thyroid gland, *Am J Surg Pathol* 33:22-34, 2009.

178. Koida S, Tsukasaki K, Tsuchiya T et al: Primary T-cell lymphoma of the thyroid gland with chemokine receptors of Th1 phenotype complicating autoimmune thyroiditis, *Haematologica* 92:e37-e40, 2007.

179. Chen HI, Akpolat I, Mody DR et al: Restricted kappa/lambda light chain ratio by flow cytometry in germinal center B cells in Hashimoto thyroiditis, *Am J Clin Pathol* 125:42-48, 2006.

180. Wang SA, Rahemtullah A, Faquin WC et al: Hodgkin's lymphoma of the thyroid: a clinicopathologic study of five cases and review of the literature, *Mod Pathol* 18:1577-1584, 2005.

181. Ansell S, Habermann T, Hoyer J et al: Primary laryngeal lymphoma, *Laryngoscope* 107:1502-1506, 1997.

182. Diebold J, Audouin J, Viry B et al: Primary lymphoplasmacytic lymphoma of the larynx: a rare localization of MALT-type lymphoma, *Ann Otol Rhinol Laryngol* 99:577-580, 1990 (review).

183. Smith M, Browne J, Teot L: A case of primary laryngeal T-cell lymphoma in a patient with acquired immunodeficiency syndrome, *Am J Otolaryngol* 17:332-334, 1996.

184. Kato S, Sakura M, Takooda S et al: Primary non-Hodgkin's lymphoma of the larynx, *J Laryngol Otol* 111:571-574, 1997.

185. Kawaida M, Fukuda H, Shiotani A et al: Isolated non-Hodgkin's malignant lymphoma of the larynx presenting as a large pedunculated tumor, *ORL* 58:171-174, 1996.

186. Korst RJ: Primary lymphoma of the subglottic airway in a patient with Sjögren's syndrome mimicking high laryngotracheal stenosis, *Ann Thorac Surg* 84:1756-1758, 2007.

187. Patiar S, Ramsden JD, Freeland AP: B-cell lymphoma of the larynx in a patient with rheumatoid arthritis, *J Laryngol Otol* 119:646-648, 2005.

188. Kania RE, Hartl DM, Badoual C et al: Primary mucosa-associated lymphoid tissue (MALT) lymphoma of the larynx, *Head Neck* 27:258-262, 2005.

189. Palenzuela G, Bernard F, Gardiner Q, Mondain M: Malignant B cell non-Hodgkin's lymphoma of the larynx in children with Wiskott Aldrich syndrome, *Int J Pediatr Otorhinolaryngol* 67:989-993, 2003.

190. Morgan K, MacLennan K, Narula A et al: Non-Hodgkin's lymphoma of the larynx (stage 1E), *Cancer* 64:1123-1127, 1989.

191. Mok J, Pak M, Chan K et al: Unusual T-and T/NK-cell non-Hodgkin's lymphoma of the larynx: a diagnostic challenge for clinicians and pathologists, *Head Neck* 23:625-628, 2001.

192. Nakamura S, Suchi T, Koshikawa T et al: Clinicopathologic study of CD56 (NCAM)-positive angiocentric lymphoma occurring in sites other than upper and lower respiratory tract, *Am J Surg Pathol* 19:284-296, 1995.

193. Isaacson P, Norton A: *Extranodal lymphomas,* Edinburgh, 1994, Churchill Livingstone.

194. Cavalot A, Preti G, Vione N et al: Isolated primary non-Hodgkin's malignant lymphoma of the larynx, *J Laryngol Otol* 115:324-326, 2001.

195. Horny H-P, Kaiserling E: Involvement of the larynx by hemopoietic neoplasms: an investigation of autopsy cases and review of the literature, *Pathol Res Pract* 191:130-138, 1995.

CHAPTER 4

Lymphomas of the Thorax

Judith A. Ferry

■ TRACHEAL LYMPHOMAS

Primary tracheal lymphoma is rare. It mainly affects older adults, both men and women, who present with dyspnea, wheezing, stridor, and/or coughing.[1,2] Rare patients have human immunodeficiency virus (HIV) infection.[3] Examination reveals a nodular or polypoid tumor with a smooth or friable surface that narrows the tracheal lumen. Diffuse mucosal abnormalities with multiple small nodules have been described.[4] Most of the few cases classified using newer lymphoma classifications have been extranodal marginal zone lymphomas of mucosa-associated lymphoid tissue (MALT lymphomas).[2,4,5] Rare high-grade lymphomas are also described. A case of extranodal natural killer (NK)/T-cell lymphoma, nasal type, that was primary in the trachea has been reported.[6] Patients usually respond well to treatment (surgery or surgery and radiation, sometimes with the addition of chemotherapy), and most are well on follow-up.[1,2,4,5] Rare patients with large thyroid lymphomas develop tracheal involvement through direct extension, with compression and luminal narrowing[7] or invasion and perforation of the trachea by the lymphoma.[8]

■ PULMONARY LYMPHOMAS

Primary Pulmonary Lymphomas

Introduction

The criteria used to define primary pulmonary lymphoma vary somewhat from one study to another. Traditionally, it has been defined as lymphoma that presents as one or more pulmonary lesions with which no clinical, pathologic, or radiographic evidence of lymphoma elsewhere has been seen in the past, at present, or for 3 months after presentation (stage IE). In some studies, cases are accepted as primary pulmonary lymphoma if staging reveals disease outside the lung, as long as the pulmonary disease predominates; such cases may show involvement of hilar lymph nodes (stage II1E) or mediastinal lymph nodes (stage II2E); direct extension to the chest wall or diaphragm[9-11]; or even more distant spread.[12]

Primary pulmonary lymphoma accounts for 0.3% of primary lung neoplasms,[13] for 3.6% of extranodal lymphomas,[14] and for fewer than 0.5% of all lymphomas.[10,15,16] Primary pulmonary lymphoma is mainly a disease of middle-aged and older adults.[9,15,17-22] Extranodal marginal zone lymphoma (MALT lymphoma) is by far the most common type, accounting for more than 70% of cases. Diffuse large B-cell lymphoma is the next most common. Other types of lymphoma are uncommon or rare (Table 4-1).[9,19-22]

Patients present with respiratory symptoms (cough, dyspnea, chest pain, hemoptysis, or wheezing) and less often with constitutional symptoms or with both respiratory and constitutional symptoms. Nearly 40% of patients are asymptomatic, and the lymphoma is an incidental finding. Most asymptomatic patients have low-grade lymphoma.[9,12,15,17-28]

Whatever the type of lymphoma, bronchial or transbronchial biopsy or computed tomography (CT)-guided transthoracic needle biopsy usually does not yield sufficient material to establish a diagnosis. Video-assisted thoracic surgery (VATS), open wedge biopsy, or lobectomy usually is required.[15,19,20,22,26]

TABLE 4-1

Pulmonary Lymphomas			
Lymphoma Type	**Clinical Features**	**Histology**	**Immunophenotype**
Marginal zone lymphoma (MZL)	Middle-aged or older adults; men ≥ women; history of smoking, autoimmune disease common; M-component relatively common *Prognosis:* Very good	Solid and interstitial mass composed of marginal zone cells, small lymphocytes, plasma cells, rare large cells; lymphoepithelial lesions; amyloid deposition in some cases; component of DLBCL in a minority	*Lymphoid cells:* CD20+, CD3−, CD5−, CD43+/−, monotypic sIg (IgM > IgG or IgA) *Plasma cells:* Monotypic or polytypic cIg
Diffuse large B-Cell lymphoma (DLBCL)	*De novo DLBCL patients:* Slightly younger than MZL patients. *Prognosis:* Good	Diffuse proliferation of large lymphoid cells	CD20+; CD3−; bcl6, bcl2, and CD10 variable
Lymphomatoid granulomatosis	Mostly middle-aged adults, men > women; underlying subtle or overt immunologic abnormality common *Prognosis:* Variable	Variable number of large atypical cells in a lymphohistiocytic background	*Large cells:* CD20+, CD30+/−, CD15−, EBV+ *Small lymphocytes:* Mostly T cells, CD4 > CD8
Classical Hodgkin's lymphoma	Young adults; rarely primary; usually accompanied by mediastinal disease *Prognosis:* Good	Reed-Sternberg cells and variants in a polymorphous background	*Tumor cells:* CD15+ (sometimes CD15−), CD30+, Pax5+, CD20 usually negative, CD3−

cIg, Cytoplasmic immunoglobulin; *EBV,* Epstein-Barr virus; *sIg,* surface immunoglobulin.

Extranodal Marginal Zone Lymphoma of Mucosa-Associated Lymphoid Tissue (MALT Lymphoma)

Clinical Features

Before marginal zone lymphoma was described, many pulmonary marginal zone lymphomas were diagnosed as pseudolymphoma, lymphoid interstitial pneumonia, lymphomatoid granulomatosis, or follicular bronchiolitis.[9,12,17] Marginal zone lymphoma almost exclusively affects adults over age 30 (the mean or median age is in the 50s or 60s in most series),[9,12,15,18,27] although rare cases in younger patients have been reported.[29,30] Men are affected about as often or slightly more often than women in most studies.[9,12,18,26,27]

Patients with pulmonary marginal zone lymphoma not infrequently have an associated immunologic abnormality. From 0[18] to 29%[15] of patients in different series have an autoimmune disease; among the more common are Sjögren's syndrome,[9,15,17] rheumatoid arthritis,[15,21,28,31] Hashimoto's thyroiditis,[12,15] and systemic lupus erythematosus.[9,15,17] A few patients have been infected by hepatitis C, a virus that may be associated with an increased risk of lymphoma.[18] A few patients are HIV positive,[29,32] and a few have developed pulmonary marginal zone lymphoma in the setting of common variable immunodeficiency.[30] Smoking is a common factor among patients who develop marginal zone lymphoma; in some series, most patients are former or active smokers.[12,22,27] In rare cases patients have concurrent carcinoma of the lung.[18]

Monoclonal serum paraproteins are relatively common[9,10,19]; they were found in 13%[17] to 43% of cases in series that have commented on this feature.[15] In studies in which the information is available, the M-component has been the same type as the immunoglobulin expressed by the lymphoma.[15] Occasional patients have had polyclonal hypergammaglobulinemia.[17,19]

Radiographic Features

Radiographic evaluation by chest x-ray film or CT scan shows a single lesion in approximately half of cases and two or more unilateral or bilateral lesions in the remainder. The lesions take the form of nodules, masses, or infiltrates that resemble consolidated lung, sometimes accompanied by air bronchograms.[9,12,15,18-23,26] Occasional cases are associated with a pleural effusion.[9,19,22]

Pathologic Features

On gross examination, the lesions are white, white-tan, gray, or gray-pink, solid, unencapsulated, poorly defined masses with a firm, fibrous, or granular cut surface. Some resemble consolidated lung with pneumonia.[11,26,29] Their histologic and immunophenotypic features are similar to those of marginal zone lymphomas in other anatomic sites. In the lung, the lymphoma usually has a solid, dense central area that effaces the normal architecture, accompanied by spread at the periphery of the lesion in an interstitial pattern with widening of alveolar septa, sometimes with formation of small nodules away from the main lesion (Figure 4-1, A). Invasion of bronchi, blood vessels, and pleura is common, and erosion of bronchial cartilage may be seen.

The lymphoma consists of a variable admixture of small lymphocytes; marginal zone cells with small, slightly irregular nuclei with pale cytoplasm; plasma cells and plasmacytoid cells; and occasional centroblasts (see Figure 4-1, B and C). Plasma cells may show a tendency to be localized toward the bronchus and may contain Dutcher bodies. Admixed reactive lymphoid follicles usually are present (see Figure 4-1, B); they often are at least partially replaced by neoplastic cells (follicular colonization).

Lymphoepithelial lesions usually are present; they may involve bronchial or bronchiolar epithelium and occasionally mucous glands (see Figure 4-1, B and C). Damage to the airways may result in significant luminal narrowing.* The infiltrate may be associated with hyaline sclerosis. Occasional cases are associated with amyloid deposition (see the following section, Marginal Zone Lymphomas Associated with Paraprotein Deposition). Necrosis is not a feature. In occasional cases, clusters of epithelioid histiocytes are seen.[15]

On immunophenotyping, the neoplastic population typically is positive for pan–B-cell antigens and monotypic surface immunoglobulin light chain and negative for CD5, CD10, CD23, and cyclin D1. CD5 co-expression by the B cells has been described in rare cases.[15] In some cases, CD43 is co-expressed by marginal zone B cells (see Figure 4-1, D to I). Plasma cells may be monotypic or polytypic.† The immunoglobulin expressed most often is IgM, with occasional IgA+ and IgG+ cases.[9] IGH is clonally rearranged.[15] The t(11;18)(q21;q21) translocation, described almost exclusively in marginal zone lymphomas and resulting in API2-MALT1 gene fusion, is more commonly found in marginal zone lymphomas arising in the lung than in nearly all other sites.[35-38] t(14;18)(q32;q21) (IGH-MALT1) and t(1;14)(p22;q32) (IGH-BCL10) also have been described in pulmonary marginal zone lymphoma but are uncommon.

Trisomy 18 occurs in a subset of cases.[38] We recently have seen a pulmonary marginal zone lymphoma with tetrasomy 18 and also trisomy 3 (see Figure 4-1, J).

Among pulmonary marginal zone lymphomas, the API2-MALT1 gene fusion is reported to be associated with an absence of underlying autoimmune disease and with typical histologic features (absence of marked plasmacytic differentiation, absence of increased large cells). This suggests that at least two separate pathways may lead to the development of pulmonary marginal zone lymphoma: one with underlying autoimmune disease and one with a

---

*References 9-11, 15, 17, 18, 26, and 33.
†References 9, 15, 18, 21, 26, and 34.

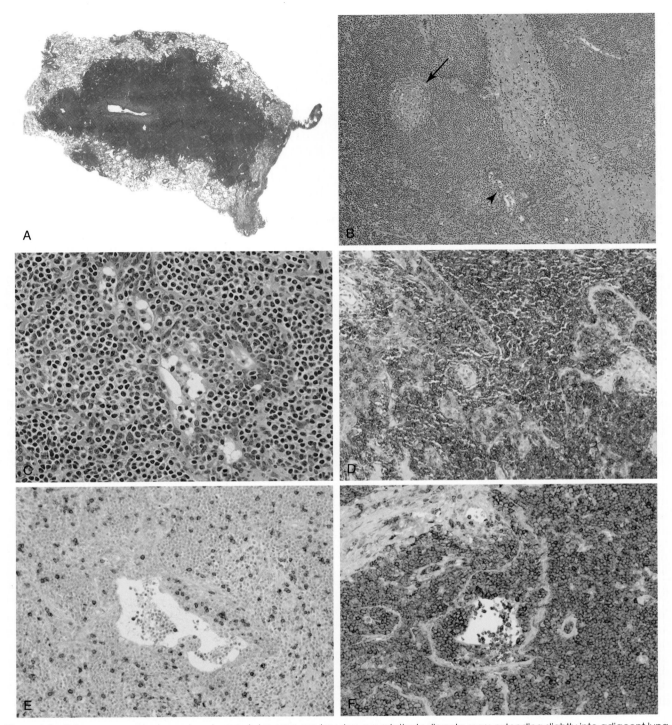

Figure 4-1   Pulmonary marginal zone lymphoma. **A,** Low-power view shows a relatively discrete mass extending slightly into adjacent lung parenchyma in an interstitial pattern. **B,** Higher power view shows a diffuse infiltrate of small lymphoid cells with one small reactive follicle *(arrow)* and a small distorted epithelial structure *(arrowhead).* **C,** Higher power view of the epithelial structure shows that it is surrounded and infiltrated by small lymphoid cells with minimally irregular nuclei with admixed plasma cells. **D** to **F,** Immunostaining shows a marked preponderance of CD20+ B cells **(D)** with only scattered T cells (CD3+) **(E);** B cells co-express CD43 **(F).** (Immunoperoxidase technique on paraffin sections.)

certain genetic abnormality acquired in the absence of an autoimmune disease.[35]

A subset of cases shows areas of diffuse large B-cell lymphoma at the time of initial diagnosis.[9,21,22] In larger series, this was found in 10%[12] to 18%[15]

of marginal zone lymphomas. Large cell lymphoma and marginal zone lymphoma usually were both present in the lung; however, in one case, the lung showed diffuse large B-cell lymphoma, and a hilar lymph node showed marginal zone lymphoma.[15]

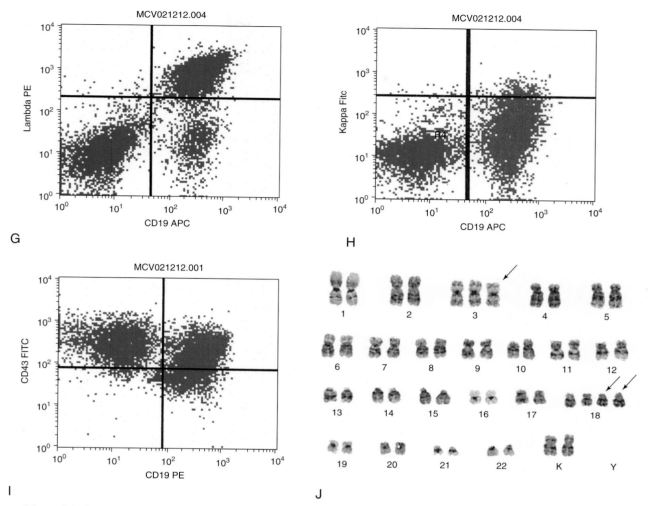

Figure 4-1, cont'd   G to I, Flow cytometric analysis reveals a CD19+ B-cell population with a marked excess of lambda light chain–positive cells **(G)** compared to kappa light chain–positive cells **(H)**. I, B cells co-express CD43. J, Cytogenetic analysis reveals trisomy 3 and tetrasomy 18; the additional chromosomes are indicated by arrows. (J, Courtesy Dr. Paola dal Cin, Brigham and Women's Hospital, Boston, Massachusetts.)

Cell of Origin

Marginal zone lymphoma is believed to arise from the marginal zone cells of the reactive organized lymphoid tissue that may develop around bronchi and bronchioles (bronchus-associated lymphoid tissue [BALT]).[17] This hyperplastic lymphoid tissue may occur in individuals with autoimmune disease and with certain immunodeficiency syndromes. In some cases, acquisition of BALT may represent a hypersensitivity reaction.[17,39] Therefore, various immunologic disorders and possibly also smoking and previous infections[20,21] could contribute to the pathogenesis of pulmonary marginal zone lymphoma by promoting the development of BALT through chronic antigenic stimulation.[21]

Staging, Treatment, and Outcome

Some studies have included only cases with lymphoma confined to the lung or those without spread beyond hilar or mediastinal lymph nodes. Studies with more liberal inclusion criteria have described cases in which staging has revealed marginal zone lymphoma with involvement of the bone marrow, skin, gastrointestinal tract, salivary gland, or spinal cord.[12,15,22,27]

Treatment has varied widely. Therapy has included surgical excision only, watchful waiting, radiation, single-agent rituximab, and anthracycline-based and non-anthracycline-based chemotherapy.* Relapses are common,[11] and recurrence in the lungs is the most common type of failure.[9,11,27] Relapses also involve the stomach,[9,11,19,27] salivary glands,[11] skin and soft tissue,[9,10] chest wall,[10] lymph nodes,[9] and bone marrow.[19] Patients treated conservatively may be alive with disease but may have few symptoms.[21] In a small number of cases, the marginal zone lymphoma may undergo histologic progression to diffuse large B-cell lymphoma,[10,18,27] which may result in the patient's death.[18]

*References 12, 15, 18, 20-22, 26, and 27.

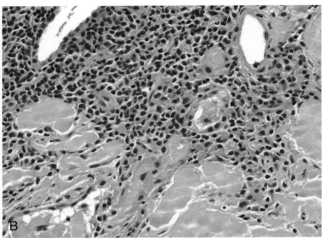

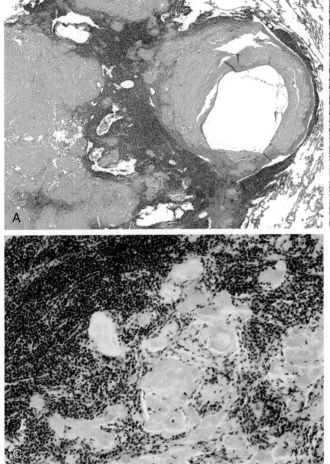

Figure 4-2   Pulmonary marginal zone lymphoma with amyloid. **A,** Large masses of amyloid are present in the stroma of the lymphoma and also replace the wall of a luminal structure, making a cystlike space. **B,** In addition to small lymphoid cells, many plasma cells are present; the plasma cells expressed monotypic cytoplasmic lambda light chain (not shown). **C,** The amyloid is positive on a Congo red stain; examination with polarized light showed apple green birefringence (not shown).

The prognosis is very good. In different series, the 5-year overall survival rate ranges from 68% to 100%,[9,12,15,19,21] and the 10-year disease-specific survival rate is 72%.[15] Despite the excellent survival rate, these patients have an ongoing risk of relapse for many years after the primary diagnosis; therefore, long-term follow-up is warranted.[9,15] Among patients with an M-component, monitoring the serum for paraprotein could help assess disease activity.[10,15]

Marginal zone lymphoma is reported to have a better prognosis than other types of pulmonary lymphomas in some studies,[11,19,21] although this result is not uniform.[20] Among patients with pulmonary marginal zone lymphoma, factors important for the prognosis have not been consistently identified. Features reported not to affect the prognosis include the stage,[12,20] systemic symptoms, autoimmune disease, distribution and number of lung lesions, nodal involvement,[15] the presence of paraprotein,[9,15] and type of therapy.[9]

Marginal Zone Lymphomas Associated with Paraprotein Deposition

Occasional cases of marginal zone lymphoma from a variety of sites are associated with stromal amyloid deposition, but this phenomenon appears to be more common in the lung (1%[40] to 6%[15] of pulmonary marginal zone lymphomas). In contrast to patients with pulmonary marginal zone lymphoma without amyloid, patients with amyloid have more often been women. They also appear to be slightly older, with a median age of approximately 70 years.[*] A few have had an autoimmune disease, including Sjögren's syndrome, rheumatoid arthritis, and immune thrombocytopenic purpura.[24,28,31]

Radiographic studies reveal multiple pulmonary nodules or masses in most cases; single lesions are uncommon. The lymphomas have histologic and immunophenotypic features similar to those of marginal zone lymphomas without amyloid, although those with amyloid usually have a prominent plasma cell component (Figure 4-2). The amyloid may be randomly distributed in the stroma of the lymphoma; it may form large masses; or it may be found in the walls of blood vessels or bronchioles. Bronchiolar involvement associated with dilatation has been described; this gives the appearance of cysts on radiographic studies.[34] The amyloid may be associated with a foreign body giant cell reaction and less often with calcification or even ossification.

---

[*]References 15, 24, 28, 31, 33, 34, and 40.

The amyloid is Congo red positive with apple green birefringence. When subtyped, the amyloid has been shown to be light chain in origin, and the light chain type has been the same as for the lymphoma.[15,34]

The prognosis appears favorable overall, although one patient died of lymphoma after large cell transformation,[33] and one study suggested that patients with marginal zone lymphoma with amyloid were more likely to die of lymphoma than those without amyloid.[15] No patient has shown evidence of systemic amyloidosis.* These patients also do not appear more likely to have a serum M-component.[33]

In the evaluation of these cases, the amyloid may be recognized and the marginal zone lymphoma overlooked, particularly on a small biopsy.[34] In cases with multiple nodules, some contain amyloid and marginal zone lymphoma, whereas others may be composed of amyloid alone.[24] The differential diagnosis of marginal zone lymphoma with amyloid includes nodular amyloidoma. In favor of marginal zone lymphoma are a predominance of B cells in any lymphoid infiltrate around the amyloid, the presence of reactive lymphoid follicles, co-expression of CD43 by B cells, and light chain restriction of lymphoid cells and/or plasma cells.[40] Other entities that may enter the differential diagnosis include pulmonary hyalinizing granuloma, silicotic nodules, pulmonary apical scars, and old infarcts.[40] None of these entities display the diagnostic features of lymphoma. Congo red stain can distinguish amyloid from collagen.

One other disorder that may mimic marginal zone lymphoma with amyloid is light chain deposition disease. One case of pulmonary marginal zone lymphoma with light chain deposition has been reported in an HIV-positive man.[32] Light chain deposition disease shows stromal deposition of material histologically resembling amyloid but without Congo red positivity or apple green birefringence. The light chain deposits are almost always kappa, in contrast to amyloid, which is more often derived from lambda light chain.

A case of pulmonary marginal zone lymphoma with massive crystal-storing histiocytosis has been reported in a 69-year-old female smoker with Graves' disease.[25] In addition to the marginal zone lymphoma, numerous histiocytes with characteristic crystalline cytoplasmic inclusions were seen. The crystals may be derived from abnormal immunoglobulin produced by the lymphoma that promotes crystallization and inhibits lysosomal degradation.

Differential Diagnosis

1. **Marginal zone lymphoma versus reactive processes.** The main difficulty in differential diagnosis is distinguishing marginal zone lymphoma from chronic inflammatory processes with a prominent component of lymphocytes and/or plasma cells, such as nodular lymphoid hyperplasia and IgG4-related sclerosing disease. In favor of lymphoma is a predominance of B cells with the morphology of marginal zone cells in a

diffuse pattern outside follicles, CD43 co-expression by the B cells, and monotypic immunoglobulin expression by lymphocytes and/or plasma cells. In favor of a reactive process is a mixture of B and T cells, with B cells predominantly in follicles. Lymphoepithelial lesions are common in lymphoid hyperplasia but less common than in marginal zone lymphoma, and the intraepithelial lymphocytes can be B or T cells, in contrast to the predominance of B cells seen in marginal zone lymphoma.[18] If a lesion has many polytypic plasma cells, fibrosis, and vascular involvement by a lymphoid infiltrate, staining for IgG and IgG4 can be performed; a high ratio of IgG4+ plasma cells to IgG+ plasma cells would support IgG4-related sclerosing disease.[41,42]

Diffuse Large B-Cell Lymphoma

Diffuse large B-cell lymphoma is the second most common type of primary pulmonary lymphoma, accounting for approximately 12% of cases.[9,11,19-21] The numbers of cases of primary pulmonary diffuse large B-cell lymphoma and diffuse large B-cell lymphoma with a component of marginal zone lymphoma, consistent with large cell transformation of the low-grade lymphoma, are roughly similar.[9,15,19-22] Some patients are HIV positive (see Pulmonary Lymphoma in HIV-Positive Patients, later in the chapter). On average, patients with diffuse large B-cell lymphoma are slightly younger than those with marginal zone lymphoma.[11,21] The radiographic findings are similar to those of marginal zone lymphoma, except that diffuse large B-cell lymphomas may have areas of necrosis, giving an appearance of cavitation.[9,11]

On gross examination, the lymphomas sometimes have areas of necrosis; these areas may take the form of a thick-walled cavity resembling an abscess. Some lymphomas are described as centroblastic and some as immunoblastic.[9] The immunophenotypic features have not been evaluated in detail in large numbers of cases, but the lymphomas express pan–B-cell antigens, and some express CD10, bcl6, and/or bcl2.[21] Most cases have been treated with chemotherapy. When relapses occur, they tend to involve the lung.[9] The lymphomas are aggressive, but complete remission and long-term survival can be achieved.[19,21] The differential diagnosis includes carcinoma, in particular small cell carcinoma. Cohesive growth and molding of tumor cells and smudging of the chromatin favor carcinoma. The diagnosis can be confirmed with immunohistochemical staining for lymphoid antigens, cytokeratin, and markers of neuroendocrine differentiation.

Lymphomatoid Granulomatosis

Introduction

Lymphomatoid granulomatosis was first described by Liebow and colleagues in 1972 as an angiocentric and angiodestructive lymphoreticular

---

*References 15, 24, 28, 31, 33, 34, and 40.

proliferation.[43] The emphasis focused on the histologic features of angiitis and granulomatosis, and the disease initially was not considered neoplastic. Over time, lymphomatoid granulomatosis came to be recognized as a lymphoproliferative disorder, and it was grouped with lethal midline granuloma/polymorphic reticulosis as an angiocentric immunoproliferative disorder. These diseases shared a tendency for extranodal involvement; angiocentric, angioinvasive growth; conspicuous necrosis; and a prominent inflammatory component with many T cells; they were considered distinctive forms of T-cell lymphoma.[44]

Advances in immunophenotyping and molecular genetic analysis subsequently showed that nearly all of the so-called angiocentric immunoproliferative disorders could be classified as one of two distinct entities: (1) extranodal NK/T-cell lymphoma, an Epstein-Barr virus (EBV)–positive lymphoma that has a predilection for midfacial localization and is of NK-cell or (less often) T-cell lineage (see Lymphomas of the Nasal Cavity and Paranasal Sinuses, in Chapter 3); or (2) lymphomatoid granulomatosis, an EBV-positive B-cell lymphoproliferative disorder with a prominent component of reactive T cells.[45,46] Some authorities then suggested that lymphomatoid granulomatosis was immunophenotypically diverse and could be of either B- or T-lineage, including T-cell cases unassociated with EBV[47]; however, this view has since fallen out of favor, and a more restricted definition of lymphomatoid granulomatosis is preferred. Lymphomatoid granulomatosis now is defined as an angiocentric, angiodestructive lymphoproliferative disease composed of EBV+ B cells and reactive T cells, with T cells usually predominating.[48] Lymphomatoid granulomatosis may involve a variety of extranodal sites and, less often, lymph nodes, but pulmonary involvement is by far the most common and most characteristic manifestation. For this reason, lymphomatoid granulomatosis is discussed under Pulmonary Lymphomas.

Clinical Features

Lymphomatoid granulomatosis mainly affects adults. Patients often are middle aged,[46,49,50] although older adults[46,49] and, in rare cases, children[49,51] also are affected. Males are affected roughly twice as often as females.[46,48,49] Although most patients who develop lymphomatoid granulomatosis are not overtly immunodeficient, an underlying immunologic abnormality is associated with an increased risk for developing lymphomatoid granulomatosis, as is the case for many EBV+ lymphoproliferative disorders.[48,50,51] Lymphomatoid granulomatosis has been reported in HIV-positive patients,[52] individuals with autoimmune disease,[46,53] patients with previous or concurrent hematologic malignancies,[49,51,54] allograft recipients,[55] and children with certain congenital immunodeficiency syndromes.[48] Rare cases of lymphomatoid granulomatosis have been described in patients receiving imatinib (a tyrosine kinase inhibitor that may be associated with severe lymphopenia) for treatment of a gastrointestinal stromal tumor (GIST).[56,57] Even in cases in which no immunodeficiency is obvious, when immunologic abnormalities are specifically sought, they often are found. They include such abnormalities as anergy, lymphopenia, defective cytotoxic T-cell activity, and impaired response to EBV.[48,50]

Patients present with respiratory symptoms, constitutional symptoms, or both. Common symptoms include fever, cough, malaise, dyspnea, weight loss, chest pain, and hemoptysis. Some patients present with neurologic symptoms related to central or peripheral nervous system involvement or skin lesions related to cutaneous involvement. A few have myalgias, arthralgias, or nonspecific gastrointestinal symptoms.[46,48-50,54-57] Very few are asymptomatic.[49]

Pulmonary involvement is seen in nearly all cases (more than 90%).[48,49] Lung lesions are bilateral in nearly 80% of cases,[49] with preferential involvement of the middle and lower lung fields.[48] Some of those presenting with unilateral lung involvement later develop bilateral lung disease.[46,49]

Radiographic studies show multiple nodules, often suggesting metastases, or consolidation.[46,49,54,55] Lobar collapse and diffuse reticulonodular infiltrates also have been described.[46,49]

On gross examination, the lesions are gray-white nodules 1 to 5 cm in diameter[52]; larger nodules frequently are necrotic.[48] On microscopic examination, the lesions are composed of a variable admixture of small lymphocytes, intermediate-sized lymphoid cells, histiocytes, plasma cells, and atypical lymphoid cells with the appearance of immunoblasts, plasmacytoid immunoblasts, and/or large bizarre cells occasionally reminiscent of Reed-Sternberg cells (Figures 4-3 and 4-4). The process is characterized by angiocentric and angiodestructive growth, which may result in coagulative necrosis, which may be extensive. Although histiocytes may be numerous, and despite the name of the disease, well-formed granulomas are not a feature. Eosinophils and neutrophils are inconspicuous.[48-50,52,55] Establishing a diagnosis may require excision of one or more nodules, rather than needle biopsy, because viable, diagnostic areas may be present only focally.

Immunophenotyping shows that the large atypical cells are B cells, with CD20 expression in nearly all cases. Large cells may co-express CD30, but they are negative for CD15. Small to medium-sized cells are mainly T cells, most of which are CD4+. Large cells are positive for EBV with in situ hybridization for Epstein-Barr virus–encoded RNA (EBER) (see Figure 4-3). The presence of EBV also may be demonstrated in some cases with an immunostain for EBV latent membrane protein (LMP).[45,46,48,52,55] The grade (1, 2, or 3) (see Figures 4-3 and 4-4) tends to correlate with the clinical behavior.[44,48] It may vary from one site to another and may rise over time.[50] The criteria for grading cases of lymphomatoid granulomatosis are shown in Table 4-2.

Clonal rearrangement of the IGH gene is demonstrable in most grade 2 and grade 3 cases, whereas

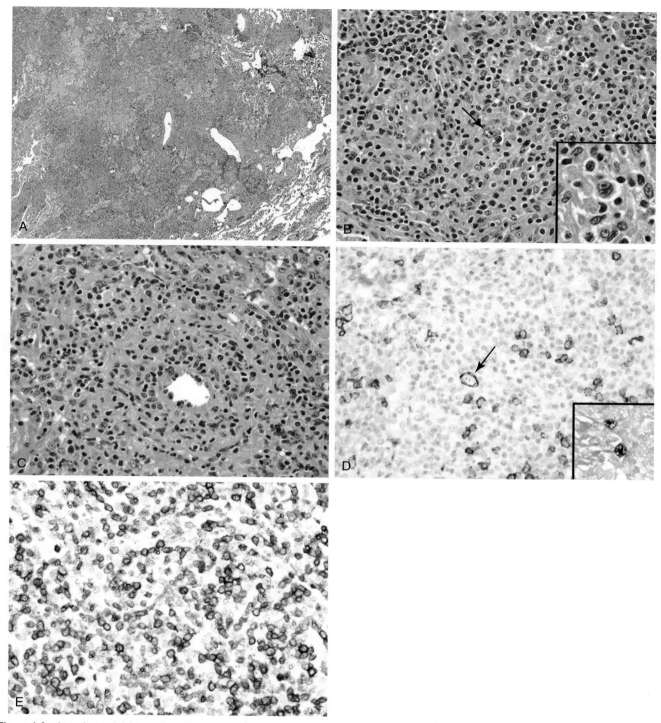

Figure 4-3   Lymphomatoid granulomatosis, grade 1 of 3. The patient presented with multiple masses in the lung. **A,** Low-power view reveals a large, nodular lesion that is mostly solid but also has entrapped air spaces. No necrosis is identified. **B,** The lesion is composed of small oval or slightly irregular lymphoid cells, bland histiocytes with abundant pink cytoplasm, and a few large lymphoid cells with large oval nuclei, vesicular chromatin, and prominent central nucleoli *(arrow)*. Rare binucleated Reed-Sternberg–like cells also are present *(inset)*. **C,** Higher power view shows a small blood vessel surrounded and infiltrated by small lymphoid cells; these were mainly T cells. **D,** Immunostaining discloses scattered B cells (CD20+), including a few large cells *(arrow)*. Rare B cells are positive for Epstein-Barr virus *(inset)*. (In situ hybridization for EBER on a paraffin section.) **E,** The B cells are present in a background rich in T cells (CD3+) (*D* and *E,* Immunoperoxidase technique on paraffin sections.)

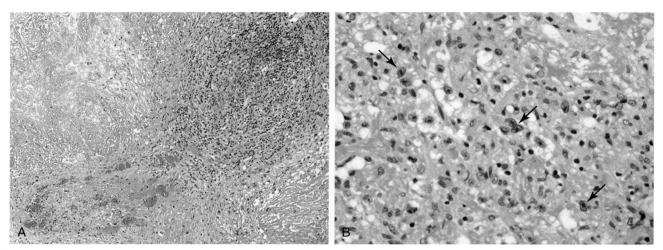

Figure 4-4   Lymphomatoid granulomatosis, grade 3 of 3. The patient was an elderly man with multiple lung nodules and a history of Crohn's disease that was treated with immunosuppressive therapy. **A,** Low-power view shows extensive necrosis and prominent angioinvasion. **B,** High-power view reveals many scattered immunoblasts *(arrows)*, which proved to be EBV+ B cells, in a background of many small T cells, histiocytes, and necrotic debris.

TABLE 4-2

Grading of Lymphomatoid Granulomatosis			
Grade	**Cellular Composition**	**Necrosis**	**EBV+ Cells**
Grade 1	Polymorphous; CD20+ large cells rare or absent	Focal or absent	<5 per hpf
Grade 2	Single or clustered CD20+ large cells in a polymorphous background	Common	Variable, but on average 5-20/hpf
Grade 3	More numerous large B cells in a polymorphous background; large cells often bizarre or Reed-Sternberg–like	Usually extensive	>50/hpf

From Pittaluga S, Wilson W, Jaffe E: Lymphomatoid granulomatosis. In Swerdlow S, Campo E, Harris N et al, editors: *WHO classification: tumours of haematopoietic and lymphoid tissues,* ed 4, pp 247-249, Lyon, 2008, IARC.
EBV, Epstein-Barr virus; *hpf,* high-power field.

clonal T cells are not detected.[45] If frozen tissue is available, Southern blot hybridization may be used to demonstrate clonal EBV. In grade 1 cases, clonality may not be found, either because of the small number of EBV+ neoplastic cells, or perhaps because, analogous to post-transplant lymphoproliferative disorders, some early cases may be polyclonal.[48] In some cases, different clones can be demonstrated in different anatomic sites, again analogous to post-transplant lymphoproliferative disorders.[58]

The differential diagnosis of lymphomatoid granulomatosis includes necrotizing infectious processes, Wegener's granulomatosis, classical Hodgkin's lymphoma, and diffuse large B-cell lymphoma. Differential features are shown in Table 4-3.

Treatment and Outcome

The clinical course of lymphomatoid granulomatosis varies. In most cases the disease has a progressive course, and the mortality rate is greater than 50% in some older series.[46,49,50] In some patients, the disease progresses to a monomorphous, EBV+ diffuse large B-cell lymphoma[48,49]; in other patients, it follows a waxing and waning course.[48] In occasional cases, when iatrogenic immunosuppression has been discontinued, the lymphomatoid granulomatosis has resolved.[51,57]

The most common cause of death is destruction of lung parenchyma, followed by central nervous system (CNS) involvement. Sepsis, sometimes related to chemotherapy, also contributes to mortality. Autopsy may reveal involvement of a wide variety of anatomic sites in addition to the commonly involved lungs, skin, and nervous system, including the spleen, liver, lymph nodes, kidneys, adrenal glands, heart and, in rare cases, the testes and eyes. The outlook, however, appears to be improving. Patients with grade 1 or grade 2 disease may respond well to interferon-α2b. Patients with grade 3 lymphomatoid granulomatosis may respond to cytotoxic chemotherapy combined with rituximab.[48] Adverse prognostic factors include a higher grade,[44,48,49] neurologic manifestations, and bilateral lung involvement.[49]

Pulmonary Lymphoma in HIV-Positive Patients

HIV-positive patients who develop primary pulmonary lymphoma are mostly men in the fourth to sixth decades of life,[52,59-61] although in rare cases women[59] and children[29] are affected. Most of these male

TABLE 4-3

Differential Diagnosis of Lymphomatoid Granulomatosis

Disease	Sites Involved	Tumor Cell Histology	Nonneoplastic Component Histology	Usual Immunophenotype of Tumor Cells	Epstein-Barr Virus
Lymphomatoid granulomatosis (LyG)	Lung most often, also CNS, skin; extranodal > nodal disease	Large cells, including immunoblasts; less often, bizarre or Reed-Sternberg–like cells	Nonneoplastic component prominent Lymphocytes, plasma cells, histiocytes; eosinophils, neutrophils, and well-formed granulomas rare or absent	CD20+, CD30+/−, CD15−	Large cells +
Granulomatous infections	Variable	Absent	Necrotizing and/or nonnecrotizing epithelioid or palisading granulomas	N/A	−
Wegener's granulomatosis	Upper respiratory tract > lung	Absent	Neutrophils; fewer lymphocytes than in LyG; histiocytes with palisading granulomas	N/A	−
Classical Hodgkin's lymphoma	Nodal > extranodal; lung disease rare without nodal disease	Reed-Sternberg cells and mononuclear variants	Lymphocytes, histiocytes, eosinophils, and/or neutrophils in varying proportions	CD15+, CD30+, CD20−	Tumor cells + or −
Diffuse large B-cell lymphoma	Nodal or extranodal	Monotonous population of large cells: centroblasts, immunoblasts, occasionally bizarre cells	Inconspicuous	CD20+	Tumor cells + or −

CNS, Central nervous system; N/A, not applicable.

patients are homosexual[59]; a few have been intravenous drug users or have acquired HIV through a blood transfusion.[59,60] The lymphomas often occur in severely immunosuppressed individuals late in the course of HIV infection.[59-61] Nearly all patients present with respiratory or constitutional symptoms.[59-61] Radiographic studies show nodules or masses, some with cavitation, in the lung.[59]

Nearly all of the lymphomas have been diffuse, high-grade, EBV+ B-cell lymphomas. When they have been described in more detail, they have been centroblastic, immunoblastic, or polymorphous in composition.[59,62] A number of cases of lymphomatoid granulomatosis also have been described (see previous section).[52] The presence of EBV sometimes has been documented using in situ hybridization for EBER and also through immunohistochemistry with antibodies to EBV-LMP.[59-61] A case of EBV+ pulmonary plasmablastic lymphoma that occurred in association with pulmonary aspergillosis has been reported (plasmablastic lymphoma is discussed in more detail in Lymphomas of the Oral Cavity, in Chapter 3).[61] Rare pulmonary marginal zone lymphomas occurring in childhood and adulthood have been described.[29,32] Immunoglobulin heavy and/or light chain genes have been clonally rearranged in cases in which this has been tested.[29,61]

Patients have a poor prognosis, usually succumbing to the lymphoma. However, concurrent opportunistic infections are common, which contribute to morbidity.[52,59] The use of optimal antiretroviral therapy may improve the prognosis and possibly prevent some lymphomas.

Rare Non-Hodgkin's Lymphomas

Rare cases of other types of lymphoma primary in the lung have been reported. These include follicular lymphoma,[9,18,20,22] Burkitt's lymphoma,[9] mantle cell lymphoma,[18,19] peripheral T-cell lymphoma not otherwise specified (NOS),[9,20] and anaplastic large cell lymphoma (ALCL).[13,21] ALCL including ALK+,[21] as well as ALCL lacking the t(2;5) translocation involving the ALK and NPM genes,[13] have been reported.

Pulmonary Hodgkin's Lymphoma

Pulmonary involvement by Hodgkin's lymphoma in the setting of systemic disease or by direct extension from bulky mediastinal disease is fairly common. In rare instances, however, classical Hodgkin's lymphoma presents as a tumor of the lung with exclusive or predominant pulmonary involvement.[22,63,64] In such cases, the presenting symptoms are similar to those of non-Hodgkin's lymphoma. On average, patients are younger than those with primary non-Hodgkin's lymphoma of the lung, as is true of patients with Hodgkin's lymphoma that presents in other sites. The lymphoma takes the form of single or multiple parenchymal masses, intrabronchial lesions, or pneumonia-like consolidation. Nodular sclerosis and mixed cellularity are the most common histologic types. The immunophenotypic features are similar to those of classical Hodgkin's lymphoma in other sites. The prognosis is favorable.[64]

The differential diagnosis is broad, and establishing a diagnosis in the lung can be difficult because of the varied reactive patterns found in the lung, such as hyperplasia of type 2 pneumocytes and the presence of many histiocytes and fibrosis; these may obscure the Hodgkin's lymphoma, which is already characterized by a relatively small number of tumor cells in a reactive background. Diagnostic considerations include lymphomatoid granulomatosis, diffuse large B-cell lymphoma, Wegener's granulomatosis, Langerhans' cell histiocytosis, carcinoma, and others.[64] Studying the histologic features and performing immunostains on the most representative area should establish a diagnosis.

Secondary Pulmonary Lymphoma

The lungs can be secondarily involved by lymphoma through direct extension from the hilus or mediastinum or through metastasis from a distant site.[65] Secondary pulmonary involvement by lymphoma is common; the lungs are involved at some time in the course of the disease in about 38% of cases of Hodgkin's lymphoma and 24% of cases of non-Hodgkin's lymphoma.[65,66] Extranodal marginal zone lymphomas arising in sites such as the ocular adnexa and the stomach can spread to involve the lung,[17,19] but Hodgkin's lymphoma, as well as a wide variety of non-Hodgkin's lymphomas of B-cell and T-cell lineage, also can involve the lung secondarily.[65] We recently have seen a case in which a patient with a history of low-grade follicular lymphoma involving lymph nodes developed dyspnea and was found to have pulmonary involvement by follicular lymphoma (Figure 4-5).

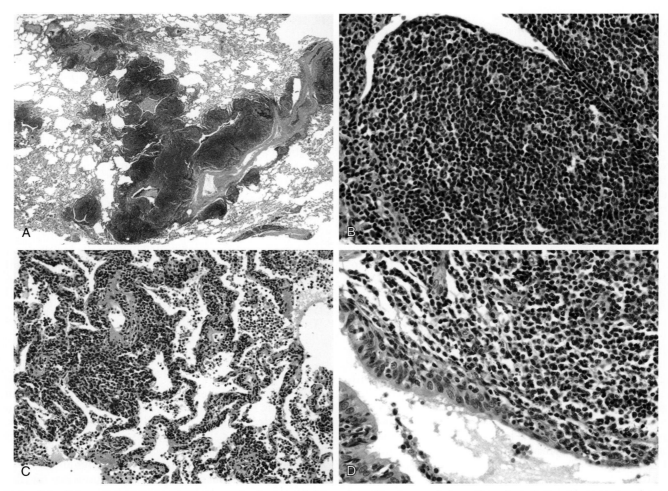

Figure 4-5   Relapsed follicular lymphoma involving the lung. **A,** Low-power view shows a lesion with preferential involvement along bronchovascular bundles. Inside the lesion are multiple cellular nodules, suggesting lymphoid follicles. **B,** Higher power view shows a single, poorly delineated follicle composed of a monotonous population of small, dark centrocytes. **C,** Extensive infiltration of atypical lymphoid cells away from the main lesion and into alveolar septae was seen; this may correlate with the patient's complaint of dyspnea. **D,** This lymphoma invaded the bronchial epithelium, mimicking the lymphoepithelial lesions characteristic of marginal zone lymphoma. Flow cytometric analysis revealed a CD10+, CD5–, monotypic kappa-positive B-cell population, as was found in the original lymph node follicular lymphoma.

■ LYMPHOMAS OF THE PLEURA AND PLEURAL CAVITY

Pleural involvement by lymphoma is common. It may occur at the time of initial presentation, but it often occurs in individuals with a past history of lymphoma.[67] Pleural involvement usually occurs with systemic disease[67] or in association with pulmonary parenchymal disease,[65] and may be of a wide variety of pathologic types.[67] In contrast, lymphoma that arises primarily in the pleural cavity is very uncommon. Diffuse large B-cell lymphoma and rare cases of follicular lymphoma[67] and marginal zone lymphoma[68] apparently primary in the pleura have been described. However, only two types of lymphoma with primary involvement of the pleura or the pleural cavity emerge as distinct entities: primary effusion lymphoma[69] and pyothorax-associated lymphoma.[70]

Primary Effusion Lymphoma

Primary effusion lymphoma, previously known as body cavity–based lymphoma, is a rare, distinctive type of human herpes virus 8+ (HHV8+) diffuse large B-cell lymphoma characterized by lymphomatous effusions involving pleural, pericardial, or peritoneal cavities unaccompanied by a solid mass.[69,71,72] (HHV8 is also known as *Kaposi's sarcoma–associated herpes virus* [KSHV]).

Clinical Features

Primary effusion lymphoma affects young and middle-aged adults, and males are affected much more often than females. Nearly all patients are HIV positive; they present late in the course of HIV infection and often are profoundly immunodeficient at the time they present with lymphoma. Occasional patients are HIV negative; these are mostly elderly individuals, often of Mediterranean origin.[73-75] The advanced age of these individuals may represent a source of immunodeficiency, and Mediterranean origin may be associated with an increased chance of harboring HHV8. Patients present with a pleural effusion, a pericardial effusion, or ascites. By definition, no discrete, contiguous lymphomatous mass is associated with the effusion. This lymphoma has a very poor prognosis, although among HIV-positive patients, the outcome may be better for those receiving highly active antiretroviral therapy (HAART).[76] Death is caused by the lymphoma, sometimes complicated by opportunistic infection or Kaposi's sarcoma or both (Table 4-4).[77]

TABLE 4-4

Clinical Features and Differential Diagnosis of Primary Effusion Lymphoma

Features	Primary Effusion Lymphoma (PEL)	Solid Lymphomas, PEL-Like	Pyothorax-Associated Lymphoma (PAL)	PEL-Like Lymphomas	Miscellaneous Lymphomas Involving Pleura, Non-PEL, Non-PAL
Synonyms and related terms	Body cavity–based lymphoma; PEL type 1	Extracavitary PEL; IBL/PBL DLBCL	DLBCL associated with chronic inflammation	KSHV/HHV8-unrelated PEL-like lymphoma; PEL types 2 and 3	N/A
Presenting symptoms	Dyspnea or abdominal distension	Fever, night sweats, and/or weight loss	Pain, cough, weight loss, fever, effusion	As for PEL	Cough, dyspnea, chest pain
Anatomic sites involved	Pleural, pericardial, or peritoneal cavity	GI tract, skin, soft tissue, lung, spleen, lymph nodes	Pleura +/− lung	As for PEL	Variable sites in addition to pleura
Pleural involvement	Effusion, no mass	N/A	Pleural mass +/− effusion	Effusion, no mass	Pleural mass or thickening; effusion common
Patients affected	*HIV positive* (majority): Young or middle aged, males >> females *HIV negative* (minority): Mostly elderly, M and F	*HIV positive* (majority): Young or middle aged, males >> females *HIV negative* (minority): Elderly	Older adults, males >> females; most have been Japanese	Mostly middle aged or older adults; males slightly > females; Subset HCV+	Varied
HIV status	Most positive, a few negative	Most positive, a few negative	Negative	Usually negative	Negative
Prognosis	Very poor	Poor; some patients develop lymphomatous effusions	Moderately poor	May be better than for PEL	Variable

DLBCL, Diffuse large B-cell lymphoma; *GI*, gastrointestinal; *HCV*, hepatitis C virus; *HHV8*, human herpes virus type 8; *HIV*, human immunodeficiency virus; *IBL*, immunoblastic; *KSHV*, Kaposi's sarcoma–associated herpes virus; *PBL*, plasmablastic; *N/A*, not applicable.

Pathologic Features

The neoplastic cells are uniform and immuno-blast-like, or pleomorphic and very large (Figure 4-6). Some are binucleated or multinucleated, and some may resemble Reed-Sternberg cells. Neoplastic cells express CD45 and activation antigens (e.g., CD30) without expression of B-cell specific markers. Despite the lack of B-cell antigens, immunoglobulin heavy and light chains are clonally rearranged, supporting a B-lineage. Occasionally, aberrant expression of T-cell–associated antigens is seen.[69]

Tumor cells usually are co-infected by EBV. Like HHV8, EBV is a gamma herpes virus; the two viruses are closely related.[71,78,79] Neoplastic cells are bcl6–, MUM1/IRF4+, and often CD138+, corresponding to a late stage in B-cell differentiation.[80] MUM1/IRF4 has been shown to downregulate cellular response to interferon, at least in vitro. MUM1/IRF4 expression by the neoplastic cells may play a role in allowing the virally infected tumor cells to escape from interferon-mediated control.[80] HHV8 also may downregulate expression of major histocompatibility complex (MHC) class I surface molecules, allowing HHV8-infected cells to escape being killed by cytotoxic T cells.[81] HHV8 also may be associated with impaired NK-cell activity.[81] These features, along with the tendency of primary effusion lymphoma to occur at a late stage in the course of HIV infection, may contribute to the very poor prognosis associated with this lymphoma.

Primary effusion lymphoma has distinctive molecular features. It frequently is associated with mutations in the 5' noncoding regions of *BCL6*,[82] as well as in the immunoglobulin gene variable (*IGV*) regions.[83] *BCL6* and *IGV* mutations are considered to indicate transition of B cells through the germinal center, and in conjunction with the immunophenotype, the genetic changes provide additional support for a late, post-germinal center stage of maturation for the neoplastic cells of primary effusion lymphoma in most cases. Gene expression profile analysis shows that primary effusion lymphoma shares features of acquired immunodeficiency syndrome (AIDS)–associated immunoblastic lymphoma and plasma cell myeloma and is quite different from other types of B-cell lymphomas.[84,85] There is, in addition, a specific set of genes unique to primary effusion lymphoma.[84] Therefore, both the immunophenotypic and genetic features indicate that the neoplastic cells of primary effusion lymphoma correspond to a late stage in B-cell differentiation. Some have proposed

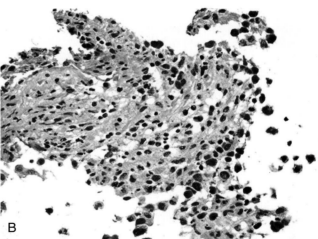

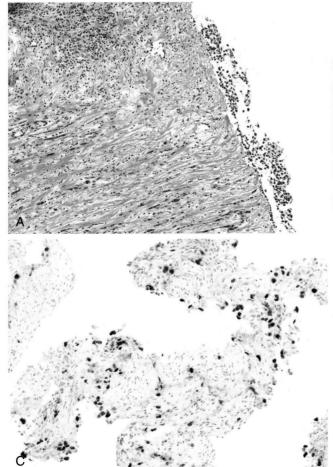

Figure 4-6   Primary effusion lymphoma in an HIV-positive man. **A,** Large cells are present in a thin layer loosely adherent to underlying fibrous tissue. **B,** Higher power view shows large, pleomorphic, discohesive lymphoid cells with irregular nuclei and scant cytoplasm scattered along the edge of the inflamed fibrous tissue, sometimes in a background of fibrin. **C,** The large cells are HHV8+. (Immunoperoxidase technique on a paraffin section.)

that HHV8, using some of the genes in the B-cell program of its host, drives the cells it occupies toward plasma cells (Table 4-5).[85]

Cases of HHV8+ lymphoma with a morphology and immunophenotypic and genetic features similar to those of primary effusion lymphoma but that produce mass lesions in lymph nodes or in extranodal sites also have been described.[79,86-88] These have been called *HHV8+* or *KSHV+ solid lymphomas; extracavitary primary effusion lymphomas*[79,87,89]; or *KSHV+ solid immunoblastic/plasmablastic diffuse large B-cell lymphomas.*[90] Some patients with "solid lymphomas" also develop HHV8+ effusion lymphomas (see Table 4-5). HHV8+ large B-cell lymphomas also can evolve from HHV8+ multicentric Castleman's disease; these lymphomas mainly affect HIV-positive patients and primarily involve the lymph nodes and spleen. They typically are composed of monotypic cytoplasmic IgM+, EBV−, HHV8+ plasmablasts.[86]

Pyothorax-Associated Lymphoma

Pyothorax-associated lymphoma is a rare EBV+ diffuse large B-cell lymphoma that arises in the setting of tuberculosis treated with iatrogenic pneumothorax, with resultant long-standing chronic pyothorax (typically longer than 20 years' duration). In the classification system established by the World Health Organization (WHO), this type of lymphoma is included in the category of diffuse large B-cell lymphoma associated with chronic inflammation.[70] The long-standing chronic, suppurative inflammation may allow EBV+ B cells to escape immune surveillance and may even promote proliferation of such cells, eventually leading to the development of lymphoma.[70,91] Because artificial pneumothorax no longer is used as a treatment for tuberculosis, pyothorax-associated lymphoma eventually may cease to exist.

Patients mostly are older adults who present with local pain, fever, weight loss, respiratory symptoms, or a combination of these. Men are affected much more often than women, and most, but not all, of these patients have been Japanese. Evaluation typically reveals a mass involving the pleura, sometimes with concurrent lung involvement, sometimes accompanied by a pleural effusion. Microscopic examination reveals a diffuse proliferation of large atypical cells, usually centroblasts and/or immunoblasts, often with plasmacytoid features, sometimes accompanied by extensive necrosis. Most cases express pan–B-cell antigens, including CD20 and CD79a, but infrequently, cases lack both of these markers. Tumor cells are also CD10−, bcl6−, IRF4/MUM1+, and may be CD138+, corresponding to a late stage in B-cell differentiation (late germinal center or post-germinal center). In situ hybridization for EBER reveals EBV in tumor cells. This lymphoma has a poor prognosis, although occasional patients have long-term survival.[70,92]

TABLE 4-5

Pathologic Features and Differential Diagnosis of Primary Effusion Lymphoma					
Features	**Primary Effusion Lymphoma (PEL)**	**Solid lymphomas, PEL-Like**	**Pyothorax-Associated Lymphoma (PAL)**	**PEL-Like Lymphomas**	**Miscellaneous Lymphomas Involving Pleura, Non-PEL, Non-PAL**
Microscopic features	Large, bizarre, pleomorphic or immunoblast-like cells dispersed in fluid	Large immunoblast-like or pleomorphic bizarre cells	Sheets of centroblasts and/or immunoblasts, often plasmacytoid	Some cases have large cells, including immunoblasts; some have Burkitt's morphology	Variable (many different types of lymphoma, DLBCL and FL most common)
HHV8	+	+	−	−	−
CD20	−	−/+	+ (occasionally −)	Usually +	Most +
MUM1/IRF4	+	+	+	N/A	Variable
CD138	+/−	+/−	+/−	−	Variable
Ig	−	−/+ (when +, lambda >> kappa)	+	+/−	Most +
CD30	+	+/−	May be +	−/+	Variable
EBV	++/−	++/−	+	May be +	Most −
IGH	Clonal	Clonal	Clonal	Clonal	BCLs clonal
Other genetic features	*IGH* and *BCL6* mutated in most cases No translocations of *BCL1, BCL2, BCL6,* or *MYC*	No translocations of *BCL1, BCL2, BCL6,* or *MYC*	*IGH* mutated	*PEL type 2: MYC* rearranged (cases typically have Burkitt's morphology) *PEL type 3: MYC* germline (typically, DLBCL morphology)	Variable

BCL, B-cell lymphoma; *DLBCL,* diffuse large B-cell lymphoma; *EBV,* Epstein-Barr virus; *FL,* follicular lymphoma; *IGH,* immunoglobulin heavy chain gene; *N/A,* not available.

Differential Diagnosis

1. **Primary effusion lymphoma versus miscellaneous other lymphomas.** Before its recognition as a distinct entity and the demonstration of its association with HHV8, primary effusion lymphoma was a poorly understood neoplasm that often caused problems in diagnosis because of its unique clinical presentation and null immunophenotype. The differential diagnosis in cases of primary effusion lymphoma includes an effusion related to pleural involvement by some other type of lymphoma. The various lymphomas other than primary effusion lymphoma that involve the pleura typically are associated with a pleural mass or diffuse pleural thickening and usually are associated with systemic disease[67]; they also lack the characteristic pathologic features of primary effusion lymphoma, particularly the presence of HHV8.

2. **Primary effusion lymphoma versus pyothorax-associated lymphoma.** In contrast to primary effusion lymphoma, pyothorax-associated lymphoma has mainly been encountered in Japan, is associated with a long-standing pyothorax related to tuberculosis, and forms a discrete pleural mass composed of large cells expressing B-cell antigens without HHV8.[70-72]

3. **Primary effusion lymphoma versus HHV8–primary effusion lymphoma–like lymphoma.** Rare cases of lymphoma presenting primarily as effusions in pleural, peritoneal, and/or pericardial cavities but lacking HHV8 have been described; these have been designated "primary effusion lymphoma–like lymphomas." Compared with primary effusion lymphoma, these HHV8-negative lymphomas affect patients who overall are older; there is less of a male preponderance, and only a minority of the patients are HIV positive. The neoplastic cells are large cells in some cases; in others, the cytomorphology is that of Burkitt's lymphoma. The subset of cases in HIV-positive patients tends to have a Burkitt's morphology. B-antigen expression is more common than in HHV8+ primary effusion lymphoma. Cases with Burkitt's morphology are associated with *MYC* rearrangement and therefore may represent true examples of Burkitt's lymphoma with an unusual anatomic distribution. The pathogenesis of a substantial subset of cases, mainly those with large cell morphology, may be related to the hepatitis C virus.[93-96] The prognosis in these rare cases is not certain but appears to be superior to that for patients with HHV8+ primary effusion lymphoma. In rare cases, apparent remissions have been reported after drainage of the effusions alone (see Tables 4-4 and 4-5).[93,97] We recently have seen the case of an elderly woman with a pleural effusion showing an HHV8– large B-cell lymphoma, with monotypic expression of immunoglobulin light chain and clonal *IGH* using polymerase chain reaction (PCR). The effusion resolved spontaneously and did not recur during 6 months of follow-up (Figure 4-7). A classification for primary effusion lymphomas (PELs) has been proposed based on the presence or absence of HHV8 and on genetic features. In this scheme, PEL type 1 includes HHV8+ cases with germline *MYC;* PEL type 2 includes HHV8– cases with rearranged *MYC;* and PEL type 3 includes HHV8– cases with germline *MYC* (Figure 4-7).[93]

■ LYMPHOMAS OF THE THYMUS

Primary Lymphomas of the Thymus

Three types of non-Hodgkin's lymphomas arise in the thymus: T-lymphoblastic lymphoma, extranodal marginal zone lymphoma, and primary mediastinal (thymic) large B-cell lymphoma. Classical Hodgkin's lymphoma, usually the nodular sclerosis type, is common in the mediastinum and sometimes arises in the thymus.[98] However, because Hodgkin's lymphoma is mainly a lymph node–based disease, discussion focuses on its importance in the differential diagnosis of mediastinal large B-cell lymphoma.

T-Lymphoblastic Leukemia/Lymphoma

Clinical Features

T-lymphoblastic leukemia/lymphoma accounts for approximately 40% of childhood lymphomas, 85% to 90% of lymphoblastic lymphomas, and 15% of pediatric acute lymphoblastic leukemias. Most patients are adolescent and young adult males, but older adults may be affected. Patients with T-lymphoblastic lymphoma present with rapidly enlarging, mediastinal (thymic) masses and/or peripheral lymphadenopathy. In the earlier literature, mediastinal T-lymphoblastic lymphoma was referred to as *Sternberg sarcoma.*[99]

Patients with T-lymphoblastic leukemia present with acute leukemia, typically with a high white blood cell count with numerous lymphoblasts. The cutoff used most commonly to establish a diagnosis of leukemia is a marrow cell population that is 25% lymphoblasts. Some patients presenting with a mediastinal mass or lymphadenopathy have marrow involvement on staging. If left untreated, most cases presenting as lymphoma progress to acute leukemia; involvement of the central nervous system is common. The tumor is rapidly fatal if left untreated, but the prognosis is favorable with optimal chemotherapy.[100-102]

Pathologic Features

T-lymphoblastic leukemia/lymphoma has a diffuse pattern of growth. The neoplastic T lymphoblasts have round or convoluted nuclei; finely dispersed chromatin; small, sometimes inconspicuous nucleoli; scant cytoplasm; and a high mitotic rate (Figure 4-8, *A* and *B*). They are morphologically

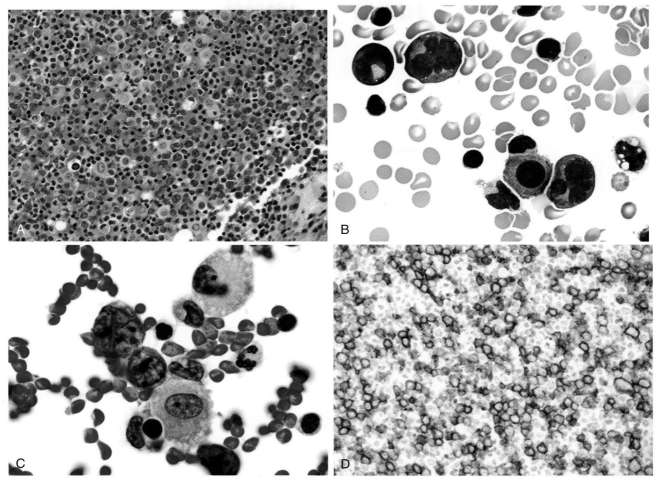

Figure 4-7   HHV8– primary effusion lymphoma–like lymphoma (primary effusion lymphoma, type 3). **A,** Cell block prepared from pleural fluid shows large atypical lymphoid cells with oval or irregular nuclei, prominent centrally or peripherally placed nucleoli, and scant cytoplasm in a background of red cells and cytologically bland histiocytes with fine chromatin and moderately abundant, pink cytoplasm. **B,** Smear stained with Wright stain shows large, highly atypical lymphoid cells with large, lobated nuclei and deep blue cytoplasm. **C,** Papanicolaou stain reveals similar large atypical cells with larger nuclei, coarser chromatin, more prominent nucleoli, and less cytoplasm than admixed histiocytes. **D** and **E,** Large atypical cells (CD20+ **(D)**) with scattered admixed small T cells (CD3+ **(E)**) are seen.

Continued

indistinguishable from B lymphoblasts. In rare cases, eosinophils may form a conspicuous part of the infiltrate; in such cases, a diagnosis of a myeloid/lymphoid neoplasm with eosinophilia and an abnormality of the *FGFR1* gene should be considered.[102]

In most cases, the neoplastic cells are CD7+, CD3+, TdT+, CD1a+/−, CD2+/−, CD5+/−, CD10+/−, CD99+, and CD4+/CD8+ (double positive) or CD4−/CD8− (double negative). They may express either TCRαβ or TCRγδ, or neither (see Figure 4-8, *C* to *G*). Cases with a leukemic presentation tend to have a more immature phenotype than those presenting as lymphoma. Tumor cells in a subset of cases express the B-cell–associated marker CD79a.[103] Myeloid-associated antigens CD13, CD33, and/or CD117 are expressed in a minority of cases, but these examples of aberrant antigen expression are not sufficient for a diagnosis of a B-lymphoblastic or myeloid neoplasm. This phenomenon does underscore the need for thorough immunophenotyping in these primitive neoplasms. Rearrangement of the T-cell receptor

(TCR) genes usually is found; *IGH* rearrangement is seen in a minority of cases.[100-102] Cytogenetic abnormalities are common, and the most frequent involve the *TCR* genes.[102] Activating mutations of *NOTCH1* play an important role in the pathogenesis of a subset of T-lymphoblastic neoplasms.[104]

Differential Diagnosis

1. **Lymphoblastic leukemia/lymphoma versus mantle cell lymphoma.** Overlap occurs in the morphology of lymphoblastic leukemia/lymphoma and that of the blastoid variant of mantle cell lymphoma. Mantle cell lymphoma can even present with a large number of circulating neoplastic cells (informally referred to as "mantle cell leukemia"). However, mantle cell lymphoma is a disease of older adults, and although bone marrow involvement is common, it often is focal, in contrast to the usual extensive diffuse involvement of the bone marrow by T-lymphoblastic leukemia. Presentation with a mediastinal mass is not typical of

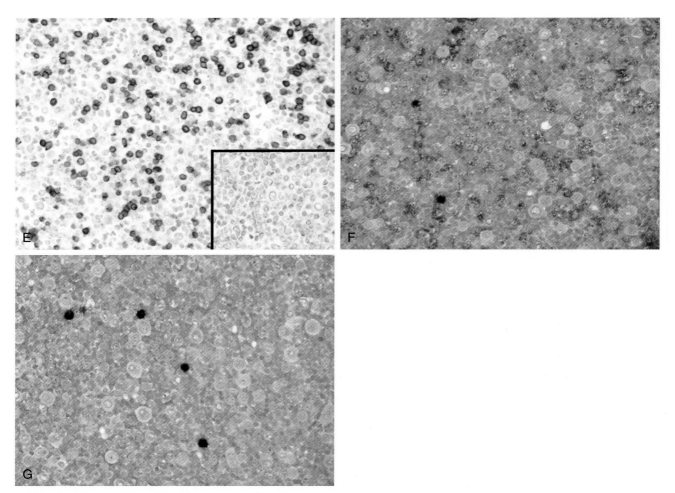

Figure 4-7, cont'd   D and E, Large atypical cells (CD20+ **(D)**) with scattered admixed small T cells (CD3+ **(E)**) are seen. An immunostain for HHV8 is negative (**E,** *inset*). (Immunoperoxidase technique on paraffin sections of the cell block.) **F** and **G,** In situ hybridization on the cell block reveals dim monotypic staining of some large cells for kappa light chain **(F)** without expression of lambda light chain **(G).**

mantle cell lymphoma, in contrast to T-lymphoblastic lymphoma. Immunophenotyping provides a definitive diagnosis (mantle cell lymphoma is CD20+, sIg+, TdT−, and cyclin D1+).

2. **Lymphoblastic leukemia/lymphoma versus acute myeloid leukemia and myeloid or monocytic sarcoma.** Cases of acute myeloid leukemia or myeloid sarcoma composed of cells with little appreciable myeloid or monocytic differentiation may mimic lymphoblastic leukemia/lymphoma. Examination of touch preps or aspirate smears can be helpful for identifying granules or Auer rods in myeloid neoplasms. Enzyme histochemical stains and immunophenotyping by flow cytometric analysis or immunohistochemistry can confirm the diagnosis by showing expression of myeloperoxidase, CD68, or lysozyme and a lack of T-cell specific markers in myeloid or monocytic neoplasms.

3. **Lymphoblastic leukemia/lymphoma versus thymomas of organoid type (WHO B1) or cortical type (WHO B2).** Thymomas of organoid type (WHO B1) or cortical type (WHO B2) contain large numbers of immature T cells that can mask the neoplastic thymic epithelial cells, leading to a misdiagnosis of lymphoblastic lymphoma. The immunophenotype of the thymic cortical-type T cells is similar to that of neoplastic T lymphoblasts (CD3dim+, TdT+, CD1a+, CD4+/CD8+ double positive). Familiarity with the variety of patterns that thymomas can assume and immunostaining for keratin to highlight epithelial cells can be very helpful in establishing a diagnosis. Making the distinction can be difficult in small biopsy specimens.

Extranodal Marginal Zone Lymphoma of Mucosa-Associated Lymphoid Tissue (MALT Lymphoma)

In 1990, Isaacson and colleagues first described marginal zone lymphoma of MALT type arising in the thymus.[105] Thymic marginal zone lymphoma is rare; only about 30 cases have been reported.[105-114] Its clinical, histologic, immunophenotypic, and genetic features differ somewhat from those of marginal zone lymphomas arising in other sites.

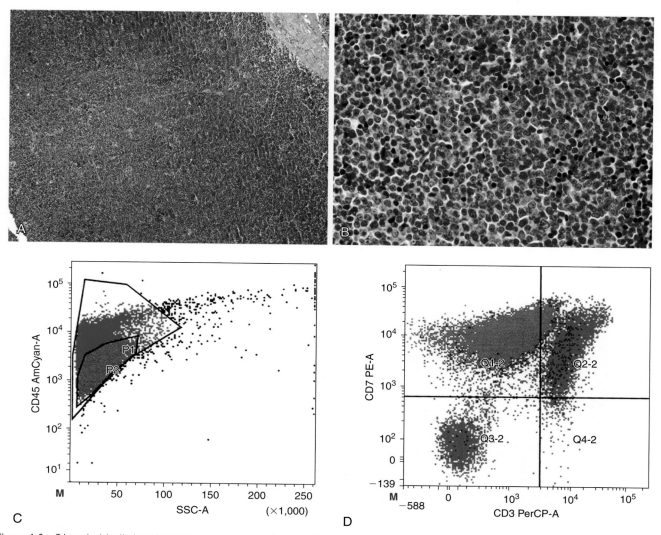

Figure 4-8   T-lymphoblastic lymphoma in a young boy with a mediastinal mass (the specimen illustrated is a cervical lymph node). **A,** Low-power view shows diffuse obliteration of the normal lymph node architecture. **B,** Higher power view shows a predominant population of medium-sized cells with fine chromatin, small nucleoli, and scant cytoplasm. **C** to **E,** Flow cytometric analysis shows a population of normal lymphocytes expressing bright CD45 *(red)* and a CD45-dim population *(green)* **(C)**. In **D,** the abnormal population expresses CD7 but not surface CD3, whereas the normal T lymphocytes appropriately express both markers.

Continued

Clinical Features

Reported cases of thymic marginal zone lymphoma describe patients who range in age from 23 to 75 years (the mean age is in the 50s). The female preponderance is marked; more than 75% of patients are women. Most reported patients by far have been Asians,[106,107,111-114] although this lymphoma affects Caucasians as well.[105,109] A strong association with autoimmune disease is seen, especially with Sjögren's syndrome. More than three fourths of patients have evidence of autoimmune disease, and Sjögren's syndrome is found in approximately half of patients.[106-110,112,114] Several patients have had rheumatoid arthritis. Two patients have had systemic lupus erythematosus,[110,113] and individual patients have had scleroderma[110] or myasthenia gravis.[110] Several patients have had poorly defined autoimmune diseases or serologic evidence of autoimmune disease in the form of positive rheumatoid factor or antinuclear antibodies, but no overt autoimmune disease.[106,111] Most patients have an abnormality of serum immunoglobulin[106-108,111,113,114]; half of these have a monoclonal protein, which is almost always IgA, although a case with an IgG M-component with hyperviscosity has been described.[108] The other half have polyclonal hypergammaglobulinemia; an increase in both IgG and IgA is most common, sometimes accompanied by increased IgM. An IgA M-component may occur in conjunction with polyclonal hypergammaglobulinemia.[114] A few patients have presented with chest or back pain or dyspnea, but the lymphomas usually have been incidental findings.

Pathologic Features

The lymphomas usually form large masses, ranging from 1.5 to 17 cm, with a mean of approximately 9 cm.[106,108] They often are described as having a

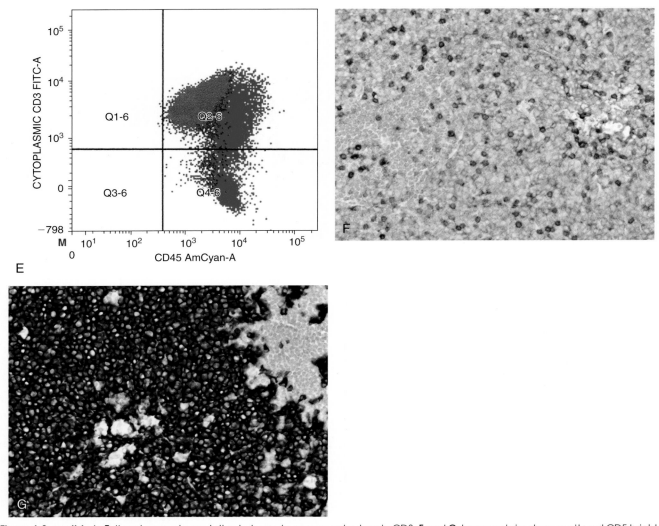

Figure 4-8, cont'd   In **E**, the abnormal population is shown to express cytoplasmic CD3. **F** and **G**, Immunostains show scattered CD5 bright–positive cells consistent with nonneoplastic T cells in a background of numerous CD5 dim neoplastic cells **(F)**. A similar pattern was seen with CD3. Neoplastic cells are CD7 bright positive **(G)**. Tumor cells also were TdT+ and negative for both CD4 and CD8 and for B-cell markers. No admixed cytokeratin-positive cells were identified. (Immunoperoxidase technique on paraffin sections.)

lobular contour and a thin, fibrous capsule.[105,111] Sectioning reveals a pink-tan, gray-white, or light tan surface that usually is solid and cystic but occasionally is homogeneously solid. The masses typically are confined to the thymus,[112-114] although in one case, in which progression to diffuse large B-cell lymphoma occurred, the lymphoma infiltrated the pericardium.[108] One report has described several cases of early thymic involvement by lymphoma arising on a background of thymic lymphoid hyperplasia, apparently without forming a discrete mass.[110]

The histologic features are very similar from case to case. The lymphomas show scattered, reactive lymphoid follicles surrounded by marginal zone cells with slightly irregular nuclei and clear cytoplasm. Also present are a few centroblasts or immunoblasts and many plasma cells and plasmacytoid cells. The marginal zone cells infiltrate the epithelium of Hassall's corpuscles to form lymphoepithelial lesions. A constant feature is the presence of cysts, even in cases that appear solid on macroscopic

examination. The cysts can vary widely in size; they usually are lined by flattened epithelium believed to be of thymic medullary origin (Figure 4-9). The cysts are filled with eosinophilic fluid and sometimes with cholesterol clefts, and the lining epithelium may be infiltrated by marginal zone cells.[105-109,111-114] In cases of early thymic involvement, the lymphoma involves and expands the medulla, with atrophy of adjacent cortex.[110] A single reported case, noted previously, showed areas of progression to diffuse large B-cell lymphoma.[108]

The immunophenotypic features overlap with those of marginal zone lymphoma that arises in other sites; the neoplastic cells are CD20+, CD79a+, CD5–, CD10–, CD23–, and CD43– and usually are bcl2+. In contrast to other marginal zone lymphomas, thymic marginal zone lymphomas reported so far uniformly show plasmacytic differentiation in the form of monotypic cytoplasmic immunoglobulin expression by plasma cells and plasmacytoid cells. The immunoglobulin expressed is almost always IgAκ or

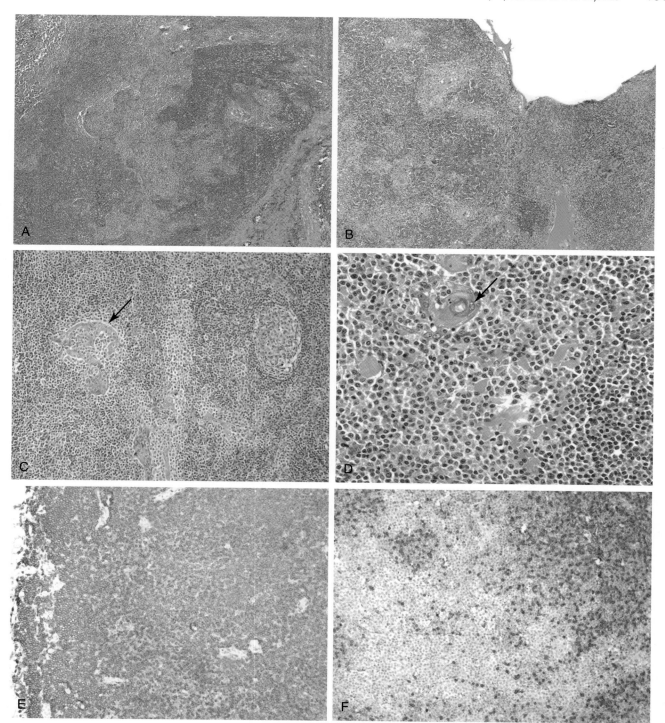

Figure 4-9 Thymic marginal zone lymphoma. **A,** The normal thymic architecture is obliterated by a dense lymphoid infiltrate with a broad, irregular band of marginal zone cells with pale cytoplasm flanked by small lymphocytes with scant cytoplasm. **B,** A cystic space is present in the lymphoma, at the upper right of the image. **C,** Bands and aggregates of pale marginal zone cells are present, focally infiltrating and disrupting a Hassall's corpuscle *(arrow).* A reactive lymphoid follicle is present on the right side of the image. **D,** Numerous marginal zone cells and plasma cells infiltrate a Hassall's corpuscle *(arrow).* **E** and **F,** Most cells, including B cells and plasma cells, are CD79a+ **(E).** Scattered CD3+ T cells also are present **(F).**

Continued

IgAλ (see Figure 4-9, *E* to *I*)[105-109,113,114]; only a few IgM+[105,108] or IgG+[106,108] cases have been described. One case was negative for myelin and lymphocyte protein (MAL), which usually is expressed in primary mediastinal large B-cell lymphoma.[109]

Immunostains for cytokeratin can be helpful for highlighting lymphoepithelial lesions.

As in other B-cell lymphomas, clonal rearrangement of the immunoglobulin heavy chain gene usually can be demonstrated.[106] However, thymic

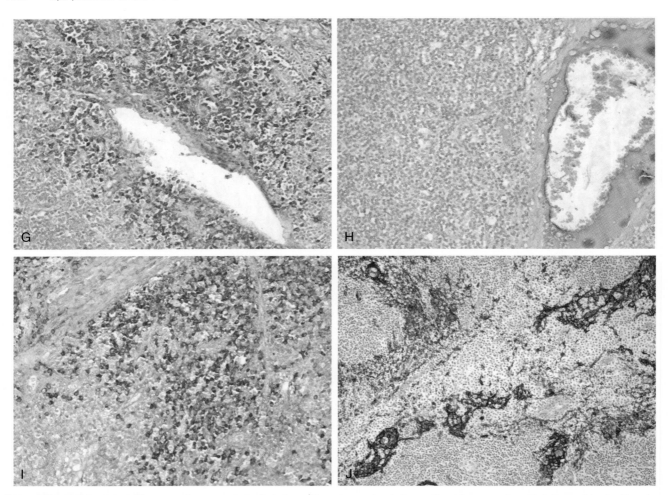

Figure 4-9, cont'd   G to I, Plasma cells are monotypic IgAκ+ with only rare lambda-positive plasma cells, which is consistent with a lymphoma with plasmacytic differentiation. Note the small cyst present in the lymphoma in **G** and **H** (kappa shown in **G,** lambda in **H,** alpha heavy chain in **I**). **J,** An immunostain for cytokeratin highlights an extensive network of epithelial cells that has been infiltrated by the lymphoma. (*E* to *J,* Immunoperoxidase technique on paraffin sections.)

marginal zone lymphomas differ from other marginal zone lymphomas with respect to their genetic and cytogenetic features. Multiple cases have been tested, and except for a single marginal zone lymphoma arising in association with a micronodular thymoma,[115] all have been negative for a fusion of the *API2* gene on chromosome 11 with the *MALT1* gene on chromosome 18.[106,109,111,114] One case was negative for a rearrangement involving *IGH* and *MALT1* genes using fluorescence in situ hybridization (FISH).[109] Thus, no evidence has been found that either of the two most common MALT lymphoma–associated translocations plays a significant role in the pathogenesis of thymic marginal zone lymphoma. Detailed studies directed at the immunoglobulin heavy chain gene have shown that the variable region (V_H) rearrangement usually has been potentially functional. V_H usage appears restricted to the V_H3 family, with nearly all cases using V_H3-30 or V_H3-23. J_H usage appears almost entirely restricted to J_H4.[115,116]

Ten cases were evaluated for evidence of somatic hypermutation, which was found in half of the cases.[107,116] In one case report, the lymphoma showed intraclonal diversity, consistent with ongoing mutation of *IGH*,[107] but in a series of nine cases, none showed evidence of ongoing *IGH* mutation.[116] The results of V_H and J_H usage suggest that thymic marginal zone lymphoma is derived from a distinct B-cell subset. B cells with V_H3-30 and V_H3-23 usage are strongly associated with autoimmune disease, which correlates with the frequent presence of autoimmune disease in patients with thymic marginal zone lymphoma. The biased usage of V_H3-30 and V_H3-23 in thymic marginal zone lymphoma is in contrast to the tendency of salivary marginal zone lymphoma, another lymphoma strongly associated with Sjögren's syndrome, to use V_H1-69.[116] Somatic hypermutation and ongoing mutation of the *IGH* gene are overall much more common in marginal zone lymphomas arising in other sites than they appear to be in thymic marginal zone lymphoma.[116] However, only small numbers of cases have been studied, and these findings should be confirmed by analysis of additional cases.

Staging, Treatment, and Outcome

Most patients have Ann Arbor stage IE disease, but involvement of regional lymph nodes is not uncommon.[105-107,109,111] A few patients have had concurrent disease in other extranodal sites, such as the salivary gland, lung, or stomach.[106] Bone marrow involvement has been described.[108] One patient with an IgGκ M-component was found to have crystal-storing histiocytosis, but no lymphoma, in her stomach.[108] Most patients are treated with surgical resection of the mass, accompanied in some cases by radiation or chemotherapy. In a few cases, the mass has only been biopsied, and patients are treated primarily with radiation or chemotherapy or both. Most patients achieve complete remission and remain free of lymphoma, but occasionally patients have spread to other extranodal sites or lymph nodes on follow-up.[105-109,112-114] Infrequently patients attain only partial remission, and one patient is known to have died of the disease.[106] Even when patients are cured of the lymphoma, the autoimmune diseases and, when present, polyclonal hypergammaglobulinemia typically persist. Follow-up was not available in the one case of large cell transformation of thymic marginal zone lymphoma.[108]

The description of one case with progression to large cell lymphoma raises the question of whether primary mediastinal (thymic) large B-cell lymphoma arises as large cell transformation of thymic marginal zone lymphoma. As discussed by Inagaki and colleagues,[106] this seems unlikely, because thymic marginal zone lymphoma has a much higher female to male ratio than mediastinal large B-cell lymphoma; on average, patients with mediastinal large B-cell lymphoma are younger; mediastinal large B-cell lymphoma is not associated with autoimmune disease, hypergammaglobulinemia, or an M-component; and the neoplastic cells of mediastinal large B-cell lymphoma usually are immunoglobulin negative. One thymic marginal zone lymphoma tested was negative for the mediastinal large B-cell lymphoma–associated marker MAL by immunostaining.[109] Therefore, although rare cases of large B-cell lymphoma arising in the thymus may represent large cell transformation of marginal zone lymphoma, the entity of primary mediastinal (thymic) large B-cell lymphoma does not appear to be related to thymic marginal zone lymphoma.

Pathogenesis and Cell of Origin

Autoimmune disease plays an important role in the genesis of most thymic marginal zone lymphomas, although the exact sequence of events is uncertain. Other marginal zone lymphomas typically arise on a background of acquired mucosa-associated lymphoid tissue. Myasthenia gravis is the condition most strongly associated with thymic acquisition of organized lymphoid tissue with reactive follicles, but thymic marginal zone lymphoma is only rarely associated with myasthenia gravis.[110] However, several cases of thymectomies showing small marginal zone lymphomas arising in lymphoid hyperplasia have been described; therefore, thymic marginal zone lymphomas, like other marginal zone lymphomas, may well arise in the setting of acquired MALT. Rare cases of marginal zone lymphoma have arisen from the lymphoid tissue associated with micronodular thymoma; some have proposed that abnormal chemokine expression by the epithelial cells of this type of thymoma recruits the lymphoid tissue characteristic of this tumor and predisposes the individual to the development of thymic lymphoma[115]; this would account for the etiology of a small subset of thymic marginal zone lymphomas.

Some researchers have suggested that thymic marginal zone lymphomas may arise from the small endogenous B-cell population normally present in the thymic medulla.[105,108] The V_H usage of the normal thymic B cells is biased toward V_H4, in contrast to that found in the lymphomas (see Pathologic Features, earlier). The V_H segments used by thymic marginal zone lymphomas are more common among peripheral blood lymphocytes,[116] which raises the question of origin from peripheral blood lymphocytes that home to the thymus, and under certain conditions undergo neoplastic transformation. The predilection of this lymphoma for Asians and its distinctive genetic features raise the question of a pathogenesis distinct from that of other marginal zone lymphomas, with racial or environmental factors, or both, possibly playing a pathogenetic role.[112]

Differential Diagnosis

1. **Thymic marginal zone lymphoma versus thymoma.** Although thymic marginal zone lymphoma is rare, it should be considered in the differential diagnosis of cystic and solid anterior mediastinal masses, particularly when the patient is Asian and has autoimmune disease, hypergammaglobulinemia, or an M-component. Cystic change is common in thymomas, but the cellular composition of most thymomas is so different from that of thymic marginal zone lymphoma that differentiating between the two usually is not difficult. Thymomas are composed of a mixture of thymic epithelial cells and lymphocytes in varying proportions. The lymphocytes are almost all T cells. Lymphoid follicles and plasma cells are very uncommon. One exception to these general rules is micronodular thymoma, a rare type of thymoma characterized by multiple small nodules of cytologically bland, spindled epithelial cells in a background of lymphoid stroma with reactive lymphoid follicles and plasma cells.[117] Micronodular thymoma and thymic marginal zone lymphoma share a number of features: They affect patients of about the same age; they present as masses of about the same size; they often have a cystic component; and they both have a conspicuous lymphoid population, including reactive lymphoid follicles and plasma cells. In contrast to marginal zone lymphoma, micronodular thymoma is not associated with autoimmune disease, does not show an Asian or female

preponderance, has a more conspicuous epithelial component composed of spindle cells rather than Hassall's corpuscles, lacks a conspicuous component of marginal zone cells, and has plasma cells that express polytypic immunoglobulin (Figure 4-10).[117] Rare cases of thymic marginal zone lymphoma arising from micronodular thymoma have been described[115]; therefore, the lymphoid component of any micronodular thymoma should be examined carefully and evaluated by immunohistochemistry and possibly molecular analysis if it is unusually prominent.

2. **Thymic marginal zone lymphoma versus lymphoid hyperplasia.** Early involvement of the thymus by a small marginal zone lymphoma may be difficult to distinguish from lymphoid hyperplasia in the medulla of the thymus. In favor of lymphoma are architectural distortion, with thymic cortical atrophy and substantial medullary expansion; conspicuous cyst formation; a conspicuous component of marginal zone cells with clear cytoplasm surrounding reactive follicles; and monotypic plasma cells. In lymphoid hyperplasia, a continuous layer of cytokeratin-positive cells is said to surround reactive follicles; this layer is disrupted in marginal zone lymphoma.[110]

Primary Mediastinal (Thymic) Large B-Cell Lymphoma

Introduction

In 1980 Lichtenstein and colleagues observed that a subset of primary mediastinal lymphomas that occurred in adults was a type distinct from the mediastinal lymphoblastic lymphoma that occurred in children.[118] This lymphoma subsequently was named *primary mediastinal (thymic) large B-cell lymphoma.* Because of its characteristic clinical and pathologic features, it has been included as a separate entity in both the Revised European-American Lymphoma (REAL) classification[119] and the subsequent WHO classification.[120] It accounts for 2% to 4% of all non-Hodgkin's lymphomas.[120]

Clinical Features

Mediastinal large B-cell lymphoma mainly affects individuals between 20 and 50 years of age[121]; in many series, the median age is in the 30s or early 40s.[121-129] Five percent of patients or fewer are older than age 60.[128,129] This lymphoma may affect young children, but such cases are uncommon.[130] A slight female preponderance is seen.[121-128,130] Almost all patients have symptoms related to the

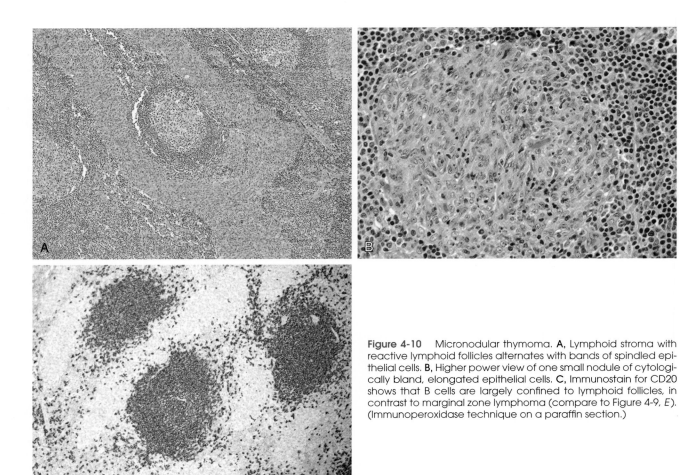

Figure 4-10   Micronodular thymoma. **A,** Lymphoid stroma with reactive lymphoid follicles alternates with bands of spindled epithelial cells. **B,** Higher power view of one small nodule of cytologically bland, elongated epithelial cells. **C,** Immunostain for CD20 shows that B cells are largely confined to lymphoid follicles, in contrast to marginal zone lymphoma (compare to Figure 4-9, *E*). (Immunoperoxidase technique on a paraffin section.)

presence of a mediastinal mass, including dyspnea, chest pain, cough, superior vena cava syndrome, or a combination of these. B symptoms (fever, sweats, weight loss) are seen in fewer than half of patients.[121,123,125-128]

Clinical and radiographic evaluation reveals an anterior superior mediastinal mass that is described as bulky (larger than 10 cm in the greatest dimension) in approximately 75% of cases.[122,125-127] Lymphoma often surrounds and invades adjacent structures, such as the pleura, pericardium, lung, mediastinal soft tissue, blood vessels, and mediastinal lymph nodes. This lymphoma may involve the supraclavicular fossa (lymph nodes or soft tissue) and occasionally even the soft tissue of the chest wall or the sternum by direct extension.[122,131-133] Lymphoma that invades the lung may penetrate bronchi and produce an endobronchial mass.[131] Invasion through the diaphragm into the liver has been described.[132] The invasive nature of this tumor frequently leads to the development of superior vena cava syndrome; neural invasion may result in hemidiaphragmatic paralysis.[121] About half of patients have a pleural or pericardial effusion.[125-128]

In most cases, the lymphoma is confined to the thoracic cavity at presentation. Approximately 70% of patients have localized disease (Ann Arbor stage I or stage II).[122,126-128] When the disease is more widespread, it tends to involve extranodal sites such as the kidneys, adrenal glands, central nervous system, and others. Marrow involvement is uncommon, occurring in no more than 5% of cases.[123,128]

Pathologic Features

Morphology

Microscopic examination reveals a diffuse infiltrate of atypical lymphoid cells that is almost always associated with sclerosis. The sclerosis can be bandlike or intercellular, or it can surround nests of cells in a compartmentalizing pattern (Figure 4-11, *A*).[132] Small and large foci of necrosis are common. Infiltration of adjacent tissues and structures may be identified microscopically (see Figure 4-11, *B*). Vascular

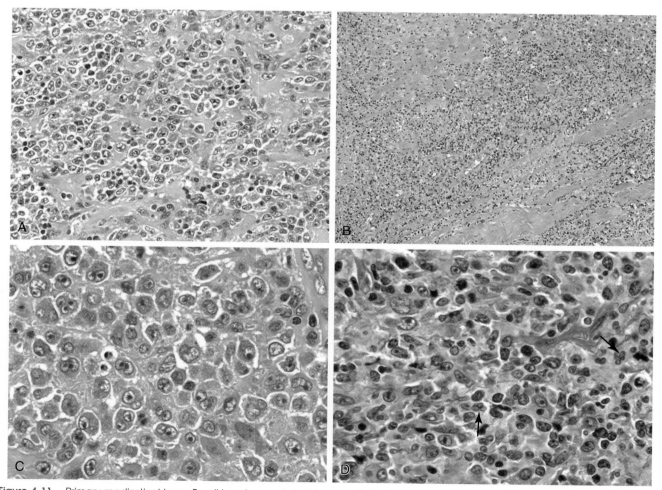

Figure 4-11   Primary mediastinal large B-cell lymphoma. **A,** In this case, delicate sclerosis delineating neoplastic large B cells into small groups (packeting or compartmentalizing sclerosis) can be seen. **B,** In another case, lymphoma extensively invades the pericardium. **C** and **D,** Cytologic features vary from one case to another. In **C,** neoplastic cells have oval, vesicular nuclei and distinct blue nucleoli; some tumor cells are binucleated. In **D,** occasional tumor cells have oval, vesicular nuclei with distinct nucleoli, but many have irregular or multilobated nuclei and inconspicuous nucleoli. Arrows indicate the multilobated cells.

Continued

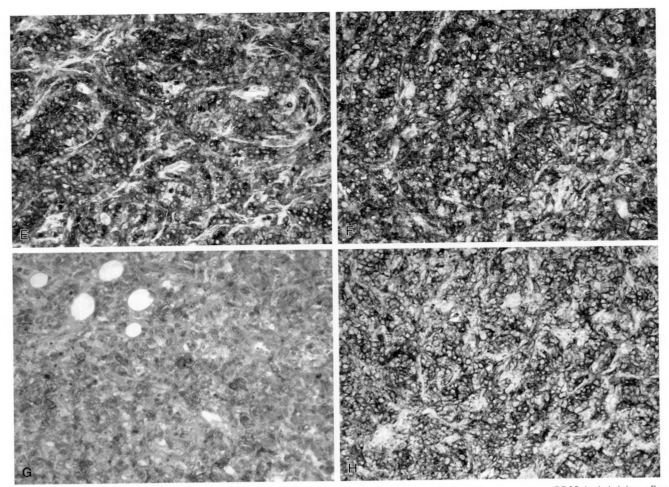

Figure 4-11, cont'd   E to H, Diffuse strong staining for CD45 **(E)** and CD20 **(F)** is seen. Neoplastic cells may express CD30, but staining often is weak, as in this example **(G)**. Neoplastic cells often are CD23+ **(H)**, as is seen in this case, although CD23 expression may be patchy.

invasion is common, mainly affecting larger blood vessels. The classic cellular composition includes a population of large cells with irregular, lobated nuclei and clear cytoplasm, which accounts for some or all of the neoplastic cells. Although the cytologic features usually are uniform from one area to another within a case, they vary from one case to another (see Figure 4-11, *C* and *D*).[131] In some cases, the neoplastic cells are centroblasts with round nuclei. A few cases are composed of anaplastic large cells. Other cases show an admixture of immunoblasts or Reed-Sternberg–like cells.[121-123,131] In a few cases, the neoplastic cells are relatively small and have been described as small centroblasts[121]; when they have clear cytoplasm, they may resemble monocytoid B cells.[131] A variable admixture of small lymphocytes and histiocytes is seen, and a few neutrophils may be present, but plasma cells and eosinophils typically are absent. In some cases, thymic remnants can be identified; an immunostain for cytokeratin can help highlight these structures.

When lymphoma infiltrates the lymph nodes, in some cases tumor cells first occupy the subcapsular sinus and may mimic metastatic carcinoma. The neoplastic cells may then spread in a perifollicular pattern and eventually replace the entire lymph node.[131] Although sclerosis typically is conspicuous when lymphoma involves mediastinal soft tissue or the lung, it is not prominent in some sites, such as lymph nodes.[131]

Immunophenotype

The neoplastic cells are diffusely positive for CD45 (leukocyte common antigen) and for pan–B-cell markers such as CD19, CD20, CD22, and CD79a. Most cases (at least 70%) lack cell surface immunoglobulin (sIg); cytoplasmic immunoglobulin (cIg) expression is rare. Interestingly, despite the lack of Ig in most cases, CD79a, the sIg co-receptor, typically is present. Tumor cells also express Oct2 and Bob1, transcription factors associated with immunoglobulin expression; therefore, lack of these factors is not the cause of the absence of Ig.[121,123,134,135] Expression of CD30 is common, but staining usually is weaker and more variable than in classical Hodgkin's lymphoma.[134-136] Most cases are bcl6+[123,136]; some cases are bcl2+.[122,136] CD10 typically is not expressed,[121,136] although in one series, nearly one third of cases were CD10+.[123] T-cell–associated antigens, including CD5, are absent,[121] as is CD21.[121,134]

In one series, CD23 was expressed by tumor cells in 70% of cases; other diffuse large B-cell lymphomas infrequently express CD23 (see Figure 4-11, *E* to *H*).[136] No evidence of EBV infection of tumor cells has been seen.[134]

Some immunophenotypic features provide clues to the pathogenesis of this lymphoma and also help set it apart as an entity distinct from other diffuse large B-cell lymphomas. In most cases, neoplastic cells express MAL, a protein normally found only in T cells. MAL localizes to the detergent-insoluble, glycolipid-enriched membrane domains involved in signal transduction and thus may be involved in lymphomagenesis.[137] Immunostains reveal staining of the plasma membrane and granular cytoplasmic staining with accentuation in the Golgi area. Other diffuse large B-cell lymphomas have been negative for MAL.[137]

An expression pattern characteristic of primary mediastinal large B-cell lymphoma for a variety of factors in pathways associated with activation and cell survival has been identified. Reticuloendotheliosis viral oncogene homolog (cREL), a member of the NFκB family of transcription factors, is a subunit of the NFκB (nuclear factor κB) heterodimer found in the cytoplasm, bound to IκB (inhibitor of NFκB) in its inactive state; upon activation, cREL is released and moves into the nucleus.[138-140] Nuclear cREL protein is reported in 65% of mediastinal large B-cell lymphomas; it may be expressed in other diffuse large B-cell lymphomas but is less common (18% in one report).[141] Tumor necrosis factor receptor–associated factors [TRAFs]) have the capacity to mediate activation of NFκB by promoting degradation of IκB, allowing NFκB to translocate to the nucleus.[142] TRAF1, an NFκB target gene, is expressed much more often in mediastinal large B-cell lymphoma than in other large B-cell lymphomas. Approximately half of mediastinal large B-cell lymphomas express both nuclear cREL and cytoplasmic TRAF1; among non-Hodgkin's lymphomas, this combination is highly specific for this type of lymphoma, and it is found only rarely in other diffuse large B-cell lymphomas.[141] This pattern of immunostaining provides strong evidence for activation of the NFκB pathway in many cases of this type of lymphoma and supports the importance of NFκB in its pathogenesis.

In its activated, phosphorylated form, signal transducer and activator of transcription 6 (STAT6) dimerizes and enters the nucleus, where it plays a role in regulating transcription and mediating interleukin 4 (IL-4)/IL-13 transcriptional effects, such as cellular proliferation. Phosphorylated STAT6 is found in the nucleus in most cases of mediastinal large B-cell lymphoma and is found only rarely in other diffuse large B-cell lymphomas.[143] STAT1 also is expressed much more often in mediastinal large B-cell lymphoma than in other large B-cell lymphomas.[140] As does STAT6, STAT1 and TRAF1 mediate the effects of IL-4/IL-13. Mediastinal large B-cell lymphoma is characterized by a distinctive chemokine receptor profile that may correlate with its

tendency to remain localized in the mediastinum for a relatively long time.[144]

Genetic and Cytogenetic Features

Primary mediastinal large B-cell lymphomas have clonally rearranged immunoglobulin heavy and light chain genes. Even though most cases lack Ig protein expression, analysis at the genetic level reveals immunoglobulin genes that appear potentially functional. They show a high load of somatic mutations with evidence of isotype switch but without ongoing somatic mutation.[145] A few cases have had missense point mutations in p53.[134,137,145] No *BCL2* rearrangement is seen, and only rare cases with *BCL6* rearrangement have been described.[140]

Mediastinal large B-cell lymphoma has characteristic cytogenetic features distinct from those of other non-Hodgkin's lymphomas. Gains of chromosomal material are much more common than losses. The most common areas showing gains include regions of chromosomes 2, 9p, 12q, and Xq. A small minority of cases show high-level amplification of the proto-oncogene *cREL*.[124,139] However, *cREL* amplification does not appear to correlate with increased NFκB activity, and activation of NFκB appears to be independent of *cREL* amplification.[139]

Gene profiling studies[133,138,140] also have shown features characteristic of primary mediastinal large B-cell lymphoma. Although the profile of mediastinal large B-cell lymphoma again is different from that of other diffuse large B-cell lymphomas, it shows substantial overlap with the profile of classical Hodgkin's lymphoma.[133,138,140] The findings of these studies, along with the immunophenotypic findings, suggest constitutive activation of the JAK/STAT pathway and the NFκB pathway,[133,138-140,143] which probably are important in the pathogenesis of this lymphoma. Elevated levels of NFκB support cell survival through promotion of antiapoptotic tumor necrosis factor alpha (TNFα) signaling. Levels of IL-13Rα (which phosphorylates JAK2 and STAT1), JAK2, and STAT1 are elevated compared with the levels seen in other diffuse large B-cell lymphomas.[140] Higher levels of MAL,[133,137] FIG1 (upregulation of which is induced by IL-4), and multiple other gene products from cytokine pathways, TNF family members, and extracellular matrix components also are present.[133,140]

A common finding among mediastinal large B-cell lymphomas is aberrant expression of certain tyrosine kinases, including JAK2, as noted previously, RON, and TIE1.[146] Activation of the PI3K/AKT pathway, possibly related to these tyrosine kinases, has been demonstrated in a subset of cases. Similar results have been found in classical Hodgkin's lymphoma but not in other B-cell lymphomas.[146] Mediastinal large B-cell lymphoma also shows a decrease in IgM and other members of the B-cell receptor (BCR) signaling cascade.

Mutations in suppressor of cytokine signaling 1 (*SOCS-1*) may play a role in activation of the JAK/STAT pathway. *SOCS-1* is involved in regulation of cellular proliferation, survival, and apoptosis through JAK/STAT signaling. *SOCS-1* downregulates the Janus kinases and provides negative feedback for STAT activity. Mutations and deletions of *SOCS-1*, which have been described in mediastinal large B-cell lymphoma, may lead to delayed degradation of JAK2 and may contribute to persistent activation of the JAK/STAT pathway.[147,148]

Cell of Origin

A small population of large B cells with dendritic processes, called *asteroid cells,* is native to the thymus. The asteroid cell may be the cell of origin for primary mediastinal large B-cell lymphoma.[120,132,136]

Treatment and Outcome

Patients typically are treated with combination chemotherapy with or without radiation therapy. This chemotherapy usually has been cyclophosphamide, doxorubicin, vincristine, and prednisone (CHOP) or more intensive third-generation regimens, such as methotrexate, doxorubicin, cyclophosphamide, vincristine, prednisone, and bleomycin (MACOP-B), or etoposide, doxorubicin, cyclophosphamide, vincristine, prednisone, and bleomycin (VACOP-B).[126-129,134] High-dose chemotherapy combined with autologous stem cell transplantation or autologous bone marrow transplantation has been used in a small number of cases; it could be considered in cases involving high-risk disease or for the treatment of relapse.[128,134]

The outcome has varied somewhat among different series. In one large study, 77% of patients achieved complete remission, 12% achieved partial remission, and the 5-year overall survival rate was 75%.[126] In another study, the 5-year overall survival rate was 87%, and the 5-year progression-free survival rate was 81%.[129] When relapse occurs, it usually happens within 1 year of completion of chemotherapy and almost always within 2 years. Patients may develop intrathoracic relapses (Figure 4-12), extrathoracic relapses, or both.[125] Extrathoracic relapses tend to involve unusual sites, such as the kidneys, adrenal glands, gastrointestinal tract, central nervous system, ovaries, breasts, and other extranodal sites, although lymph nodes may be involved as well.[125,135] The sites of involvement and the strong tendency for relapse within a short period after treatment are additional features that distinguish primary mediastinal large B-cell lymphoma from other diffuse large B-cell lymphomas.[126]

A poor prognosis has been associated with older age, male gender, bulky disease, poor performance status, higher stage disease, pleural effusion, and pericardial effusion.[125,128,134] Microscopic features, including cell size, sclerosis, and necrosis, appear to have no influence on the prognosis.[125,131] Failure to respond to initial therapy is associated with a poor prognosis, as is the occurrence of relapse; in either scenario, patients usually succumb to lymphoma within a year.[121,123,125-127] Some studies have reported superior outcomes with MACOP-B and similar

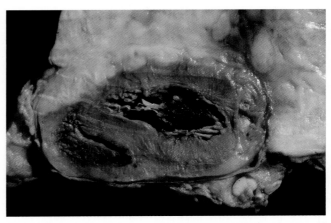

Figure 4-12   Primary mediastinal large B-cell lymphoma at autopsy. Yellow-white lymphoma partially surrounds the heart and deeply invades the myocardium. The patient also had multiple extrathoracic sites of disease, including the kidneys, liver, and bowel.

regimens compared with CHOP,[127,128] but this issue is controversial.[134] The addition of involved field radiation has been associated with a better outcome,[127] but the benefits of radiation must be balanced against the increased risk of breast cancer in young women and the risk of cardiac and pulmonary toxicity. The impact of rituxan in the treatment of this disease remains to be determined.[135]

Differential Diagnosis

1. **Primary mediastinal large B-cell lymphoma versus other diffuse large B-cell lymphomas.** Diffuse large B-cell lymphomas other than mediastinal large B-cell lymphoma may arise elsewhere and secondarily involve the mediastinum. Mediastinal large B-cell lymphoma has characteristic histologic features, but they are not specific, and distinguishing primary mediastinal large B-cell lymphoma from other large B-cell lymphomas involving the mediastinum may be difficult. Mediastinal large B-cell lymphoma is more likely than other diffuse large B-cell lymphomas to affect younger individuals and females and to present with bulky disease.[122,133] Mediastinal large B-cell lymphoma also is much more likely to attain a large size within the thoracic cavity before dissemination. As noted, mediastinal large B-cell lymphomas are more likely to spread to unusual extranodal sites when they do disseminate. They also have distinctive immunohistochemical, cytogenetic, and genetic features. Diffuse large B-cell lymphomas other than mediastinal large B-cell lymphoma are more likely to involve lymph nodes than thymus. In practice, when a specimen obtained from the anterior mediastinum shows histologic and immunophenotypic features compatible with mediastinal large B-cell lymphoma, we make a diagnosis of diffuse large B-cell lymphoma consistent with mediastinal large B-cell lymphoma and include a note stating that if the patient has a large mediastinal mass and if this represents most or all of

the patient's disease, the findings support a diagnosis of mediastinal large B-cell lymphoma. Gene expression profiling studies suggest that a few cases otherwise compatible with mediastinal large B-cell lymphoma have a molecular signature that is distinct from other cases in this category and more like that of other diffuse large B-cell lymphomas; therefore, they may not represent true examples of mediastinal large B-cell lymphoma.[133] As methods improve, criteria for the diagnosis of this disease likely will be refined.

The distinction between other diffuse large B-cell lymphomas and mediastinal large B-cell lymphoma may be important, because some investigators advocate more aggressive chemotherapy for patients with the mediastinal type. Relapses of mediastinal large B-cell lymphoma almost all occur early, whereas other diffuse large B-cell lymphomas may relapse many years after diagnosis.[126]

2. **Primary mediastinal large B-cell lymphoma versus classical Hodgkin's lymphoma.** Classical Hodgkin's lymphoma, particularly the nodular sclerosis type, shares many features with mediastinal large B-cell lymphoma. Both lymphomas tend to affect younger adults, with some female preponderance, and to produce mediastinal neoplasms characterized by a prominent sclerosis. Hodgkin's lymphoma usually arises in lymph nodes; however, in the mediastinum, approximately half of cases involve the thymus and nearly one fourth are confined to the thymus at presentation; therefore, a subset of cases clearly arises in the thymus.[98] The cell of origin is a B cell for both lymphomas. Mediastinal large B-cell lymphoma is composed of large atypical cells (some of which may resemble Reed-Sternberg cells) that usually lack immunoglobulin and may express CD30. In addition, the two lymphomas have similar cytogenetic abnormalities, including frequent gains in 2p13-p16 and 9p24 (location of *REL* and *JAK2*, respectively).[148] The gene expression profile of mediastinal large B-cell lymphoma is more like that of classical Hodgkin's lymphoma than like the profiles of other diffuse large B-cell lymphomas.[133,140] As in mediastinal large B-cell lymphoma, the neoplastic cells of classical Hodgkin's lymphoma show evidence of activation of the NFκB pathway, indicated by nuclear cREL and bright cytoplasmic TRAF1 expression in most cases.[142] Both may also have mutations in *SOCS-1,* which may play a role in their pathogenesis.[148] Rare cases of synchronous and metachronous lymphomas with one component consisting of mediastinal large B-cell lymphoma and a second component consisting of classical Hodgkin's lymphoma have been described.[149] These observations have led to the idea that mediastinal large B-cell lymphoma and nodular sclerosis classical Hodgkin's lymphoma are closely related entities, possibly sharing a common cell of origin and a common or similar pathogenesis.

With so many similarities, it is not surprising that in some cases, distinguishing mediastinal large B-cell lymphoma from mediastinal nodular sclerosis classical Hodgkin's lymphoma may be difficult. In favor of Hodgkin's lymphoma are an admixture of many reactive cells, especially eosinophils; neoplastic cells with an appearance convincing for Reed-Sternberg cells and variants; CD15 expression by tumor cells; diffuse bright CD30 expression by tumor cells; absence or weak, variable expression of B-cell antigens (CD20 and CD79a) on tumor cells; and absence of CD45 on tumor cells (Figure 4-13). Patients with mediastinal Hodgkin's lymphoma also seem to present with less severe symptoms related to the presence of a mass than those with mediastinal large B-cell lymphoma.

3. **Primary mediastinal large B-cell lymphoma versus mediastinal gray-zone lymphoma.** The term "B-cell lymphoma, unclassifiable, with features intermediate between diffuse large B-cell lymphoma and classical Hodgkin's lymphoma," or, informally, "gray-zone lymphoma," has been used to describe lymphomas with features intermediate between those of diffuse large B-cell lymphoma and classical Hodgkin's lymphoma in which subclassification is difficult. Gray-zone lymphomas most often are found in the mediastinum.[149,150] The typical histologic appearance is sheets of tumor cells that are more pleomorphic than in the usual mediastinal large B-cell lymphoma and that often resemble Hodgkin's cells, including lacunar variants. Reactive cells are more sparse than is usually seen in classical Hodgkin's lymphoma, but a mixed infiltrate, including eosinophils, may be present. Necrosis may be present, but it lacks the neutrophils often seen in Hodgkin's lymphoma with necrosis.[150] The immunophenotype usually is intermediate between classical Hodgkin's lymphoma and diffuse large B-cell lymphoma. CD45 and CD30 usually are positive, and CD15, Oct2, Bob1, and Pax5 are positive in most cases. B-cell markers such as CD20 and CD79a are often positive. ALK and immunoglobulin are not expressed.[150] Possible examples of gray-zone lymphomas include a lymphoma with morphology consistent with mediastinal large B-cell lymphoma but with an immunophenotype more like that of Hodgkin's lymphoma, and, conversely, a lymphoma with the morphology suggesting classical Hodgkin's lymphoma but with diffuse, strong CD20 expression. Another example of gray-zone lymphoma is one in which both the morphology and immunophenotype are intermediate between those typically associated with classical Hodgkin's lymphoma and mediastinal large B-cell lymphoma (Figure 4-14).

4. **Primary mediastinal large B-cell lymphoma versus thymoma.** Thymic epithelial neoplasms, particularly well-differentiated thymic carcinoma (WHO type B3), may mimic mediastinal large B-cell lymphoma on routinely stained sections. Cohesive growth and nested tumor cells with

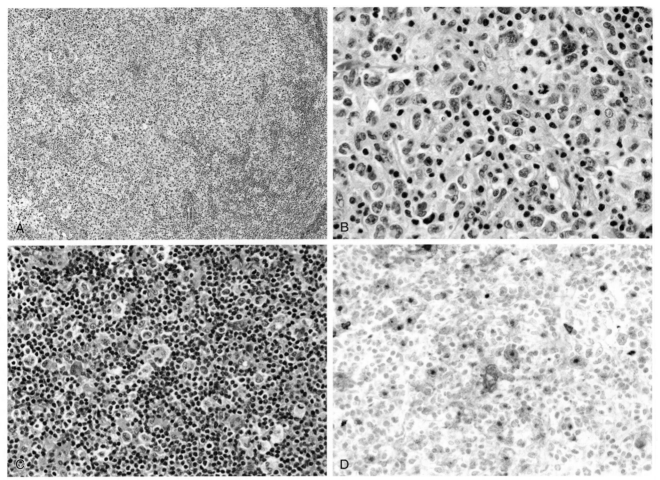

Figure 4-13   Nodular sclerosis classical Hodgkin's lymphoma, syncytial variant. **A,** In this case, neoplastic cells are abundant, forming a pale sheet that occupies much of the image. The numerous neoplastic cells could suggest a non-Hodgkin's lymphoma. **B,** Higher power view shows that the neoplastic cells include multinucleated and wreathlike forms, more in keeping with classical Hodgkin's lymphoma. **C,** In some areas, reactive cells, including many small lymphocytes and scattered eosinophils, are more numerous, and the appearance is more typical of classical Hodgkin's lymphoma. **D** to **G,** Immunophenotyping shows that the large atypical cells are positive for CD15 (**D,** membrane and Golgi pattern) and CD30 (**E,** membrane and Golgi pattern) and negative for CD45 (**F**) and CD20 (**G**).

distinct cell membranes and perivascular spaces favor thymoma (Figure 4-15). Immunophenotyping shows cytokeratin expression by the neoplastic cells and often an admixture of immature T cells (CD1a+, TdT+).

5. **Primary mediastinal large B-cell lymphoma versus germinoma.** Extragonadal germ cell tumors with the pathologic features of a seminoma are known as *germinomas.* A significant subset of these rare neoplasms presents as localized mediastinal masses. The age of affected patients overlaps with that of patients who develop mediastinal large B-cell lymphoma, but germinoma is seen virtually exclusively in males. It has an excellent prognosis.[151]

Microscopic examination reveals nests or sheets of large polygonal cells with large, oval nuclei that often are flattened along one edge; prominent nucleoli; and abundant, pale, glycogen-rich cytoplasm. The tumor is accompanied by a variably prominent lymphoid stroma, often with lymphoid follicles

and epithelioid granulomas (Figure 4-16). The histologic features are distinctive, but a certain amount of overlap exists with the morphology of mediastinal large B-cell lymphoma, and a definitive diagnosis may be difficult from a small biopsy sample. Immunophenotyping and special stains can establish a diagnosis, because the neoplastic germ cells are PLAP+ and Oct4+ (Figure 4-16, *C*), negative for lymphoid markers, and have PAS+ cytoplasm.

■ CARDIAC LYMPHOMAS

Primary Cardiac Lymphomas

Primary cardiac lymphoma, or lymphoma that arises in the heart, is rare. Cardiac neoplasms are quite uncommon, and only 1% to 2% of them are lymphomas. A diagnosis of primary cardiac lymphoma can be entertained only if the lymphoma is entirely or nearly entirely confined to the heart.[152-154]

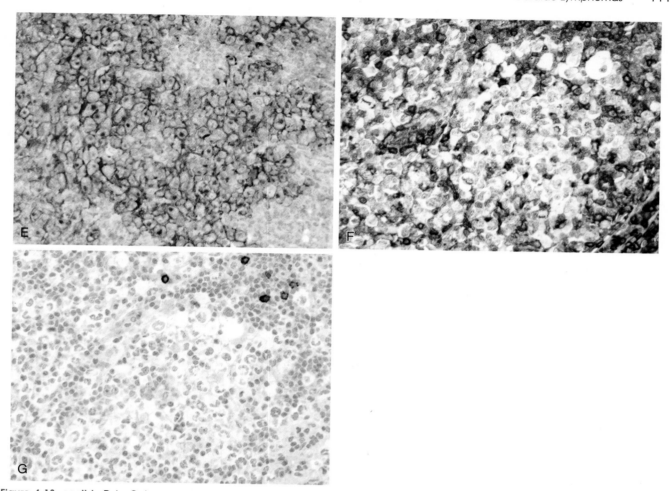

Figure 4-13, cont'd   D to G, Immunophenotyping shows that the large atypical cells are positive for CD15 (**D,** membrane and Golgi pattern) and CD30 (**E,** membrane and Golgi pattern) and negative for CD45 (**F**) and CD20 (**G**). (Immunoperoxidase technique on paraffin sections.) Compare to Figure 4-11, *E - G.*

Clinical Features

Primary cardiac lymphoma occurs in two clinical settings: (1) rarely and sporadically in immunocompetent patients and (2) infrequently in immunodeficient patients. Immunodeficiency is a significant risk factor for the development of primary cardiac lymphoma. In one review, nearly half of all patients with primary cardiac lymphoma were immunosuppressed, most often because of HIV infection, followed by iatrogenic immunosuppression in allograft recipients (Figure 4-17).[155] Cardiac lymphoma in immunocompetent individuals mainly affects older adults, and men and women are affected roughly equally.[152,153,155-158] Rare cases in children have been described.[159,160] Affected HIV-positive patients overall are younger, and a pronounced male preponderance is seen.[155] Presenting signs and symptoms vary from one patient to another and are deceptively nonspecific. They include chest pain, dyspnea, congestive heart failure, syncope, arrhythmias, and even complete atrioventricular block. Pericardial effusion is common and may be associated with tamponade.[153,155,158,161,162] Constitutional symptoms are uncommon (Table 4-6).

The lymphomas often form large masses, which ranged from 4 to 8.3 cm in one series.[158] They most often involve the myocardium, sometimes with extension to the pericardium. Involvement of valves is rare,[154] although rare cases of lymphoma arising in association with prosthetic cardiac valves have been described, which raises the question of whether lymphoma could be a rare complication of valvular replacement.[163-165] The lymphomas often involve more than one chamber of the heart, but the right side of the heart is involved more often than the left side, and the site most commonly involved is the right atrium. Left atrial involvement is uncommon,[155,158,161,166] although a case of lymphoma presenting with involvement of a left atrial myxoma has been reported,[163] and we have seen two such cases in our department (unpublished results).

Tumor localization can be defined by echocardiogram, CT scan, and/or magnetic resonance imaging (MRI). Transesophageal echocardiography is an especially sensitive technique for identifying these lesions.[167] The diagnosis may be based on examination of samples from an open biopsy done during thoracotomy, a transvenous endomyocardial

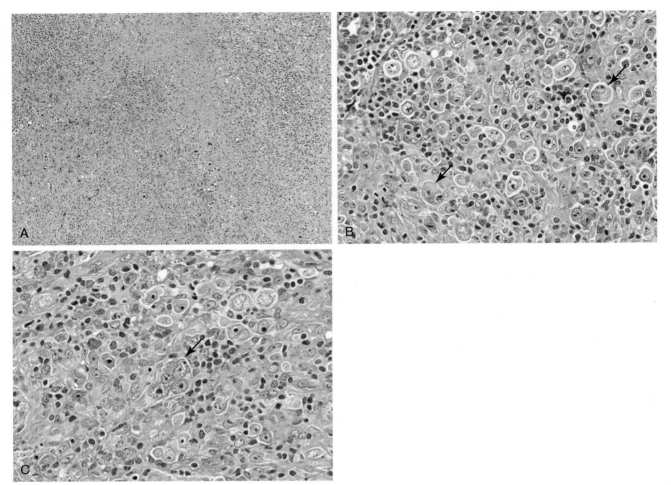

Figure 4-14   Mediastinal gray-zone lymphoma. **A,** Low-power view shows an atypical lymphohistiocytic infiltrate surrounding an area of necrosis. **B** and **C,** High-power view shows very large atypical lymphoid cells, including some binucleated forms (**B,** *arrows*) and multinucleated forms (**C,** *arrow*) in a background of lymphocytes and histiocytes. In contrast to typical Reed-Sternberg cells and variants, the nucleoli are blue rather than red and paranucleolar haloes are inconspicuous. Eosinophils are absent. Immunophenotyping showed that the large cells were CD20+ (diffuse, strong staining), Pax5+ (stronger staining than usual for Hodgkin's lymphoma), bcl6+, and CD15–, which is compatible with a diffuse large B-cell lymphoma; however, there was diffuse strong expression of CD30, dim to absent CD79a expression, and expression of Oct2 but not Bob1, which is more in keeping with classical Hodgkin's lymphoma. In this case, therefore, both the morphology and immunophenotype are intermediate between classic Hodgkin's lymphoma and diffuse large B-cell lymphoma.

biopsy, or an ultrasound-guided biopsy done during transesophageal echocardiography, or on cytologic examination of pericardial fluid. The cytologic features of pericardial effusions in these cases are not always diagnostic; a negative result does not exclude lymphoma.[155,157,166-168]

Historically the prognosis has been considered poor; diagnosis often was delayed and made only postmortem, and when chemotherapy was initiated, it could be accompanied by fatal arrhythmias.[153] The prognosis appears to be improving for more recent cases because of improvements in imaging, earlier diagnosis, and improvements in therapy, including careful monitoring of cardiac function at the beginning of therapy. Patients treated promptly with combination chemotherapy with or without radiation therapy may respond well and achieve complete remission.[152,154,158,161,169] The lymphomas arising in association with prosthetic cardiac valves appear to have a favorable prognosis, in some cases without

additional therapy after replacement of the valve involved by the lymphoma.[163,164]

Pathologic Features

Among both immunocompetent and immunodeficient patients, the lymphomas are nearly all the diffuse large B-cell type; their immunophenotypic features have not been extensively studied but appear similar to those found in other sites.[*] A CD20+, CD10+, bcl6+, bcl2+, and CD5– diffuse large B-cell lymphoma has been described; this case and one other showed a *BCL2* rearrangement—consistent with follicle center origin of at least some primary cardiac lymphomas.[158] The lymphomas involving prosthetic valves also have usually been the diffuse large B-cell type[163]; the few cases evaluated have been EBV+ (as determined by in situ hybridization for EBER) with

---

*References 153, 155, 158, 161, 162, and 168-170.

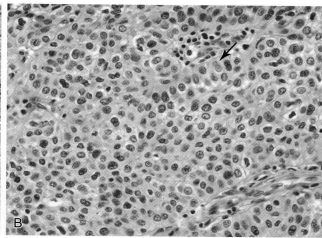

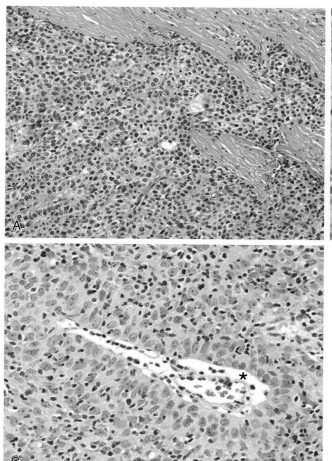

Figure 4-15   Well-differentiated thymic carcinoma (WHO classification, type B3 thymoma). **A,** Cohesive growth is conspicuous in this invasive focus at the periphery of the tumor. **B,** Higher power view shows many neoplastic cells with distinct cell borders and palisading along a blood vessel *(arrow)*, features that tend to exclude lymphoma. **C,** A perivascular space (*) within the thymoma is surrounded by palisading neoplastic epithelial cells.

a non-germinal center phenotype (CD20+, CD10–, bcl6+/–, bcl2+/–, MUM1/IRF4+).[164] The previously reported lymphoma involving an atrial myxoma also was a diffuse large B-cell lymphoma,[163] as were the two myxoma-associated lymphomas seen in our department; both had, in addition, the unusual feature of plasmacytic differentiation, and although the patients had no known immunodeficiency, the lymphomas both were EBV+ (Figure 4-18). Rare cases of primary cardiac low-grade B-cell lymphoma[158] and T-cell lymphoma (T-lymphoblastic[166] and ALK+ anaplastic large cell lymphoma[171]) have been reported. B-lymphoblastic lymphoma and Burkitt's lymphoma have been described in children (see Table 4-6).[159,160]

Differential Diagnosis

Because of the rarity of cardiac lymphoma and the nonspecific nature of the presenting signs, the diagnosis rarely is suspected before biopsy (or, in some cases, autopsy). Clinically it can mimic much more common, nonneoplastic causes of cardiac dysfunction. Once a mass has been identified radiographically, the combination of a right-sided tumor and high levels of lactate dehydrogenase (LDH), particularly in an immunocompromised patient, is suspicious for lymphoma. The most common mass lesion

that arises in the heart is a myxoma; in contrast to the preferential right atrial involvement shown by cardiac lymphoma, myxomas typically involve the left atrium.

Secondary Cardiac Lymphoma

Secondary involvement of the heart by lymphoma is much more common than primary cardiac lymphoma.[152,172] In one large autopsy series, 16% of patients with lymphoma had cardiac involvement.[173] In most cases the cardiac involvement was clinically silent, but 32% showed significant cardiac dysfunction attributable to lymphoma, including heart failure, tamponade, arrhythmias, and sudden death. Primary sites included both lymph nodes and a variety of extranodal sites, although most of the extranodal primary sites were in the head and neck.[173] Lymphoma secondarily involving the heart may involve any of its layers,[174,175] but epicardial involvement is almost uniformly seen, and myocardial and endocardial involvement is seen in only a subset of cases.[173] This is in contrast to primary cardiac lymphoma, which more consistently involves the myocardium.

B-cell, T-cell, and NK-cell lymphomas, and less often Hodgkin's lymphoma, may involve the heart

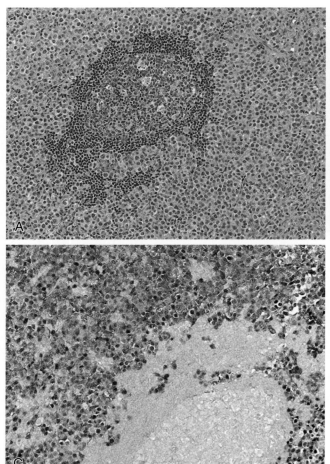

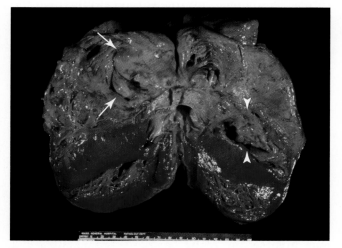

Figure 4-16 Mediastinal germinoma. **A,** Neoplastic germ cells surround a reactive lymphoid follicle. The cohesive growth of the tumor cells as they invade the follicle tends to exclude lymphoma. **B,** The neoplastic cells are large and have oval nuclei, fine chromatin, distinct nucleoli, and abundant, clear to light pink cytoplasm. A lymphoid follicle is in the lower right corner. **C,** Neoplastic germ cells are Oct4+ (immunoperoxidase technique on a paraffin section); they were also PLAP+ and CD117 (ckit)+, and negative for lymphoid markers (not shown).

Figure 4-17 Cardiac lymphoma in a renal allograft recipient. The heart has been bisected to reveal yellow-tan tumor extensively involving the right atrium *(arrows)* and the right ventricle, with tumor protruding into the cavity of the right ventricle *(arrowheads).* The left ventricle, at the bottom of the image, is spared. Microscopic examination revealed a diffuse large B-cell lymphoma (monomorphous post-transplantation lymphoproliferative disorder). (From Case Records of the Massachusetts General Hospital, Case 4-1985, *N Engl J Med* 312:226-237, 1985.)

TABLE 4-6

Principal Features of Primary Cardiac Lymphoma	
Frequency	**Rare**
Patients affected	*Immunocompetent patients:* Older adults; children (rare); slight male preponderance. *Immunodeficient patients:* HIV-positive patients, transplant recipients; marked male preponderance.
Clinical manifestations	Chest pain, heart failure, syncope, arrhythmias, pericardial effusion.
Distribution of tumor	Usually right side of the heart, especially right atrium; myocardium usually involved; cardiac valves typically spared.
Pathologic features	Diffuse large B-cell lymphoma predominates; other lymphomas rare.
Response to therapy and outcome	Many cases respond well to chemotherapy; outcome may be favorable with prompt diagnosis and optimal treatment.

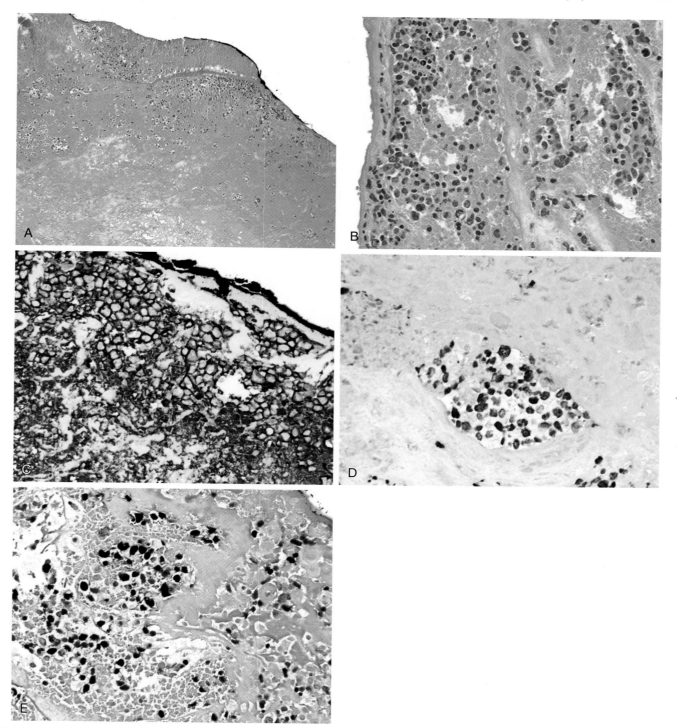

Figure 4-18   Diffuse large B-cell lymphoma involving a left atrial myxoma. This patient died several weeks after excision of the myxoma and had not received additional treatment for lymphoma. A complete autopsy did not reveal any residual lymphoma, confirming a diagnosis of lymphoma primary in this site. **A,** Scattered clusters of atypical lymphoid cells are seen in the hypocellular matrix of the myxoma. **B,** High-power view shows an area with large atypical, somewhat pleomorphic lymphoid cells. **C** and **D,** The large atypical lymphoid cells are CD20+ **(C)** and MUM1/IRF4+ **(D)** (immunoperoxidase technique on paraffin sections). Tumor cells also expressed monotypic cytoplasmic kappa light chain. **E,** In situ hybridization for Epstein-Barr virus (EBER probe) shows positive staining of the lymphoid cells.

secondarily. Among B-cell lymphomas, the diffuse large B-cell type is most common. We have seen an HIV-positive male who presented with cranial neuropathies and a mass in the region of the cerebellar-pontine angle that was considered suspicious for lymphoma, but who also had a cardiac mass. Endomyocardial biopsy revealed an HHV8+ diffuse large B-cell lymphoma. Large atypical cells similar to those seen in the heart also were identified in the cerebrospinal fluid (Figure 4-19).

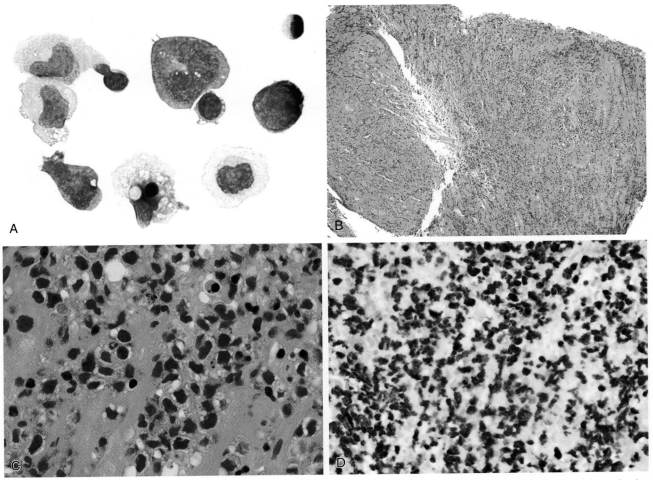

Figure 4-19   HHV8+ diffuse large B-cell lymphoma. **A,** A few highly atypical lymphoid cells with irregular nuclei and deep blue cytoplasm are present in the cerebrospinal fluid. Also present are a few monocytes with abundant, pale cytoplasm and small lymphocytes. (Wright stain, oil immersion.) **B,** Endomyocardial biopsy specimen shows tissue with an extensive interstitial cellular infiltrate. **C,** Higher power view shows that the cells are pleomorphic large lymphoid cells that resemble those in the cerebrospinal fluid. **D,** Tumor cells are positive for HHV8; they also expressed MUM1/IRF4 but were negative for CD20 (not illustrated). (Immunoperoxidase technique on a paraffin section.)

A variety of T-cell and NK-cell lymphomas have been seen, including peripheral T-cell lymphoma NOS, adult T-cell leukemia/lymphoma, anaplastic large cell lymphoma, Sézary syndrome, and extranodal NK/T-cell lymphoma, nasal type. Compared with B-cell lymphomas, a higher proportion of T- or NK-cell lymphomas appears to involve the heart secondarily. NK- or T-cell lymphomas also appear more likely to be associated with symptomatic cardiac disease in this setting. Hematogenous dissemination is the most common mode of spread to the heart, but mediastinal lymphoma, particularly primary mediastinal large B-cell lymphoma, may involve the heart by direct extension (see Figure 4-12).[173,176]

As for primary cardiac lymphoma, establishing a premortem diagnosis of secondary cardiac involvement by lymphoma may be challenging.[173] Because the presenting symptoms of cardiac lymphoma are nonspecific, some have suggested that, in patients with a history of lymphoma, the possibility of cardiac involvement by lymphoma should be considered whenever these patients develop symptoms related to the heart.[172]

■ LYMPHOMAS OF THE BREAST

Primary Lymphomas of the Breast

Introduction

Primary lymphoma of the breast usually is defined as lymphoma involving one or both breasts, with or without ipsilateral axillary lymph node involvement, without evidence of disease elsewhere at presentation, in a patient without a previous history of lymphoma. Tissue should be adequate for pathologic examination, and the lymphoma should be seen close to mammary tissue,[177] although some have relaxed the latter criterion if the diagnostic specimen is obtained through a needle biopsy.[178] Some authorities also accept cases in which staging reveals more distant lymph node or bone marrow involvement as long as, clinically, the primary or major manifestation of the lymphoma is the breast.[179]

The breast is an uncommon primary site for lymphoma, possibly because of the sparsity of endogenous lymphoid tissue at this site. Primary lymphoma of the breast accounts for 0.1% to 0.15%[179-182] of all malignant neoplasms of the breast, for 0.34% to 0.85% of all non-Hodgkin's lymphomas,[179,181,183-185] and for fewer than 2% of all extranodal non-Hodgkin's lymphomas.[179]

Clinical Features

Most patients are middle-aged or elderly women, although occasionally young women (and in rare cases, adolescents) are affected.[177,180,186-189] In most series, the median age is in the sixth or seventh decade.[178,181-185,190-198] Approximately 2% of patients with primary breast lymphoma are males.[178,181-185,191-198] Occasionally the disease affects pregnant or lactating women (see Lymphoma of the Breast in Pregnancy and Lactation, later in the chapter). In rare cases patients have previous breast carcinoma.[177]

Most patients present with a palpable breast mass with or without ipsilateral axillary lymphadenopathy.* The lesions typically are painless but in a few cases are painful.[197,199] A few patients have been asymptomatic, and the lymphoma was detected by mammography; lymphomas detected initially by routine mammography typically are low-grade lymphomas.[181,187,188,190] Constitutional symptoms are uncommon; they were found in 0[183,190,192,194,200] to 4%[196] of patients in different series. Patients presented with bilateral disease in 0 to 25% of cases in different series. Overall, slightly fewer than 10% of primary breast lymphomas are bilateral.† A few patients have a history of autoimmune disease, diabetes mellitus, or mastitis.[179,181,182,192] Several HIV-positive patients have developed lymphoma presenting with involvement of the breast.[202] However, most patients have no underlying illness, and specific factors predisposing to lymphoma of the breast have not been identified.[178,185,201]

On physical examination, patients usually have discrete, mobile masses. The overlying skin is involved infrequently; it may be thickened,[197] erythematous, or inflamed,[180,203] mimicking inflammatory carcinoma. Skin retraction and nipple discharge are virtually never found. The proportion of cases with ipsilateral axillary lymphadenopathy varies widely among series, ranging from 11%[187] to about 50%.

Mammographic Features

Although most breast lymphomas are not initially detected by mammography, they do have characteristic radiographic features. The most common finding is a solitary lesion with irregular or indistinct borders, in most cases lacking microcalcifications. In some cases, the lymphoma has a round border, potentially mimicking a benign condition. Less commonly, primary lymphoma of the breast manifests as multiple lesions or as diffuse, unilateral or bilateral enlargement of the breast.[178,192,197] In some cases of diffuse large B-cell lymphoma, routine mammograms obtained several months before the patients were found to have lymphoma were negative, probably because these aggressive lymphomas have a relatively rapid rate of growth.[185]

Pathologic Features and Clinicopathologic Correlates

In most series, diffuse large B-cell lymphoma is the most common type, comprising 43% to 94% of cases in different series and approximately 60% of cases overall.* The remainder are mainly low-grade extranodal marginal zone or follicular lymphomas. However, recent studies suggest that low-grade B-cell lymphomas may be more prevalent, with marginal zone lymphoma the more common, followed by follicular lymphoma.[182,188] In different series, extranodal marginal zone lymphoma accounts for 0 to 50% of cases and for approximately 20% of cases overall.† Follicular lymphomas account for approximately 6% of primary breast lymphomas. It is possible that a larger number of low-grade lymphomas are being detected because of identification of asymptomatic lesions by mammography,[188] and because with the wider recognition of marginal zone lymphomas and the greater variety of immunostains for paraffin sections, pathologists now are better able to recognize and diagnose these lymphomas. Burkitt's lymphoma is uncommon, and T-cell lymphoma is rare (Table 4-7).[178,188]

Although breast lymphomas may appear circumscribed grossly, on microscopic examination they often show some invasion into surrounding tissues at the periphery of the mass.[187] The neoplastic cells infiltrate around and within mammary ducts and lobules, sometimes obliterating these structures. In a few cases, the histologic changes of lymphocytic mastitis are described in association with primary breast lymphoma.[201,205]

Diffuse Large B-cell Lymphoma

Diffuse large B-cell lymphoma affects women (and a few men) over a wide age range, including some young patients.[181,189,192,196,198] The lesions range from 1 to 20 cm in greatest dimension, with a median size of 4 to 5 cm. A few patients have diffuse breast enlargement.‡ On average, therefore, these lymphomas are larger than carcinomas of the breast. They have been described as discrete, hard, rubbery,[193]

---

*References 178, 181, 183, 192, 194, and 197.
†References 177, 180, 182, 184, 185, 193, 194, 196, 198, 200, and 201.

*References 178, 180-184, 189, 190, 194, 195, and 204.
†References 178-184, 187, 190, 194, 195, and 204.
‡References 184, 185, 192, 194, 196, and 198.

TABLE 4-7

Principal Features of Primary Lymphoma of the Breast

Type of Lymphoma	Patients Affected	Histology	Usual Immunophenotype	Genetic and Cytogenetic Features	Clinical Behavior
Diffuse large B-cell lymphoma	Adults, females >> males, broad age range; few pregnant	Diffuse proliferation of large lymphoid cells; CB more common than IB	CD45+, CD20+, CD10 usually –; bcl6+/–, bcl2, and MUM1/IRF4 usually +; Ki67 high; non-GC > GC	No MALT1 rearrangements; possible NFκB activation in a minority	Aggressive; CNS, opposite breast most common sites of relapse; best outcomes with CHOP or CHOP-like chemotherapy +/– RT.
Extranodal marginal zone lymphoma (MZL)	Middle-aged or older adults; females >> males	Marginal zone B cells, plasma cells variable; reactive follicles may be present; LELs often not prominent	CD45+, CD20+, CD5–, CD10–, CD23–, CD43+/–, bcl2+/–, cyclin D1–, clg+/–	No MALT1 rearrangements; trisomy 3, 12, or 18 in a minority	Good prognosis; localized extranodal relapses possible. Few show large cell transformation. Few die of lymphoma.
Follicular lymphoma (FL)	Middle-aged or older women	Similar to lymph node FL	CD45+, CD20+, CD10+, CD5–, CD23–, CD43–, bcl2+, cyclin D1–, sIg+	N/A	Prognosis less favorable than for MZL; behavior similar to that of nodal FL.
Burkitt's lymphoma	Young or middle-aged females, few older women, some pregnant or lactating	Diffuse infiltrate of medium-sized round cells, many mitoses, starry sky	CD45+, CD20+, CD10+, bcl6+, bcl2–, Ki67 ~ 100%*	Translocation of MYC with IGH [t(8;14)], less often with IGK or IGL*	Very aggressive; disease often is widespread.
Anaplastic large cell lymphoma associated with implant	Women with saline or silicone implants for cosmetic purposes or after mastectomy; lymphoma occurs years after implantation; seroma rather than discrete mass	Large atypical, pleomorphic cells in background of inflammation and sclerosis	CD45+, CD30+, ALK–, some T antigen(s) commonly expressed; EMA usually +, EBV–, HHV8–	TCR: Clonal IGH: Polyclonal	Very good prognosis. Systemic spread is uncommon.

CB, Centroblastic; CHOP, cytoxan, doxorubicin, vincristine, prednisone; cIg, monotypic cytoplasmic immunoglobulin; CNS, central nervous system; EBV, Epstein-Barr virus; GC, germinal center immunophenotype; IB, immunoblastic; IGH, immunoglobulin heavy chain gene; IGK, immunoglobulin kappa light chain gene; IGL, immunoglobulin lambda light chain gene; LELs, lymphoepithelial lesions; non-GC, non-germinal center immunophenotype; RT, radiation therapy; sIg, monotypic surface immunoglobulin; TCR, T-cell receptor.
*Based on Burkitt's lymphoma in other sites. Immunophenotypic and cytogenetic features often are not given in detail in reported cases of mammary Burkitt's lymphoma.

soft, or fleshy masses[180] that sometimes enlarge rapidly.[177,193,203]

The lymphomas are composed of a diffuse infiltrate of large lymphoid cells (Figure 4-20). When these diffuse large B-cell lymphomas have been subclassified, most are centroblastic, a minority are immunoblastic,[178,180,195,206] and rare cases are diffuse large B-cell lymphoma, anaplastic variant, co-expressing CD30.[185] A few cases of diffuse large B-cell lymphoma have had a component of extranodal marginal zone lymphoma, consistent with large cell transformation of the low-grade lymphoma.[196,198] A case of intravascular large B-cell lymphoma presenting with breast involvement has been reported.[207]

The lymphomas are CD45+ and CD20+, and rare CD5+ cases are seen.[198] CD10 is expressed in a small minority; bcl6 is expressed in approximately half of cases; bcl2 is expressed in most cases; and MUM1/IRF4 is expressed in nearly all cases.[178,182,192,198,200] Most cases have a non-germinal center immunophenotype (CD10−, bcl6+, MUM1/IRF4+, or CD10−, bcl6−) (see Figure 4-20, C to F), and a minority has a germinal center phenotype (CD10+, bcl6+ or CD10−, bcl6+, MUM1/IRF4−).[178] The proliferation index is fairly high (60% to 95% in one series) (see Figure 4-20, G).[198] Immunostaining for p50 and p65 has shown nuclear localization of p50 in a minority of cases, which suggests NFκB activation in a subset of cases.[206] In situ hybridization for Epstein-Barr virus using a probe for EBER is typically negative.[198]

Genetic and cytogenetic features have not been extensively studied. The available data show no evidence of *MALT1* rearrangement, similar to mammary marginal zone lymphoma.[206] *IGH* variable region gene mutational analysis has shown a mutation frequency of 1% to 10%, usually without ongoing somatic mutation. In conjunction with the results of immunophenotyping, these findings suggest that neoplastic cells usually correspond to a post-germinal center stage of differentiation. Evaluation of V_H family usage appears to show preferential use of V_H4 and V_H3. Although only a few cases have been studied, all V_H4 cases used V_H4-34.[198] The findings suggest a nonrandom pattern of V_H usage.

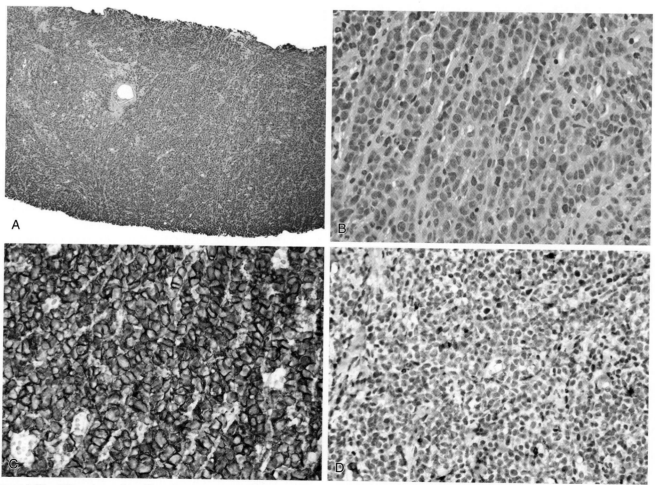

Figure 4-20   Diffuse large B-cell lymphoma of the breast with a non-germinal center immunophenotype. **A,** Core biopsy specimen showing replacement of tissue by a dense, diffuse cellular infiltrate. **B,** Higher power view shows large atypical, discohesive lymphoid cells with an Indian file–like pattern; interspersed apoptotic debris also is present. The large cells are B cells, strongly positive for CD20 **(C),** accompanied by a few interspersed small T cells **(D).**

Continued

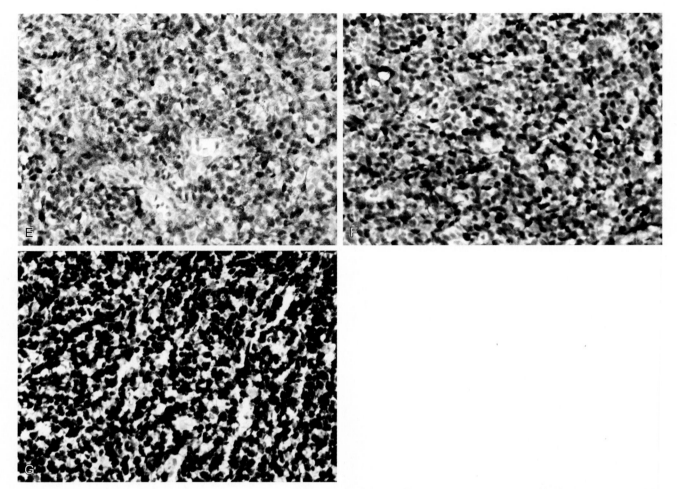

Figure 4-20, cont'd Most of the large B cells were bcl6+ **(E)** and MUM1/IRF4+ **(F)** and were negative for CD10 (not shown), which is consistent with a non-germinal center immunophenotype. The proliferation fraction, as assessed by Ki67, is high **(G)**. (Immunoperoxidase technique on paraffin sections.)

Staging, Treatment, and Outcome

Most large studies of diffuse large B-cell lymphoma primary in the breast include only cases with lymphoma confined to the breast (Ann Arbor stage I) or with spread to ipsilateral axillary lymph nodes (stage II).[185,196] The relative proportion of stage I and stage II cases varies among series, but overall more than 60% of patients have stage I disease. Most of the remainder have stage II disease, and a few have stage IV (bilateral breast) disease.[*]

Currently, patients with diffuse large B-cell lymphoma typically are treated with doxorubicin-based combination chemotherapy, accompanied in some cases by radiation therapy. Rituxan has been administered to a few patients, who appear to have benefited from this therapy.[200]

Relapses may involve lymph nodes and a wide variety of extranodal sites; among the latter, the central nervous system (CNS) and the ipsilateral and contralateral breast are most common.[†] CNS involve-ment is associated with a very poor prognosis[191,195]; for this reason, some authorities advocate the addition of CNS prophylaxis to the treatment regimen.[192,195]

A variety of clinical and pathologic features affects the prognosis. Patients treated only with local therapy have a worse outcome than those who receive combination chemotherapy.[182,184,191,192,196] In some studies, the addition of radiation is associated with a decreased risk of local relapse and an improved prognosis.[184,191,196] Mastectomy does not improve survival; obtaining a large enough biopsy sample for optimal pathologic evaluation is the only surgery needed.[192,194,196] Men and women have a similar prognosis.[196] Diffuse large B-cell lymphoma arising from marginal zone lymphoma and de novo diffuse large B-cell lymphoma do not show obvious differences in outcome.[196] In a number of studies, the tumor size and stage (stage I or stage II) did not affect the prognosis,[191,192,196] although other investigators have described a poorer outcome for those with stage II disease compared with patient who have stage I disease.[189] A trend for a worse outcome for patients with bilateral disease has been observed.[196] Some have described a worse outcome

---

[*]References 183, 191-193, 195, 196, 198, and 204.
[†]References 180, 183, 184, 189, 191, 192, 195, 196, 198, and 206.

for younger patients (under age 45 years)[189]; others have not noted this. Some have suggested a better outcome for patients with CD10+, bcl6+ lymphomas compared to those with CD10–, bcl6– lymphomas[192] and a worse outcome for those with a non-germinal center immunophenotype.[178] A 10-year overall survival rate of up to approximately 80% for optimally treated patients has been reported,[191] although most other series report less favorable outcomes.[178,196]

Extranodal Marginal Zone Lymphoma of Mucosa-Associated Lymphoid Tissue (MALT Lymphoma)

Clinical Features

Marginal zone lymphoma of the breast was first reported by Lamovec in 1987.[180] Marginal zone lymphoma mainly affects middle-aged and older women and, in rare cases, men.[179-181,183,187,204]

Pathologic Features

A description of features on gross examination is available in only a few cases; the lymphomas have ranged from about 1 to 7 cm, with a median size of about 4 cm.[180,183,187,204] Their histologic features are similar to those in other sites. The lymphomas are composed of small to medium cells with slightly irregular nuclei and a variable amount of pale cytoplasm. Reactive follicles, sometimes with follicular colonization, and plasmacytic differentiation, sometimes accompanied by Dutcher bodies, are found in some cases. Sclerosis typically is absent. Infiltration of epithelial structures by lymphocytes may be seen, but prominent, well-formed lymphoepithelial lesions tend to be less conspicuous than in marginal zone lymphomas involving some other sites.[178,181,187,206] Amyloid deposition in association with marginal zone lymphoma with plasmacytic differentiation has been described.[180]

The immunophenotypic features are similar to those found in other sites. The neoplastic cells are CD45+, CD20+, CD5–, CD10–, CD23–, CD43+/–, bcl2+/–, and cyclin D1–, with monotypic cytoplasmic immunoglobulin in cases with plasmacytic differentiation.[182] The cytogenetic features have not been studied extensively, but fluorescence in situ hybridization (FISH) studies have been consistently negative for rearrangements of *MALT1*.[206,208] In a minority of cases, trisomy 3, trisomy 12, and trisomy 18 each have been identified.[208] The absence of nuclear p50 and p65 expression indicates lack of NFκB activation.[206] The genetic defects leading to the development of marginal zone lymphoma of the breast are uncertain, and its etiology is not understood. Some have suggested that the lymphoma may arise from mucosa-associated lymphoid tissue acquired during lactation.[182]

Staging, Treatment, and Outcome

Most patients present with Ann Arbor stage I disease. A minority have involvement of ipsilateral axillary lymph nodes (stage II), and rare patients have more distant spread.[178,179,181-183,195] Treatment has varied; some patients have been treated with surgery only, some with radiation, and others with chemotherapy. Patients with marginal zone lymphoma typically remain well after treatment or develop relapses that usually are extranodal (the same or the opposite breast, subcutis, larynx, or chest wall) but occasionally involve lymph nodes as well, although usually without generalized disease.[179,180,204] Progression to diffuse large B-cell lymphoma has been reported.[180,187] A small proportion of patients dies of lymphoma, sometimes after large cell transformation.[187] In one study, the median disease-free survival time was 31 months, and the median overall survival time was 118 months.[178] Mammary marginal zone lymphoma, therefore, behaves in a manner similar to that of marginal zone lymphoma in other sites.[179,180,187,195]

Follicular Lymphoma

Follicular lymphoma affects middle-aged and older women.[183,187,204] Detailed information on the pathology is available in only a limited number of cases, but the tumors appear to range from 1.5 to 6 cm, with a median size of about 2 cm.[183,187,204] The histologic and immunophenotypic features are similar to those of nodal follicular lymphomas. Follicular lymphomas of all three grades have been reported.[187,188,192,194] Single cell epithelial infiltration has been described, which could be mistaken for lymphoepithelial lesions.[182] Neoplastic follicles typically are CD45+, CD20+, CD10+, CD5–, CD23–, CD43–, bcl2+, cyclin D1–, and monotypic immunoglobulin light chain positive.[182] Patients present with disease involving the breast, sometimes accompanied by axillary nodal involvement. Occasional patients have more widespread disease.[181-183,187,195,204] The prognosis does not appear to be as favorable as for those with marginal zone lymphoma; a number of patients had died of lymphoma or were alive with disease at the last follow-up.[187,195]

Burkitt's Lymphoma

Lymphomas classified as Burkitt's lymphoma or Burkitt-like lymphoma are found mainly in young or middle-aged women,[181,194,195,209] who are sometimes pregnant or postpartum (see Lymphoma of the Breast in Pregnancy and Lactation, later in the chapter).[181,194,195] Some patients are from Africa, consistent with endemic Burkitt's lymphoma,[210] although Burkitt's lymphoma also is encountered in Western countries.[209] (The pathologic features of Burkitt's lymphoma are discussed in detail in Chapter 5, under Lymphomas of the Gastrointestinal Tract.)

T-Cell Lymphomas

Primary breast lymphoma of T-lineage is uncommon, accounting for only about 2% to 3% of cases.[178,181,193] As with most other breast lymphomas, patients typically present with unilateral and occasionally with bilateral masses. Some of these lymphomas are ALK– anaplastic large cell lymphoma (ALCL, ALK–) that arises in association with breast implants (see Lymphoma of the Breast in Association with Implants, later in the chapter). Other types of lymphoma seen include ALCL with ALK+; peripheral T-cell lymphoma NOS, including both CD4+ and CD8+ cases; T-lymphoblastic lymphoma[178,181,199,211-213]; and subcutaneous panniculitis-like T-cell lymphoma.[204] Despite aggressive therapy in at least some cases, the lymphomas often disseminate and result in death. Based on the small number of cases, the prognosis appears poor; the behavior of these lymphomas overall is more aggressive than that of B-cell lymphomas in this site. An exception is ALCL that arises in association with implants, which has a good prognosis.

Other Rare Lymphomas

Rare cases of B-lymphoblastic lymphoma[178] that presented with localized involvement of the breast have been reported. Rare cases of classical Hodgkin's lymphoma also have occurred in this setting, typically with concurrent lymph node involvement, which suggests that the breast involvement actually was secondary.[178]

Lymphoma of the Breast in Pregnancy and Lactation

Lymphoma rarely presents in the breast in women who are pregnant or breast-feeding, but when it does, it has distinctive features. This phenomenon first received attention in cases of endemic Burkitt's lymphoma that resulted in dramatic, bilateral mammary enlargement,[214] although the breasts can be involved by lymphoma outside this clinical setting as well. As would be expected, almost all patients are in their 20s or 30s. Patients have been from Africa, the United States, Europe, and Asia.[*] They tend to present with rapidly enlarging breast masses that may be bilateral and extremely large. Some patients have localized disease,[222] but staging not infrequently reveals widespread disease involving a variety of extranodal sites (female genital tract, kidneys, CNS, and others), as well as lymph nodes in some cases.[215-217,219,221]

The lymphomas almost all have appeared to be aggressive B-cell lymphomas classified as Burkitt's lymphoma (or as small noncleaved cell lymphoma)[203,209,215-218,221] or diffuse large B-cell lymphoma,[†] although pathologic findings often have not been described in detail, and immunophenotyping studies sometimes are limited or were not performed at all. Most patients have died within a year of diagnosis; others, however, have been well 1 to 20 years later.[177,178,218,222] One well-documented case of ALCL including ALK+, which initially had been misinterpreted as adenocarcinoma on the basis of a fine needle aspiration cytology specimen, has been reported without follow-up.[223] ALCL including ALK– arising adjacent to an implant and diagnosed during pregnancy has been reported; this patient was treated and was well after 9 months of follow-up.[224] (See the next section, Lymphoma of the Breast in Association with Implants). Mediastinal T-lymphoblastic lymphoma[220] and mediastinal large B-cell lymphoma[225] presenting during pregnancy with breast masses have been described.

In all cases in which infants were delivered, including some that were born prematurely, the infants were well, whenever that information was given.[177,218-221,225]

The reason for the massive involvement of the breasts and poor outcome in this setting is uncertain. Possibilities include the hypervascularity that may characterize the breast during pregnancy and lactation,[216] immune modulation or decreased immune surveillance related to pregnancy,[217] and homing of neoplastic cells to hormonally stimulated tissue.[216] Another possible factor is delay in establishing a diagnosis or instituting therapy because of pregnancy.[183]

Lymphoma of the Breast in Association with Implants

Lymphoma has rarely arisen adjacent to breast implants used either for cosmetic purposes or for reconstruction after mastectomy for carcinoma.[204,224,226-228] This scenario accounts for only a small proportion of breast lymphomas; only 2% of cases in each of two large series of lymphoma involving the breast arose in association with an implant.[178,204] Despite the distinctive clinical and pathologic features of lymphoma in this setting, no convincing evidence has emerged in large epidemiologic studies to indicate an increased risk of non-Hodgkin's lymphoma in association with breast implants.[229] The implants studied have been the saline and silicone types; however, even saline implants typically have a silicone capsule, which has led to speculation about a role for silicone in the pathogenesis of lymphoma through an immunologic mechanism.[224,226,230-233] The interval from insertion of the implant to diagnosis of lymphoma has ranged from 1 to 23 years, with a median interval of about 7 to 8 years.[204,209,224,234-238] Curiously, in contrast to the marked preponderance of B-cell lymphomas among breast lymphomas in general, most lymphomas arising in patients with implants have been ALCL, ALK–.

Most patients with ALCL present with swelling related to a seroma adjacent to the implant, sometimes accompanied by tenderness or pain, and by erythema and warmth or ulceration of the overlying skin; however, a discrete mass often is absent.[204,224,226-228,234-238]

Microscopic examination reveals large atypical, pleomorphic, mitotically active cells with oval or indented nuclei, prominent nucleoli, and moderately abundant cytoplasm. often accompanied by

---

[*]References 177, 178, 183, 196, 203, 209, and 215-221.
[†]References 178, 183, 196, 209, 219, and 222.

a mixed inflammatory infiltrate composed of lymphocytes, plasma cells, histiocytes, and sometimes eosinophils, neutrophils, and giant cells in a sclerotic background (Figure 4-21).[227,234,238] Neoplastic cells may form a thin layer between necrotic material adjacent to the implant and surrounding fibrosis.[226] Refractile silicone may be identified adjacent to the infiltrate (Figure 4-21, A).[238] Cytologic examination of fluid from the seroma may reveal large numbers of neoplastic cells (Figure 4-21, D). The lymphomas have been CD30+, ALK−, and CD45+, with variable expression of T-cell antigens, often with loss of one or more pan–T-cell antigens. Expression of epithelial membrane antigen (EMA) is common. Cytotoxic granule proteins, such as TIA1 and granzyme B, often are expressed. EBV and HHV8 are absent.* Clonal rearrangement of the TCRγ chain gene usually can be demonstrated, whereas clonal B-cells are not found.[224,226,235,238]

Patients typically present with localized disease.[224,226,236] Treatment has varied but usually has included removal of the implant, with or without additional therapy[224,235,236,238] Follow-up is uneventful in most cases,[224,236-238] although in one case progression to systemic involvement occurred.[235] In a few cases, patients have presented with disease that has spread beyond the breast; the prognosis for these cases is uncertain.[209] Some investigators have suggested that ALCL in this setting is reminiscent of primary cutaneous ALCL (see Chapter 11), rather than systemic ALCL with ALK−, which is an aggressive lymphoma with a poor prognosis.[224] In contrast to most cases of primary cutaneous ALCL, however, these lymphomas often have been EMA+. Primary cutaneous ALCL secondarily involving the breast in association with an implant also has been described.[228]

Establishing a diagnosis may be problematic. The manner of presentation can lead to a clinical impression of inflammation, infection, or a leaking implant. The associated inflammation may obscure the neoplastic population. The neoplastic lymphoid cells may be mistaken for carcinoma, particularly in women previously treated for breast carcinoma. Familiarity with the rare occurrence of ALCL arising in association with a breast implant can help the pathologist establish a diagnosis.

Other types of lymphoma rarely involve the breast in association with an implant. In one remarkable case, a 46-year-old woman developed an HHV8+ primary effusion lymphoma in an artificial cavity adjacent to the capsule of a silicone breast implant. The lymphoma had anaplastic cytologic features; expressed CD30, CD45, and CD43; lacked other B- and T-cell–associated markers; and showed clonal rearrangement of the immunoglobulin heavy chain gene.[73] Four cases of mycosis fungoides/Sézary syndrome (beginning in three cases in the skin overlying the implant),[231,233] and one case each of follicular lymphoma[230] and lymphoplasmacytic lymphoma[232] have affected patients with breast implants. The

two B-cell lymphomas were widespread at presentation and likely did not represent primary breast lymphomas.[230,232]

Differential Diagnosis

The diagnosis of lymphoma of the breast is almost never suspected preoperatively. The clinical impression typically is carcinoma but also may be fibroadenoma or phyllodes tumor.[203] A number of problems in the differential diagnosis of lymphoma of the breast may arise, particularly when the specimen submitted is small or a diagnosis is requested on frozen section.

1. **Extranodal versus lymph node lymphoma.** Differentiating lymphoma in a low axillary or intramammary lymph node from a lymphoma involving the breast parenchyma itself is important and occasionally can be difficult, particularly on a small biopsy specimen. The area with the lymphoid infiltrate should be examined for evidence of an underlying lymph node, such as a discrete capsule, patent sinuses, or areas of residual, uninvolved lymph node, confirming nodal involvement; finding the infiltrate in continuity with ducts or lobules indicates breast parenchymal involvement.

2. **Diffuse large B-cell lymphoma and other aggressive lymphomas versus carcinoma.** Differentiating lymphoma from carcinoma may be difficult, especially in cases of lobular carcinoma with discohesive cells growing in Indian file[192]; lymphoma occasionally can mimic this pattern of growth (see Figure 4-20, B). In some instances, mastectomy and axillary lymph node dissection have been performed because of a mistaken diagnosis of carcinoma.[200] Careful study of the histologic features should raise the consideration of lymphoma. Cohesive growth or lumen formation by the tumor and ductal or lobular carcinoma in situ favor a diagnosis of carcinoma. A basic panel of immunostains, with antibodies to cytokeratin and B- and T-cell–associated markers, should establish a diagnosis.

3. **Lymphoepithelioma-like carcinoma and medullary carcinoma versus lymphoma.** Both lymphoepithelioma-like carcinoma and medullary carcinoma of the breast are associated with a dense lymphoid infiltrate; in this setting, neoplastic cells may be obscured by the lymphoid infiltrate or mistaken for large lymphoid cells. Lymphoepithelioma-like carcinoma produces an ill-defined mass with infiltrative borders. Neoplastic cells can be found as single cells, cords, nests, or sheets associated with a dense lymphoid infiltrate that may contain reactive follicles.[239] Medullary carcinoma takes the form of a well-circumscribed mass containing neoplastic epithelial cells with high nuclear grade and numerous mitoses growing in a syncytial pattern in a background of numerous lymphoid cells.[203] Careful examination of well-prepared slides is important in establishing a diagnosis. Atypical lobular hyperplasia and lobular

---

*References 224, 226-228, 234, 235, 237, and 238.

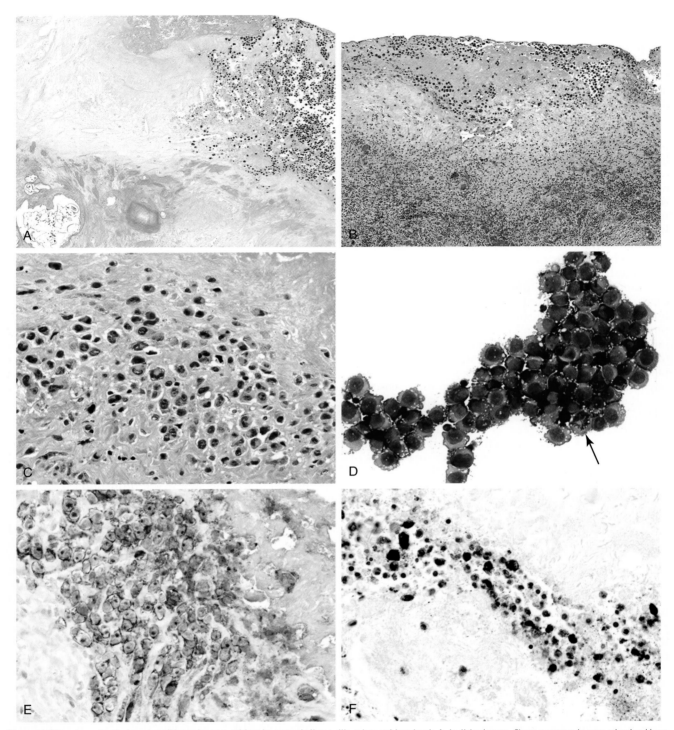

Figure 4-21   Anaplastic large cell lymphoma arising in association with a breast implant. **A,** In this dense, fibrous capsule are atypical lymphoid cells *(right)* and entrapped fragments of pale silicone *(lower left)*. **B,** Large atypical lymphoid cells are present in the fibrous capsule along the upper edge of the tissue; a prominent chronic inflammatory cell infiltrate, in the bottom half of the image, could obscure the neoplastic infiltrate. **C,** Higher power view shows large atypical cells with oval and indented nuclei, prominent nucleoli, and moderately abundant, eosinophilic cytoplasm. The cells with indented, C-shaped nuclei have the appearance of the hallmark cells characteristic of anaplastic large cell lymphoma. **D,** Fluid from an aspirated specimen shows large atypical cells with moderately abundant, basophilic, vacuolated cytoplasm. The arrow indicates a mitotic figure. (Wright stain.) **E** and **F,** Tumor cells are strongly positive for CD30 **(E)** and epithelial membrane antigen (EMA) **(F)**; they also were positive for CD4 and CD43 but were negative for Alk1 and many other lymphoid and nonlymphoid markers (not illustrated). (Immunoperoxidase technique on paraffin sections.)

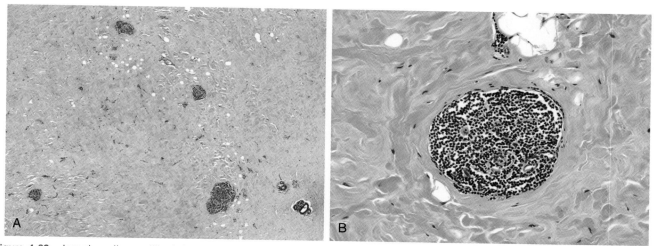

Figure 4-22   Lymphocytic mastitis. **A,** Low-power view shows dense, hypocellular, fibrous tissue with scattered small, discrete lymphoid aggregates. **B,** High-power view shows a tightly circumscribed perivascular aggregate of small lymphocytes.

carcinoma in situ have been reported in association with lymphoepithelioma-like carcinoma; atypical epithelium in lobules may provide a clue to the diagnosis of carcinoma rather than lymphoma.[239] Immunostains for cytokeratin and lymphoid-associated antigens can delineate reactive and neoplastic components in cases of carcinoma. Unlike in the nasopharynx, lymphoepithelioma-like carcinoma in the breast is negative for EBV; therefore, staining for EBV is not helpful.[239]

4. **Low-grade lymphoma versus reactive lymphoid infiltrate.** Dense reactive lymphoid infiltrates that may mimic lymphoma are unusual in the breast. One condition that may cause difficulty in differential diagnosis is diabetic mastopathy. This is an uncommon, reactive, fibroinflammatory process mainly encountered in women but also occasionally seen in men, who typically have long-standing type I diabetes mellitus. A few patients have had type II diabetes mellitus. The condition also may occur in patients with other immunologic disorders and in those who otherwise are well; in these cases, the condition may be referred to as "autoimmune mastopathy" or "lymphocytic mastitis." It usually presents as a unilateral, palpable breast mass (or less often as bilateral palpable breast masses) in young or middle-aged women, although older women may be affected.[210,240,241] Some patients have recurrences, which may be unilateral or bilateral.[240] Microscopic examination reveals a perilobular and/or periductal infiltrate of small lymphocytes and a variable number of plasma cells. The infiltrate may also be perivascular and may invade small blood vessels. Reactive lymphoid follicles may be present. Some cases show lobular atrophy and dense, keloidal fibrosis, sometimes with reactive epithelioid fibroblasts (Figure 4-22). Immunophenotyping reveals that the lymphocytes are predominantly B cells with varying numbers of T cells. Lymphoepithelial lesions composed of B cells are found in some cases. No clonal B-cell population is identified

through immunophenotyping or PCR.[210,241] The tight perilobular or periductal distribution, lack of cytologic atypia, and lack of clonal B cells, as well as the characteristic sclerosis, help distinguish this disorder from lymphoma.

In the differential diagnosis of marginal zone lymphoma and chronic inflammation, in favor of lymphoma are the presence of large numbers of B cells with the morphology of marginal zone cells outside follicles and monotypic immunoglobulin expression by the lymphoid cells or by admixed plasma cells. In distinguishing follicular hyperplasia from follicular lymphoma, criteria similar to those for follicular proliferations in lymph nodes can be used.

Secondary Lymphoma of the Breast

Secondary lymphoma of the breast includes cases of lymphoma that relapses in the breast and cases that present with widespread disease with involvement of the breast, such that the breast is unlikely to be the primary site. Lymphoma is thought to be the most common type of neoplasm to involve the breast secondarily.[242] In a number of studies that have included any lymphoma involving the breast, more secondary lymphomas have been seen than primary lymphomas,[178,181,187,243] which suggests that secondary involvement of the breast by lymphoma is more common than primary lymphoma of the breast. As for primary lymphoma, most patients are women, but a few men are affected.[178,181,187,204,243] Patients often present with a mass,[204] although radiologic evaluation more often reveals multicentric disease in the breast,[178,197] and the lesions tend to be smaller than in cases of primary breast lymphoma.[197]

Almost all are B-cell lymphomas, of a variety of types. The most common are diffuse large B-cell lymphoma, follicular lymphoma, and marginal zone lymphoma.* Less commonly, small lymphocytic

---

*References 178, 181, 187, 189, 204, and 243.

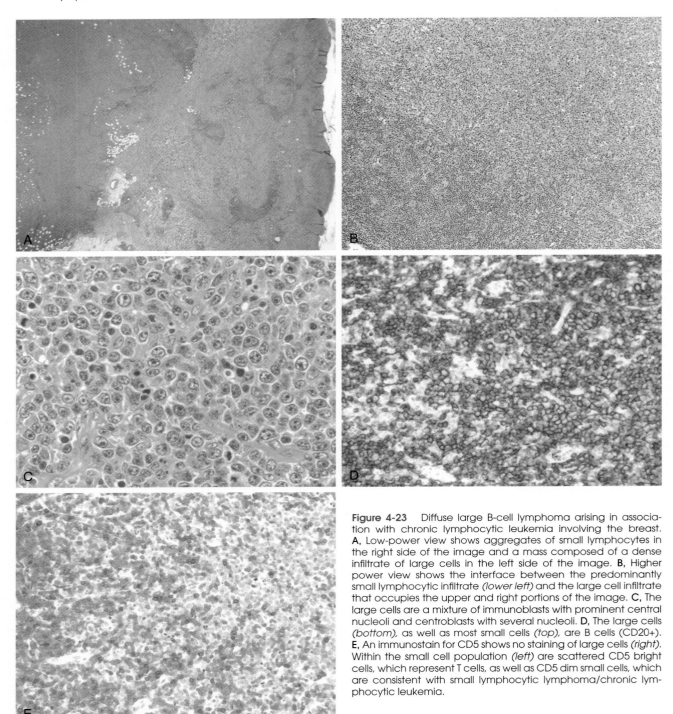

Figure 4-23 Diffuse large B-cell lymphoma arising in association with chronic lymphocytic leukemia involving the breast. **A,** Low-power view shows aggregates of small lymphocytes in the right side of the image and a mass composed of a dense infiltrate of large cells in the left side of the image. **B,** Higher power view shows the interface between the predominantly small lymphocytic infiltrate *(lower left)* and the large cell infiltrate that occupies the upper and right portions of the image. **C,** The large cells are a mixture of immunoblasts with prominent central nucleoli and centroblasts with several nucleoli. **D,** The large cells *(bottom)*, as well as most small cells *(top)*, are B cells (CD20+). **E,** An immunostain for CD5 shows no staining of large cells *(right)*. Within the small cell population *(left)* are scattered CD5 bright cells, which represent T cells, as well as CD5 dim small cells, which are consistent with small lymphocytic lymphoma/chronic lymphocytic leukemia.

lymphoma/chronic lymphocytic leukemia, mantle cell lymphoma, and B-lymphoblastic lymphoma involve the breast secondarily.[178,187,188,244] We have seen a case in which the breast was the site of Richter's transformation in a patient with a history of chronic lymphocytic leukemia. The breast was involved by small lymphocytic lymphoma/chronic lymphocytic leukemia in addition to diffuse large B-cell lymphoma (Figure 4-23). Cases of ALCL including ALK+, ALCL/ALK−, and primary cutaneous ALCL involving the breast at relapse or in the setting of widespread disease have been described.[178,228] Rare cases of peripheral T-cell lymphoma,[187,189,243] T-lymphoblastic lymphoma,[178] and classical Hodgkin's lymphoma[178] have been described. One case of mantle cell lymphoma initially was interpreted as probable diffuse large B-cell lymphoma on a breast biopsy specimen, although staging revealed widespread disease, and additional evaluation confirmed a diagnosis of mantle cell lymphoma.[244]

Several cases of adult T-cell leukemia/lymphoma have been reported in a study from Brazil, where the incidence of human T-lymphocyte virus 1 (HTLV-1) infection is relatively high.[204] We have seen a case of hairy cell leukemia that spread to involve the breast; without knowledge of the patient's history, distinguishing the leukemia from marginal zone lymphoma or even lobular carcinoma could have been difficult.[227] A case of EBV+ NK-cell lymphoma presenting with widespread disease, including breast involvement, has been described.[245]

The primary sites for the marginal zone lymphomas tend to be the salivary glands, the ocular adnexa, and soft tissue.[187] Primary sites for other types of lymphoma have varied but often have been lymph nodes. In rare cases, the B-lymphoblastic lymphomas have occurred in patients with chronic myelogenous leukemia who had developed lymphoblastic blast crisis.[178]

The outcome for patients with secondary lymphoma of the breast tends to be worse overall than for patients with primary lymphoma.[189] However, patients with marginal zone lymphoma may have isolated relapses in the breast, as well as other extranodal relapses, with a favorable outcome.[187] Patients with marginal zone lymphoma with large cell transformation may succumb to the disease.[178]

REFERENCES

1. Fidias P, Wright C, Harris N et al: Primary tracheal non-Hodgkin's lymphoma: a case report and review of the literature, *Cancer* 77:2332-2338, 1996.
2. Kaplan M, Pettit C, Zukerberg L, Harris N: Primary lymphoma of the trachea with morphologic and immunophenotypic characteristics of low-grade B-cell lymphoma of mucosa-associated lymphoid tissue, *Am J Surg Pathol* 16:71-75, 1992.
3. Louie BE, Harlock J, Hosein A, Miller JD: Laser therapy for an obstructing primary tracheal lymphoma in a patient with AIDS, *Can Respir J* 12:86-88, 2005.
4. Kang JY, Park HJ, Lee KY et al: Extranodal marginal zone lymphoma occurring along the trachea and central airway, *Yonsei Med J* 49:860-863, 2008.
5. Okubo K, Miyamoto N, Komaki C: Primary mucosa-associated lymphoid tissue (MALT) lymphoma of the trachea: a case of surgical resection and long term survival, *Thorax* 60:82-83, 2005.
6. Gaitonde S, Attele A, Abutalib SA et al: Extranodal natural killer/T-cell lymphoma, nasal type, in a patient with a constitutional 11q terminal deletion disorder, *Acta Haematol* 118:42-46, 2007.
7. Lee J, Won JH, Kim HC, Soh EY: Emergency dilation by self-expandable tracheal stent for upper airway obstruction in a patient with a giant primary thyroid lymphoma, *Thyroid* 19:193-195, 2009.
8. Jaremko JL, Rawat B, Naik S: Oesophageal and tracheal perforation in thyroid B-cell lymphoma, *Australas Radiol* 51(suppl):B193-B195, 2007.
9. Li G, Hansmann M, Zwingers T, Lennert K: Primary lymphomas of the lung: morphological, immunohistochemical and clinical features, *Histopathology* 16:519-531, 1990.
10. L'Hoste RJ Jr, Filippa DA, Lieberman PH, Bretsky S: Primary pulmonary lymphomas: a clinicopathologic analysis of 36 cases, *Cancer* 54:1397-13406, 1984.
11. Saltzstein SL: Pulmonary malignant lymphomas and pseudolymphomas: classification, therapy, and prognosis, *Cancer* 16:928-955, 1963.
12. Stefanovic A, Morgenszstern D, Fong T, Lossos IS: Pulmonary marginal zone lymphoma: a single centre experience and review of the SEER database, *Leuk Lymphoma* 49:1311-1320, 2008.
13. Rush W, Andriko J, Taubenberger J et al: Primary anaplastic large cell lymphoma of the lung: a clinicopathologic study of five patients, *Mod Pathol* 13:1285-1292, 2000.
14. Freeman C, Berg J, Cutler S: Occurrence and prognosis of extranodal lymphomas, *Cancer* 29:252-260, 1972.
15. Kurtin P, Myers J, Adlakha H et al: Pathologic and clinical features of primary pulmonary extranodal marginal zone B-cell lymphoma of MALT type, *Am J Surg Pathol* 25:997-1008, 2001.
16. Rosenberg SA, Diamond HD, Jaslowitz B, Craver LF: Lymphosarcoma: a review of 1269 cases, *Medicine* 40:31-84, 1961.
17. Addis B, Hyjek E, Isaacson P: Primary pulmonary lymphoma: a reappraisal of its histogenesis and its relationship to pseudolymphoma and lymphoid interstitial pneumonia, *Histopathology* 13:1-17, 1988.
18. Begueret H, Vergier B, Parrens M et al: Primary lung small B-cell lymphoma versus lymphoid hyperplasia, *Am J Surg Pathol* 26:76-81, 2002.
19. Cordier J, Chailleux E, Lauque D et al: Primary pulmonary lymphomas: a clinical study of 70 cases in nonimmunocompromised patients, *Chest* 103:201-208, 1993.
20. Ferraro P, Trastek V, Adlakha H et al: Primary non-Hodgkin's lymphoma of the lung, *Ann Thorac Surg* 69:993-997, 2000.
21. Kim JH, Lee SH, Park J et al: Primary pulmonary non-Hodgkin's lymphoma, *Jpn J Clin Oncol* 34:510-514, 2004.
22. Graham BB, Mathisen DJ, Mark EJ, Takvorian RW: Primary pulmonary lymphoma, *Ann Thorac Surg* 80:1248-1253, 2005.
23. Zinzani PL, Tani M, Gabriele A et al: Extranodal marginal zone B-cell lymphoma of MALT-type of the lung: single-center experience with 12 patients, *Leuk Lymphoma* 44:821-824, 2003.
24. Kawashima T, Nishimura H, Akiyama H et al: Primary pulmonary mucosa-associated lymphoid tissue lymphoma combined with idiopathic thrombocytopenic purpura and amyloidoma in the lung, *J Nippon Med Sch (Nihon Ika Daigaku zasshi)* 72:370-374, 2005.
25. Fairweather PM, Williamson R, Tsikleas G: Pulmonary extranodal marginal zone lymphoma with massive crystal storing histiocytosis, *Am J Surg Pathol* 30:262-267, 2006.
26. Xu HY, Jin T, Li RY et al: Diagnosis and treatment of pulmonary mucosa-associated lymphoid tissue lymphoma, *Chin Med J* 120:648-651, 2007.
27. Arkenau HT, Gordon C, Cunningham D et al: Mucosa associated lymphoid tissue lymphoma of the lung: the Royal Marsden Hospital experience, *Leuk Lymphoma* 48:547-550, 2007.
28. Nakamura N, Yamada G, Itoh T et al: Pulmonary MALT lymphoma with amyloid production in a patient with primary Sjögren's syndrome, *Intern Med* 41:309-311, 2002.
29. Teruya-Feldstein J, Temeck B, Sloas M et al: Pulmonary malignant lymphoma of mucosa-associated lymphoid tissue (MALT) arising in a pediatric HIV-positive patient, *Am J Surg Pathol* 19:357-363, 1995.
30. Aghamohammadi A, Parvaneh N, Tirgari F et al: Lymphoma of mucosa-associated lymphoid tissue in common variable immunodeficiency, *Leuk Lymphoma* 47:343-346, 2006.
31. Satani T, Yokose T, Kaburagi T et al: Amyloid deposition in primary pulmonary marginal zone B-cell lymphoma of mucosa-associated lymphoid tissue, *Pathol Int* 57:746-750, 2007.
32. Bhargava P, Rushin JM, Rusnock EJ et al: Pulmonary light chain deposition disease: report of five cases and review of the literature, *Am J Surg Pathol* 31:267-276, 2007.
33. Lim J, Lacy M, Kurtin P et al: Pulmonary marginal zone lymphoma of MALT type as a cause of localised pulmonary amyloidosis, *J Clin Pathol* 54:642-646, 2001.
34. Lantuejoul S, Moulai N, Quetant S et al: Unusual cystic presentation of pulmonary nodular amyloidosis associated with MALT-type lymphoma, *Eur Respir J* 30:589-592, 2007.

35. Okabe M, Inagaki H, Ohshima K et al: API2-MALT1 fusion defines a distinctive clinicopathologic subtype in pulmonary extranodal marginal zone B-cell lymphoma of mucosa-associated lymphoid tissue, *Am J Pathol* 162:1113-1122, 2003.

36. Streubel B, Simonitsch-Klupp I, Mullauer L et al: Variable frequencies of MALT lymphoma–associated genetic aberrations in MALT lymphomas of different sites, *Leukemia* 18:1722-1726, 2004.

37. Ye H, Liu H, Attygalle A et al: Variable frequencies of t(11;18)(q21;q21) in MALT lymphomas of different sites: significant association with CagA strains of *H. pylori* in gastric MALT lymphoma, *Blood* 102:1012-1018, 2003.

38. Remstein ED, Dogan A, Einerson RR et al: The incidence and anatomic site specificity of chromosomal translocations in primary extranodal marginal zone B-cell lymphoma of mucosa-associated lymphoid tissue (MALT lymphoma) in North America, *Am J Surg Pathol* 30:1546-1553, 2006.

39. Nicholson AG, Wotherspoon AC, Diss TC et al: Reactive pulmonary lymphoid disorders, *Histopathology* 26:405-412, 1995.

40. Dacic S, Colby TV, Yousem SA: Nodular amyloidoma and primary pulmonary lymphoma with amyloid production: a differential diagnostic problem, *Mod Pathol* 13:934-940, 2000.

41. Yamashita K, Haga H, Kobashi Y et al: Lung involvement in IgG4-related lymphoplasmacytic vasculitis and interstitial fibrosis: report of 3 cases and review of the literature, *Am J Surg Pathol* 32:1620-1626, 2008.

42. Shrestha B, Sekiguchi H, Colby TV et al: Distinctive pulmonary histopathology with increased IgG4-positive plasma cells in patients with autoimmune pancreatitis: report of 6 and 12 cases with similar histopathology, *Am J Surg Pathol* 33:1450-1462, 2009.

43. Liebow A, Carrington C, Friedman P: Lymphomatoid granulomatosis, *Hum Pathol* 3:457-558, 1972.

44. Lipford E, Margolich J, Longo D et al: Angiocentric immunoproliferative lesions: a clinicopathologic spectrum of postthymic T cell proliferations, *Blood* 5:1674-1681, 1988.

45. Guinee D, Jaffe E, Kingma D et al: Pulmonary lymphomatoid granulomatosis: evidence for a proliferation of Epstein-Barr virus infected B lymphocytes with a prominent T-cell component and vasculitis, *Am J Surg Pathol* 18:753-764, 1994.

46. Nicholson A, Wotherspoon A, Diss T et al: Lymphomatoid granulomatosis: evidence that some cases represent Epstein-Barr virus–associated B-cell lymphoma, *Histopathology* 29:317-324, 1996.

47. Myers JL, Kurtin PJ, Katzenstein A-LA et al: Lymphomatoid granulomatosis: evidence of immunophenotypic diversity and relationship to Epstein-Barr virus infection, *Am J Surg Pathol* 19:1300-1312, 1995.

48. Pittaluga S, Wilson W, Jaffe E: Lymphomatoid granulomatosis. In Swerdlow S, Campo E, Harris N et al, editors: *WHO classification: tumours of haematopoietic and lymphoid tissues,* ed 4, Lyon, 2008, IARC.

49. Katzenstein A, Carrington C, Liebow A: Lymphomatoid granulomatosis: a clinicopathologic study of 152 cases, *Cancer* 43:360-373, 1979.

50. Jaffe ES, Wilson WH: Lymphomatoid granulomatosis: pathogenesis, pathology and clinical implications, *Cancer Surv* 30:233-248, 1997.

51. Cuadra-Garcia I, Proulx G, Wu C et al: Sinonasal lymphoma: a clinicopathologic analysis of 58 cases from the Massachusetts General Hospital, *Am J Surg Pathol* 23:1356-1369, 1999.

52. Haque A, Myers J, Hudnall S et al: Pulmonary lymphomatoid granulomatosis in acquired immunodeficiency syndrome: lesions with Epstein-Barr virus infection, *Mod Pathol* 11:347-356, 1998.

53. Kameda H, Okuyama A, Tamaru J et al: Lymphomatoid granulomatosis and diffuse alveolar damage associated with methotrexate therapy in a patient with rheumatoid arthritis, *Clin Rheumatol* 26:1585-1589, 2007.

54. Muller FM, Lewis-Jones S, Morley S et al: Lymphomatoid granulomatosis complicating other haematological malignancies, *Br J Dermatol* 157:426-429, 2007.

55. Joseph R, Chacko B, Manipadam MT et al: Pulmonary lymphomatoid granulomatosis in a renal allograft recipient, *Transpl Infect Dis* 10:52-55, 2008.

56. Salmons N, Gregg RJ, Pallalau A et al: Lymphomatoid granulomatosis in a patient previously diagnosed with a gastrointestinal stromal tumour and treated with imatinib, *J Clin Pathol* 60:199-201, 2007.

57. Yazdi AS, Metzler G, Weyrauch S et al: Lymphomatoid granulomatosis induced by imatinib treatment, *Arch Dermatol* 143:1222-1223, 2007.

58. Swerdlow S, Webber S, Chadburn A, Ferry J: Post-transplant lymphoproliferative disorders. In Swerdlow S, Campo E, Harris N et al, editors: *WHO classification: tumours of haematopoietic and lymphoid tissues,* ed 4, Lyon, 2008, IARC.

59. Ray P, Antoine M, Mary-Krause M et al: AIDS-related primary pulmonary lymphoma, *Am J Respir Crit Care Med* 158:1221-1229, 1998.

60. Corti M, Villafane MF, Trione N et al: Primary pulmonary AIDS-related lymphoma, *Rev Inst Med Trop Sao Paulo* 47:231-234, 2005.

61. Lin Y, Rodrigues GD, Turner JF, Vasef MA: Plasmablastic lymphoma of the lung: report of a unique case and review of the literature, *Arch Pathol Lab Med* 125:282-285, 2001.

62. Bazot M, Cadranel J, Benayoun S et al: Primary pulmonary AIDS-related lymphoma: radiographic and CT findings, *Chest* 116:1282-1286, 1999.

63. Habermann T, Ryu J, Inwards J, Kurtin P: Primary pulmonary lymphoma, *Semin Oncol* 26:307-315, 1999.

64. Rodriguez J, Tirabosco R, Pizzolitto S et al: Hodgkin lymphoma presenting with exclusive or preponderant pulmonary involvement: a clinicopathologic study of 5 new cases, *Ann Diagn Pathol* 10:83-88, 2006.

65. Costa MB, Siqueira SA, Saldiva PH et al: Histologic patterns of lung infiltration of B-cell, T-cell, and Hodgkin lymphomas, *Am J Clin Pathol* 121:718-726, 2004.

66. Berkman N, Breuer R, Kramer M, Polliack A: Pulmonary involvement in lymphoma, *Leuk Lymphoma* 20:229-237, 1995.

67. Vega F, Padula A, Valbuena JR et al: Lymphomas involving the pleura: a clinicopathologic study of 34 cases diagnosed by pleural biopsy, *Arch Pathol Lab Med* 130:1497-1502, 2006.

68. Mitchell A, Meunier C, Ouellette D, Colby T: Extranodal marginal zone lymphoma of mucosa-associated lymphoid tissue with initial presentation in the pleura, *Chest* 129:791-794, 2006.

69. Said J, Cesarman E: Primary effusion lymphoma. In Swerdlow S, Campo E, Harris N et al, editors: *WHO classification: tumours of haematopoietic and lymphoid tissues,* ed 4, Lyon, 2008, IARC.

70. Chan J, Aozasa K, Gaulard P: DLBCL associated with chronic inflammation. In Swerdlow S, Campo E, Harris N et al, editors: *WHO classification: tumours of haematopoietic and lymphoid tissues,* ed 4, Lyon, 2008, IARC.

71. Cesarman E, Chang Y, Moore PS et al: Kaposi's sarcoma–associated herpes virus–like DNA sequences in AIDS-related body cavity–based lymphomas, *N Engl J Med* 332:1186-1191, 1995.

72. Nador R, Cesarman E, Chadburn A et al: Primary effusion lymphoma: a distinct clinicopathologic entity associated with the Kaposi's sarcoma–associated herpes virus, *Blood* 88:645-656, 1996.

73. Said JW, Tasaka T, Takeuchi S et al: Primary effusion lymphoma in women: report of two cases of Kaposi's sarcoma herpes virus–associated effusion-based lymphoma in human immunodeficiency virus–negative women, *Blood* 88:3124-3128, 1996.

74. Ferry J, Harris N: *Atlas of lymphoid hyperplasia and lymphoma,* Philadelphia, 1997, Saunders.

75. Klepfish A, Sarid R, Shtalrid M et al: Primary effusion lymphoma (PEL) in HIV-negative patients: a distinct clinical entity, *Leuk Lymphoma* 41:439-443, 2001.

76. Boulanger E, Gerard L, Gabarre J et al: Prognostic factors and outcome of human herpesvirus 8–associated primary effusion lymphoma in patients with AIDS, *J Clin Oncol* 23:4372-4380, 2005.

77. Carbone A, Gloghini A: AIDS-related lymphomas: from pathogenesis to pathology, *Br J Haematol* 130:662-670, 2005.

78. Cesarman E, Knowles D: Kaposi's sarcoma–associated herpesvirus: a lymphotropic human herpesvirus associated with Kaposi's sarcoma, primary effusion lymphoma and multicentric Castleman's disease, *Semin Diagn Pathol* 14:54-66, 1997.

79. Chadburn A, Hyjek E, Mathew S et al: KSHV-positive solid lymphomas represent an extra-cavitary variant of primary effusion lymphoma, *Am J Surg Pathol* 28:1401-1416, 2004.

80. Carbone A, Gloghini A, Cozzi MR et al: Expression of MUM1/IRF4 selectively clusters with primary effusion lymphoma among lymphomatous effusions: implications for disease histogenesis and pathogenesis, *Br J Haematol* 111:247-257, 2000.

81. Sirianni MC, Libi F, Campagna M et al: Downregulation of the major histocompatibility complex class I molecules by human herpesvirus type 8 and impaired natural killer cell activity in primary effusion lymphoma development, *Br J Haematol* 130:92-95, 2005.

82. Gaidano G, Capello D, Cilia AM et al: Genetic characterization of HHV-8/KSHV-positive primary effusion lymphoma reveals frequent mutations of BCL6: implications for disease pathogenesis and histogenesis, *Gen Chrom Canc* 24:16-23, 1999.

83. Hamoudi R, Diss TC, Oksenhendler E et al: Distinct cellular origins of primary effusion lymphoma with and without EBV infection, *Leuk Res* 28:333-338, 2004.

84. Klein U, Gloghini A, Gaidano G et al: Gene expression profile analysis of AIDS-related primary effusion lymphoma (PEL) suggests a plasmablastic derivation and identifies PEL-specific transcripts, *Blood* 101:4115-4121, 2003.

85. Jenner RG, Boshoff C: The molecular pathology of Kaposi's sarcoma–associated herpesvirus, *Biochim Biophys Acta* 1602:1-22, 2002.

86. Isaacson P, Campo E, Harris N: Large B-cell lymphoma arising in HHV8-associated multicentric Castleman's disease. In Swerdlow S, Campo E, Harris N et al, editors: *WHO classification: tumours of haematopoietic and lymphoid tissues*, ed 4, Lyon, 2008, IARC.

87. Carbone A, Gloghini A, Vaccher E et al: Kaposi's sarcoma–associated herpesvirus/human herpesvirus type 8–positive solid lymphomas: a tissue-based variant of primary effusion lymphoma, *J Mol Diagn* 7:17-27, 2005.

88. DePond W, Said J, Tasaka T et al: Kaposi's sarcoma–associated herpesvirus and human herpesvirus 8 (KSHV/HHV8)–associated lymphoma of the bowel: report of two cases in HIV-positive men with secondary effusion lymphomas, *Am J Surg Pathol* 21:719-724, 1997.

89. Carbone A, Gloghini A, Vaccher E et al: KSHV/HHV-8 associated lymph node based lymphomas in HIV seronegative subjects: report of two cases with anaplastic large cell morphology and plasmablastic immunophenotype, *J Clin Pathol* 58:1039-1045, 2005.

90. Deloose ST, Smit LA, Pals FT et al: High incidence of Kaposi sarcoma–associated herpesvirus infection in HIV-related solid immunoblastic/plasmablastic diffuse large B-cell lymphoma, *Leukemia* 19:851-855, 2005.

91. Aozasa K: Pyothorax-associated lymphoma, *J Clin Exp Hematop* 46:5-10, 2006.

92. Petitjean B, Jardin F, Joly B et al: Pyothorax-associated lymphoma: a peculiar clinicopathologic entity derived from B cells at late stage of differentiation and with occasional aberrant dual B- and T-cell phenotype, *Am J Surg Pathol* 26:724-732, 2002.

93. Ichinohasama R, Miura I, Kobayashi N et al: Herpes virus type 8–negative primary effusion lymphoma associated with PAX-5 gene rearrangement and hepatitis C virus: a case report and review of the literature, *Am J Surg Pathol* 22:1528-1537, 1998.

94. Ascoli V, Lo Coco F, Mecucci C: Herpes virus 8–negative primary effusion lymphoma associated with hepatitis C virus, *Am J Surg Pathol* 24:157-158, 2000.

95. Carbone A, Gloghini A: PEL and HHV8-unrelated effusion lymphomas: classification and diagnosis, *Cancer* 114:225-227, 2008.

96. Kobayashi Y, Kamitsuji Y, Kuroda J et al: Comparison of human herpes virus 8 related primary effusion lymphoma with human herpes virus 8 unrelated primary effusion lymphoma–like lymphoma on the basis of HIV: report of 2 cases and review of 212 cases in the literature, *Acta Haematol* 117:132-144, 2007.

97. Terasaki Y, Okumura H, Saito K et al: HHV-8/KSHV-negative and CD20-positive primary effusion lymphoma successfully treated by pleural drainage followed by chemotherapy containing rituximab, *Intern Med* 47:2175-2178, 2008.

98. Keller A, Castleman B: Hodgkin's disease of the thymus gland, *Cancer* 33:1615-1623, 1974.

99. Palutke M, Tranchida L: T-cell lymphoma: report of a case, *Am J Clin Pathol* 64:26-33, 1975.

100. Chetty R, Pulford K, Jones M et al: SCL-Tal-1 expression in T-acute lymphoblastic leukemia: an immunohistochemical and genotypic study, *Hum Pathol* 26:994-998, 1995.

101. Sheibani K, Winberg C, Burke J: Lymphoblastic lymphoma expressing natural killer cell–associated antigens: a clinicopathologic study of six cases, *Leuk Res* 11:371-377, 1987.

102. Borowitz M, Chan J: T lymphoblastic leukaemia/lymphoma. In Swerdlow S, Campo E, Harris N et al, editors: *WHO classification: tumours of haematopoietic and lymphoid tissues*, ed 4, Lyon, 2008, IARC.

103. Hashimoto M, Yamashita Y, Mori N: Immunohistochemical detection of CD79a expression in precursor T cell lymphoblastic lymphoma/leukaemias, *J Pathol* 197:341-347, 2002.

104. Grabher C, von Boehmer H, Look AT: Notch 1 activation in the molecular pathogenesis of T-cell acute lymphoblastic leukaemia, *Nature Reviews* 6:347-359, 2006.

105. Isaacson P, Chan J, Tang C, Addis B: Low-grade B-cell lymphoma of mucosa-associated lymphoid tissue arising in the thymus: a thymic lymphoma mimicking myoepithelial sialadenitis, *Am J Surg Pathol* 14:342-351, 1990.

106. Inagaki H, Chan J, Ng J et al: Primary thymic extranodal marginal zone B-cell lymphoma of mucosa-associated lymphoid tissue type exhibits distinctive clinicopathological and molecular features, *Am J Pathol* 160:1435-1443, 2002.

107. Kamimura K, Nakamura N, Ishibashi T et al: Somatic hypermutation of immunoglobulin heavy chain variable region genes in thymic marginal zone B-cell lymphoma of MALT type of a patient with Sjögren's syndrome, *Histopathology* 40:294-304, 2002.

108. Lorsbach R, Pinkus G, Shahsafaei A, Dorfman D: Primary marginal zone lymphoma of the thymus, *Am J Clin Pathol* 113:784-791, 2000.

109. Ortonne N, Copie-Bergman C, Remy P et al: Mucosa-associated lymphoid tissue lymphoma of the thymus: a case report with no evidence of MALT1 rearrangement, *Virchows Arch* 446:189-193, 2005.

110. Parrens M, Dubus P, Danjoux M et al: Mucosa-associated lymphoid tissue of the thymus: hyperplasia vs lymphoma, *Am J Clin Pathol* 117:51-56, 2002.

111. Shimizu K, Ishii G, Nagai K et al: Extranodal marginal zone B-cell lymphoma of mucosa-associated lymphoid tissue (MALT lymphoma) in the thymus: report of four cases, *Jpn J Clin Oncol* 35:412-416, 2005.

112. Kinoshita N, Ashizawa K, Abe K et al: Mucosa-associated lymphoid tissue lymphoma of the thymus associated with Sjögren's syndrome: report of a case, *Surg Today* 38:436-439, 2008.

113. Maeda A, Hayama M, Nakata M et al: Mucosa-associated lymphoid tissue lymphoma in the thymus of a patient with systemic lupus erythematosus, *Gen Thorac Cardiovasc Surg* 56:288-291, 2008.

114. Sakamoto T, Yamashita K, Mizumoto C et al: MALT lymphoma of the thymus with Sjögren's syndrome: biphasic changes in serological abnormalities over a 4-year period following thymectomy, *Int J Hematol* 89:709-713, 2009.

115. Strobel P, Marino M, Feuchtenberger M et al: Micronodular thymoma: an epithelial tumour with abnormal chemokine expression setting the stage for lymphoma development, *J Pathol* 207:72-82, 2005.

116. Yoshida M, Okabe M, Eimoto T et al: Immunoglobulin VH genes in thymic MALT lymphoma are biased toward a restricted repertoire and are frequently unmutated, *J Pathol* 208:415-422, 2006.

117. Suster S, Moran C: Micronodular thymoma with lymphoid B-cell hyperplasia: clinicopathologic and immunohistochemical study of eighteen cases of a distinctive morphologic variant of thymic epithelial neoplasm, *Am J Surg Pathol* 23:955-962, 1999.

118. Lichtenstein A, Levine A, Taylor C et al: Primary mediastinal lymphoma in adults, *Am J Med* 68:509-514, 1980.

119. Harris NL, Jaffe ES, Stein H et al: A revised European-American classification of lymphoid neoplasms: a proposal from the International Lymphoma Study Group, *Blood* 84:1361-1392, 1994.

120. Gaulard P, Stein H, Harris N et al: Primary mediastinal (thymic) large B-cell lymphoma. In Swerdlow S, Campo E, Harris N et al, editors: *WHO classification: tumours of haematopoietic and lymphoid tissues,* ed 4, Lyon, 2008, IARC.

121. Al-Sharabati M, Chittal S, Duga-Neulat I et al: Primary anterior mediastinal B-cell lymphoma, *Cancer* 67:2579-2587, 1991.

122. Cazals-Hatem D, Lepage E, Brice P et al: Primary mediastinal large B-cell lymphoma: a clinicopathologic study of 141 cases compared with 916 nonmediastinal large B-cell lymphomas—a GELA ("Groupe d'Etude des Lymphomes de l"Adulte") study, *Am J Surg Pathol* 20:877-888, 1996.

123. de Leval L, Ferry J, Falini B et al: Expression of bcl-6 and CD10 in primary mediastinal large cell lymphoma: evidence for derivation from germinal center B cells? *Am J Surg Pathol* 25:1277-1282, 2001.

124. Joos S, Otano-Joos M, Ziegler S et al: Primary mediastinal (thymic) B-cell lymphoma is characterized by gains of chromosomal material including 9p and amplification of the REL gene, *Blood* 87:1571-1578, 1996.

125. Lazzarino M, Orlandi E, Paulli M et al: Treatment outcome and prognostic factors for primary mediastinal (thymic) B-cell lymphoma: a multicenter study of 106 patients, *J Clin Oncol* 15:1646-1653, 1997.

126. Savage KJ, Al-Rajhi N, Voss N et al: Favorable outcome of primary mediastinal large B-cell lymphoma in a single institution: the British Columbia experience, *Ann Oncol* 17:123-130, 2006.

127. Todeschini G, Secchi S, Morra E et al: Primary mediastinal large B-cell lymphoma (PMLBCL): long-term results from a retrospective multicentre Italian experience in 138 patients treated with CHOP or MACOP-B/VACOP-B, *Br J Cancer* 90:372-376, 2004.

128. Zinzani P, Martelli M, Bertini M et al: Induction chemotherapy strategies for primary mediastinal large B-cell lymphoma with sclerosis: a retrospective multinational study on 426 previously untreated patients, *Haematologica* 87:1258-1264, 2002.

129. De Sanctis V, Finolezzi E, Osti MF et al: MACOP-B and involved-field radiotherapy is an effective and safe therapy for primary mediastinal large B cell lymphoma, *Int J Radiat Oncol Biol Phys* 72:1154-1160, 2008.

130. Burkhardt B, Zimmermann M, Oschlies I et al: The impact of age and gender on biology, clinical features and treatment outcome of non-Hodgkin lymphoma in childhood and adolescence, *Br J Haematol* 131:39-49, 2005.

131. Paulli M, Strater J, Gianelli U et al: Mediastinal B-cell lymphoma: a study of its histomorphologic spectrum based on 109 cases, *Hum Pathol* 30:178-187, 1999.

132. Addis B, Isaacson P: Large cell lymphoma of the mediastinum: a B-cell tumor of probable thymic origin, *Histopathology* 10:379-390, 1986.

133. Rosenwald A, Wright G, Leroy K et al: Molecular diagnosis of primary mediastinal B cell lymphoma identifies a clinically favorable subgroup of diffuse large B-cell lymphoma related to Hodgkin lymphoma, *J Exp Med* 198:851-862, 2003.

134. Aisenberg AC: Primary large cell lymphoma of the mediastinum, *Semin Oncol* 26:251-258, 1999.

135. Savage KJ: Primary mediastinal large B-cell lymphoma, *Oncologist* 11:488-495, 2006.

136. Calaminici M, Piper K, Lee AM, Norton AJ: CD23 expression in mediastinal large B-cell lymphomas, *Histopathology* 45:619-624, 2004.

137. Copie-Bergman C, Gaulard P, Maouche-Chretien L et al: The MAL gene is expressed in primary mediastinal large B-cell lymphoma, *Blood* 94:3567-3575, 1999.

138. Calvo KR, Traverse-Glehen A, Pittaluga S, Jaffe ES: Molecular profiling provides evidence of primary mediastinal large B-cell lymphoma as a distinct entity related to classic Hodgkin lymphoma: implications for mediastinal gray zone lymphomas as an intermediate form of B-cell lymphoma, *Adv Anat Pathol* 11:227-238, 2004.

139. Feuerhake F, Kutok JL, Monti S et al: NFκB activity, function, and target-gene signatures in primary mediastinal large B-cell lymphoma and diffuse large B-cell lymphoma subtypes, *Blood* 106:1392-1399, 2005.

140. Savage K, Monti S, Kutok J et al: The molecular signature of mediastinal large B-cell lymphoma differs from that of other diffuse large B-cell lymphomas and shares features with classical Hodgkin lymphoma, *Blood* 102:3871-3879, 2003.

141. Rodig S, Savage K, LaCasce A et al: Expression of TRAF1 and nuclear c-Rel distinguishes primary mediastinal large cell lymphoma from other types of diffuse large B-cell lymphoma, *Am J Surg Pathol* 31:106-112, 2007.

142. Rodig SJ, Savage KJ, Nguyen V et al: TRAF1 expression and c-Rel activation are useful adjuncts in distinguishing classical Hodgkin lymphoma from a subset of morphologically or immunophenotypically similar lymphomas, *Am J Surg Pathol* 29:196-203, 2005.

143. Guiter C, Dusanter-Fourt I, Copie-Bergman C et al: Constitutive STAT6 activation in primary mediastinal large B-cell lymphoma, *Blood* 104:543-549, 2004.

144. Rehm A, Anagnostopoulos I, Gerlach K et al: Identification of a chemokine receptor profile characteristic for mediastinal large B-cell lymphoma, *Int J Cancer* 125:2367-2374, 2009.

145. Leithauser F, Bauerle M, Huynh M, Moller P: Isotype-switched immunoglobulin genes with a high load of somatic hypermutation and lack of ongoing mutational activity are prevalent in mediastinal B-cell lymphoma, *Blood* 98:2762-2770, 2001.

146. Renne C, Willenbrock K, Martin-Subero JI et al: High expression of several tyrosine kinases and activation of the PI3K/AKT pathway in mediastinal large B cell lymphoma reveals further similarities to Hodgkin lymphoma, *Leukemia* 21:780-787, 2007.

147. Melzner I, Weniger M, Bucur A et al: Biallelic deletion within 16p13.13 including SOCS-1 in Karpas 1106P mediastinal B-cell lymphoma line is associated with delayed degradation of JAK2 protein, *Int J Cancer* 118:1941-1944, 2006.

148. Weniger MA, Melzner I, Menz CK et al: Mutations of the tumor suppressor gene SOCS-1 in classical Hodgkin lymphoma are frequent and associated with nuclear phospho-STAT5 accumulation, *Oncogene* 25:2679-2684, 2006.

149. Traverse-Glehen A, Pittaluga S, Gaulard P et al: Mediastinal gray zone lymphoma: the missing link between classic Hodgkin's lymphoma and mediastinal large B-cell lymphoma, *Am J Surg Pathol* 29:1411-1421, 2005.

150. Jaffe E, Stein H, Swerdlow S et al: B-cell lymphoma, unclassifiable, with features intermediate between diffuse large B-cell lymphoma and classical Hodgkin lymphoma. In Swerdlow S, Campo E, Harris N et al, editors: *WHO classification: tumours of haematopoietic and lymphoid tissues,* ed 4, Lyon, 2008, IARC.

151. Schantz A, Sewall W, Castleman B: Mediastinal germinoma: a study of 21 cases with an excellent prognosis, *Cancer* 30:1189-1194, 1972.

152. Gowda RM, Khan IA: Clinical perspectives of primary cardiac lymphoma, *Angiology* 54:599-604, 2003.

153. Rolla G, Bertero M, Pastena G et al: Primary lymphoma of the heart: a case report and review of the literature, *Leuk Res* 26:117-120, 2002.

154. Kaplan LD, Afridi NA, Holmvang G, Zukerberg LR: Case records of the Massachusetts General Hospital—weekly clinicopathological exercises: case 31-2003: a 44-year-old man with HIV infection and a right atrial mass, *N Engl J Med* 349:1369-1377, 2003.

155. Chim C, Chan A, Kwong Y, Liang R: Primary cardiac lymphoma, *Am J Hematol* 54:79-83, 1997.

156. Ikeda H, Nakamura S, Nishimaki H et al: Primary lymphoma of the heart: case report and literature review, *Pathol Int* 54:187-195, 2004.

157. Saito T, Tamaru J, Kayao J et al: Cytomorphologic diagnosis of malignant lymphoma arising in the heart: a case report, *Acta Cytol* 45:1043-1048, 2001.

158. Nascimento AF, Winters GL, Pinkus GS: Primary cardiac lymphoma: clinical, histologic, immunophenotypic, and genotypic features of 5 cases of a rare disorder, *Am J Surg Pathol* 31:1344-1350, 2007.

159. Bassi D, Lentzner BJ, Mosca RS, Alobeid B: Primary cardiac precursor B lymphoblastic lymphoma in a child: a case report and review of the literature, *Cardiovasc Pathol* 13:116-119, 2004.

160. Meshref M, Sassolas F, Schell M et al: Primary cardiac Burkitt lymphoma in a child, *Pediatr Blood Cancer* 42:380-383, 2004.

161. Dawson M, Mariani J, Taylor A et al: The successful treatment of primary cardiac lymphoma with a dose-dense schedule of rituximab plus CHOP, *Ann Oncol* 17:176-177, 2006 (letter).

162. Nagano M, Uike N, Suzumiya J et al: Successful treatment of a patient with cardiac lymphoma who presented with a complete atrioventricular block, *Am J Hematol* 59:171-174, 1998.

163. Bagwan IN, Desai S, Wotherspoon A, Sheppard MN: Unusual presentation of primary cardiac lymphoma, *Interact Cardiovasc Thorac Surg*, 9:127-129, 2009.

164. Miller DV, Firchau DJ, McClure RF et al: Epstein-Barr virus–associated diffuse large B-cell lymphoma arising on cardiac prostheses, *Am J Surg Pathol* 34:377-384, 2010.

165. Durrleman N, El-Hamamsy I, Demaria R et al: Cardiac lymphoma following mitral valve replacement, *Ann Thorac Surg* 79:1040-1042, 2005.

166. Giunta R, Cravero R, Granata G et al: Primary cardiac T-cell lymphoma, *Ann Hematol* 83:450-454, 2004.

167. Jurkovich D, deMarchena E, Bilsker M et al: Primary cardiac lymphoma diagnosed by percutaneous intracardiac biopsy with combined fluoroscopic and transesophageal echocardiographic imaging, *Catheter Cardiovasc Interv* 50:226-233, 2000.

168. Saotome M, Yoshitomi Y, Kojima S, Kuramochi M: Primary cardiac lymphoma: a case report, *Angiology* 53:239-241, 2002.

169. Anghel G, Zoli V, Petti N et al: Primary cardiac lymphoma: report of two cases occurring in immunocompetent subjects, *Leuk Lymphoma* 45:781-788, 2004.

170. Begueret H, Labouyrie B, Dubus P et al: Primary cardiac lymphoma in an immunocompetent woman, *Leuk Lymphoma* 31:423-428, 1998.

171. Lim Z, Grace R, Salisbury J et al: Cardiac presentation of ALK positive anaplastic large cell lymphoma, *Eur J Haematol* 75:511-514, 2005.

172. Sanna P, Bertoni F, Zucca E et al: Cardiac involvement in HIV-related non-Hodgkin's lymphoma: a case report and short review of the literature, *Ann Hematol* 77:75-78, 1998.

173. Chinen K, Izumo T: Cardiac involvement by malignant lymphoma: a clinicopathologic study of 25 autopsy cases based on the WHO classification, *Ann Hematol* 84:498-505, 2005.

174. Meng Q, Lai H, Lima J et al: Echocardiographic and pathological characteristics of cardiac metastasis in patients with lymphoma, *Oncol Rep* 9:85-88, 2002.

175. Ito M, Nakagawa A, Tsuzuki T et al: Primary cardiac lymphoma: no evidence for an etiologic association with Epstein-Barr virus, *Arch Pathol Lab Med* 120:555-559, 1996.

176. Fuchida S-I, Yamada N, Uchida R et al: Malignant lymphoma presenting as a cardiac tumor and superior vena cava syndrome successfully treated by haploidentical stem cell transplantation, *Leuk Lymphoma* 46:1517-1521, 2005.

177. Wiseman C, Liao K: Primary lymphoma of the breast, *Cancer* 29:1705-1712, 1972.

178. Talwalkar SS, Miranda RN, Valbuena JR et al: Lymphomas involving the breast: a study of 106 cases comparing localized and disseminated neoplasms, *Am J Surg Pathol* 32:1299-1309, 2008.

179. Hugh J, Jackson F, Hanson J, Poppema S: Primary breast lymphoma: an immunohistologic study of 20 new cases, *Cancer* 66:2602-2611, 1990.

180. Lamovec J, Jancar J: Primary malignant lymphoma of the breast: lymphoma of the mucosa-associated lymphoid tissue, *Cancer* 60:3033-3041, 1987.

181. Domchek SM, Hecht JL, Fleming MD et al: Lymphomas of the breast: primary and secondary involvement, *Cancer* 94:6-13, 2002.

182. Farinha P, Andre S, Cabecadas J, Soares J: High frequency of MALT lymphoma in a series of 14 cases of primary breast lymphoma, *Appl Immunohistochem Mol Morphol* 10:115-120, 2002.

183. Cabras MG, Amichetti M, Nagliati M et al: Primary non-Hodgkin's lymphoma of the breast: a report of 11 cases, *Haematologica* 89:1527-1528, 2004.

184. Lin Y, Guo XM, Shen KW et al: Primary breast lymphoma: long-term treatment outcome and prognosis, *Leuk Lymphoma* 47:2102-2109, 2006.

185. Vigliotti ML, Dell'olio M, La Sala A, Di Renzo N: Primary breast lymphoma: outcome of 7 patients and a review of the literature, *Leuk Lymphoma* 46:1321-1327, 2005.

186. Liu M, Hsieh C, Wang A et al: Primary breast lymphoma: a pooled analysis of prognostic factors and survival in 93 cases, *Ann Saudi Med* 25:288-293, 2005.

187. Mattia A, Ferry J, Harris N: Breast lymphoma: a B-cell spectrum including the low grade B-cell lymphoma of mucosa associated lymphoid tissue, *Am J Surg Pathol* 17:574-587, 1993.

188. Wang LA, Harris NL, Ferry JA: Lymphoma of the breast and the role of mammography in the detection of low-grade lymphomas, *Mod Pathol* 17:276A, 2004.

189. Lin YC, Tsai CH, Wu JS et al: Clinicopathologic features and treatment outcome of non-Hodgkin lymphoma of the breast: a review of 42 primary and secondary cases in Taiwanese patients, *Leuk Lymphoma* 50:918-924, 2009.

190. Lyons J, Myles J, Pohlman B et al: Treatment and prognosis of primary breast lymphoma: a review of 13 cases, *Am J Clin Oncol* 23:334-336, 2000.

191. Aviles A, Delgado S, Nambo MJ et al: Primary breast lymphoma: results of a controlled clinical trial, *Oncology* 69:256-260, 2005.

192. Fruchart C, Denoux Y, Chasle J et al: High grade primary breast lymphoma: is it a different clinical entity? *Breast Cancer Res Treat* 93:191-198, 2005.

193. Uesato M, Miyazawa Y, Gunji Y, Ochiai T: Primary non-Hodgkin's lymphoma of the breast: report of a case with special reference to 380 cases in the Japanese literature, *Breast Cancer (Tokyo, Japan)* 12:154-158, 2005.

194. Vignot S, Ledoussal V, Nodiot P et al: Non-Hodgkin's lymphoma of the breast: a report of 19 cases and a review of the literature, *Clin Lymphoma* 6:37-42, 2005.

195. Ribrag V, Bibeau F, El Weshi A et al: Primary breast lymphoma: a report of 20 cases, *Br J Haematol* 115:253-256, 2001.

196. Ryan G, Martinelli G, Kuper-Hommel M et al: Primary diffuse large B-cell lymphoma of the breast: prognostic factors and outcomes of a study by the International Extranodal Lymphoma Study Group, *Ann Oncol* 19:233-241, 2008.

197. Sabate JM, Gomez A, Torrubia S et al: Lymphoma of the breast: clinical and radiologic features with pathologic correlation in 28 patients, *Breast J* 8:294-304, 2002.

198. Yoshida S, Nakamura N, Sasaki Y et al: Primary breast diffuse large B-cell lymphoma shows a non-germinal center B-cell phenotype, *Mod Pathol* 18:398-405, 2005.

199. Kebudi A, Coban A, Yetkin G et al: Primary T-lymphoma of the breast with bilateral involvement, unusual presentation, *Int J Clin Pract* 95-98, 2005.

200. Pisani F, Romano A, Anticoli Borza P et al: Diffuse large B-cell lymphoma involving the breast: a report of four cases, *J Exp Clin Cancer Res* 25:277-281, 2006.

201. Aozasa K, Ohsawa M, Saeki K et al: Malignant lymphoma of the breast: immunologic type and association with lymphocytic mastopathy, *Am J Clin Pathol* 97:699-704, 1992.

202. Chanan-Khan A, Holkova B, Goldenberg AS et al: Non-Hodgkin's lymphoma presenting as a breast mass in patients with HIV infection: a report of three cases, *Leuk Lymphoma* 46:1189-1193, 2005.

203. Jeon H, Akagi T, Hoshida Y et al: Primary non-Hodgkin's malignant lymphoma of the breast, *Cancer* 70:2451-2459, 1992.

204. Gualco G, Bacchi CE: B-cell and T-cell lymphomas of the breast: clinical-pathological features of 53 cases, *Int J Surg Pathol* 16:407-413, 2008.

205. Rooney N, Snead D, Goodman S, Webb A: Primary breast lymphoma with skin involvement arising in lymphocytic lobulitis, *Histopathology* 24:81-84, 1994.

206. Talwalkar SS, Valbuena JR, Abruzzo LV et al: MALT1 gene rearrangements and NFκB activation involving p65 and p50 are absent or rare in primary MALT lymphomas of the breast, *Mod Pathol* 19:1402-1408, 2006.

207. Monteiro M, Duarte I, Cabecadas J, Orvalho ML: Intravascular large B-cell lymphoma of the breast, *Breast* 14:75-78, 2005.

208. Joao C, Farinha P, da Silva MG et al: Cytogenetic abnormalities in MALT lymphomas and their precursor lesions from different organs: a fluorescence in situ hybridization (FISH) study, *Histopathology* 50:217-224, 2007.

209. de Jong D, Vasmel WL, de Boer JP et al: Anaplastic large-cell lymphoma in women with breast implants, *JAMA* 300:2030-2035, 2008.

210. Brogi E, Harris N: Lymphomas of the breast: pathology and clinical behavior, *Semin Oncol* 26:357-364, 1999.

211. Vakiani E, Savage DG, Pile-Spellman E et al: T-cell lymphoblastic lymphoma presenting as bilateral multinodular breast masses: a case report and review of the literature, *Am J Hematol* 80:216-222, 2005.

212. Aguilera NS, Tavassoli FA, Chu WS, Abbondanzo SL: T-cell lymphoma presenting in the breast: a histologic, immunophenotypic and molecular genetic study of four cases, *Mod Pathol* 13:599-605, 2000.

213. Briggs JH, Algan O, Stea B: Primary T-cell lymphoma of the breast: a case report, *Cancer Invest* 21:68-72, 2003.

214. Burkitt D, Wright D: *Burkitt's lymphoma,* Edinburgh, 1970, E & S Livingstone.

215. Antic N, Colovic M, Cemerikic V et al: Disseminated Burkitt's-like lymphoma during pregnancy, *Med Oncol* 17:233-236, 2000.

216. Armitage JO, Feagler JR, Skoog DP: Burkitt lymphoma during pregnancy with bilateral breast involvement, *JAMA* 237:151, 1077.

217. Durodola JI: Burkitt's lymphoma presenting during lactation, *Int J Gynaecol Obstet* 14:225-231, 1976.

218. Miyoshi I, Yamamoto K, Saito T, Taguchi H: Burkitt lymphoma of the breast, *Am J Hematol* 81:147-148, 2006.

219. Sherer DM, Stimphil RG, Santoso P et al: Stage IV large B cell lymphoma presenting as gigantomastia and pulmonary hypertension, *Obstet Gynecol* 103:1061-1064, 2004.

220. Vandenberghe G, Claerhout F, Amant F: Lymphoblastic lymphoma presenting as bilateral gigantomastia in pregnancy, *Int J Gynaecol Obstet* 91:252-253, 2005.

221. Windom KW, McDuffie RS Jr: Non-Hodgkin's lymphoma presenting with gigantomastia in pregnancy, *Obstet Gynecol* 93:852, 1999.

222. Kirkpatrick A, Bailey D, Weizel H: Bilateral primary breast lymphoma in pregnancy: a case report and literature review, *Can J Surg* 39:333-335, 1996.

223. Iyengar P, Reid-Nicholson M, Moreira AL: Pregnancy-associated anaplastic large-cell lymphoma of the breast: a rare mimic of ductal carcinoma, *Diagn Cytopathol* 34:298-302, 2006.

224. Roden AC, Macon WR, Keeney GL: Seroma-associated primary anaplastic large-cell lymphoma adjacent to breast implants: an indolent T-cell lymphoproliferative disorder, *Mod Pathol* 21:455-463, 2008.

225. Shulman LN, Hitt RA, Ferry JA: Case records of the Massachusetts General Hospital: case 4-2008: a 33-year-old pregnant woman with swelling of the left breast and shortness of breath, *N Engl J Med* 358:513-523, 2008.

226. Wong AK, Lopategui J, Clancy S et al: Anaplastic large cell lymphoma associated with a breast implant capsule: a case report and review of the literature, *Am J Surg Pathol* 32:1265-1268, 2008.

227. Farkash E, Ferry J, Harris N et al: Rare lymphoid malignancies of the breast: a report of two cases illustrating potential diagnostic pitfalls, *J Hematopathol* 2:237-44, 2009.

228. Miranda RN, Lin L, Talwalkar SS et al: Anaplastic large cell lymphoma involving the breast: a clinicopathologic study of 6 cases and review of the literature, *Arch Pathol Lab Med* 133:1383-1390, 2009.

229. Lipworth L, Tarone RE, McLaughlin JK: Breast implants and lymphoma risk: a review of the epidemiologic evidence through 2008, *Plast Reconstr Surg* 123:790-793, 2009.

230. Cook PD, Osborne BM, Connor RL, Strauss JF: Follicular lymphoma adjacent to foreign body granulomatous inflammation and fibrosis surrounding silicone breast prosthesis, *Am J Surg Pathol* 19:712-717, 1995.

231. Duvic M, Moore D, Menter A, Vonderheid EC: Cutaneous T-cell lymphoma in association with silicone breast implants, *J Am Acad Dermatol* 32:939-942, 1995.

232. Kraemer DM, Tony HP, Gattenlohner S, Muller JG: Lymphoplasmacytic lymphoma in a patient with leaking silicone implant, *Haematologica* 89:ELT01, 2004.

233. Sendagorta E, Ledo A: Sézary syndrome in association with silicone breast implant, *J Am Acad Dermatol* 33:1060-1061, 1995.

234. Fritzsche FR, Pahl S, Petersen I et al: Anaplastic large-cell non-Hodgkin's lymphoma of the breast in periprosthetic localisation 32 years after treatment for primary breast cancer: a case report, *Virchows Arch* 449:561-564, 2006.

235. Gaudet G, Friedberg JW, Weng A et al: Breast lymphoma associated with breast implants: two case-reports and a review of the literature, *Leuk Lymphoma* 43:115-119, 2002.

236. Newman MK, Zemmel NJ, Bandak AZ, Kaplan BJ: Primary breast lymphoma in a patient with silicone breast implants: a case report and review of the literature, *J Plast Reconstr Aesthet Surg* 61:822-825, 2008.

237. Olack B, Gupta R, Brooks GS: Anaplastic large cell lymphoma arising in a saline breast implant capsule after tissue expander breast reconstruction, *Ann Plast Surg* 59:56-57, 2007.

238. Sahoo S, Rosen PP, Feddersen RM et al: Anaplastic large cell lymphoma arising in a silicone breast implant capsule: a case report and review of the literature, *Arch Pathol Lab Med* 127:e115-e118, 2003.

239. Sanati S, Ayala AG, Middleton LP: Lymphoepithelioma-like carcinoma of the breast: report of a case mimicking lymphoma, *Ann Diagn Pathol* 8:309-315, 2004.

240. Ely KA, Tse G, Simpson JF et al: Diabetic mastopathy: a clinicopathologic review, *Am J Clin Pathol* 113:541-545, 2000.

241. Valdez R, Thorson J, Finn WG et al: Lymphocytic mastitis and diabetic mastopathy: a molecular, immunophenotypic, and clinicopathologic evaluation of 11 cases, *Mod Pathol* 16:223-228, 2003.

242. Vizcaino I, Torregrosa A, Higueras V et al: Metastasis to the breast from extramammary malignancies: a report of four cases and a review of literature, *Eur Radiol* 11:1659-1665, 2001.

243. Duncan VE, Reddy VV, Jhala NC et al: Non-Hodgkin's lymphoma of the breast: a review of 18 primary and secondary cases, *Ann Diagn Pathol* 10:144-148, 2006.

244. Windrum P, Morris TC, Catherwood MA et al: Mantle cell lymphoma presenting as a breast mass, *J Clin Pathol* 54:883-886, 2001.

245. Lima M, Goncalves C, Teixeira MA et al: Aggressive natural-killer cell lymphoma presenting with skin lesions, breast nodule, suprarenal masses and life-threatening pericardial and pleural effusions, *Leuk Lymphoma* 42:1385-1391, 2001.

CHAPTER 5

Lymphomas of the Esophagus, Gastrointestinal Tract, Hepatobiliary Tract, and Pancreas

Judith A. Ferry

LYMPHOMAS OF THE ESOPHAGUS

Primary Esophageal Lymphomas

Primary esophageal lymphoma is rare, accounting for 0.2% of extranodal non-Hodgkin's lymphomas[1] and fewer than 1% of tumors of the esophagus.[2] The esophagus is the least common primary site for lymphoma in the alimentary tract.[1] Patients with primary esophageal lymphoma are predominantly middle-aged or older adults, and men are affected more often than women.[2-8] Patients usually present with dysphagia, chest pain, and/or weight loss and occasionally with fever.[2,6-11] In rare cases, esophageal lymphoma has been an incidental finding.[5]

Evaluation reveals a mass that may be submucosal, smooth, polypoid, or fungating and circumferential or longitudinal. Ulceration sometimes is seen. The lesion may result in diffuse mural thickening and often in stenosis.[2-5,7-11] Because many of the lymphomas have not been classified according to the system established by the World Health Organization (WHO), the subtype often is uncertain. However, the most common types have included diffuse large cell lymphomas (frequently, no immunophenotyping has been done, but B-lineage has been documented in some cases to establish a diagnosis of diffuse large B-cell lymphoma [Figure 5-1][11,12]) and low-grade lymphomas that are extranodal marginal zone lymphomas of mucosa-associated lymphoid tissue (MALT lymphomas)[13-15] or that are most likely extranodal marginal zone lymphomas.[2,4,7]

Several patients with diffuse large cell lymphoma have been HIV positive.[9] One patient had a history of hepatitis C viral infection and of pure red cell aplasia related to large granular lymphocyte leukemia that was treated with cytoxan before the diffuse large cell lymphoma developed.[3] Studies have reported patients with marginal zone lymphoma with mixed connective tissue disease,[15] with autoimmune thyroiditis, and with gastritis associated with *Helicobacter pylori* infection.[5] One patient with esophageal marginal zone lymphoma had concurrent pulmonary marginal zone lymphoma.[16] Rare cases of primary

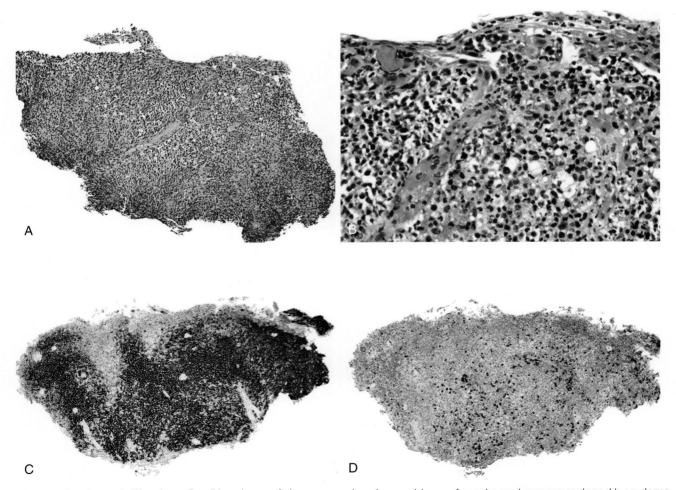

Figure 5-1   Esophageal diffuse large B-cell lymphoma. **A,** Low-power view shows a biopsy of esophageal mucosa replaced by a dense cellular infiltrate. **B,** Higher power view shows large atypical lymphoid cells in a background of apoptotic debris and scattered inflammatory cells. A small amount of squamous epithelium remains on the surface of the tissue. An immunostain for CD20 **(C)** shows diffuse strong staining of numerous cells throughout most of the tissue. A few scattered CD3+ T cells **(D)** also are present. (Immunoperoxidase technique on paraffin sections.)

esophageal T-cell lymphoma[2,6,10,17] and a case of a probable low-grade follicular lymphoma[8] have been reported.

Information on outcome is limited, but patients often respond well to therapy, and the prognosis appears relatively good.[6-7,11] In some cases, however, patients have died of lymphoma or of complications of therapy,[2-3,9] including a patient who died when a tracheoesophageal fistula developed.[7]

Secondary Esophageal Involvement by Lymphoma

Secondary involvement of the esophagus by lymphoma that arises elsewhere, whether by direct extension from adjacent structures or by spread from distant sites, also is unusual but is more common than primary esophageal lymphoma.[2,3] In one large series, 1.5% of all non-Hodgkin's lymphomas involved the esophagus, but all 19 cases arose elsewhere and involved the esophagus secondarily. In most of the 19 cases, esophageal involvement was identified at autopsy.[18] The most common primary sites were the stomach and adjacent lymph nodes.

Several cases of esophageal involvement by mantle cell lymphoma and follicular lymphoma with the endoscopic picture of multiple lymphomatous polyposis have been described; the immunophenotypic and genetic features were similar to those of these types of lymphomas in other sites. These lymphomas also showed gastric and intestinal involvement.[19,20] A case has been reported of anaplastic large cell lymphoma, ALK+, with extensive lymph nodal involvement; it presented initially as an esophageal mass with a tracheoesophageal fistula.[21] An isolated esophageal relapse of Hodgkin's lymphoma 13 years after initial diagnosis has been reported.[7] A patient with esophageal involvement by chronic lymphocytic leukemia in the form of mucosal nodularity has been reported; esophageal involvement developed late in the course of disease, a few months before death.[22]

■ LYMPHOMAS OF THE GASTROINTESTINAL TRACT

Introduction

The gastrointestinal tract is the most common primary site for extranodal lymphomas; up to 20% of all non-Hodgkin's lymphomas arise in this site. The stomach is most often involved, followed by the small intestine and ileocecal region and then by the colon.[23,24] In a few cases, lymphoma presents with multifocal involvement of different portions of the gastrointestinal tract.[24,25]

Anatomic Distribution and Pathologic Types of Lymphoma

The stomach is the primary site in approximately two-thirds of cases of gastrointestinal lymphoma.[23,24]

Extranodal marginal zone lymphoma of mucosa-associated lymphoid tissue (MALT lymphoma) and diffuse large B-cell lymphoma are the most common types.[26] Other types of lymphoma are uncommon, but occasional cases of follicular lymphoma, Burkitt's lymphoma, mantle cell lymphoma, and peripheral T-cell lymphoma involve the stomach.

Most of the remaining cases of gastrointestinal lymphoma arise in the small intestine or the ileocecal region. The ileum is more commonly affected than the duodenum or jejunum.[23,24,27-29] The large intestine is the primary site less often than is the small intestine.[24,28-30] The cecum is the most common site of involvement in the large intestine, followed by the rectum; other portions of the colon are only rarely affected.[23,31]

The most common type of intestinal lymphoma overall is diffuse large B-cell lymphoma. The proportion of other types of lymphoma varies in different series, depending on the patients' age, ethnic background, and country of origin. These other lymphomas include marginal zone lymphoma (including immunoproliferative small intestinal disease), Burkitt's lymphoma, mantle cell lymphoma, follicular lymphoma, peripheral T-cell lymphomas, and extranodal natural killer (NK)/T-cell lymphoma, nasal type.[23,25,27,29,32-34] Lymphomas that arise in the ileocecal region are almost all diffuse high-grade B-cell lymphomas, either diffuse large B-cell lymphoma or Burkitt's lymphoma.[25,31] Appendiceal lymphomas are uncommon; subtypes encountered include diffuse large B-cell lymphoma, Burkitt's lymphoma,[32,35,36] rare cases of extranodal marginal zone lymphoma,[36] and peripheral T-cell lymphoma.[37] Anal lymphomas are rare and usually are diffuse large B-cell lymphomas.[38]

A variety of lymphomas can present with multifocal gastrointestinal involvement, including mantle cell lymphoma, follicular lymphoma, enteropathy-associated T-cell lymphoma, marginal zone lymphoma, and diffuse large B-cell lymphoma.[25,31]

Presenting Manifestations

Patients present with abdominal pain, anorexia or weight loss, obstruction, a palpable mass, diarrhea, nausea or vomiting, fever, perforation, and/or bleeding, with some variation, depending on the type of lymphoma and the portion of the gastrointestinal tract involved. Bulky lymphomas that arise in the ileocecal area may be associated with intussusception.* Patients with appendiceal lymphoma typically present with right lower quadrant abdominal pain that mimics acute appendicitis.[35,43] Infrequently the lymphoma is an incidental finding. Symptoms characteristic of different types of lymphoma are noted in the corresponding sections.

---

*References 24, 25, 27, 28, 32, and 39-42.

Predisposing Factors

Multiple predisposing factors are involved in the development of gastrointestinal lymphoma: *H. pylori* infection (see Gastric Marginal Zone Lymphoma of Mucosa-Associated Lymphoid Tissue [MALT Lymphoma]), *Campylobacter jejuni* infection (see Immunoproliferative Small Intestinal Disease), celiac disease (see Enteropathy-Associated T-Cell Lymphoma), and a variety of inherited and acquired immunodeficiency syndromes.

HIV infection is an important risk factor for the development of gastrointestinal lymphoma. Lymphoma is the second most common malignancy in HIV-positive patients, after Kaposi's sarcoma. The risk of lymphoma in HIV-positive patients has been estimated to be 50 to 60 times higher than for HIV-negative individuals.[44,45] The proportion of extranodal lymphomas is higher among HIV-positive patients than in the general population, and the gastrointestinal tract is the extranodal site most often affected; roughly one third of all HIV-associated, non-Hodgkin's lymphomas arise in this site.[45] However, the introduction of highly active antiretroviral therapy (HAART) in recent years appears to be associated with a decreased risk of lymphoma, including gastrointestinal lymphoma.[46] The occurrence of lymphoma in different parts of the gastrointestinal tract in HIV-positive patients is the opposite of that seen in HIV-negative patients: the colon and anorectal area are affected most often, followed by the small intestine; the stomach is the least often involved.[45] The lymphomas are almost all high-grade B-cell lymphomas.

Iatrogenically immunosuppressed allograft recipients have an increased risk of lymphoma compared to the general population. Many cases of posttransplantation lymphoproliferative disorder (PTLD) arise in extranodal locations, and the gastrointestinal tract is among the most common of these. A statistically increased risk for gastrointestinal lymphoma has been documented among allograft recipients.[46] The small intestine is affected more often than the stomach or colon.[47]

PTLDs are classified as (1) early lesions, (2) polymorphic PTLDs, (3) monomorphic PTLDs, (4) plasmacytoma-like lesions, and (5) T-cell rich large B-cell lymphoma/Hodgkin's lymphoma–like lesions (Table 5-1).[48] The polymorphic and monomorphic PTLDs of B-lineage are most likely to be encountered in the gastrointestinal tract.[47,49,50] A few gastrointestinal PTLDs have been T-lineage (monomorphic T-PTLD).[51]

Lymphoma rarely arises in association with inflammatory bowel disease. Patients with inflammatory bowel disease appear to have no definite increased risk for lymphoma.[52] However, patients with severe inflammatory bowel disease treated with immunomodulatory agents do appear to have an increased risk for lymphoma,[53] estimated at four times that of the general population in one study.[54] Whether lymphomagenesis is related to therapy or to the severity of the inflammatory bowel disease, or to a combination of these factors, is uncertain.[53,54] Lymphoma in patients with inflammatory bowel disease has characteristic features; this reinforces the theory that even though lymphoma is rare in inflammatory bowel disease, it is a distinct entity. Intestinal lymphomas in patients with ulcerative colitis almost always involve areas of active inflammation; they also are more often multifocal and more often distally located in the colon.[55] Most cases are diffuse large B-cell lymphoma, and they often are positive for the Epstein-Barr virus (EBV), which supports the hypothesis that lymphomagenesis is related to immune dysregulation.[56,57]

Gastrointestinal lymphomas that arise in association with Crohn's disease affect the small intestine or colon (or both) in areas affected by Crohn's disease. Most cases are diffuse large B-cell lymphomas. Classical Hodgkin's lymphomas also have been described in this setting (see Hodgkin's Lymphoma of the Gastrointestinal Tract, later in the chapter).[56-58]

A number of cases of hepatosplenic T-cell lymphoma have been described in patients with inflammatory bowel disease who were treated with a combination of infliximab, a tumor necrosis factor alpha blocking agent (TNFα), and other immunosuppressive medication[59] (see Lymphomas of the Spleen, Chapter 6).

Various genetically determined immunodeficiency syndromes are associated with an increased risk for lymphoma, including gastrointestinal lymphoma. X-linked lymphoproliferative disorder (Purtilo's disease), a rare, X-linked recessive disorder that affects young boys, is characterized by a selective immunodeficiency for EBV. Upon exposure to EBV, these children develop severe, often fatal, infectious mononucleosis or malignant lymphoma. In most cases, the lymphomas affect the gastrointestinal tract, and the ileocecal area most often is affected. These are aggressive, EBV+, B-lineage lymphomas that can be classified as Burkitt's lymphoma or diffuse large B-cell lymphoma.[60,61] Wiskott-Aldrich syndrome also is associated with an increased incidence of lymphoma. The risk of lymphoma approaches 100% by 30 years of age. The small intestine is the second most common site of involvement by lymphoma, after the central nervous system.[62]

Common variable immunodeficiency (CVID) is an immunodeficiency syndrome that usually presents in adulthood but sometimes does so in childhood. It is characterized by decreased levels of one or more classes of immunoglobulin, manifested by recurrent sinopulmonary infections, chronic lung disease, autoimmune disorders, and susceptibility to infection by a variety of pathogens, including *Giardia* organisms, cytomegalovirus, and certain bacteria.[63] Patients with CVID have an increased risk of non-Hodgkin's lymphomas, some of which involve the gastrointestinal tract. The occurrence of gastric diffuse large B-cell lymphoma in association with CVID has been reported.[64] Rare cases of small intestinal lymphoma (usually diffuse large B-cell lymphoma) also have been reported in patients with CVID, in a

TABLE 5-1

Post-Transplantation Lymphoproliferative Disorders

Category	Common Anatomic Sites	Morphology	Immunophenotype	Epstein-Barr Virus*	Genetic Features
Early lesion: Plasmacytic hyperplasia	Lymph nodes, tonsils	Architecture preserved; many plasma cells, lymphocytes, few immunoblasts	Mix of polytypic B cells, polytypic plasma cells, and T cells	Often present	Clonal B cells usually absent
Early lesion: Infectious mononucleosis (IM)–like lesion	Lymph nodes, tonsils	Architecture preserved; paracortical expansion with immunoblasts in a polymorphic background (as for IM in nontransplant patients)	Mix of polytypic B cells, polytypic plasma cells, and T cells	EBV+ immunoblasts	Clonal B cells often absent; small clonal or oligoclonal B-cell populations may be found
Polymorphic PTLD	GI tract and other extranodal sites; lymph nodes	Architecture effaced by polymorphic mix of small and medium-sized lymphoid cells, plasma cells, immunoblasts, with or without large bizarre cells and with or without necrosis	Polytypic, monotypic, or mixture of polytypic and monotypic B cells and/or plasma cells	Numerous EBV+ cells	Clonal B cells, often in polyclonal background
Monomorphic PTLD: B-cell neoplasms	GI tract and other extranodal sites; lymph nodes	DLBCL most common; Burkitt's lymphoma less often	Similar to DLBCL and Burkitt's lymphoma in nontransplant patients	Usually present	Clonal B cells
Monomorphic PTLD: T-cell neoplasms	Lymph nodes and/or extranodal sites	Peripheral T-cell lymphoma NOS; hepatosplenic T-cell lymphoma; others	Similar to these lymphomas in nontransplant patients	Variable	Clonal T cells
Classical Hodgkin-type PTLD	Rare, data limited	As in classical Hodgkin's lymphoma in nontransplant patients	Similar to Hodgkin's lymphoma in nontransplant patients	EBV+ Reed-Sternberg and Hodgkin cells	Clonal population may not be found

DLBCL, Diffuse large B-cell lymphoma; *EBV*, Epstein-Barr virus; *GI*, gastrointestinal; *NOS*, not otherwise specified; *PTLD*, post-transplantation lymphoproliferative disorder.
*As determined by in situ hybridization using Epstein-Barr virus–encoded RNA.

background of nodular lymphoid hyperplasia.[65,66] A case of rectal diffuse large B-cell lymphoma that presented as an exacerbation of inflammatory bowel disease in a patient with CVID has been described.[63]

Primary Gastrointestinal Lymphomas

Gastric Marginal Zone Lymphoma of Mucosa-Associated Lymphoid Tissue (MALT Lymphoma)

Clinical Features

The stomach is the most common primary site for extranodal marginal zone lymphoma of mucosa-associated lymphoid tissue (MALT lymphoma). Gastric marginal zone lymphoma overall affects men slightly more often than women. Most patients are

middle-aged or older adults, and a median age in the sixth or seventh decade is seen in most series. Infrequently, young adults and adolescents are affected.[67-79] Patients often present with epigastric pain or dyspepsia; nausea and vomiting, bleeding, and weight loss are less common.[79,80] The symptoms may suggest gastritis or peptic ulcer disease rather than lymphoma.[81]

Pathologic Features

Gross and Microscopic Features

On endoscopy or on gross examination of a resection specimen, the lymphoma takes the form of erosions, flat areas of ulceration, mucosal granularity, thickened mucosal folds, or a diffusely infiltrative, ill-defined lesion (Figure 5-2). Superficial lesions

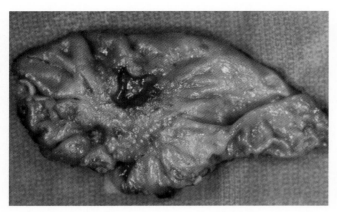

Figure 5-2 Gastric marginal zone lymphoma (MALT lymphoma), partial gastrectomy specimen. The stomach shows a central area of peptic ulceration. The surrounding gastric wall is thickened, with nodularity and loss of the normal mucosal folds. Proximal and distal margins were involved by lymphoma.

(confined to the mucosa or submucosa) are more common than large exophytic or deeply invasive masses. In some cases, the appearance suggests gastritis.* The lymphomas usually involve one portion of the stomach but occasionally may involve the stomach in a multifocal or diffuse pattern.[73,81,82,84] When the lymphomas are superficially invasive, the lymph nodes usually are not involved. Invasion into the muscularis propria or deeper is associated with a greater risk of nodal involvement.[77]

Microscopic examination reveals a diffuse or vaguely nodular infiltrate of marginal zone B cells, small to medium-sized cells with oval to slightly irregular nuclei, dispersed chromatin, and inconspicuous nucleoli, often with distinct rims of clear cytoplasm (Figures 5-3 and 5-4). In some cases, neoplastic lymphoid cells have scant cytoplasm and resemble small lymphocytes.[69] In about one third of cases, the lymphoma shows plasmacytic differentiation (see Figure 5-3). This usually takes the form of a bandlike infiltrate of plasma cells superficially in the lamina propria beneath the surface epithelium, with the neoplastic marginal zone cells deep to the plasma cell layer. The plasma cells may resemble normal plasma cells or may have cytoplasm with globular or crystalline inclusions or nuclei with Dutcher bodies (see Figure 5-3, C). Small clusters of neoplastic cells usually can be identified infiltrating and disrupting gastric glands to form lymphoepithelial lesions (see Figure 5-4, B and C). Intact reactive lymphoid follicles or remnants of reactive follicles usually can be found in the lymphoma (see Figure 5-3), often with infiltration and replacement by neoplastic cells (follicular colonization) (see Figure 5-4).

The cells colonizing the follicles usually are marginal zone cells, but plasma cells or large cells also may colonize follicles. Sometimes follicles are not recognizable on routinely stained sections, but evidence of pre-existing follicles can be found using antibodies to follicular dendritic cells (CD21 or CD23)

*References 33, 46, 67, 68, 70, 73, and 80-83.

(see Figure 5-4, F). Small numbers of large cells (centroblasts or immunoblasts) may be scattered among the marginal zone cells[33,81]; however, the presence of many large cells in a solid or sheetlike pattern indicates histologic progression to diffuse large B-cell lymphoma. In such cases, a diagnosis of diffuse large B-cell lymphoma arising in association with marginal zone lymphoma should be rendered.[85]

Biopsy specimens frequently show evidence of infection with *H. pylori.* The organism can be detected on routinely stained sections in some cases or with special stains (e.g., Giemsa [Figure 5-5], thiazine, or Steiner stain) or with immunohistochemistry using antibodies to *H. pylori.* Evidence of *H. pylori* infection also can be detected using the rapid urease test, urea breath test, tissue culture, or serology.[70] The frequency of *H. pylori* positivity varies among studies; in some series, 80% to 100% of cases are reported to harbor *H. pylori,* whereas in other studies, only a minority of cases show evidence of the organism.[67,84] *H. pylori* is more likely to be found with lymphomas that are superficial (confined to the mucosa or submucosa), are confined to the stomach, and lack areas of progression to diffuse large B-cell lymphoma[67,86]; this suggests that lymphomas that are larger and/or have a component of diffuse large B-cell lymphoma are less likely to depend on *H. pylori* for persistence and growth. In addition, the use of proton pump inhibitors may reduce the number of *H. pylori* bacteria present, leading to false-negative results.[46]

Immunophenotypic Features

Immunophenotyping shows CD20+, CD5−, CD10−, bcl6−, monotypic surface immunoglobulin (sIg)+ B cells. In cases with plasmacytic differentiation, plasma cells express monotypic cytoplasmic immunoglobulin (cIg) (see Figure 5-3, E to K). The immunoglobulin expressed most often is IgM, but in some cases IgA or IgG is expressed. The neoplastic cells usually are bcl2+, although occasionally bcl2 expression may be lost, particularly in colonized follicles. CD21 and CD23 stain follicular dendritic meshworks, which may be irregular or disrupted (see Figure 5-4, F). B cells co-express CD43 in up to about one third of cases. An immunostain for cytokeratin can highlight lymphoepithelial lesions. The proliferation fraction, as measured with antibody Ki67, is low, although it characteristically is high in residual reactive follicle centers.[77,81,82,87] In contrast to marginal zone lymphoma, the large cell lymphomas that arise from them occasionally express bcl6 and have a high proliferation fraction although they are CD10−.[76,81]

Genetic and Cytogenetic Features

As in other B-cell lymphomas, immunoglobulin heavy and light chain genes are clonally rearranged. Sequence analysis of the immunoglobulin genes has shown somatic hypermutation, sometimes with intraclonal variation, consistent with ongoing somatic hypermutation.[88] Despite the somatic hypermutation, in most cases no isotype class switch

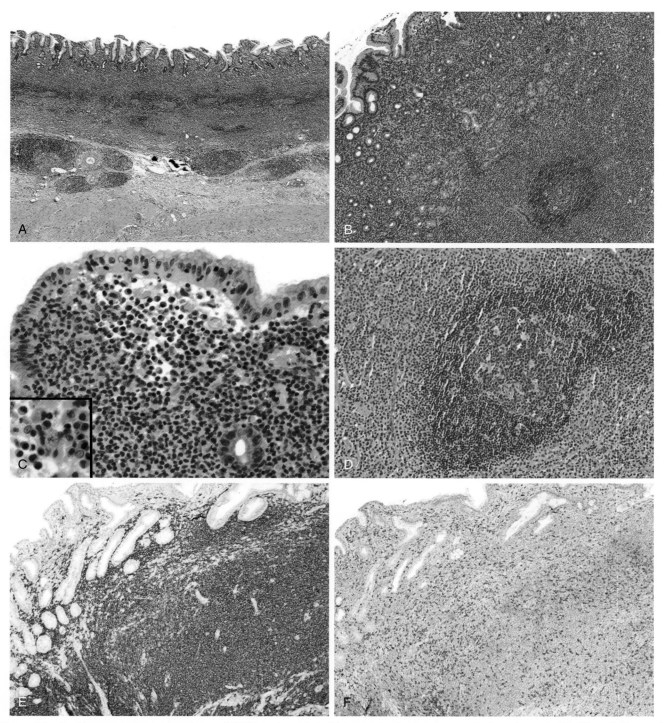

Figure 5-3 Gastric marginal zone lymphoma (MALT lymphoma). In this example, the lymphoma displays plasmacytic differentiation and contains admixed reactive follicles. **A,** A broad band of lymphoid cells occupies the mucosa and much of the submucosa. **B,** A diffuse infiltrate of marginal zone cells fills the mucosa. Note the reactive lymphoid follicle with a mantle composed of cells slightly smaller and darker than the surrounding marginal zone cells *(lower right)*. **C,** Many mature plasma cells are present in the superficial portion of the lamina propria. A plasma cell with multiple cytoplasmic inclusions of immunoglobulin is seen *(inset)*. **D,** A reactive lymphoid follicle with a dark mantle and a distinct follicle center is surrounded by marginal zone cells with pale cytoplasm. **E,** An immunostain for CD20 shows that most lymphoid cells are B cells, present in a diffuse pattern. **F,** A few scattered T cells (CD3+) are present.

Continued

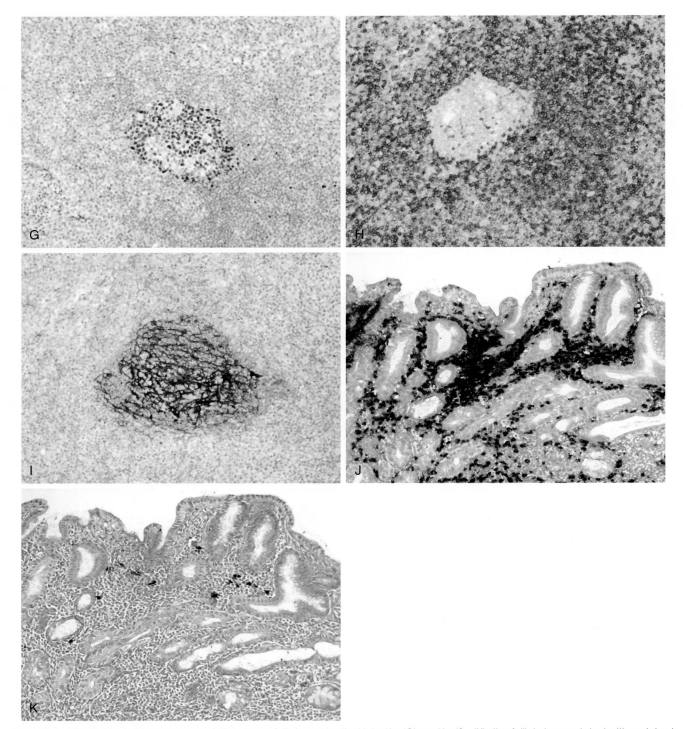

Figure 5-3, cont'd **G** to **I**, A small reactive follicle has a follicle center that is bcl6+ **(G)** and bcl2– **(H)**; the follicle is associated with an intact CD21+ dendritic meshwork **(I)**. The lymphoma is bcl2+, bcl6–. (Immunoperoxidase technique on paraffin sections.) **J** and **K**, Plasma cells in the superficial lamina propria express monotypic kappa light chain, with only a few lambda-positive plasma cells. (In situ hybridization on paraffin sections.)

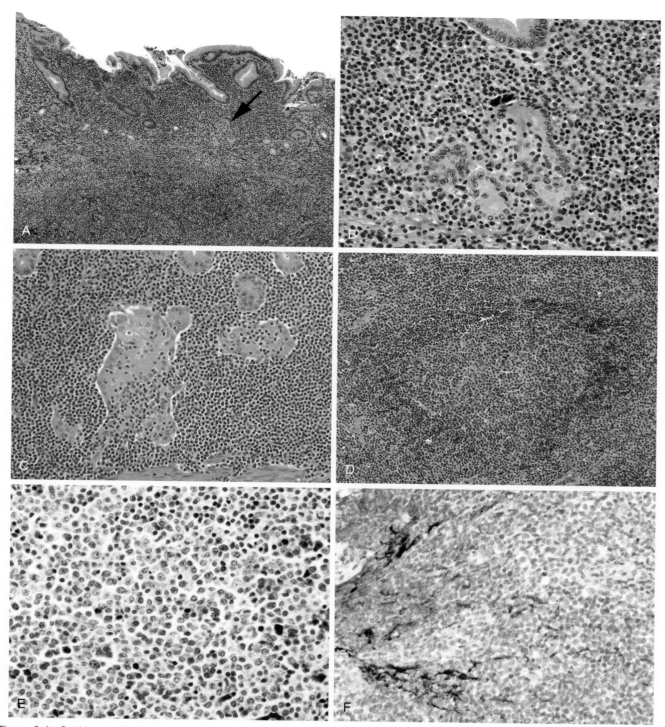

Figure 5-4 Gastric marginal zone lymphoma (MALT lymphoma) with lymphoepithelial lesions and prominent follicular colonization. **A,** A dense infiltrate of marginal zone cells replaces much of the gastric tissue, with focal lymphoepithelial lesion formation *(arrow)*. **B,** Higher power view shows a lymphoepithelial lesion composed of clusters of lymphoid cells with clear cytoplasm infiltrating and disrupting a gastric gland. **C,** These lymphoepithelial lesions are associated with prominent distortion and eosinophilic change of the epithelium. **D,** A lymphoid follicle has been invaded and replaced by marginal zone cells and plasmacytoid cells (follicular colonization). An attenuated, partially disrupted mantle of small lymphocytes remains. The appearance is more monomorphous than that of the intact reactive follicle in Figure 5-3, *D.* **E,** The plasmacytoid nature of many of the cells in the colonized follicle is evident with Giemsa staining. **F,** A distorted CD21+ dendritic meshwork is present in the lymphoma. (Immunoperoxidase technique on paraffin sections.)

occurs; that is, most gastric marginal zone lymphomas express IgM rather than IgG or IgA.[88] Biased usage of IGV$_H$1-69 has been described; use of this gene segment has been associated with production of autoantibodies and polyreactive antibodies (with the ability to bind multiple antigens, including autoantigens and foreign antigens). Accordingly, the antibodies produced by the neoplastic B cells sometimes are reported to have specificity for a variety of autoantigens[88,89] and some foreign antigens, including *H. pylori*.[88]

Translocation t(11;18)(q21;q21) is the most common cytogenetic abnormality in gastric marginal zone lymphoma,[90] although different studies have shown wide variation in its frequency, ranging from approximately 5%[91] to 40% of cases; a number of studies have shown a frequency on the order of about 20% to 30% of cases.[68,69,90,92] This translocation, which involves the *API2* gene on chromosome 11 and the *MALT1* gene on chromosome 18, is believed to confer a survival advantage on the neoplastic cells. Most marginal zone lymphomas that fail to regress with *H. pylori* eradication therapy

harbor the t(11;18), whereas t(11;18) is consistently absent in cases that regress with such therapy. This translocation tends to be associated with a higher proportion of cases lacking *H. pylori* and with higher stage disease.[68,90,91,93,94]

The reason for the variation in frequency of t(11;18) is uncertain. Possibilities include factors related to the genetic makeup of different patient populations; the prevalence of *H. pylori* or different strains of *H. pylori* in different geographic locales; differences in the types of specimens studied (biopsy samples with small, superficial lymphomas versus resection specimens with larger, deeply invasive lymphomas); the inclusion of cases of marginal zone lymphoma that secondarily involve the stomach,[91] and factors related to technique. Despite the frequency of t(11;18) [*API2/MALT1*] in gastric marginal zone B-cell lymphoma, it is virtually absent in gastric diffuse large B-cell lymphoma; this suggests t(11;18) may block transformation of marginal zone lymphoma to large B-cell lymphoma.[95-97]

A cytogenetic abnormality much less often associated with gastric marginal zone lymphoma is t(1;14)(p22;q32), involving the genes for *BCL10* and immunoglobulin heavy chain (*IGH*). Like t(11;18), t(1;14) is associated with failure of lymphoma to regress with antibiotics. t(1;14) is associated with strong nuclear expression of the bcl10 protein; t(11;18) is associated with moderate nuclear expression of bcl10. Some cases lacking both translocations demonstrate moderate bcl10 expression; therefore, expression of the protein does not appear to be specific for a certain cytogenetic change.[98] Rare cases with t(14;18) involving genes for *IGH* and *MALT1*[90,92] and rare cases with t(3;14) involving *FOXP1* and *IGH*[68] have been documented. Table 5-2 presents the clinical and pathologic correlates of the translocations that may be seen in gastric marginal zone lymphoma. Trisomy 3,[96] trisomy 18,[91,92] and extra copies of the *MALT1* gene on chromosome 18[68] and of the *FOXP1* gene on chromosome 3[68] also are relatively common.

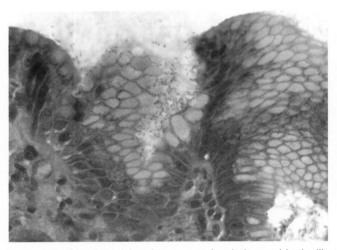

Figure 5-5 Giemsa staining shows many bacteria consistent with *Helicobacter pylori* in this gastric pit.

TABLE 5-2

Clinical and Pathologic Correlates of Translocations in Gastric Marginal Zone Lymphoma		
Cytogenetic Abnormality	**Genes Involved**	**Clinical and Pathologic Correlates**
t(11;18)(q21;q21)	*API2, MALT1*	• Higher stage • *Helicobacter pylori* less likely to be present • Failure to regress with HPET • Most composed of lymphoid cells with abundant, clear cytoplasm; some composed of small cells with scant cytoplasm • Prominent plasmacytic differentiation uncommon • Moderate nuclear expression of bcl10 • No progression to DLBCL
t(1;14)(p22;q32)	*BCL10, IGH*	• Failure to regress with HPET • Strong nuclear expression of bcl10
t(14;18)(q32;q21)	*IGH, MALT1*	• Rare, no known correlates
t(3;14)(p14.1;q32)	*FOXP1, IGH*	• Rare, no known correlates

DLBCL, Diffuse large B-cell lymphoma; *HPET, Helicobacter pylori* eradication therapy.

Translocations involving $BCL6$[99] (including $BCL6$/IGH) and MYC,[81,95,97,100,101] as well as p53 inactivation and allelic loss[33] and p16 deletion,[97] may play a role in the progression of gastric marginal zone lymphoma to diffuse large B-cell lymphoma.

Pathogenesis

In most cases gastric marginal zone lymphoma arises on a background of gastritis with a component of acquired mucosa associated-lymphoid tissue induced by *H. pylori* infection. Persistent infection and chronic antigenic stimulation lead to the appearance of a clonal population of B cells. The T cells in the infiltrate have strain-specific reactivity for *H. pylori* and appear to promote proliferation of B cells.[89] B cells may express polyreactive antibodies with specificity that includes *H. pylori*–associated antigens; therefore, in some cases, *H. pylori* may directly stimulate B cells to proliferate.[88]

In the early phases of the disease, the B cells require *H. pylori* and the T cells to proliferate. Accordingly, in this phase, the lymphoma remains localized and may respond to antibiotic therapy directed against *H. pylori*.[85,102] Over time, the clonal B cells accumulate genetic changes that may result in autonomous growth, leading to a histologically low-grade lymphoma that does not regress with *H. pylori* eradication therapy and that may spread beyond the stomach.

Only a small proportion of individuals with *H. pylori* gastritis go on to develop marginal zone lymphoma. Factors that may play a role in the pathogenesis of this lymphoma include the *H. pylori* strain involved, patient characteristics, or environmental factors. Certain polymorphisms in the T-cell regulatory gene cytotoxic T-lymphocyte antigen 4 (*CTLA4*) could be associated with an increased or a decreased risk of marginal zone lymphoma.[103] An increased risk of gastric marginal zone lymphoma with certain polymorphisms of genes involved in an inflammatory response and antioxidative capacity has been described; individuals with alterations in the inflammatory response to *H. pylori* and diminished antioxidative capacity appear more likely to develop lymphoma.[78,104]

Some cases have shown no evidence of *H. pylori* infection,[84] even when studied by histology, immunohistochemistry, urease test, and/or serology.[94] In these cases, it is not known whether infection had been present previously and had resolved after the lymphoma attained autonomous growth or whether other, as yet unrecognized etiologic agents are involved in gastric marginal zone lymphoma. A few *H. pylori*–negative marginal zone lymphomas (as well as a small proportion of cases of chronic gastritis) are caused by *Helicobacter* species other than *H. pylori*, such as *H. heilmannii*.[105,106]

Staging, Treatment, and Outcome

Staging reveals disease confined to the stomach in about 58% to 88% of cases.* Most of the remaining cases have regional lymph node involvement. In occasional

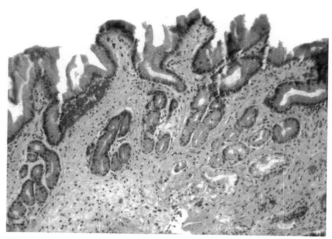

Figure 5-6 Complete histologic regression of gastric marginal zone lymphoma; the gastric mucosa has a hypocellular, empty-appearing lamina propria that contains only a few plasma cells and stromal cells.

cases more widespread disease is seen,[68,76,82,107,108] with involvement of another MALT site, especially the small intestine or colon, but also the lungs, kidneys, salivary glands, thyroid, ocular adnexa, and others; a few patients have had bone marrow involvement.* The lymphoma is indolent and may remain localized for years, even without specific therapy.[33]

In 1993 Wotherspoon and colleagues[102] documented the remarkable observation of regression of gastric marginal zone lymphoma when antibiotics were used to eradicate *H. pylori*. Their findings were confirmed by many others, and the response rates typically ranged from 60% to 90%.[70-72,79,80,110,111] Complete histologic regression of lymphoma after *H. pylori* eradication therapy is characterized by a lamina propria with a distinctive empty appearance, basal aggregates of small lymphocytes, and scattered plasma cells (Figure 5-6). Partial regression shows areas of empty lamina propria with foci of atypical lymphoid cells and/or lymphoepithelial lesions.[111] The interval to histologic regression may be prolonged, ranging from 1 month to approximately 3 years (median is 5 to 15 months).[74,79,82,111]

Features associated with failure of regression include invasion beyond the submucosa, spread beyond the stomach, the absence of *H. pylori*, and the presence of t(11;18) or t(1;14).† The presence of a component of diffuse large B-cell lymphoma also makes regression less likely. However, some observers have described complete regression of a subset of cases of diffuse large B-cell lymphoma arising in association with marginal zone lymphoma confined to the stomach with antibiotic therapy alone.[95,112-115] Regression appears more likely when the lymphoma is superficial (i.e., confined to the mucosa or submucosa), as may be documented on endoscopic ultrasound.[95,112-114] Regression also is unlikely if *H. pylori* fails to respond to the antibiotics used.[112] The diffuse large B-cell

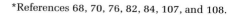

*References 68, 70, 76, 82, 84, 107, and 108.

*References 24, 33, 82, 84, 90, and 109.
†References 33, 79, 82, 83, 93, 112, and 113.

lymphomas that regress completely appear to have a durable, complete remission that lasts for years.[112] Some authorities suggest that treatment of gastric diffuse large B-cell lymphoma with *Helicobacter* eradication therapy should be undertaken only if meticulous clinical, histologic, and radiographic evaluation and endoscopic follow-up can be performed.[114]

One group found that although most cases of concurrent marginal zone lymphoma and diffuse large B-cell lymphoma are clonally related, in a minority of cases the two components appear to represent two distinct, unrelated clones. The two components responded in the same manner to *H. pylori* eradication therapy when they were clonally related. In contrast, in most cases in which the two components were not clonally related, a discordant response to *H. pylori* eradication therapy was seen; usually, the marginal zone lymphoma responded to therapy, but the diffuse large B-cell lymphoma did not.[115]

Even with complete histologic regression of marginal zone lymphoma, many patients have a persistent clonal B-cell population detected by polymerase chain reaction (PCR), and this population may persist for years.[33,71,82,108,111] Histologic regression is considered the gold standard for effective therapy; molecular evidence of clonality alone does not warrant additional therapy. Microdissection studies suggest that the clonal B cells reside in basal lymphoid aggregates.[111] A minority of patients have relapse of lymphoma, which may be precipitated by *H. pylori* reinfection.[72,79] If the lymphoma does not respond to or relapses after *H. pylori* eradication, other modalities may be used, such as surgery, radiation therapy, and/or chemotherapy[67,70,82-84,110,111]; complete remission usually can be attained. Surgical resection does not appear to improve the outcome, compared with other modalities, and may be avoided to reduce the morbidity of therapy.[26]

Gastric marginal zone lymphoma has an excellent prognosis,[26,108] with a 5-year disease-specific survival rate of at least 90%[*] and a 10-year survival rate of 80% to 90%.[70,79,83] A few patients die of lymphoma, sometimes after transformation to diffuse large B-cell lymphoma.[79] Some investigators have found that marginal zone lymphoma with a component of diffuse large B-cell lymphoma has a prognosis similar to that of marginal zone lymphoma alone[26,116]; in some studies in which this was the case, most patients with a component of diffuse large B-cell lymphoma were treated with aggressive combination chemotherapy with or without rituximab, and the more aggressive therapy may have eliminated the difference in natural history between marginal zone lymphoma with and without a component of diffuse large B-cell lymphoma.[26,116]

Differential Diagnosis

1. **Marginal zone lymphoma versus gastritis.** Histologic features in favor of lymphoma include the presence of a dense, destructive lymphoid

---

*References 33, 75, 76, 79, 107, and 116.

TABLE 5-3

Histologic Differential Diagnosis of Gastric Marginal Zone Lymphoma (MALT Lymphoma): Wotherspoon Score		
Score	**Diagnosis**	**Histologic Features**
0	Normal	Scattered plasma cells in lamina propria No lymphoid follicles
1	Chronic active gastritis (CAG)	Small clusters of lymphocytes in lamina propria No lymphoid follicles No lymphoepithelial lesions
2	CAG with florid lymphoid follicle formation	Prominent lymphoid follicles with surrounding mantle zone and plasma cells No lymphoepithelial lesions
3	Suspicious lymphoid infiltrate, probably reactive	Lymphoid follicles surrounded by small lymphocytes that infiltrate diffusely in the lamina propria and occasionally into epithelium
4	Suspicious lymphoid infiltrate, probably lymphoma	Lymphoid follicles surrounded by marginal zone cells that infiltrate diffusely in the lamina propria and into epithelium in small groups
5	Marginal zone lymphoma	Dense, diffuse infiltrate of marginal zone cells in lamina propria with prominent lymphoepithelial lesions

From Wotherspoon A, Doglioni C, Diss T et al: Regression of primary low-grade B-cell gastric lymphoma of mucosa-associated lymphoid tissue type after eradication of *Helicobacter pylori*, *Lancet* 342:575-577, 1993.

infiltrate with loss of glands, cytologic atypia of the infiltrating cells (having the appearance of marginal zone B cells rather than normal small lymphocytes), frequent lymphoepithelial lesions, and Dutcher bodies. Immunohistochemical studies can help establish a diagnosis. Demonstration of monotypic immunoglobulin light chain expression by either lymphoid cells or plasma cells confirms a diagnosis of lymphoma. A diffuse infiltrate of B cells and co-expression of CD43 by B cells both favor a diagnosis of lymphoma. The criteria devised by Wotherspoon and colleagues[102] can be used to arrive at a diagnosis and to assess regression of the lymphoma after *H. pylori* eradication therapy based on histologic features (Table 5-3).

Rare cases of severe gastritis related to EBV infection have been described[117]; pathologic changes include diffuse thickening of the gastric wall and a dense, diffuse infiltrate of small and medium-sized T cells (CD8 more than CD4) and occasional large, EBV-infected B cells. The infiltrate may be associated with lymphoepithelial lesion formation and ulceration. Clues to the diagnosis include the presence of other clinical and pathologic manifestations of infectious mononucleosis and the mixed nature of the infiltrate, which has a composition similar to that found in other tissues involved by infectious mononucleosis.

2. **Marginal zone lymphoma versus other histologically low-grade B-cell lymphomas.** Although marginal zone lymphoma is much more common than follicular lymphoma or mantle cell lymphoma in the stomach, either may present in the stomach and mimic marginal zone lymphoma (see the sections on follicular lymphoma and mantle cell lymphoma of the gastrointestinal tract, later in the chapter). Marginal zone lymphoma is composed of CD5–, CD10– B cells with relatively abundant, clear cytoplasm and may show plasmacytic differentiation. A few scattered large transformed cells may be admixed. Mantle cell lymphoma is composed of a monotonous population of small to medium-sized CD5+, cyclin D1+ B cells, usually with scant cytoplasm, without a component of plasma cells or large cells. Follicular lymphoma usually has a more distinct follicular architecture than either marginal zone lymphoma or mantle cell lymphoma and is composed of CD10+, bcl6+ B cells with nuclei that usually are more angulated and cytoplasm that usually is scant compared to marginal zone cells.

3. **Marginal zone lymphoma versus marginal zone lymphoma with progression to diffuse large B-cell lymphoma.** Sheets or solid aggregates of large lymphoid cells of B-lineage found outside follicles in a background of marginal zone lymphoma represent large cell transformation.[85] Before a diagnosis of focal large cell transformation is rendered, it is important to exclude the possibility that the large cells are residual reactive germinal center cells (common) or neoplastic large cells confined to colonized follicles (uncommon). Diffuse large B-cell lymphomas arising from marginal zone lymphomas may express bcl6, although CD10 expression is not expected; reactive germinal centers usually express both CD10 and bcl6. Immunohistochemical stains for CD21 or CD23 can demonstrate whether a follicular dendritic network associated with aggregates of large cells is present.

4. **Poorly preserved high-grade lymphoma versus low-grade B-cell lymphoma.** In a small biopsy sample of an aggressive lymphoma with artifactual degenerative change, cellular shrinkage and distortion may lead to a misdiagnosis of low-grade lymphoma. The presence of apoptotic debris or mitotic figures suggests an aggressive lymphoma. Staining with the proliferation marker Ki67 can help distinguish between low- and high-grade lymphomas. Clinical information, such as the endoscopic appearance of the tumor, also can provide a clue to the diagnosis, because a higher grade lymphoma is more likely to form a large, bulky mass than is a marginal zone lymphoma or other low-grade lymphoma.[33]

5. **Plasmacytoma versus marginal zone lymphoma.** In the gastrointestinal tract, most neoplasms with a prominent plasmacytic component are marginal zone lymphomas with plasmacytic differentiation. In favor of lymphoma are the presence of a component of B lymphocytes, reactive lymphoid follicles, lymphoepithelial lesions, and IgM+ expression (although expression of other heavy chains does not exclude marginal zone lymphoma). A pure population of plasma cells expressing CD138 and monotypic IgA or IgG raises the question of plasmacytoma. A history of plasma cell myeloma would heighten the suspicion for plasmacytoma. Involvement of the gastrointestinal tract by a true plasma cell neoplasm is uncommon, however, and the diagnosis should be made with caution.

Gastric Diffuse Large B-Cell Lymphoma

Clinical Features

Gastric diffuse large B-cell lymphoma may arise in association with marginal zone lymphoma, consistent with large cell transformation of the low-grade lymphoma (see Gastric Marginal Zone Lymphoma of Mucosa-Associated Lymphoid Tissue [MALT Lymphoma]), whereas other gastric large B-cell lymphomas arise de novo; the proportion of cases in the two categories varies among series.[*]

When only small biopsy samples showing diffuse large B-cell lymphoma are available for examination, excluding an underlying marginal zone lymphoma (or other low-grade B-cell lymphoma) definitively may be difficult because of sampling artifact. Also, the large B-cell lymphoma may have obliterated any underlying low-grade lymphoma.

This section focuses on gastric diffuse large B-cell lymphoma that apparently arises de novo. Gastric diffuse large B-cell lymphoma is mainly a disease of older adults, and the mean or median age is in the seventh decade; very few patients are children or young adults. Males are affected slightly more often than females.[†] Patients may have a palpable mass on physical examination.[33]

Pathologic Features

On gross or endoscopic examination, the lymphomas are usually single (but occasionally multiple) mass-forming, ulcerated lesions that usually are transmurally invasive and may invade adjacent viscera (Figure 5-7).[33,73,95] Small, superficial lesions are uncommon.[95] Any portion of the stomach (upper, middle, or lower third) may be involved, and occasionally more than one portion is involved.[73]

---

*References 24, 73, 75, 76, 99, 107, and 116.
†References 73, 75-77, 95, 116, 118, and 119.

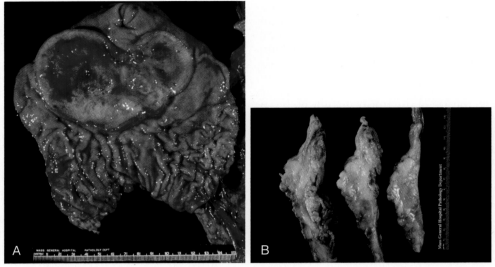

Figure 5-7 Gastric diffuse large B-cell lymphoma, gastrectomy specimen. **A,** A large, heart-shaped ulcer with raised edges occupies a large portion of the stomach. The surrounding mucosa shows no definite abnormality. **B,** Cross section shows a fleshy, light tan tumor transmurally involving the wall of the stomach with prominent thickening of the gastric wall.

Microscopic examination reveals a diffuse proliferation of large cells with round, oval, irregular, or lobated nuclei, distinct nucleoli, and a narrow but distinct rim of cytoplasm (Figure 5-8, *A* and *B*). Immunophenotyping reveals CD20+ B cells (Figure 5-8, *C*) that express monotypic sIg and occasionally cIg and that co-express CD43 in about half of cases.[107] The proportion of lymphomas expressing CD10, bcl6, and MUM1/IRF4 varies in different series, but CD10 is expressed in fewer than half of cases and is expressed less often than bcl6 or MUM1/IRF4.[76,99,119]

Immunophenotyping shows that roughly one fourth to one half of cases are the germinal center B-cell type (CD10+ or CD10–, bcl6+, MUM1–),[120] and one half to three fourths are the non-germinal center B-cell type (CD10–, bcl6+, MUM1+ or CD10–, bcl6–).[95,99,119] A case has been reported of a young man with *ALK+ diffuse large B-cell lymphoma* of the stomach with a t(2;17)(p23;q23), yielding CLTC (Clathrin) *ALK* gene fusion.[121]

Immunoglobulin heavy and light chains are clonally rearranged. Cytogenetic analysis often reveals a karyotype with complex abnormalities.[122] *BCL2* rearrangement is less common, and *MYC* rearrangement and abnormalities of the *BCL6* are more common than in diffuse large B-cell lymphoma arising in the lymph nodes.[100] *BCL6* abnormalities include both translocation and somatic hypermutation.[99] In one study, gastric lymphomas with germline *BCL6* were more likely to present in an advanced stage and showed a trend for decreased complete remission and worse survival.[123] Translocations involving *MALT1* on chromosome 18 and *FOXP1* on chromosome 3 are uncommon; they were detected in 0 and 2% of cases of gastric diffuse large B-cell lymphoma, respectively, in one large series.[95] Extra copies of genetic material in the area of the *BCL2* and *MALT1* genes on chromosome 18 and of *BCL6* and *FOXP1* on chromosome 3, suggesting partial or complete

trisomy 18 and trisomy 3, are found in a subset of cases.[95] Some diffuse large B-cell lymphomas (36% in one series) harbor translocations involving *IGH*, often with an unknown partner.[95]

Staging, Treatment, and Outcome

In most cases,[76,107,118] patients present with stage I or stage II disease. Patients with stage II disease usually outnumber those with stage I disease, and stage IIe1 disease is more common than stage IIe2 disease.[75,76,107] In a minority of patients, staging reveals more widespread disease that involves more distant lymph nodes, other extranodal sites, and/or bone marrow.[116] Patients have been treated with surgery, radiation, and/or chemotherapy. A modest number of cases have been treated with *H. pylori* eradication therapy (HPET). In contrast to diffuse large B-cell lymphoma arising in association with marginal zone lymphoma, in which a subset of cases may respond to HPET, de novo diffuse large B-cell lymphomas are unlikely to respond to HPET (see Gastric Marginal Zone Lymphoma of Mucosa-Associated Lymphoid Tissue [MALT Lymphoma]).[95]

The 5-year survival rate varies from one series to another but overall is approximately 65%.[33] Pathologic features that affect the prognosis have varied from series to series. In one study, large B-cell lymphoma associated with marginal zone lymphoma had a 5-year survival rate of 92%, and CD10+ large B-cell lymphoma had a 5-year survival rate of 89%; on the other hand, CD10– large B-cell lymphoma without a low-grade component had a 5-year survival rate of only 30%.[76] In another study, patients with marginal zone lymphoma with a component of diffuse large B-cell lymphoma had a 5-year overall survival rate of 84%, whereas those with pure diffuse large B-cell lymphoma had a 5-year overall survival rate of 45%.[116] In a study of localized gastric lymphoma, patients with diffuse large B-cell lymphoma

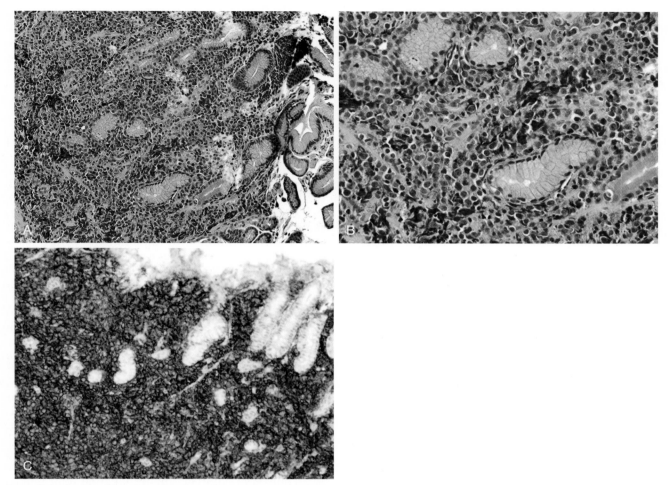

Figure 5-8 Gastric diffuse large B-cell lymphoma, biopsy specimen. **A,** A dense, destructive cellular infiltrate involves the gastric mucosa. **B,** Higher power view shows large atypical lymphoid cells with oval to irregular, dark nuclei and scant cytoplasm infiltrating among gastric glands. **C,** The large lymphoid cells are diffusely positive for CD20. (Immunoperoxidase technique on a paraffin section.)

with associated marginal zone lymphoma had a slightly but not significantly better outcome than those without an underlying marginal zone lymphoma, although the survival rate was excellent in both groups (100% and 91% cause-specific survival rate, respectively at 42 months).[26]

In another study, large B-cell lymphoma associated with a component of marginal zone lymphoma or with lymphoepithelial lesions formed by small cells had a 5-year cause-specific survival rate of 84%, compared with 64% for de novo large B-cell lymphoma. The presence of lymphoepithelial lesions formed by large lymphoid cells was not associated with a better prognosis.[75] Some studies report that gastric diffuse large B-cell lymphomas with a germinal center immunophenotype have a better prognosis than those with a non-germinal center immunophenotype[99] and that those with bcl6 protein expression have a better overall survival rate,[95] but this result has not been uniform. Others have not found a survival advantage with a germinal center immunophenotype or with expression of CD10 or bcl6.[119] Superior overall survival and event-free survival have been reported for cases with translocations involving *IGH* compared with cases without *IGH* translocations.[95]

Younger patients have a better prognosis.[95] A worse prognosis is associated with deeper invasion of the gastric wall and higher stage disease.[95] Patients with stage Ie or IIe1 having a better outcome than those with IIe2 or higher.[76,107] Surgical resection does not appear to improve the survival of patients also receiving chemotherapy and radiation.[26] In one study of high-grade gastric lymphoma, four features were identified as independent factors for an unfavorable outcome: age over 60 years, male gender, high lactate dehydrogenase (LDH) level, and ascites.[118] Survival worsened as the number of these factors present increased.[118]

Differential Diagnosis

Poorly differentiated carcinoma may be composed of discohesive-appearing cells and may form few or no glands, thereby entering the differential diagnosis of diffuse large B-cell lymphoma. Lymphoid cells may show artifactual vacuolar change and mimic signet ring cells. At least focal cohesive growth and the formation of even rare glands favor carcinoma.

A basic panel of immunohistochemical stains can help establish a diagnosis.

Intestinal Marginal Zone Lymphoma of Mucosa-Associated Lymphoid Tissue (MALT Lymphoma)

Clinical Features

Approximately 3% of all primary gastrointestinal lymphomas are intestinal marginal zone lymphomas.[24] Patients are mostly older adults, although a few younger adults and, in rare cases, adolescents are affected.[32,92,124,125] The male to female ratio varies among series, with some showing a male preponderance,[32,124] some reporting a female preponderance,[125] and others reporting similar numbers of men and women affected.[92] Patients present most often with abdominal pain. They may also have bleeding or a change in bowel habits; a minority have diarrhea; and a small subset has constitutional symptoms.[124,126]

Pathologic Features

The lymphomas may be located in any portion of the small or large intestine,[92,124] but the most commonly involved sites are the ileocecal area[124] and the rectum.[31,125,126] In approximately 15% of cases, marginal zone lymphoma involves the intestines in a multifocal or diffuse pattern.[124,125] Gross or endoscopic examination reveals raised or polypoid masses, sometimes with ulceration.[32,39,127] Infrequently the lymphomas have the appearance of multiple small, slightly raised lesions with erosion and erythema,[128,129] similar to gastric marginal zone lymphoma. Most cases are transmurally invasive,[32] although in a subset of cases, the lymphoma is detected when it is only superficially invasive.[39,125] In one series, roughly half of cases were invasive only of the submucosa.[125] In a few cases, the lymphoma has the appearance of multiple lymphomatous polyposis[19] (see Mantle Cell Lymphoma of the Gastrointestinal Tract, later in the chapter).

The histologic and immunophenotypic features of marginal zone lymphoma in the intestine are similar to those seen in the stomach (Figure 5-9),[27,32,81] although lymphoepithelial lesions may be found in only a minority of cases.[126]

Cytogenetic changes overlap with those that may be seen in gastric marginal zone lymphoma, although the results vary somewhat from series to series. The t(11;18) [API2/MALT1] translocation that may be found in gastric marginal zone lymphomas is present in approximately 19% of cases of intestinal marginal zone lymphomas overall,[34,91,92,125,126] with a range of 12%[92] to 41%.[91] Lymphomas with t(11;18) are reported to form larger tumors and to be associated with higher stage disease.[125] Lymphomas that secondarily involve the intestine (usually spread from a gastric primary lymphoma) have an even higher frequency of t(11;18), consistent with the tendency of this translocation to be associated with higher stage disease.[92] The t(1;14) [BCL10/IGH] translocation is uncommon or absent in intestinal marginal zone lymphomas.[91,92] The t(14;18) [IGH/MALT1] translocation has not been identified,[91] although tests have been done to detect it in a limited number of cases. Trisomy 3 and trisomy 18 both are encountered with some frequency in intestinal marginal zone lymphoma.[91,92]

Staging, Treatment, and Outcome

In most cases, the disease is localized to the bowel with or without mesenteric lymph node involvement. Distant spread is found in a minority of cases on staging[39,81,125]; sites that may be involved include the stomach, Waldeyer's ring, lungs, omentum and, in rare cases, liver, or bone marrow.[124,126,130] Treatment has varied but usually consists of surgery with or without chemotherapy. Rare patients with intestinal marginal lymphoma have responded to antibiotic therapy,[39,127,128,131] which suggests that H. pylori[128] or other microorganisms[129] play a role in the pathogenesis of at least a subset of these lymphomas.

On follow-up, lymphomas may have spread to lymph nodes or to a variety of extranodal sites, such as the lungs, stomach, bladder, and breasts.[130] In one study, 80% of patients with intestinal marginal zone lymphoma were alive and well at last follow-up.[32] In two other studies, the 5-year overall survival rates were 87% and 86%, respectively, and the 5-year progression-free survival rates were 65% and 54%, respectively.[124,126] In one additional study, only 1 of 47 patients was known to have died of lymphoma.[125] The prognosis is worse for patients older than age 60 and those with higher stage disease.[124] In one analysis, a subset of colorectal marginal zone lymphomas had a CpG island methylator phenotype (CIMP); those positive for CIMP had higher stage disease and a much worse progression-free survival rate.[126]

Overall, intestinal marginal zone lymphoma is an indolent disease that responds well to therapy but that may have frequent relapses, similar to marginal zone lymphomas in other sites.[124] The prognosis is favorable, although less so than for gastric marginal zone lymphoma. However, among intestinal lymphomas, marginal zone lymphoma has the best prognosis.[27,39]

Immunoproliferative Small Intestinal Disease

Introduction

In 1962 Azar described the spectrum of malignancies encountered in the Department of Pathology of the American University of Beirut.[132] He noted a high prevalence of lymphoma in patients from Lebanon and neighboring Arab countries. Over time, it became apparent that some of these were a distinctive type of small intestinal lymphoproliferative disorder that was designated immunoproliferative small intestinal disease (IPSID). IPSID occurs mainly in the Middle East and in countries surrounding the Mediterranean, but occasional cases in South Africa, the Far East, Europe, and the Western Hemisphere have been described. The disease's geographic

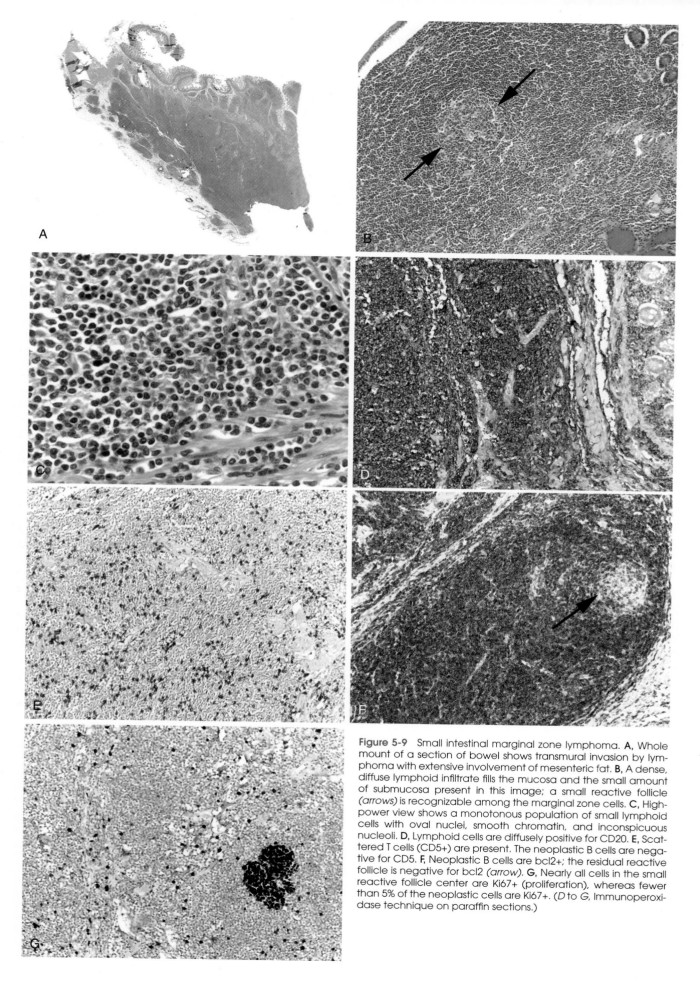

Figure 5-9 Small intestinal marginal zone lymphoma. **A,** Whole mount of a section of bowel shows transmural invasion by lymphoma with extensive involvement of mesenteric fat. **B,** A dense, diffuse lymphoid infiltrate fills the mucosa and the small amount of submucosa present in this image; a small reactive follicle *(arrows)* is recognizable among the marginal zone cells. **C,** High-power view shows a monotonous population of small lymphoid cells with oval nuclei, smooth chromatin, and inconspicuous nucleoli. **D,** Lymphoid cells are diffusely positive for CD20. **E,** Scattered T cells (CD5+) are present. The neoplastic B cells are negative for CD5. **F,** Neoplastic B cells are bcl2+; the residual reactive follicle is negative for bcl2 *(arrow)*. **G,** Nearly all cells in the small reactive follicle center are Ki67+ (proliferation), whereas fewer than 5% of the neoplastic cells are Ki67+. (*D* to *G,* Immunoperoxidase technique on paraffin sections.)

distribution has led to the alternative designation of "Mediterranean lymphoma."[133-135]

Previously, early phases of IPSID were thought to represent an inflammatory disorder, and only when progression to diffuse large B-cell lymphoma was seen was IPSID thought to be neoplastic. However, molecular studies revealed clonal lymphoid cells even in early stage cases,[136] and with the description of extranodal marginal zone lymphoma as an entity, IPSID came to be recognized as an uncommon type of intestinal marginal zone lymphoma with distinctive clinical and pathologic features.

Clinical Features

On average, patients with IPSID are younger than patients with most other types of gastrointestinal lymphoma. Most patients are adolescents or young adults; smaller numbers of children and middle-aged or older individuals are affected. Some investigators report that males and females are affected equally; other series have shown a slight male preponderance.[137,138] IPSID is more prevalent in groups with lower socioeconomic status, poor hygiene, malnutrition, and increased instances of infectious enteritis and intestinal parasitic infections.[138] Genetic predisposition may play a role in the development of IPSID, because there appears to be an association with certain human leukocyte antigen (HLA) types and with blood group B.[133] *C. jejuni* has been identified in some cases of IPSID and may be related to its pathogenesis, analogous to the association between *H. pylori* and gastric marginal zone lymphoma[139,140]; however, the other host and environmental factors described previously also likely play a role in the development of IPSID.[138] The incidence of this disease appears to be declining in some countries because of improvements in living conditions.[137,138,141]

Patients present with long-standing abdominal pain, malabsorption, diarrhea, and weight loss.[133,134,141,142] Obstruction, bleeding, and perforation are uncommon,[134] although perforation has been described in cases that have undergone large cell transformation.[141] Analogous to gastric marginal zone B-cell lymphoma, in the early phase of the disease, the lymphoma may respond to broad-spectrum antibiotics. Over time, with invasion of the muscularis propria and/or transformation to a high-grade lymphoma, the lymphoma becomes aggressive.[33] The prognosis overall has been poor,[141] but patients with high-grade lymphoma who are treated with combination chemotherapy that includes doxorubicin appear to have a better prognosis.[133,138,141,142]

Laboratory Abnormalities

In most cases, an unusual and highly distinctive laboratory abnormality is seen: the serum contains free alpha heavy chains without associated light chain. Cases of IPSID with this abnormality have been called "alpha heavy chain disease." The paraprotein is an alpha$_1$ heavy chain with an internal deletion of V_H and C_H1.[138,142] Free alpha heavy chains also can be detected in intestinal fluid, urine, and saliva. IPSID apparently develops in patients with recurrent or persistent intestinal infections, leading to chronic antigenic stimulation of IgA-secreting intestinal lymphoid tissue, with the eventual emergence of a clonal B-cell population. It is hypothesized that this population acquires mutations leading to the production of alpha heavy chain with the internal deletion described previously and loss of this population's ability, in most cases, to synthesize light chain.[142] Some cases show pathologic changes otherwise typical of IPSID in which free alpha heavy chain is not secreted; some of these lymphomas instead produce intact IgA or other classes of immunoglobulin, and a serum paraprotein may or may not be present. Some have proposed that these cases also be considered to represent IPSID.[141]

Pathologic Features

As its name suggests, IPSID mainly affects the small intestine, although in rare cases concurrent involvement of the stomach and colon may be seen. The abnormalities involve the proximal small intestine, the entire small intestine or, in rare cases, the ileum alone.[134] Mesenteric lymphadenopathy is common.[81,134,135,142] The classic finding in IPSID is a dense, continuous, bandlike mucosal lymphoplasmacytic infiltrate that is uninterrupted along the length of the involved portions of the small intestine.[134,135,142] The extent of the infiltrate correlates with the severity of malabsorption. The histologic features are similar to those of marginal zone lymphomas in other extranodal sites, except that IPSID shows consistently marked plasmacytic differentiation.

In the earliest phases, lymphoma is confined to the small intestinal mucosa and mesenteric lymph nodes. The infiltrate consists predominantly of plasma cells (Figure 5-10). Marginal zone B cells may be inconspicuous on routinely stained sections.[81] Villous blunting or villous atrophy may be present. With time, the infiltrate invades beyond the muscularis mucosae. Reactive lymphoid follicles surrounded and colonized by neoplastic marginal zone cells become more conspicuous, and scattered large atypical immunoblasts may be seen. Total or subtotal villous atrophy is seen. Eventually, in some cases, the disease progresses to a diffuse large B-cell lymphoma that takes the form of one or more bulky intestinal masses. The neoplastic cells may be immunoblasts, plasmacytoid immunoblasts, or large, pleomorphic, bizarre cells. The staging system proposed for IPSID differs from that used for other gastrointestinal lymphomas (Table 5-4).[141]

Immunohistochemical analysis usually shows expression of alpha heavy chain without light chain in the plasmacytic population. In a minority of cases, monotypic light chain is expressed. Molecular genetic analysis has shown clonal rearrangement of immunoglobulin heavy and light chains, even in early cases responsive to antibiotic therapy.[81,133]

Differential Diagnosis

The clinical differential diagnosis is broad; it includes chronic infectious enteritis, parasitic infections, celiac disease, tropical sprue, other types of

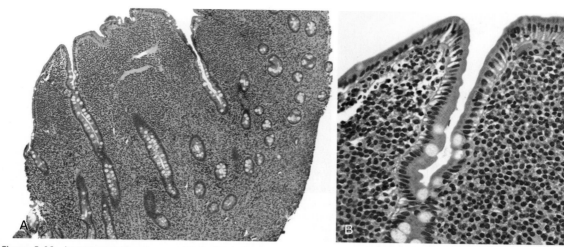

Figure 5-10   Immunoproliferative small intestinal disease. **A,** A densely cellular infiltrate fills the lamina propria with marked distortion of the normal villous architecture. **B,** The infiltrate consists of small, mature plasma cells. The surface epithelium is well preserved, without increased intraepithelial lymphocytes. A Dutcher body can be seen *(inset).* The plasma cells expressed alpha heavy chain unaccompanied by light chain.

TABLE 5-4

Staging of Immunoproliferative Small Intestinal Disease	
Stage	**Features**
A	Within the bowel, lymphoplasmacytic infiltrate confined to mucosa, with or without mesenteric lymph nodal involvement
B	Extension below muscularis mucosae
C	Lymphomatous masses, high-grade transformation

lymphoma,[133] and inflammatory bowel disease. The differential diagnosis on pathologic evaluation is similar to that of marginal zone lymphoma with marked plasmacytic differentiation in other sites. The failure of plasma cells to express light chains may lead to diagnostic difficulty until stains for heavy chains are performed and plasma cells are shown to express alpha heavy chain exclusively. The small intestinal localization and the villous blunting may raise the question of celiac disease, but celiac disease mainly affects individuals of northwestern European descent. Celiac disease is characterized by total villous atrophy (in contrast to the villous broadening seen in early stage IPSID), elongated crypts, intraepithelial T lymphocytosis, and surface epithelial damage.[142] High-grade lymphomas may be found in association with either, but the lymphoma that complicates celiac disease is a T-cell lymphoma prone to cause multifocal ulceration and perforation.

Intestinal Diffuse Large B-Cell Lymphoma

Clinical Features

Most patients with intestinal diffuse large B-cell lymphoma are middle-aged or older adults; the median age is the 60s.[119,143] Occasional patients are HIV positive; these are mostly young or middle-aged adults.[45,144] A few cases occur in younger adults or children. Among adults, a slight male preponderance is seen; in children, almost all patients are boys. In a minority of cases, patients present with intussusception or perforation.[27,119,125,143]

The sites most commonly involved are the ileum and the cecum. The jejunum, duodenum, and segments of the colon distal to the cecum are affected less often. In occasional cases the lymphoma is multicentric within the intestines. Lymphoma infrequently arises in the appendix. Lymphoma in children is almost exclusively found in the ileocecal area.[32,40,42,125,143] Lymphoma in HIV-positive patients tends to be located more distally in the intestines, including cases involving the anorectal area.[45,144]

Pathologic Features

On gross examination, the tumors are similar to[39] or larger than[40] low-grade lymphomas. They typically are raised or infiltrative, ulcerated lesions that usually are transmurally invasive (Figure 5-11).[27,125] Most are composed of centroblasts, often with an admixture of immunoblasts and/or multilobated large lymphoid cells; a minority are composed mainly of immunoblasts.[27,32] As noted in the discussion of predisposing factors for gastrointestinal lymphoma, individuals with inflammatory bowel disease may have an increased risk of intestinal lymphoma. Figure 5-12 illustrates an EBV+ diffuse large B-cell lymphoma presenting as a rectal mass that developed in a patient with Crohn's disease who was treated with a combination of immunosuppressive and immunomodulatory agents. The presence of EBV strongly suggests that the lymphoma was related to the underlying inflammatory bowel disease and its treatment.

HIV-positive patients may have diffuse large B-cell lymphomas with features indistinguishable from those in the general population, but these patients also have a higher frequency of lymphomas

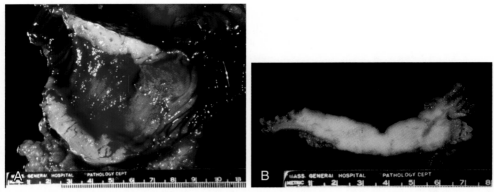

Figure 5-11   Small intestinal diffuse large B-cell lymphoma. **A,** The bowel has been opened to reveal mural thickening by light yellow tumor with mucosal flattening. Normal mucosal folds are seen in uninvolved bowel *(upper left)*. **B,** Cross section of the fixed specimen shows homogeneous white tumor expanding and replacing the wall of the bowel.

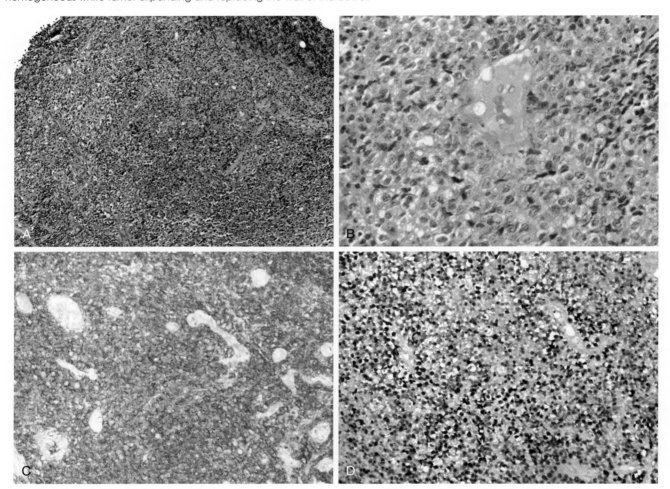

Figure 5-12   Diffuse large B-cell lymphoma, EBV+, presenting as a rectal mass in a patient with Crohn's disease. **A,** In this fragment, tissue has been replaced by a dense infiltrate of lymphoid cells. **B,** The infiltrate is composed of large lymphoid cells with oval to slightly irregular, vesicular nuclei; sometimes with small nucleoli; and a moderate amount of pale cytoplasm with indistinct cell borders. **C,** The atypical cells are diffusely positive for CD20. (Immunoperoxidase technique on a paraffin section.) Only a few scattered T cells were identified (not illustrated). **D,** Neoplastic cells are EBV+. (In situ hybridization for EBER on a paraffin section.)

composed almost entirely of immunoblasts. *Plasmablastic lymphoma* of the oral cavity type has been described in the gastrointestinal tract; it occurs most often in the anorectal area[145,146] and is strongly associated with HIV infection. In some cases, plasmablastic lymphoma is composed of a monotonous population of large cells, whereas in other cases, morphologic evidence of plasmacytic differentiation is seen. Figure 5-13 shows an example of plasmablastic lymphoma with plasmacytic differentiation that occurred in a patient not known to be HIV positive (see Lymphomas of the Oral Cavity in Chapter 3

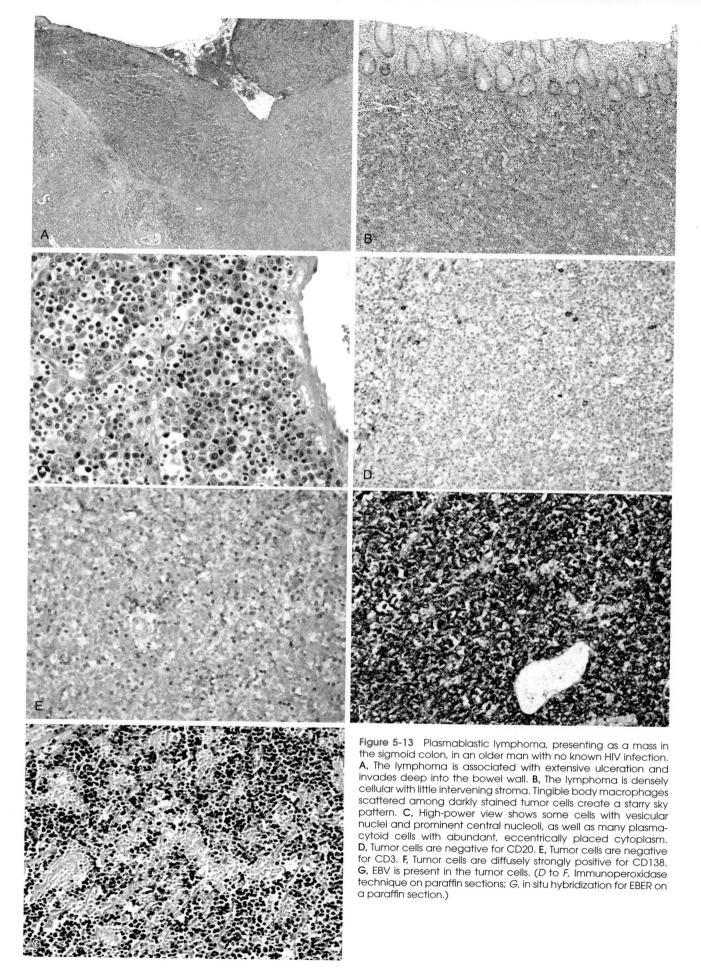

Figure 5-13 Plasmablastic lymphoma, presenting as a mass in the sigmoid colon, in an older man with no known HIV infection. **A,** The lymphoma is associated with extensive ulceration and invades deep into the bowel wall. **B,** The lymphoma is densely cellular with little intervening stroma. Tingible body macrophages scattered among darkly stained tumor cells create a starry sky pattern. **C,** High-power view shows some cells with vesicular nuclei and prominent central nucleoli, as well as many plasmacytoid cells with abundant, eccentrically placed cytoplasm. **D,** Tumor cells are negative for CD20. **E,** Tumor cells are negative for CD3. **F,** Tumor cells are diffusely strongly positive for CD138. **G,** EBV is present in the tumor cells. (*D* to *F,* Immunoperoxidase technique on paraffin sections; *G,* in situ hybridization for EBER on a paraffin section.)

for detailed discussion of plasmablastic lymphoma). Several cases of human herpes virus 8–positive (HHV8+) large B-cell lymphomas with features similar to those seen in primary effusion lymphoma have presented as intestinal tumors in HIV-positive patients; these have been called "HHV8+ solid lymphomas" or "extracavitary primary effusion lymphomas." In some of these cases, patients later developed lymphomatous effusions.[147,148] (HHV8+ lymphomas are discussed in detail under Lymphomas of the Pleura and Pleural Cavity in Chapter 4.)

The WHO Classification recently defined *EBV+ diffuse large B-cell lymphoma of the elderly* as an EBV+ clonal B-cell lymphoproliferation that occurs in patients older than age 50 who have had no known immunodeficiency or previous lymphoma.[149] The etiology is believed to be related to the deterioration of immunity that may occur with advancing age. In most cases, patients present with extranodal disease, sometimes accompanied by lymph node involvement. The gastrointestinal tract is among the more common extranodal sites where this lymphoma may be encountered.

In some cases, the composition of the lymphoma may be monomorphous, with a predominance of large atypical lymphoid cells that may have the appearance of immunoblasts or Reed-Sternberg cells and variants. In other cases, the composition may be more polymorphous, showing B cells of a range of stages of maturation (including some large atypical cells), as well as reactive cells, including histiocytes, small lymphocytes, and plasma cells although eosinophilis typically are absent. Geographic necrosis may be present. The tumor cells usually are CD20+ and/or CD79a+ and often are CD30+ and MUM1/IRF4+, but CD15–. By definition, EBV is present. Figure 5-14 illustrates an EBV+ diffuse large B-cell lymphoma of the elderly involving the bowel in the form of multiple nodules in the wall of the duodenum.

In some intestinal diffuse large B-cell lymphomas, a component of marginal zone lymphoma is found, consistent with large cell transformation of the marginal zone lymphoma. The proportion of cases with an underlying low-grade lymphoma varies substantially from one series to another, ranging

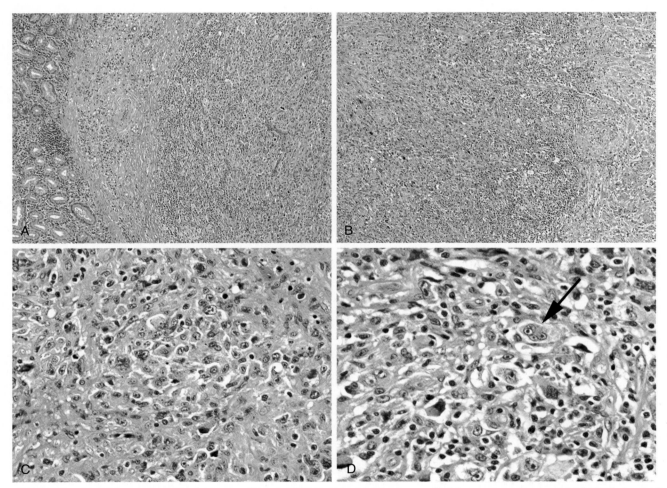

Figure 5-14 EBV+ diffuse large B-cell lymphoma of the elderly involving the duodenum. **A,** A large area with a cellular infiltrate beneath the duodenal mucosa is shown. **B,** A large cellular nodule present deep in the duodenal wall; as in *A,* a peripheral rim of small lymphocytes is present around an area with atypical cells and fibrosis. **C,** High-power view shows many large atypical lymphoid cells with oval, slightly irregular or lobated nuclei, vesicular chromatin, and distinct nucleoli. **D,** Another field shows more admixed reactive cells. A multinucleated, Reed-Sternberg–like cell is present *(arrow).*

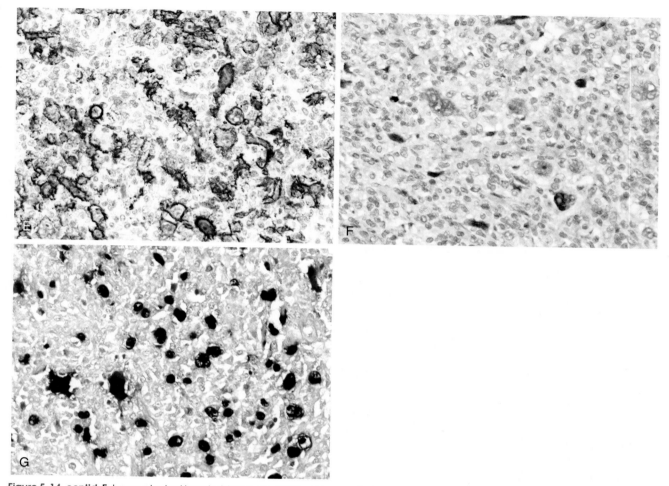

Figure 5-14, cont'd *E,* Large atypical lymphoid cells are CD20+. *F,* Large atypical cells are CD30+ (dim). *G,* Large B cells are positive for EBV. (*E* and *F,* Immunoperoxidase technique on paraffin sections; *G,* in situ hybridization for EBER on a paraffin section.)

from 10% to more than 50% of diffuse large B-cell lymphomas.[27,32,39,125] The immunophenotypic and genotypic features overlap with those found in gastric diffuse large B-cell lymphoma. Intestinal diffuse large B-cell lymphomas are only rarely CD5+.[119] The proportion of cases expressing CD10 has varied among series, ranging from 23%[143] to 64%.[119] Most cases are positive for bcl6, bcl2, and MUM1/IRF4.[119,143] Some authors have reported that most intestinal diffuse large B-cell lymphomas have a non-germinal center immunophenotype,[143] but others have found a predominance of a germinal center phenotype.[119] CD138 is not typically expressed except in cases of plasmablastic lymphoma.[119]

Cytogenetic analysis has demonstrated a heterogeneous assortment of chromosomal translocations in intestinal diffuse large B-cell lymphoma. Translocations involving *BCL6* or *IGH* are found in nearly 30% of cases overall.[34,143] A few cases (fewer than 10%) have *MYC* rearrangement.[34,143] *IGH/BCL2* fusion is uncommon.[34,143] Although the t(11;18) translocation involving *API2* and *MALT1* is considered to be exclusively associated with extranodal marginal zone lymphoma, it has been described in one case of intestinal diffuse large B-cell lymphoma.[34]

Staging, Treatment, and Outcome

Regional lymph node involvement at presentation is common.[32,42,125,143] In most cases, the lymphoma is confined to the bowel with or without regional lymph node involvement; a minority of patients present with more widespread disease.[125,143] After a diagnosis has been established by a biopsy sample or resection specimen, patients usually are treated with combination chemotherapy, as for diffuse large B-cell lymphoma in other sites. Intestinal diffuse large B-cell lymphoma is relatively aggressive. The 5-year overall survival rate ranges from 25% to 67%.[33,81,119,125,143] Perforation is associated with a high mortality rate.[143] Diffuse large B-cell lymphoma that arises in association with marginal zone lymphoma may have a better outcome than de novo diffuse large B-cell lymphoma.[39]

Differential Diagnosis

The differential diagnosis is similar to that for gastric diffuse large B-cell lymphoma. In addition, the differential diagnosis may include the hyperplastic lymphoid tissue that may be found in the intestines. Hyperplastic lymphoid tissue normally is found in the terminal ileum (Peyer's patches),

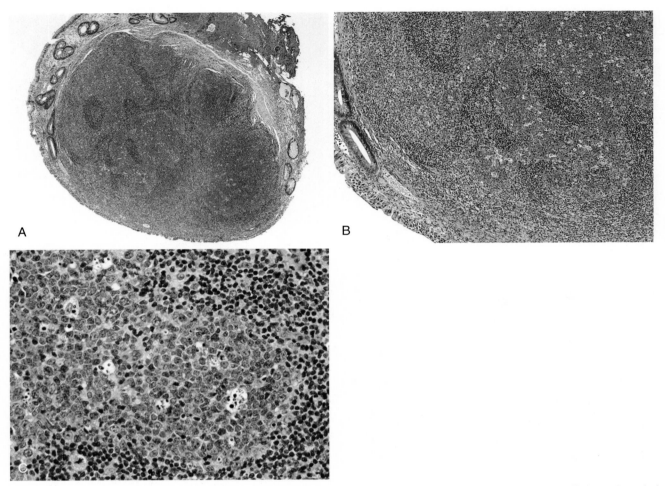

Figure 5-15   Rectal tonsil. **A,** Low-power view shows a discrete, raised lesion composed of organized lymphoid tissue with large, irregularly shaped lymphoid follicles. The overlying mucosa is thinned centrally. **B,** Slightly higher power view shows a serpiginously shaped, floridly hyperplastic lymphoid follicle. The overlying epithelium shows reactive changes. **C,** High-power view shows part of one follicle composed of many actively proliferating large lymphoid cells, with interspersed tingible body macrophages, surrounded by small lymphocytes.

but it occasionally arises in other parts of the intestine. Lymphoid polyps (polypoid lesions composed of reactive lymphoid tissue) may develop in the colon and when large and prominent can suggest lymphoma. The "rectal tonsil" is a large, discrete nodule of organized lymphoid tissue with reactive follicles, often showing florid hyperplasia that is found in the lamina propria or submucosa of the rectum. Overlying cryptitis, mild architectural distortion, intraepithelial lymphocytes, and lymphoepithelial lesions are seen in some cases (Figure 5-15).[150] In lymphoid follicular proctitis, a condition characterized by congested, nodular mucosa and often associated with rectal bleeding, reactive lymphoid tissue, including lymphoid follicles, is found in the distal portion of the gastrointestinal tract.[151]

In any of these types of hyperplastic lymphoid tissue, large reactive follicles with active follicle centers containing many large cells, tingible body macrophages, and frequent mitoses may be seen. In some cases, follicular architecture may be difficult to detect without immunostaining for follicular

dendritic cells, and the appearance may suggest a diffuse, high-grade lymphoma.[150] Familiarity with these entities and delineation of the lymphoid components with immunostains for B- and T-cell markers and markers for follicular dendritic cells, showing large B cells mostly confined to follicles, can prevent overdiagnosis as lymphoma.

Mantle Cell Lymphoma of the Gastrointestinal Tract

Clinical Features

Mantle cell lymphoma affects middle-aged or older adults. Almost all patients are 50 years of age or older, and the median age is approximately 60 years. Men are affected much more often than women.[19,40,81,152,153] The lymphoma often takes the form of innumerable polyps, so-called multiple lymphomatous polyposis, a term devised by Cornes[154] to describe lymphoma with the appearance of multiple sessile or pedunculated gastrointestinal polyps. Patients with multiple

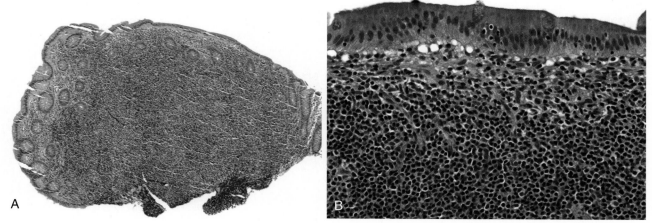

Figure 5-16   Mantle cell lymphoma. **A,** A polypoid fragment of colonic mucosa has been mostly replaced by a large infiltrative nodule of lymphoid cells. **B,** The neoplastic mantle cells are slightly larger and have slightly finer chromatin than do normal lymphocytes.

lymphomatous polyposis present with abdominal pain, diarrhea, bloody stool, and weight loss.[19] Any portion of the gastrointestinal tract can be affected,[39,81] and frequently the lymphoma affects multiple sites, including the stomach, small intestine, colon and, in rare cases, even the esophagus.[19] Appendiceal involvement by mantle cell lymphoma in the form of multiple lymphomatous polyposis has been described.[35] In rare cases patients have involvement of the entire gastrointestinal tract from esophagus to rectum.[20]

Among patients presenting with gastrointestinal involvement by mantle cell lymphoma, mesenteric lymph nodes usually are involved by lymphoma,[81] and staging frequently reveals widespread disease away from the gastrointestinal tract. Conversely, in patients diagnosed with mantle cell lymphoma in sites away from the gastrointestinal tract, when upper and lower endoscopy is performed, gastrointestinal tract involvement has been found in nearly all patients, even when endoscopic findings are normal or only subtly abnormal.[155] Although mantle cell lymphoma usually responds to combination chemotherapy, relapses are common, and the median survival is 3 to 5 years.[153]

Pathologic Features

On gross or endoscopic examination, multiple lymphomatous polyposis has the appearance of multiple, fleshy white nodules involving the mucosa, sometimes with superficial submucosal involvement. Mantle cell lymphoma also (and less commonly) may take the form of a discrete mass or an ulcerated lesion.[33] Microscopic examination in cases of multiple lymphomatous polyposis shows a bandlike infiltrate or multiple ill-defined nodules of atypical lymphoid cells that usually are slightly larger and more irregular than normal lymphocytes and have inconspicuous nucleoli and scant cytoplasm (Figure 5-16). Less often, the lymphoma has a mantle zone pattern, with neoplastic cells confined to the mantles of reactive follicles. Single

epithelioid histiocytes may be scattered among the neoplastic cells. Remnants of reactive follicle centers can be identified within some nodules. The lymphoma may displace and obliterate glands, but formation of true lymphoepithelial lesions is not a feature.[81,152]

Occasionally some deviation is seen from the classic histologic picture of mantle cell lymphoma. In the small cell variant, the neoplastic cells may be small and round, potentially mimicking small lymphocytic lymphoma/chronic lymphocytic leukemia. In the marginal zone–like variant, the neoplastic cells have abundant, pale cytoplasm, and the lymphoma may be mistaken for marginal zone lymphoma (Figure 5-17).[153] Aggressive variants of mantle cell lymphoma include the blastoid variant, in which neoplastic cells have finely dispersed chromatin and a high mitotic rate, resembling lymphoblasts (Figure 5-18), and the pleomorphic variant, in which neoplastic cells are relatively large and pleomorphic, often with recognizable nucleoli, potentially mimicking diffuse large B-cell lymphoma. In contrast to other histologically low-grade B-cell lymphomas, mantle cell lymphoma does not undergo transformation to diffuse large B-cell lymphoma; however, over time, mantle cell lymphoma with the typical appearance may progress to one of the aggressive variants.[153]

Immunophenotyping typically shows CD20+, CD5+, CD43+, CD10−, CD23−, bcl2+, cyclin D1+ B cells expressing bright monotypic surface immunoglobulin, IgMD type; lambda light chain is expressed more frequently than kappa light chain (see Figure 5-18, *C* to *F*). Less often, dim expression of CD23 may be seen, or CD5 may not be expressed (see Figure 3-19). With antibodies to follicular dendritic cells (e.g., CD21), an underlying follicular dendritic meshwork can almost always be demonstrated; in most cases, the meshwork is expanded or disrupted rather than intact and orderly. In aggressive variants of mantle cell lymphoma (see Figure 5-18), the proliferation fraction may be high (see Figure 5-18, *G*). The

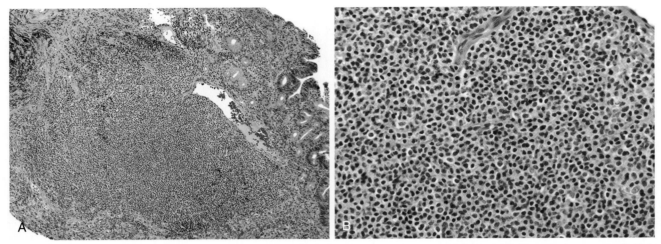

Figure 5-17   Mantle cell lymphoma, marginal zone–like. **A,** Neoplastic mantle cells form a nodule beneath the colonic mucosa. **B,** Higher power view shows small to medium-sized lymphoid cells with abundant, clear to pale pink cytoplasm, closely mimicking marginal zone lymphoma.

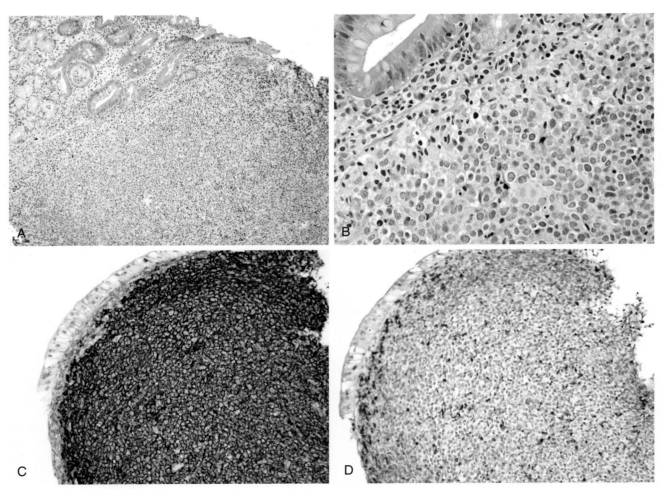

Figure 5-18   Mantle cell lymphoma, blastoid variant, involving the duodenum. **A,** Atypical lymphoid cells form a dense infiltrate adjacent to the duodenal mucosa. **B,** Higher power view shows medium-sized to large neoplastic cells with oval nuclei and finely dispersed chromatin, closely mimicking lymphoblasts (compare to size of small lymphocytes at upper left of image). Neoplastic cells are CD20+ **(C),** with a few scattered CD3+ T cells **(D).**

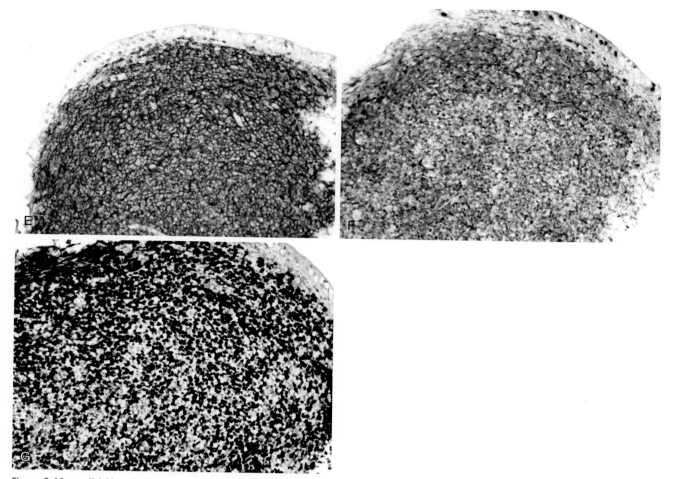

Figure 5-18, cont'd Neoplastic B cells co-express CD5 **(E)** and cyclin D1 **(F)**; 80% to 90% of cells are Ki67+ (proliferation, **G**). The immunophenotype is similar to that of other mantle cell lymphomas except that a higher proportion of cells is Ki67+ in the aggressive variants. (Immunoperoxidase technique on paraffin sections.)

underlying genetic abnormality is t(11;14)(q13;q32), a translocation involving *BCL1* and *IGH* that leads to overexpression of cyclin D1 mRNA and then of cyclin D1 protein. Expression of α4β7, the mucosal homing receptor, has been associated with gastrointestinal involvement.[19,81,156]

Differential Diagnosis

1. **Mantle cell lymphoma versus other lymphomas.** On occasion, lymphomas other than the mantle cell type can be associated with the picture of lymphomatous polyposis. Follicular lymphoma[19,33,39]; marginal zone lymphoma[19]; and even rare T-cell lymphomas, particularly adult T-cell leukemia/lymphoma (human T-cell leukemia virus type 1 [HTLV-1]+),[157,158] can have the appearance of multiple lymphomatous polyposis. A case of diffuse large B-cell lymphoma, probably of the plasmablastic type, that presented as multiple lymphomatous polyposis has been reported in an HIV-positive male.[159] Cases of the small cell variant and the marginal zone–like variant of mantle cell lymphoma can be especially easy to misinterpret as other types of B-cell lymphomas.

The diagnosis usually can be established with careful study of hematoxylin and eosin (H&E)-stained slides accompanied by immunohistochemistry. The distinction is important because of the inferior prognosis for mantle cell lymphoma compared with most other B-cell lymphomas in the differential diagnosis.

2. **Mantle cell lymphoma versus reactive lymphoid infiltrates.** Subtle, early involvement of the gastrointestinal mucosa by mantle cell lymphoma may be easy to mistake for a chronic inflammatory process. The presence of a dense, monotonous infiltrate with some cytologic atypia can raise the index of suspicion for lymphoma. If the patient is known to have mantle cell lymphoma in another anatomic site, the index of suspicion for gastrointestinal involvement should be raised even if lymphoid infiltrates are not strikingly atypical on routine sections. When neoplastic mantle cells are confined to the mantles of reactive follicles, they may be difficult to recognize as abnormal; immunophenotyping with antibody to cyclin D1 readily highlights the neoplastic population.

Follicular Lymphoma of the Gastrointestinal Tract

Introduction

Follicular lymphoma of the gastrointestinal tract is uncommon, accounting for fewer than 4% of all lymphomas primary in this site.[29] In one large series, 3% of gastric B-cell lymphomas were follicular lymphomas.[73] However, gastrointestinal follicular lymphoma has distinctive clinical and pathologic features; accordingly, primary intestinal follicular lymphoma is designated a variant of follicular lymphoma in the WHO Classification.[160]

Clinical Features

Most patients are middle-aged or older adults, and the mean[161-163] and/or median age is in the 50s.[29,163-166] Most series report a female preponderance.[29,161,164,167,168] Patients present with abdominal pain, less often with diarrhea,[163,167] and in rare cases with jaundice.[169] In some cases, follicular lymphoma is an incidental finding[162,163]; this is particularly common when endoscopy is performed as part of a routine checkup.[162] The small intestine most often is involved. A number of studies describe a marked predilection for the duodenum.[29,161,165-168] This is a striking observation, because among gastrointestinal lymphomas, the duodenum is a particularly uncommon primary site. A few other studies have shown more frequent involvement of the ileum.[163,164] Occasionally the jejunum, stomach, and colorectum may be affected.[166,167] Follicular lymphoma can involve multiple portions of the small intestine simultaneously.[162,167]

The most common endoscopic appearance is multiple small, whitish polyps and granularity or nodularity of the mucosa, sometimes with the picture of multiple lymphomatous polyposis.[19,161,162,166] Although the term "multiple lymphomatous polyposis" is most closely associated with mantle cell lymphoma, it is interesting that in the first report using this term, the illustrations of case 1 appear to show a follicular lymphoma.[154] Less often the lymphoma takes the form of a large, discrete, deeply invasive mass.[163,169] Ulceration

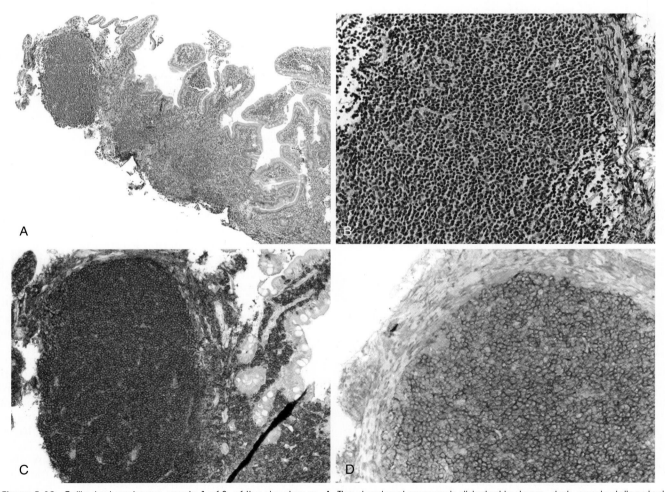

Figure 5-19   Follicular lymphoma, grade 1 of 3, of the duodenum. **A,** The duodenal mucosa is distorted by large, dark, poorly delineated nodules of lymphoid cells; increased numbers of small lymphocytes are present in the stroma of the villi. **B,** Higher power view of the large nodule in the upper left of *A* shows a monotonous population of small, slightly irregular lymphoid cells. The atypical cells are CD20+ **(C)** and co-express CD10 **(D)**

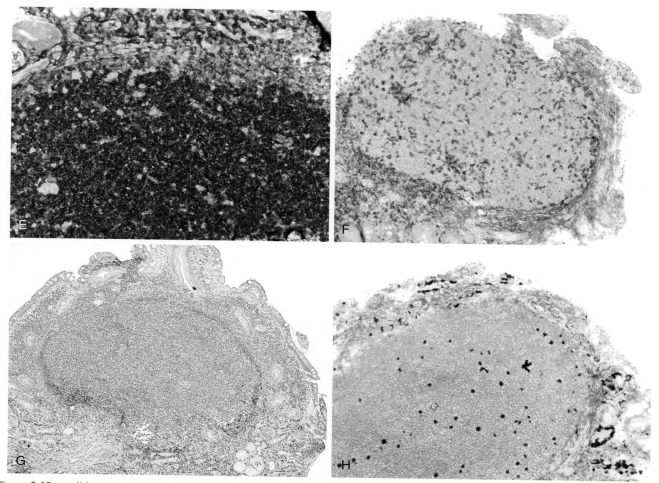

Figure 5-19, cont'd and bcl2 **(E)** but not CD5 **(F)**; CD5 highlights a small population of interspersed T cells. **G,** The CD21+ dendritic mesh-work associated with this neoplastic follicle is well preserved only at the periphery of the follicle. **H,** Ki67 (proliferation) highlights fewer than 5% of cells in the neoplastic follicle, which correlates with the lymphoma's low grade. (*C* to *H,* Immunoperoxidase technique on paraffin sections.)

is unusual but has been described.[164] Lymphomas arising near the ampulla of Vater sometimes invade subjacent pancreas.[163,169] The lymphoma often is confined to the bowel wall but may show regional lymph node involvement.[166,169,170] The bone marrow is involved in a few cases,[162] but overall, intestinal follicular lymphoma tends to present at a lower stage than follicular lymphoma of the lymph nodes.[170]

Pathologic Features

The pathologic features described vary somewhat from one series to another. In most series, the cases are almost uniform. They typically are grade 1 of 3 follicular lymphomas with an entirely follicular pattern and with an immunophenotype similar to that found in nodal follicular lymphomas (CD20+, CD10+, bcl2+, bcl6+, CD5−, MUM1/IRF4−, cyclin D1−, with a small percent of Ki67+ cells) (Figures 5-19 and 5-20).[29,164-168,170,171] Molecular and cytogenetic studies show clonal immunoglobulin heavy and light chain genes and *BCL2* rearrangement in most cases so analyzed.[164,170-172]

Some series include cases of follicular lymphoma that deviate from the typical picture; for example, those that are grade 2 or grade 3 of 3, that have diffuse areas, and/or that lack expression of CD10, bcl6, or bcl2.[19,161,163,167,170] Rare cases negative for *BCL2* rearrangement have been reported.[19]

In contrast to follicular lymphoma of the lymph nodes, α4β7, the mucosal homing receptor, is frequently expressed in gastrointestinal follicular lymphoma, which suggests an origin from local, antigen-responsive B cells.[173] Preferential expression of IgA was described in one study, although others have found IgM to be expressed most frequently.[163] According to one study, in contrast to follicular lymphomas of the lymph nodes, in duodenal follicular lymphomas, follicular dendritic cell meshworks are concentrated around the periphery of the follicle and lost centrally,[170] so that the dendritic meshworks appear hollow. Also in contrast to lymph node follicular lymphomas, intestinal follicular lymphomas are reported to lack activation-induced cytidine deaminase (AID), although they still have ongoing somatic hypermutation, the

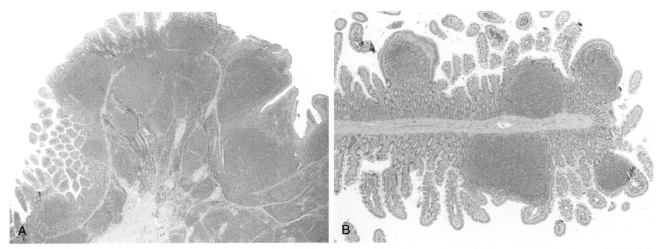

Figure 5-20   Follicular lymphoma, grade 1 of 3, small intestine. **A,** This lymphoma forms a large lesion composed of crowded follicles. **B,** Individual neoplastic follicles involve small intestinal mucosa away from the main mass.

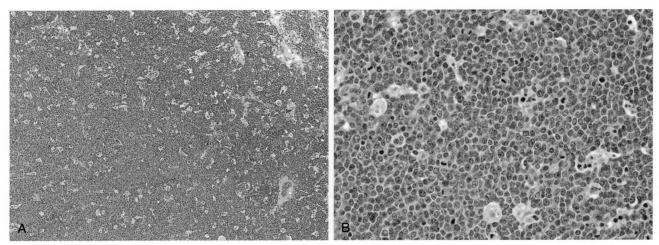

Figure 5-21   Burkitt's lymphoma in an African patient (endemic Burkitt's lymphoma) with a large abdominal mass. **A,** The tissue has been replaced by a dense infiltrate of basophilic cells with a starry sky pattern, related to pale tingible body macrophages, with little or no intervening fibrous stroma. **B,** High-power view shows relatively uniform, medium-sized cells with oval nuclei, stippled chromatin, and small nucleoli. Mitoses are numerous. Tingible body macrophages are interspersed.

mechanism for which is uncertain.[170] Biased usage of immunoglobulin heavy chain variable region genes (*IGVH*) has been described, with disproportionate use of V_H4, particularly V_H4-34.[166,170] Possible preferential use of V_H5-51 also has been reported.[170] Usage of V_H4 and V_H5 is more common than in lymph node follicular lymphoma.[170] These observations also suggest a role for antigen in the pathogenesis of this lymphoma.[166,170]

Outcome

Gastrointestinal follicular lymphoma has a good prognosis. It typically displays indolent behavior and a good response to therapy. Some patients have persistent lymphoma, and some experience relapse within or beyond the gastrointestinal tract.[163,167] Large cell transformation has been described.[164] A patient with low-grade gastrointestinal follicular lymphoma seen at our hospital had high-grade

transformation and an aggressive clinical course; cytogenetic analysis revealed concurrent *BCL2* and *MYC* rearrangements.[174] Rare patients succumb to the lymphoma.[19,164,165,168]

Although studies vary to some degree, the results taken together suggest that a high proportion of duodenal lymphomas are follicular lymphoma and that a high proportion of gastrointestinal follicular lymphomas arise in the small intestine, with a disproportionate number arising in the duodenum. The combination of origin in the gastrointestinal tract, the tendency to remain localized to that site, disrupted follicular dendritic meshworks, expression of α4β7, and skewed V_H gene usage, suggesting antigen selection, are features that duodenal follicular lymphoma shares with marginal zone lymphoma, although the histology and most immunophenotypic features are similar to those of nodal follicular lymphoma.

Burkitt's Lymphoma of the Gastrointestinal Tract

Clinical Features

Burkitt's lymphoma is a highly aggressive, rapidly growing lymphoma with characteristic histologic, immunophenotypic, and genetic features. According to the WHO,[175] Burkitt's lymphoma has three clinical variants: (1) the endemic type, (2) the sporadic type, and (3) the immunodeficiency-associated type. Involvement of the ileocecal region is the most common manifestation of sporadic Burkitt's lymphoma. Although gastrointestinal involvement occasionally is seen with endemic (see Figure 5-21) and immunodeficiency-associated Burkitt's lymphoma, presentation with disease outside the gastrointestinal tract is more common. Infrequently, sites in the gastrointestinal tract other than the ileocecal area are involved, including the stomach[176] and more distal portions of the colon. In one large series, only 1% of gastric B-cell lymphomas were Burkitt's lymphomas.[73] Sporadic Burkitt's lymphoma mainly affects children and young adults; a male preponderance is seen overall, and among children the male preponderance is striking.[27,175] Most patients with immunodeficiency-associated Burkitt's lymphoma are HIV positive, some are iatrogenically immunosuppressed, and a few have an underlying congenital immunodeficiency.[62,176] In some cases, staging reveals disease beyond the gastrointestinal tract. Young, immunocompetent patients with Burkitt's lymphoma who are treated with appropriate high-intensity, short-duration chemotherapy have an excellent prognosis.[177]

Pathologic Features

On gross inspection, the tumors usually are bulky, exophytic lesions, sometimes with ulceration.[39] Microscopic examination reveals a diffuse infiltrate of uniform, medium-sized cells with round nuclei, stippled chromatin, three or four small nucleoli, and distinct rims of deeply basophilic cytoplasm. Numerous tingible body macrophages are seen, resulting in a starry sky pattern. The mitotic rate is very high. Sclerosis typically is absent within the lymphoma. Except for the tingible body macrophages, interspersed reactive cells are very infrequent (see Figures 5-21 and 5-22). In some cases, the nuclei of the neoplastic cells show greater pleomorphism, and nucleoli are fewer in number but tend to be more prominent; previously, these cases were referred to as "atypical Burkitt's lymphoma." However, because the cases otherwise are similar to the more classic-appearing Burkitt's lymphoma, and to prevent confusion, these cases now are also called "Burkitt's lymphoma," without any special designation.

In cases of Burkitt's lymphoma with plasmacytoid differentiation, the neoplastic cells have eccentric basophilic cytoplasm and often a single central nucleolus; this variant is most often encountered in immunodeficient patients.[175]

Immunophenotyping reveals monotypic IgM+, CD20+, CD10+, bcl6+, CD5−, bcl2− B cells with a proliferation fraction of nearly 100% (see Figure 5-22, C to F). Expression of CD10 and bcl6 is strong and diffuse. Cytogenetic analysis reveals t(8;14), t(2;8), or t(8;22), corresponding to translocations involving the *MYC* gene and either the immunoglobulin heavy chain gene or kappa or lambda light chain gene; this cytogenetic finding is a hallmark of Burkitt's lymphoma. The karyotype usually is simple, with the translocation involving *MYC* present as the sole abnormality or accompanied by very few other abnormalities. EBV is found in about one third of sporadic and immunodeficiency-associated Burkitt's lymphomas and in essentially all endemic Burkitt's lymphoma.[175]

Differential Diagnosis

The main problem in the differential diagnosis of Burkitt's lymphoma is distinguishing it from other high-grade B-cell lymphomas. When Burkitt's lymphoma occurs in a young boy as a mass in the ileocecal region and has the usual histologic and immunophenotypic features, diagnosis is straightforward. When it occurs in adults, among whom Burkitt's lymphoma is relatively uncommon, careful evaluation of the histology, immunophenotype, and cytogenetics is required to establish a diagnosis. *MYC* rearrangement, while characteristic of Burkitt's lymphoma, is not specific for Burkitt's lymphoma; the same is true of the immunophenotype of Burkitt's lymphoma. High-grade B-cell lymphomas that may mimic Burkitt's lymphoma but that are not true Burkitt's lymphoma may have an inferior response to treatment and a worse prognosis than Burkitt's lymphoma. The WHO Classification has defined a category of high-grade B-cell lymphoma with features intermediate between Burkitt's lymphoma and diffuse large B-cell lymphoma.[178] Included in this category are so-called "double hit" lymphomas, with concurrent *BCL2* and *MYC* translocations; these lymphomas may closely mimic Burkitt's lymphoma, but they have a very poor prognosis.[174]

Florid reactive follicular hyperplasia also may enter the differential diagnosis of Burkitt's lymphoma, if the tissue submitted is a small biopsy sample and follicular architecture is not apparent, because the histologic features of the dark zone of a reactive follicle overlap with those of Burkitt's lymphoma, and the immunophenotype also is similar. Table 5-5 presents features that can be helpful in the differential diagnosis.

Enteropathy-Associated T-Cell Lymphoma

Introduction

An association between malabsorption and intestinal lymphoma was recognized in the first half of the twentieth century. Analysis of the lymphomas arising in association with celiac disease suggested that they were a distinctive type. Initially, they were

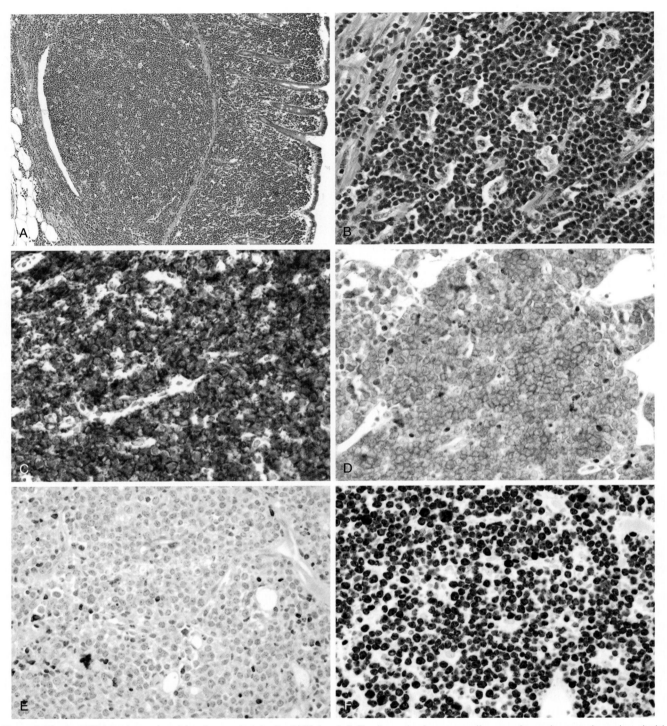

Figure 5-22   Burkitt's lymphoma involving the gastrointestinal (GI) tract. **A,** The ileocolectomy resection specimen shows a dense lymphoid infiltrate filling the lamina propria and invading deeply into the subjacent bowel wall. **B,** Medium-sized, relatively uniform lymphoid cells with many interspersed tingible body macrophages infiltrate muscularis. Neoplastic B cells are CD20+ **(C),** CD10+ **(D),** and bcl2– **(E);** nearly all cells are Ki67+ **(F).** (*C* to *F,* Immunoperoxidase technique on paraffin sections.)

thought to be a form of malignant histiocytosis, but later studies showed that the neoplastic cells were T cells and the neoplasms thus were peripheral T-cell lymphomas.[179,180] The disease now is called *enteropathy-associated T-cell lymphoma (EATL)*[181,182]; it was referred to previously as *enteropathy-type intestinal T-cell lymphoma*[183] and *intestinal T-cell lymphoma.*[184]

In the WHO Classification, this entity is defined as a lymphoma that arises from the intraepithelial T lymphocytes, typically associated with changes of enteropathy.[182] The pathogenesis is thought to be related to chronic antigenic stimulation by gluten in patients with gluten-sensitive enteropathy, or celiac disease. A monomorphic variant, also known

TABLE 5-5

Differential Diagnosis of Burkitt's Lymphoma

Type of Lymphoma	Clinical Features	Morphology	Usual Immunophenotype	Cytogenetics
Burkitt's lymphoma	Gastrointestinal (GI) tract most common site of sporadic Burkitt's lymphoma; higher proportion of lymphomas in children than in adults; males affected more than females; rapidly growing masses	Uniform or slightly pleomorphic medium-sized cells, deep blue cytoplasm, starry sky pattern	CD20+, CD10+, CD5−, bcl6+, bcl2−, TdT−, monotypic sIg+, Ki67 ~ 100%	Simple karyotype with t(8;14), t(2;8) or t(8;22) (*MYC* and *IGH* or *IGL*); no *BCL2* or *BCL6* translocation
Diffuse large B-Cell lymphoma	Adults affected more often than children; nodal or extranodal; sometimes large mass lesions, often localized	Large oval, irregular, or lobated nuclei; scant cytoplasm	CD20+, CD10−/+, bcl6+/−, bcl2+/−, monotypic sIg+/−	*BCL2* and *BCL6* abnormalities common; *MYC* abnormal in a minority
High-grade B-Cell lymphoma with "double-hit"	Affects adults, some with previous low-grade follicular lymphoma; aggressive lymphomas; very poor prognosis	May resemble Burkitt's or diffuse large B-cell lymphoma or may have intermediate features	May be similar to Burkitt's lymphoma but often bcl2+, Ki67 < 100%	Concurrent *MYC* and *BCL2* translocations; karyotype often complex
B-lymphoblastic lymphoma/ leukemia	Children affected more often than adults; leukemia seen more often than lymphoma	Small to medium-sized cells with fine chromatin, variable size and shape	CD19+, CD20−/+, CD10+, TdT+, sIg−	Variable, often hyperdiploid; *MYC* rearrangement rare
Mantle cell lymphoma, blastoid variant	Middle-aged and older adults affected, males more than females; usually widespread disease in nodes and other sites; GI tract involvement common	Medium-sized to large lymphoblast-like or pleomorphic cells with scant cytoplasm	CD20+, CD5+, CD10−, bcl6−, bcl2+, cyclin D1+, monotypic sIg+	t(11;14) (*BCL1* and *IGH*)
Florid follicular hyperplasia	Can be seen in Peyer's patches and elsewhere in GI tract	Large, irregular follicles with many blast cells and mitoses	CD20+, CD10+, bcl6+, bcl2−, Ki67 ~ 100%, CD21+, CD23+ dendritic meshworks, polytypic Ig expression	No clonal abnormalities

as *enteropathy-associated T-cell lymphoma, type 2*, may arise independent of celiac disease. Although the higher risk for lymphoma among patients with celiac disease is greatest for primary gastrointestinal lymphomas of T-lineage, a large population-based study revealed an increased risk for B-cell lymphoma and for lymphoma arising outside the gastrointestinal tract as well.[185] Enteropathy-associated T-cell lymphoma is uncommon; in one large study, it accounted for 13% of all small intestinal lymphomas.[186]

Clinical Features

Enteropathy-associated T-cell lymphoma occurs almost exclusively in adults; the mean or median age is in the 50s or 60s in most series. More than 90% of patients are over age 50. Young adults are only occasionally affected. In contrast to celiac disease, in which most patients are women, enteropathy-associated T-cell lymphoma has a slight male preponderance.[186-190] Because the pathogenesis of this lymphoma is closely linked to celiac disease, it is

more frequently encountered among individuals of northern European descent, among whom celiac disease is more prevalent.[187]

Patients with enteropathy-associated T-cell lymphoma (EATL) often have a history of celiac disease, which may be of long or short duration.[187] Strict, long-term adherence to a gluten-free diet markedly reduces the risk for the development of lymphoma, whereas poor compliance with a gluten-free diet is associated with a significant risk for lymphoma.[190,191] Patients with celiac disease responsive to a gluten-free diet may progress to develop refractory celiac disease (discussed later) and then to enteropathy-associated T-cell lymphoma (secondary EATL).[189]

In contrast, other patients with enteropathy-associated T-cell lymphoma have no previous history of celiac disease (de novo EATL); they often present acutely with symptoms related to the lymphoma. In some of these cases, histologic evidence of enteropathy is seen, which suggests that the patient had subclinical celiac disease. Even when no histologic evidence of enteropathy is identified, the presence of antibodies to gliadin or endomysium or the HLA types associated with celiac disease (HLA-DQ2 or DQ8) usually can be found.[182,189]

Patients with enteropathy-associated T-cell lymphoma present with abdominal pain, weight loss, diarrhea, vomiting, fever, night sweats, or a combination of these findings. In some cases, patients present with intestinal perforation or obstruction. Among patients with a history of celiac disease, symptoms may suggest worsening celiac disease, with loss of response to a gluten-free diet.[27,187,192] The lymphoma most often affects the proximal small intestine.[186] The jejunum is most frequently affected, followed by the ileum and the duodenum. In some cases the lymphoma is multifocal, affecting both the proximal and distal small intestine. A few patients present with gastric involvement. Colonic involvement is uncommon. In rare cases patients present with disease outside the gastrointestinal tract.[182,186,190,192]

The diagnosis usually is established on a resection specimen rather than a biopsy sample[186] because of the location of the disease and the frequent presentation with ulceration and perforation.

Pathologic Features

Enteropathy-associated T-cell lymphoma may produce single or multiple intestinal lesions in the form of plaques, nodules, or strictures with circumferential ulceration and sometimes perforation. Large, bulky masses are uncommon.[27,187]

Most cases are enteropathy-associated T-cell lymphoma, type 1, which is characterized by a diffuse infiltrate of atypical lymphoid cells associated with ulceration and a variable admixture of inflammatory cells, often with many histiocytes and other reactive cells. Occasionally eosinophils are numerous; in such cases, peripheral eosinophilia may be seen.[193] The reactive cells sometimes are so prominent they obscure the neoplastic population, particularly if only a biopsy sample is submitted for diagnosis.

The appearance of the neoplastic cells varies from one case to another. They often are moderately pleomorphic and medium to large (Figure 5-23), but they may have a bizarre anaplastic appearance.

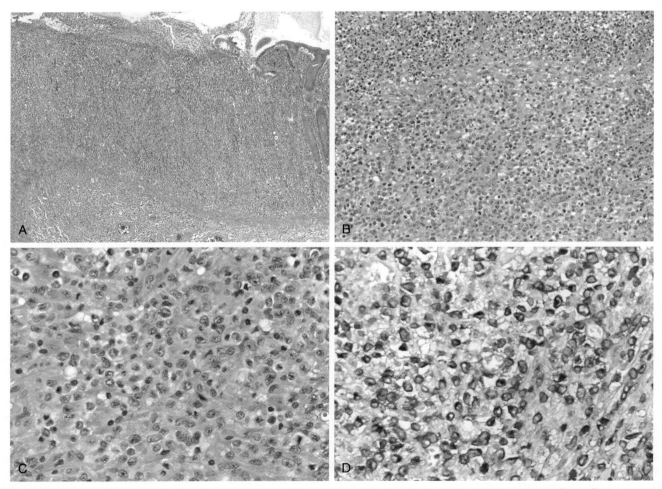

Figure 5-23   Enteropathy-associated T-cell lymphoma, type 1, in a patient with abdominal pain. **A,** A dense cellular infiltrate fills the mucosa and invades the wall of the small bowel. No large exophytic lesion was identified. **B,** An infiltrate of atypical lymphoid cells is present beneath an ulcerated surface. **C,** High-power view shows medium-sized to large atypical lymphoid cells with oval or irregular nuclei, with scattered histiocytes and eosinophils admixed. Atypical lymphoid cells are CD3+ **(D)**

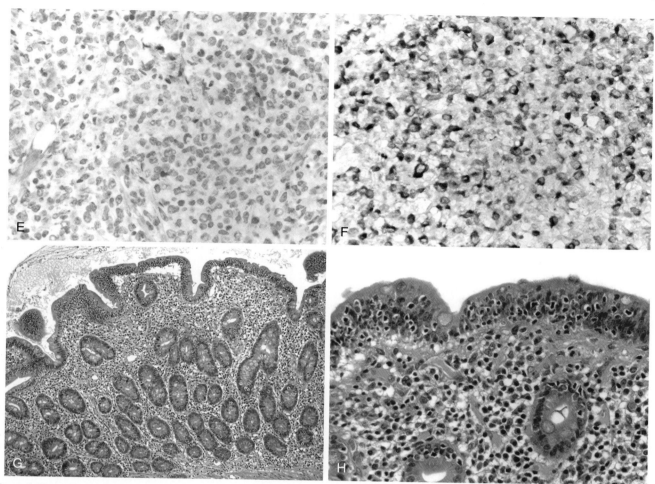

Figure 5-23, cont'd CD5– (**E**), and perforin+ (**F**). They also were granzyme B+ and CD30+/– and were negative for CD20, CD4, CD8, and CD56 (not illustrated), consistent with abnormal T cells with a cytotoxic phenotype. (*D* to *F*, Immunoperoxidase technique on paraffin sections.) **G,** The adjacent mucosa shows changes of celiac disease, with villous blunting, crypt hyperplasia, increased lymphocytes and plasma cells in the lamina propria, and loss of mucin. **H,** High-power view shows marked increase in numbers of intraepithelial lymphocytes.

Intravascular clusters of neoplastic cells sometimes are found. Changes of celiac disease, including increased numbers of intraepithelial lymphocytes, villous atrophy, crypt hyperplasia, and a lympho-plasmacytic infiltrate in the lamina propria, often are seen in the mucosa away from the lymphoma (Figure 5-23, *G* and *H*).[142,180,182,187]

In a minority of cases, the tumor cells are medium-sized and relatively uniform and have smooth, dark chromatin and clear cytoplasm (the monomorphic variant of enteropathy-associated T-cell lymphoma, or enteropathy-associated T-cell lymphoma, type 2). The monomorphic variant shows less conspicuous fibrosis and necrosis and fewer admixed inflammatory cells (Figure 5-24).

The histologic changes of enteropathy often are conspicuous, but the monomorphic variant may occur without an association with celiac disease.[182] Some enteropathy-associated T-cell lymphomas may arise from intraepithelial lymphocytes driven to neoplastic transformation by other, as yet undefined types of chronic antigenic stimulation.[194] Whether some specific cause other than celiac disease can

result in enteropathy-associated T-cell lymphoma or whether some cases truly arise sporadically is uncertain.

In the more common enteropathy-associated T-cell lymphoma, type 1, immunophenotyping usually shows neoplastic cells expressing cytoplasmic CD3, CD7, and CD103. CD5 expression often is lost. In most cases, CD4 and CD8 are both absent (see Figure 5-23, *D* and *E*). A few cases are CD8+, but CD4 expression is rare. CD56 typically is not expressed.[181,182,188] Most cases are thought to be α/β T-cell in origin, although a few cases of γ/δ T-cell origin have been described.[183] CD30 is expressed by some lymphomas with anaplastic morphology. The neoplastic cells have a cytotoxic phenotype; they express TIA-1 and sometimes granzyme B and perforin (see Figure 5-23, *F*).[180,181,195] The cytotoxic nature of the neoplastic cells and of the intraepithelial cells from which they arise could be responsible for the mucosal damage, including villous atrophy, ulceration, and necrosis, that is seen with celiac disease and lymphoma. CD103 is expressed by intestinal intraepithelial lymphocytes and by a subset of lamina propria lymphocytes. Among lymphomas, its expression is nearly unique for enteropathy-associated T-cell lymphoma,[196] except that CD103 also is expressed by hairy cell leukemia. Rare cases with CD20 co-expression by neoplastic T cells have been reported.[197]

The monomorphic variant typically is composed of CD3+, CD4–, CD8+, CD56+ αβ T cells (see Figure 5-24, E to H). The intraepithelial lymphocytes in the adjacent mucosa usually have the same immunophenotype as that of the lymphoma, whether it is the more common type or the monomorphic variant (see Figure 5-24, E to F).[182] p53 protein is detected in most enteropathy-associated T-cell lymphomas,[198] although loss of heterozygosity of the p53 locus is not consistently detected,[198,199] and p53 mutations appear to be uncommon.[198]

Molecular genetic studies have shown clonal rearrangement of T-cell receptor (TCR) beta and gamma chain genes.[182,188,195,200] EBV typically is absent from tumor cells, although its presence was reported in a series of cases of enteropathy-associated T-cell lymphoma in Mexican patients.[201]

Enteropathy-associated T-cell lymphomas have frequent genetic imbalances. The most common abnormality is amplification of chromosome 9q34, a region containing the NOTCH1 and ABL1 genes, both of which are important in the regulation of hematopoiesis and thus potentially important in the pathogenesis of a subset of enteropathy-associated T-cell lymphoma.[199,202] Loss of heterozygosity at chromosome 9p21, a region harboring tumor suppressor genes p14/p15/p16, also is relatively common; cases with loss of genetic material in this area show loss of p16 protein expression, which suggests that this genetic change is functionally significant.[198]

Mesenteric lymph nodes are almost always enlarged, although they are not always involved by lymphoma. In lymph nodes partially involved by lymphoma, the lymphoma may be found in sinuses or in the paracortex.[81] Enlarged nodes may show nonspecific reactive changes, edema, or mesenteric lymph node cavitation. In the latter condition, the lymph nodes may be markedly enlarged and show cystic change, such that the lymph node consists of

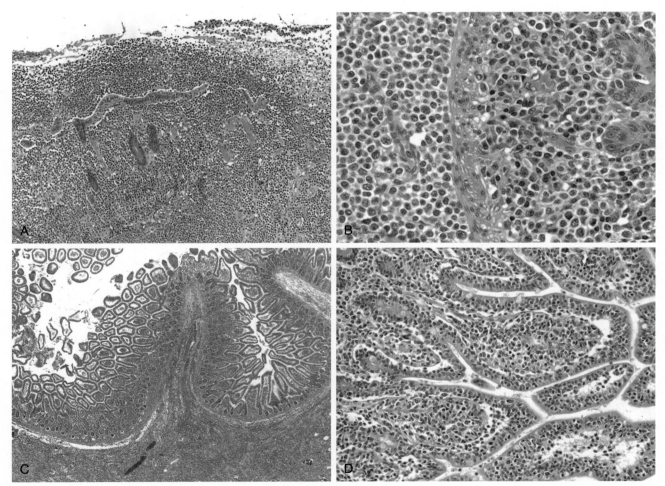

Figure 5-24 Enteropathy-associated T-cell lymphoma, type 2. The patient presented with a small intestinal perforation. **A,** A dense infiltrate of neoplastic lymphoid cells replaces most of the wall of the bowel. **B,** High-power view shows small to medium-sized, relatively monotonous lymphoid cells with oval to slightly irregular lymphoid cells, stippled chromatin, and pale cytoplasm. **C,** In this area, mucosa overlying the lymphoma shows preservation of villous architecture. **D,** Although villous blunting is not conspicuous, there is a striking increase in intraepithelial lymphocytes.

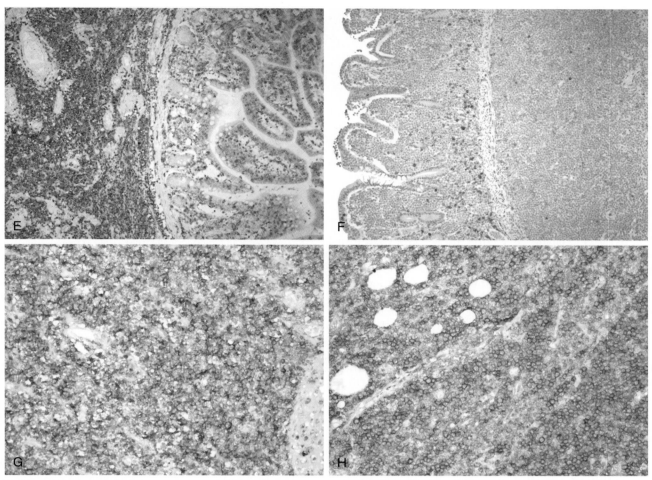

Figure 5-24, cont'd The lymphoma and also the intraepithelial lymphocytes are positive for CD2 **(E)** and CD3 (not shown) and negative for CD5 **(F)**. The lymphoma is CD8+ **(G)** and CD56+ **(H)**, as were the intraepithelial lymphocytes (not shown).

a thickened capsule and a thin rim of lymphoid tissue surrounding clear or turbid fluid that most likely represents lymph.[203] Mesenteric lymph node cavitation is not specific for EATL; it also can be related to severe malnutrition. In the latter case, upon correction of the malnutrition, the lymph node changes may regress.[192]

Staging, Treatment, and Outcome

Lymphoma is confined to the abdomen at presentation in approximately three-fourths of cases.[187,188] Mesenteric lymph nodes often are involved by lymphoma. Staging reveals more distant spread in a minority of cases to sites such as the bone marrow or liver. EATL has a worse prognosis than any other small intestinal lymphoma.[27] The administration of therapy is complicated by the severe malnutrition from which many of these patients suffer, and patients frequently are unable to complete the planned regimen of chemotherapy.[187-189] Chemotherapy also may be complicated by perforation, gastrointestinal bleeding, or sepsis.[187] In one study of 31 patients, 84% of the patients died of the lymphoma or of complications of therapy.[187] In another study, the median survival was 3 months, and 70%

of patients had died within 6 months.[188] In a third study, the 2-year survival rate for patients with de novo enteropathy-associated T-cell lymphoma was 20%; about 15% patients with secondary enteropathy-associated T-cell lymphoma survived for 2 years.[189] However, in most studies, a few patients were long-term survivors, which suggests that combination chemotherapy, sometimes followed by autologous stem cell transplantation,[204] is effective in a subset of cases.[187,188] Intestinal perforation as a result of lymphoma is the most common cause of death, but in some cases dissemination of disease to lymph nodes and a wide variety of extranodal sites, including the liver, spleen, brain, heart, bone marrow, lungs, kidneys, thyroid, and others, contributes to mortality.[180,187] Unlike with B-cell lymphomas, the prognosis for these T-cell lymphomas is independent of the cytology of the neoplastic cells; all behave in an aggressive manner.[182]

Complicated Celiac Disease: Refractory Celiac Disease and Ulcerative Jejunitis

Refractory celiac disease (RCD) and ulcerative jejunitis are serious, potentially fatal forms of celiac disease. Refractory celiac disease, or refractory sprue, is characterized by worsening malabsorption and failure to respond to a gluten-free diet. Biopsy samples typically show changes with the appearance of celiac disease. Ulcerative jejunitis, or ulcerative jejunoileitis, is defined as showing histologically benign mucosal ulcers in a patient with celiac disease (Table 5-6). Patients with refractory celiac disease or ulcerative jejunitis have an increased risk of developing enteropathy-associated T-cell lymphoma, which suggests a relationship between enteropathy-associated T-cell lymphoma and complicated celiac disease.[179,189,192]

Normal jejunal intraepithelial lymphocytes are predominantly TCRαβ T cells with a variable admixture of TCRγδ T cells. The αβ T cells are mostly surface CD3 (sCD3)+, CD5+, predominantly CD8+ T cells, whereas the γδ T cells are sCD3+, CD5 dim or negative, and CD8+/−, with few CD56+ T cells. Therefore, depending on the proportion of αβ and γδ T cells, the immunophenotype of the intraepithelial lymphocytes is somewhat variable.[188,195,204,205] Many patients with refractory celiac disease have an abnormal TCRαβ population of intraepithelial lymphocytes that are sCD3−, cytoplasmic CD3 (cCD3)+, CD7+, CD4−, and CD8− or CD8+ (Figure 5-25).[206] This immunophenotype overlaps with that found in most enteropathy-type T-cell lymphomas (sCD3−, cCD3+, CD4−, CD8−).

Molecular genetic analysis has shown that clonal T cells are present in refractory celiac disease and in ulcerative jejunitis in most cases.[192,195,200,204,207] When lymphoma follows refractory celiac disease or ulcerative jejunitis, the same clone is found in the lymphoma, in the histologically benign disorders,[200,204,207] and in the mucosa surrounding the lymphoma.[195] Intestinal tissue from individuals without celiac disease or with celiac disease responsive to a gluten-free diet do not harbor clonal T cells.[192,195,200,207]

Relying on paraffin section immunohistochemistry to determine whether an abnormal T-cell population is present may be problematic, because this technique does not readily distinguish between sCD3 and cCD3 staining. If large numbers of reactive TCRγδ T cells are present, the mucosa may appear to show aberrant loss of CD5 and increased numbers of CD4/CD8 double-negative T cells.[205,206] Also, in cases of enteropathy-associated T-cell lymphomas composed of CD56+, CD8+ T cells, the clonal intraepithelial lymphocytes may be CD8+; therefore, the number of CD4/CD8 double-negative T cells may not be increased in the surrounding mucosa to hint at the presence of an abnormal population.[195]

Flow cytometry may be better suited to defining abnormal T-cell populations, because it can detect the absence of sCD3.[206] Refractory celiac disease has been subclassified as type I and type II. In type I, no immunophenotypically abnormal T-cell population is detected, whereas in type II, an abnormal T-cell population (sCD3−, cCD3+, CD4−, CD8−, CD7+) is found (see Table 5-6).[189,206] Patients with

TABLE 5-6

Enteropathy-Associated T-Cell Lymphoma and Related Conditions

Condition	Description
Enteropathy-associated T-cell lymphoma (EATL)	T-cell lymphoma derived from intraepithelial T cells (IELs), associated with enteropathy
Celiac disease	Gluten-sensitive enteropathy or celiac sprue, characterized by villous blunting, crypt hyperplasia, lymphoplasmacytic infiltrate of lamina propria, and increased IELs
De novo EATL	EATL that occurs without a previous recognized history of celiac disease
Secondary EATL	EATL that evolves from celiac disease, usually refractory celiac disease
Refractory celiac disease (RCD)	Celiac disease that is unresponsive to a gluten-free diet
RCD type I	RCD without a detectable immunophenotypically abnormal IEL population
RCD type II	RCD with an immunophenotypically abnormal IEL population
Ulcerative jejunitis	Histologically benign ulcers in a patient with celiac disease; patients may have RCD clinically

RCD type I appear to have a low-risk of progression to enteropathy-associated T-cell lymphoma and are reported to have a good prognosis when treated with prednisone and azathioprine.[189] In contrast, patients with RCD type II have a high risk of progression to lymphoma. Most of these patients eventually succumb to lymphoma or to severe malnutrition related to malabsorption.[189] The optimal treatment for RCD type II has yet to be determined.

Intraepithelial TCRγδ T cells may play a role in the regulation of celiac disease. An increase in γδ T cells is seen in patients with active celiac disease compared with individuals without celiac disease.[205,206] In celiac disease, interleukin 15 (IL-15) is secreted by enterocytes and antigen-presenting cells after exposure to gliadin. IL-15–stimulated intraepithelial TCRαβ T cells in celiac disease appear to have cytotoxic activity that damages the intestinal mucosa. TCRγδ T cells are thought to play a role in suppressing the cytotoxic programming of the TCRαβ T cells, thus serving as regulatory T cells. However, without withdrawal of gliadin, the γδ T cells may be overwhelmed and fail to function properly, leading to increased mucosal damage and worsening malabsorption.[205] Patients with RCD type II have been shown to have fewer TCRγδ T cells than patients with other forms of celiac disease, which perhaps correlates with the emergence of an abnormal population of TCRαβ T cells.[206]

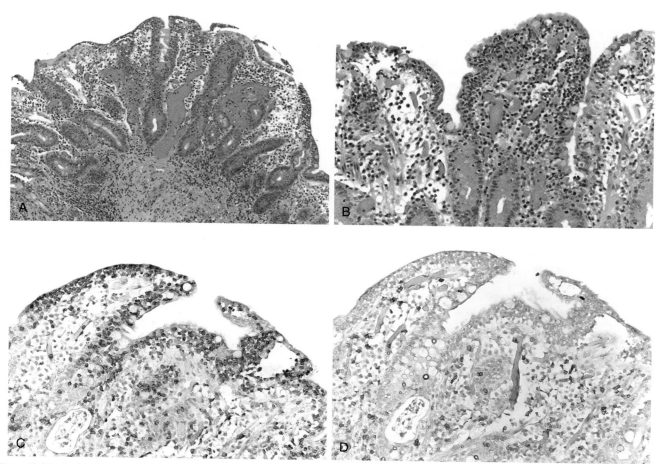

Figure 5-25 Celiac disease with an abnormal population of intraepithelial T cells. **A,** The small intestinal mucosa shows villous blunting and crypt hyperplasia. **B,** Intraepithelial lymphocytes have increased conspicuously. The intraepithelial lymphocytes are CD3+ **(C)** and CD5– **(D)**; they also were negative for CD4 and CD8 (not shown). T cells in the lamina propria express both CD3 and CD5. Molecular studies revealed a clonal T-cell population.

This information suggests that refractory celiac disease and ulcerative jejunitis are neoplastic or preneoplastic disorders. Alternative designations of low-grade or cryptic enteropathy-associated T-cell lymphoma,[192] epitheliotropic lymphoma, or intraepithelial lymphoma[198] have been suggested.

Differential Diagnosis

1. **Enteropathy-associated T-cell lymphoma versus nonneoplastic ulceration.** Enteropathy-associated T-cell lymphoma usually does not form a large mass, and numerous inflammatory cells may be admixed, potentially obscuring the neoplastic population. These features may lead to a diagnosis of an inflammatory ulcer rather than lymphoma. Careful examination of routine sections and immunostains for atypical cells, as well as molecular genetic studies in selected cases, should lead to the diagnosis. Any ulcerated lesion in a patient with clinical or histologic evidence of celiac disease should be viewed with suspicion.
2. **Enteropathy-associated T-cell lymphoma versus diffuse large B-cell lymphoma.** Diffuse large B-cell lymphoma is the most common type of small intestinal lymphoma, and the appearance of the neoplastic cells may not be helpful in distinguishing between B- and T-cell lymphoma. However, in contrast to enteropathy-associated T-cell lymphoma, diffuse large B-cell lymphoma tends to be found distally, in the ileum, and it is multifocal less often than enteropathy-associated T-cell lymphoma. B-cell lymphomas produce larger, exophytic masses.[27,181] Changes of celiac disease should be absent. Immunohistochemical studies readily distinguish B- and T-cell lymphomas.
3. **Enteropathy-associated T-cell lymphoma, monomorphic variant, versus marginal zone lymphoma.** Enteropathy-associated T-cell lymphoma, monomorphic variant, is composed of a monotonous population of small to medium cells with clear cytoplasm that may mimic marginal zone lymphoma. A history of celiac disease that would provide a clue to the diagnosis may be absent. A basic panel of immunostains using B- and T-cell markers can exclude marginal zone lymphoma. The distinction is critical, because marginal zone

lymphoma has a much better prognosis than enteropathy-associated T-cell lymphoma.

4. **Enteropathy-associated T-cell lymphoma versus extranodal NK/T-cell lymphoma, nasal type.** Nasal-type NK/T-cell lymphomas occasionally metastasize to the intestine, and nasal-type extranodal NK/T-cell lymphomas rarely arise in the intestine (see Extranodal NK/T-Cell Lymphoma, Nasal Type, later in the chapter). The pathologic features of enteropathy-associated T-cell lymphoma show some overlap with those of nasal-type extranodal NK/T-cell lymphoma. Both tend to produce ulcerated lesions without formation of a large mass, and both can be composed of neoplastic cells that vary in size from case to case. Both express some T-cell–associated antigens. Consequently, problems in differential diagnosis may arise. However, in NK/T-cell lymphomas, CD56 is nearly always expressed, and the presence of EBV is virtually universal; in enteropathy-associated T-cell lymphomas, CD56 is expressed in only a minority of cases, and EBV typically is absent. Histologic and/or serologic evidence of celiac disease strongly favors enteropathy-associated T-cell lymphoma. The presence of a clonal T-cell population also supports a diagnosis of enteropathy-associated T-cell lymphoma, because most extranodal NK/T-cell lymphomas are of NK-cell origin and do not rearrange their T-cell receptors gene.

5. **Enteropathy-associated T-cell lymphoma versus peripheral T-cell lymphoma not otherwise specified (NOS).** Peripheral T-cell lymphoma NOS may arise in the intestine.[193] The presence of a T-cell lymphoma in the absence of clinical or histologic evidence of enteropathy, antigliadin and antiendomysial antibodies, or celiac disease–associated HLA types suggests a diagnosis of peripheral T-cell lymphoma NOS (see the following section).

6. **Enteropathy-associated T-cell lymphoma versus anaplastic large cell lymphoma.** Some enteropathy-associated T-cell lymphomas are CD30+. Unless CD30 expression is diffuse and strong, cytologic features are characteristic, and no evidence of underlying celiac disease is seen, a diagnosis of anaplastic large cell lymphoma should not be made. Expression of Alk1 in addition to CD30 supports a diagnosis of ALK+ anaplastic large cell lymphoma and would not be expected in enteropathy-associated T-cell lymphoma.

Peripheral T-Cell Lymphomas of the Gastrointestinal Tract

Gastrointestinal peripheral T-cell lymphomas are rare. With the exception of enteropathy-associated T-cell lymphoma, they appear to be more common in Asian countries than in the West. In one large European series of localized gastric lymphomas, only 1% were peripheral T-cell lymphomas.[26] In a study from Korea, 6.5% of high-grade primary gastric lymphomas were T-cell lymphomas.[118] In another Asian series, approximately 13% of intestinal lymphomas were T-cell lymphomas.[31]

Peripheral T-cell lymphoma NOS is the most common type of gastrointestinal T-cell lymphoma, aside from enteropathy-associated T-cell lymphoma.[31,208] Patients with gastric T-cell lymphoma are mostly adults; the age range is broad, and a male preponderance is seen.[208,209] The lymphomas can affect any portion of the stomach and sometimes are multifocal. They may take the form of ulcerated, exophytic, or superficial, spreading lesions. In most cases the neoplastic cells are large, whereas in other cases the neoplastic cells are medium sized.

The immunophenotype is variable. CD3 is almost always expressed. Tumor cells may be CD4+, CD8+, or CD4/CD8 double negative, with variable expression of CD5, CD30, and cytotoxic granule proteins, typically without evidence of EBV in tumor cells.[209] An unusual case of peripheral T-cell lymphoma involving the stomach at presentation has been reported; in this case, after therapy an isolated recurrence in the stomach developed with an appearance that mimicked lymphocytic gastritis.[210] Rare cases of primary gastric T-cell lymphoma are EBV+.[211] Staging sometimes reveals widespread disease, and the prognosis is unfavorable.[208] A 5-year survival rate of 54% was found in one study of primary gastric T-cell lymphoma; a better prognosis was associated with medium-sized neoplastic cells and early stage disease.[209]

The histologic and immunophenotypic features of intestinal peripheral T-cell lymphoma NOS are variable. Overall, their prognosis is worse than for intestinal B-cell lymphomas.[31] There are uncommon but well-documented cases of intestinal T-cell lymphomas composed of small to medium cells that are CD8+, CD56+, and express cytotoxic granule proteins, similar to the monomorphic variant of enteropathy-associated T-cell lymphoma (see the preceding section); however, these cases lacked both histologic evidence of enteropathy and evidence of underlying celiac disease. These lymphomas appear to be more common in Asia.[212]

There have been rare cases of a distinctive small intestinal T-cell lymphoma that affects young to older adults without celiac disease; that is composed of CD4+ small lymphoid cells, often with admixed eosinophils and epithelioid histiocytes; and that sometimes is associated with peripheral blood eosinophilia. The neoplastic cells express CD2, CD3, and CD5, in addition to CD4, and lack expression of CD103 and cytotoxic granule proteins, in contrast to enteropathy-associated T-cell lymphoma. Patients may have only partial remission after treatment, or they may have relapses, but the lymphoma tends to behave in an indolent manner, and survival can be long. This type of lymphoma is hypothesized to arise from CD4+ $\alpha\beta$ T cells of the lamina propria.[213]

Adult T-cell leukemia/lymphoma is a peripheral T-cell neoplasm caused by the retrovirus HTLV-1.[214] Among patients with adult T-cell leukemia/

lymphoma, gastrointestinal involvement in the setting of widespread disease is fairly common. Primary gastrointestinal adult T-cell leukemia/lymphoma is rare.[215,216] In some instances, patients present initially with disease related to gastrointestinal involvement, although staging usually reveals more extensive disease.[157,217,218] The stomach is the portion most commonly involved, followed by the colon and the small intestine.[158] In rare instances the esophagus is involved.[218] Concurrent involvement of more than one segment of the gastrointestinal tract is fairly common (e.g., esophagus and stomach,[218] stomach and ileum,[217] duodenum and stomach, duodenum and colon[157]).

Among patients with the lymphoma form or the acute form of adult T-cell leukemia/lymphoma, 30% have gastric involvement.[219] Among patients who die with adult T-cell leukemia/lymphoma, 70% have gastrointestinal involvement.[158] Adults are affected over a broad age range, with a median age in the 50s. Men and women are affected roughly equally.[215] Gastroscopy most often reveals multiple ulcers in cases with gastric involvement. Other findings include giant folds, polypoid lesions, and diffuse erosions.[215,219] Intestinal involvement by adult T-cell leukemia/lymphoma can produce lesions that are polypoid or ulcerated[217] and can even take the form of multiple lymphomatous polyposis.[157] As in other sites, the lymphoma is composed of atypical T cells that may have lobulated nuclei. Neoplastic cells are CD4+, CD7− T cells. Serology is positive for HTLV-1+, and tumor cells have monoclonal integration of proviral DNA.[215]

Adult T-cell leukemia/lymphoma has a poor prognosis overall, but gastrointestinal involvement is associated with an even worse prognosis.[215,219] Most patients succumb to the disease.[158,217,218] The small minority of patients presenting with primary disease localized to the gastrointestinal tract may achieve complete remission and have prolonged survival when treated appropriately.[215]

Other T-cell lymphomas, including rare gastric,[208] small intestinal,[220] and rectal[221] CD30+ anaplastic large cell lymphomas of T-lineage, have been reported. One of the small intestinal anaplastic large cell lymphomas was ALK+.[220]

A few cases of gastrointestinal peripheral T-cell lymphoma have arisen after solid organ transplantation (monomorphic T-lineage post-transplantation lymphoproliferative disorder), usually many years after transplantation and usually involving the small intestine but rarely involving the stomach. Some have been EBV+.[51]

Extranodal NK/T-Cell Lymphoma, Nasal Type, of the Gastrointestinal Tract

Nasal-type extranodal NK/T-cell lymphoma infrequently involves the gastrointestinal tract. This type of lymphoma may secondarily involve the gastrointestinal tract from a primary site that most often is in the upper aerodigestive tract; less often, it may arise in the gastrointestinal tract. In any case, this lymphoma is more often encountered in Asian countries. It almost always affects adults, most of whom are young or middle aged (the median age is in the fifth decade).[212,222,223] Thus these patients are overall slightly younger than patients with most other types of gastrointestinal lymphoma.

Patients present with abdominal pain or gastrointestinal bleeding, sometimes accompanied by constitutional symptoms.[222,223] The bleeding may be massive. Depending on the portion of the gastrointestinal tract involved, patients may have hematemesis, melena, or hematochezia. The lymphomas also may be associated with obstruction or perforation. Involvement of the intestine, usually the small intestine, is more common than gastric or esophageal involvement.[212,222,223] The lesions typically are ulcerated and/or infiltrative and do not form a large mass. The size of the neoplastic cells can vary from one case to another; the lymphomas can be composed of small to medium-sized, medium-sized, or medium to large-sized pleomorphic cells.

The usual immunophenotype is sCD3−, cCD3+, CD2+, CD5−, CD7+, CD56+, CD30+/−, and B antigen negative, with EBV in tumor cells, best demonstrated with in situ hybridization for Epstein-Barr virus–encoded ribonucleic acid (RNA) (EBER). Even when these lymphomas appear to be primary in the gastrointestinal tract, staging may reveal more widespread disease.[222] The prognosis is very poor[222,223]; survival usually is less than 1 year.[212] A few cases have been associated with a hemophagocytic syndrome.[212]

The differential diagnosis of this type of lymphoma with enteropathy-associated T-cell lymphoma is discussed in the earlier section on enteropathy-associated T-cell lymphoma. Extranodal NK/T-cell lymphoma is discussed in greater detail under Lymphomas of the Nasal Cavity and Paranasal Sinuses in Chapter 3.

Differential Diagnosis

1. **Extranodal NK/T-cell lymphoma versus NK-cell enteropathy.** Rare cases of an atypical NK-cell, or possibly NK-like T-cell, lymphoproliferative lesion of unknown etiology, referred to as *NK-cell enteropathy*[224a], *lymphomatoid gastropathy*[224b] and *indolent CD56-positive T-cell lymphoproliferative disorder*[224c] have been described in patients with a persistent, atypical lymphoid infiltrate involving the gastrointestinal tract but in whom the clinical course is much more indolent than that of extranodal NK/T-cell lymphoma.[224a, 224b, 224c] Patients are adults without celiac disease who have multiple small, ulcerated lesions often described as superficial, involving one or more portions of the gastrointestinal tract. Biopsy samples show a diffuse infiltrate of medium-sized to large atypical lymphoid cells with acute inflammation and glandular destruction. The immunophenotype is consistent with NK lineage: cCD3+, CD5−, CD7+, CD4−, CD8−, CD56+, TIA1, perforin and/or granzyme B+ (Figure 5-26). In contrast

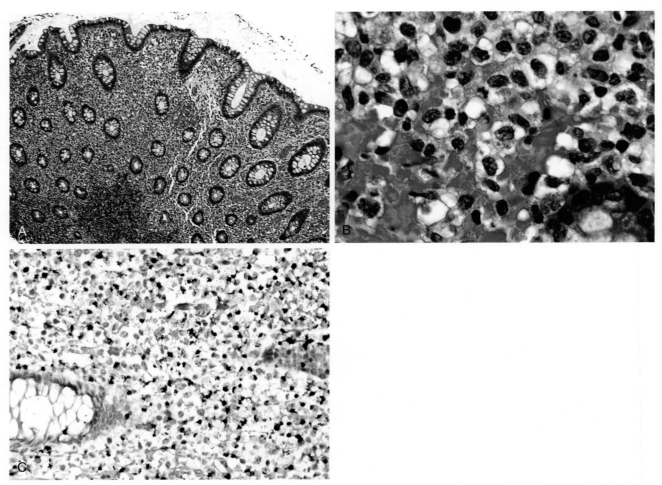

Figure 5-26 NK-cell enteropathy. **A**, Low-power view shows colonic mucosa with an atypical lymphoid infiltrate expanding the lamina propria in an interstitial pattern. Ulceration was present in other areas. **B**, The infiltrate in the lamina propria consists of medium-sized lymphoid cells with oval or slightly indented nuclei with multiple red cytoplasmic granules in a paranuclear location. (Oil immersion.) **C**, Note the intense staining for granzyme B, corresponding to the cytoplasmic granules and consistent with cytotoxic granules. (Immunoperoxidase technique on a paraffin section.) Lymphoid cells also were CD3+ and CD56+ and negative for CD20, CD4, CD5, CD8, CD30, and EBV (not shown).

to extranodal NK/T-cell lymphoma, the atypical cells are negative for EBV. T-cell lymphoma, possibly of γδ lineage, also can be considered in the differential diagnosis, but clonal rearrangement of TCR genes is not demonstrated. Follow-up in some cases has been short; although the mucosal lesions often persist, patients have otherwise been well.[224a] These observations suggest caution in rendering a diagnosis of NK/T-cell lymphoma in the absence of EBV, particularly if the lesions are small and superficial on endoscopy.

Hodgkin's Lymphoma of the Gastrointestinal Tract

Introduction

Rare cases of Hodgkin's lymphoma arising in the gastrointestinal tract have been reported; fewer than 0.5% of all cases of Hodgkin's lymphoma arise in the gastrointestinal tract.[225] All reported cases have been classical Hodgkin's lymphoma. Because of the rarity of Hodgkin's lymphoma in this site, strict criteria for diagnosis should be used. For a diagnosis of primary gastrointestinal Hodgkin's lymphoma, the gastric or intestinal lesion should predominate. Adjacent lymph nodes may be involved, but substantial hepatic or splenic disease should be absent. A variety of other neoplastic and nonneoplastic disorders can mimic gastrointestinal Hodgkin's lymphoma, and these must be excluded before a diagnosis is made.

Clinical Features

Based on the small number of cases of primary gastrointestinal Hodgkin's lymphoma reported, this lymphoma appears to affect adults over a broad age range, and a male preponderance is seen. In the general population, the sites involved, in descending order, are the stomach, small intestine, and colon. Some patients have had long-standing inflammatory bowel disease, almost always Crohn's disease, that was treated with immunosuppressive therapy.[225-227] In such cases the Hodgkin's lymphoma preferentially affects portions of the small intestine or colon

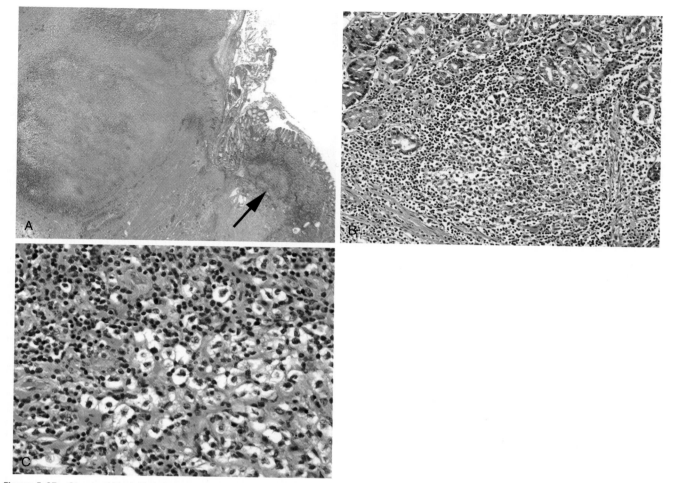

Figure 5-27 Classical Hodgkin's lymphoma involving the stomach at relapse. **A,** This gastrectomy specimen shows ulceration with large cellular nodules surrounded by fibrosis deep to the ulcer base, as well as a small cellular nodule invading the mucosa *(arrow).* **B,** A loose aggregate of large atypical cells with admixed eosinophils and surrounded by small lymphocytes involves the gastric mucosa. **C,** Many of the large atypical cells have the morphology of lacunar cells. Many eosinophils also are present.

(or both) involved by the inflammatory bowel disease. On occasion, some other form of underlying immunologic abnormality has been present, such as human immunodeficiency virus (HIV) infection[228] or another inflammatory condition.[225,229] Hodgkin's lymphoma that arose in the stomach as a secondary neoplasm in a patient with chronic lymphocytic leukemia has been reported.[230] Relapse of classical Hodgkin's lymphoma in the gastrointestinal tract has been described, but this is also uncommon (Figure 5-27).[231]

Patients with gastric or duodenal Hodgkin's lymphoma present with upper abdominal pain, weight loss, or poor appetite. Endoscopy reveals one or more ulcers.[230,232-234] Patients with intestinal lymphoma have hematochezia, pain, nausea, vomiting, or diarrhea; in some cases, patients have perforation. In patients with Crohn's disease, the symptoms may mimic exacerbation of the original disease.[225,226]

Although by convention the bulk of the tumor is in the gastrointestinal tract at presentation, staging often reveals regional nodal involvement[226,234] and occasionally more distant spread.[225] Patients have a favorable prognosis, with good response to therapy in many cases.[225-227,229,232-234]

Pathologic Features

Hodgkin's lymphoma takes the form of lesions that often are ulcerated, transmural, and multifocal,[225,227,230,233,234] sometimes accompanied by an exophytic, polypoid component.[233] In Crohn's disease, areas with fissures and pre-existing severe inflammation typically are involved.[225,227] Classical Hodgkin's lymphoma of mixed cellularity and nodular sclerosis subtypes have been reported. Immunophenotyping shows that Reed-Sternberg cells and variants are CD15+, CD30+, focally or weakly CD20+ or CD20−, CD3−,* Pax5 dim+, MUM1/IRF4+,[232] CD79a−, and CD45−,[225,232,233] typical of classical Hodgkin's lymphoma. Neoplastic cells have almost always been positive for EBV using in situ hybridization[225,227,228,232] and immunohistochemistry for latent membrane protein (EBV-LMP).[225,230,233]

Among patients with Crohn's disease, the occurrence of Hodgkin's lymphoma in areas of inflamed

---

*References 225-227, 229, 230, 233, 235, and 236.

bowel suggests that the tumor is pathogenetically related to the chronic inflammatory process. The history of azathioprine or prednisone therapy seen in most Crohn's disease–associated cases and the presence of EBV in cases with and without inflammatory bowel disease suggest that immune dysregulation plays a role in the pathogenesis of gastrointestinal Hodgkin's lymphoma.[225] However, recent observations suggest that some cases previously reported as gastrointestinal Hodgkin's lymphoma in the setting of inflammatory bowel disease may not represent Hodgkin's lymphoma, but rather examples of *EBV+ mucocutaneous ulcer* (discussed below, under Differential Diagnosis).[237]

Differential Diagnosis

Lesions that mimic Hodgkin's lymphoma are more common than true examples of Hodgkin's lymphoma involving the gastrointestinal tract. Hodgkin's lymphoma should be diagnosed only in the setting of classic histologic and immunophenotypic features and after its mimics have been carefully excluded.

1. **Non-Hodgkin's lymphomas versus classical Hodgkin's lymphoma.** As in other sites, the differential diagnosis of classical Hodgkin's lymphoma in the gastrointestinal tract includes non-Hodgkin's lymphomas such as anaplastic large cell lymphoma and diffuse large B-cell lymphoma. The most common lymphoma in the gastrointestinal tract overall is diffuse large B-cell lymphoma. In cases in which neoplastic B cells are unusually bizarre and pleomorphic, a diagnosis of Hodgkin's lymphoma may be considered. EBV+ diffuse large B-cell lymphoma of the elderly (discussed previously) may be especially problematic to distinguish from Hodgkin's lymphoma (see Figure 5-14).[149] Cases in which Reed-Sternberg–like cells are conspicuous and admixed reactive cells are abundant can mimic classical Hodgkin's lymphoma. A higher proportion of cases of EBV+ diffuse large B-cell lymphoma of the elderly than cases of Hodgkin's lymphoma has gastrointestinal involvement.[238] The frequent expression of CD30 and the constant presence of EBV strengthen the resemblance to gastrointestinal classical Hodgkin's lymphoma. Classical Hodgkin's lymphoma is more likely to have an admixture of eosinophils. EBV+ diffuse large B-cell lymphoma of the elderly has more consistent expression of B-cell antigen or antigens than Hodgkin's lymphoma and lacks CD15.[149,238] Strict adherence to criteria for a diagnosis of Hodgkin's lymphoma are required in the gastrointestinal tract, and in other extranodal sites, to prevent misdiagnosis.

2. **Classical Hodgkin's lymphoma versus Hodgkin's lymphoma–like lymphoid proliferations related to immunosuppression.** Lymphoid proliferations related to immunosuppression sometimes contain Reed-Sternberg–like cells and may mimic classical Hodgkin's lymphoma, including EBV+ diffuse large B-cell lymphoma of the elderly (discussed earlier in this chapter). Also in this group are a variety of lymphoid proliferations that range from reactive to overtly neoplastic. Post-transplantation lymphoproliferative disorders of early, polymorphic, and less often monomorphic types may have scattered Reed-Sternberg–like cells (see Table 5-1).[48] Other types of iatrogenic immunosuppression, especially treatment with methotrexate, may be associated with lymphoproliferative disorders that may mimic classical Hodgkin's lymphoma.[239] Although rare, true examples of Hodgkin's lymphoma arise among iatrogenically immunosuppressed patients; these cases should be distinguished from Hodgkin's lymphoma–like lymphoid proliferations that may arise in this setting.

   EBV+ mucocutaneous ulcer is a recently described lymphoproliferative disorder that occurs in patients with underlying immunosuppression of various causes, including advanced age and iatrogenic immunosuppression.[237] Patients have ulcerated lesions of the skin or mucosal sites, including the oral cavity, tonsils, or gastrointestinal tract. Distinguishing this disorder from Hodgkin's lymphoma may be difficult, because the lesional cells sometimes resemble Reed-Sternberg cells and variants and have an immunophenotype that overlaps with that of Hodgkin's lymphoma (CD30+, CD15–/+, CD45+/–, CD20+/–, Pax5+, MUM1/IRF4+), with an inflammatory background of reactive cells. However, EBV+ mucocutaneous ulcer is characterized by well-circumscribed superficial lesions with a conspicuous rim of CD8+ T cells at the base of the lesions. The lymphoid cells present often include immunoblasts, medium-sized lymphoid cells with angulated nuclei and apoptotic cells with a plasmacytoid appearance, in addition to Reed-Sternberg–like cells. Eosinophils are seen in occasional cases but are much less common than in classical Hodgkin's lymphoma. In contrast, classical Hodgkin's lymphoma typically shows large atypical cells with the appearance of Reed-Sternberg cells and variants in a background of small, cytologically bland lymphocytes, histiocytes, eosinophils, and/ or plasma cells. Apoptotic debris is not usually present. Hodgkin's lymphoma is more likely to produce a large mass; involvement in the form of small superficial ulcers is uncommon. The distinction is important, because EBV+ mucocutaneous ulcer usually behaves in an indolent manner, without progression to disseminated disease and with some spontaneous remissions. Individuals with other forms of lymphoproliferative disorders related to iatrogenic immunosuppression also have sometimes experienced regression of the lymphoproliferative disorder on reduction of the immunosuppressive therapy.[239]

3. **Poorly differentiated carcinoma versus classical Hodgkin's lymphoma.** Carcinomas composed of large, bizarre, anaplastic cells may enter the differential diagnosis of Hodgkin's lymphoma. The two tumors usually can be differentiated on routine sections. However, if immunohistochemistry is

used, it should be noted that, like Reed-Sternberg cells, some carcinomas are CD15+ and CD45−. An immunohistochemical panel that includes cytokeratin can help establish a diagnosis.

4. **Nonneoplastic ulcer versus classical Hodgkin's lymphoma.** Gastrointestinal Hodgkin's lymphoma is associated with ulceration and, as in other sites, with a prominent component of reactive cells. Because of sampling artifact, small mucosal biopsy samples may not be diagnostic and may be interpreted as benign.[232,233,235] Clinical information may be helpful, because the ulcers may appear malignant on endoscopy; however, in some cases a diagnosis has not been established until a resection specimen was obtained.[232,233]

Secondary Involvement of the Gastrointestinal Tract by Lymphoma

A variety of lymphomas can involve the gastrointestinal tract in the setting of widespread disease; a number of these have been noted in the corresponding previous sections on different types of lymphoma. In addition, individuals with chronic lymphocytic leukemia often have widespread involvement of many lymph nodes and extranodal sites and may develop involvement of the gastrointestinal tract. Symptoms related to gastrointestinal chronic lymphocytic leukemia may be subtle; the leukemia may be an incidental finding in specimens removed for unrelated reasons. A wide variety of types of lymphoma also can relapse in the gastrointestinal tract. Diffuse large B-cell lymphomas that arise in Waldeyer's ring tend to spread to the gastrointestinal tract. When gastric diffuse large B-cell lymphomas relapse, approximately half of the relapses involve the gastrointestinal tract.[240] As noted previously, classical Hodgkin's lymphoma rarely involves the gastrointestinal tract at the time of relapse. We have seen the case of a patient with nodular sclerosis classical Hodgkin's lymphoma who achieved complete remission but later developed a relapse with extensive gastric involvement (see Figure 5-27).[231]

■ HEPATIC LYMPHOMAS

Primary Hepatic Lymphomas

Introduction

Primary hepatic lymphoma, or lymphoma that arises in and is entirely or nearly entirely confined to the liver, is an uncommon but well-documented entity. Of all non-Hodgkin's lymphomas, 0.016% are primary hepatic lymphomas, as are 0.4% of extranodal lymphomas.[1] An estimated 4.3% of primary hepatic malignancies are lymphoma.[241] Hepatic lymphomas often are associated with an underlying infectious process, some other source of ongoing chronic inflammation, or an immunologic abnormality,[242,243] including HIV infection[244] and iatrogenic immunosuppression

in allograft recipients.[245,246] Some investigators suggest that hepatic lymphoma has been increasing in frequency in recent years,[243,247] although it also is possible that more cases of primary hepatic lymphoma are being recognized because of improvements in radiographic techniques. In earlier reports, the diagnosis sometimes was made only at autopsy.[243,248]

The relationship between lymphoma and hepatitis C virus (HCV) is controversial, and findings in various studies differ; however, some show a significantly increased prevalence of HCV infection in patients with primary hepatic lymphoma, which suggests that HCV may play a role in lymphomagenesis.[249,250] Examined from the opposite point of view, in a study of HCV-infected patients with lymphoma, the liver was the second most frequently involved extranodal site, after the spleen.[251] Interestingly, hepatic involvement by lymphoma was more common when HCV-positive patients had cirrhosis or hepatitis.[251] Although lymphomas in HCV-positive patients usually are low-grade B-cell lymphomas, primary hepatic lymphomas in these patients usually are the diffuse large B-cell type.[249,250,252,253]

The pathogenesis of HCV-associated lymphomas is not well understood. HCV is an RNA virus believed to be both hepatotropic and lymphotropic, although lymphomas in HCV-infected individuals do not contain HCV.[252] Lymphomagenesis may be related to chronic antigenic stimulation directly by HCV or indirectly through hepatic damage related to HCV. Another consideration is that HCV may transiently infect lymphocytes and alter them, leaving them more susceptible *to neoplastic transformation, a so-called* "hit-and-run" mechanism. HCV infection of lymphocytes is associated with an increased frequency of somatic mutation of the immunoglobulin heavy chain gene variable region *(IGHV)*. HCV also is associated with increased mutation frequency of *BCL6,* of the tumor suppressor gene *p53,* and of the proto-oncogene beta-catenin.[254] The increased mutational load induced by HCV in these critical genes could well play a role in lymphomagenesis.

Diffuse Large B-Cell Lymphoma

Clinical Features

Most primary hepatic lymphomas are diffuse large B-cell lymphomas.[248,250,252,255] In one large series, diffuse large B-cell lymphoma accounted for 71% of primary hepatic lymphomas.[250] As noted previously, most hepatic lymphomas that arise in association with HCV are diffuse large B-cell lymphomas.[250,252] As in other sites, diffuse large B-cell lymphoma also is the most common hepatic lymphoma among HIV-positive patients (see Figure 5-27).[244,256] Most cases occur in middle-aged or older adults, with occasional cases in young adults and rare cases in adolescents.[241] The median age is in the sixth decade. A modest male preponderance is seen among immunocompetent patients.[241,249,250,252,255] Patients who have HIV infection are younger and are almost exclusively male, in contrast to patients who are HIV negative.[244,255]

Patients present with abdominal pain, sometimes with constitutional symptoms. On physical examination, patients often have hepatomegaly or a palpable mass. Only a minority of patients are jaundiced.[248-250,252,255,257] Lactate dehydrogenase (LDH) frequently is elevated, and hepatic aminotransferases also may be elevated; however, alpha fetoprotein (AFP) and carcinoembryonic antigen (CEA) levels usually are normal.[242,248,249,255] A case of a man with HCV infection, cirrhosis, and diffuse large B-cell lymphoma involving the liver who presented with lactic acidosis and hypoglycemia has been reported.[253]

In many cases (and in a majority of cases in some series), patients have some other disease, often in the form of an immunodeficiency or chronic stimulation of the immune system. The disorders include HIV infection[244,249,255,256]; hepatitis B virus (HBV)[242] or HCV[252,253] infection, sometimes associated with chronic active hepatitis or cirrhosis[249,252,253]; previous Hodgkin's lymphoma[255]; and others. HCV is more prevalent among patients with primary hepatic lymphoma and more likely to play an important role in its pathogenesis than is HBV.[249]

Some series have accepted only cases confined to the liver as primary hepatic lymphoma.[250] In other series with more liberal criteria for a diagnosis of primary hepatic lymphoma, staging may reveal spread to sites such as the bone marrow in a minority of cases.[241,248] Patients with diffuse large B-cell lymphoma have a relatively good prognosis.[249] In one review of primary hepatic lymphoma in which most cases were diffuse large B-cell lymphoma, the 2-year survival rate was estimated to be 66%. No deaths caused by lymphoma were recorded for those who survived for 2 years or longer.[242] In another series, in which diffuse large B-cell lymphoma was by far the most common type, 70% of patients had a sustained complete remission.[250] In one other large series, in which 96% of cases were diffuse large cell lymphomas (lineage not determined in all cases), the cause-specific survival rate at 5 years was 87%.[249]

HCV does not appear to be a poor prognostic factor.[249] All four patients with diffuse large B-cell lymphoma in one series, three of whom had chronic active hepatitis related to HCV, were alive and free of lymphoma after treatment with combination chemotherapy 28 to 102 months later.[252] In another series, all five patients with follow-up, one of whom was HCV positive, were alive and well 11 to 34 months after treatment with combination chemotherapy.[241] Among HIV-positive patients, the outcome is significantly worse.[244]

Pathologic Features

In nearly all cases, the lymphoma either forms a large solitary mass or multiple nodules. In about 5% of cases, diffuse hepatic enlargement without a discrete mass is seen.[241,242,248-250,255] A single dominant lesion may be present, accompanied by satellite nodules.[241] Multiple lesions appear to be more common among HIV-infected individuals than among immunocompetent patients.[244]

The lymphomas take the form of unencapsulated, beige, firm tumors.[241] The lesions usually are contained within the liver, but invasion into adjacent structures, including the gallbladder and adrenal glands, has been described.[241] Diffuse large B-cell lymphomas are composed of a diffuse, destructive infiltrate of large atypical lymphoid cells, often with the appearance of centroblasts and often with extensive necrosis (Figure 5-28).[241,248,250,255] Lymphomas with diffuse hepatic enlargement may show prominent sinusoidal involvement.[248] Sclerosis is infrequent.[248]

Diffuse large B-cell lymphomas express CD45, CD20, and CD79a. The immunophenotype has not been studied in detail, but expression of CD10 is

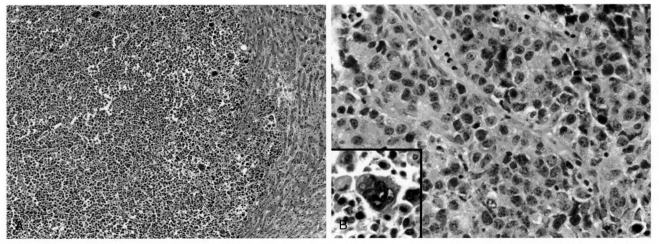

Figure 5-28 Primary hepatic diffuse large B-cell lymphoma in an HIV-positive man. **A,** Low-power view of the liver shows a large lesion composed of atypical lymphoid cells. Lymphoma formed multiple large nodules within the hepatic parenchyma and was confined to the liver. **B,** The lymphoma is composed of large atypical lymphoid cells with occasional bizarre cells *(inset)*. The lymphoma was CD20+ and negative for CD5, CD10, and EBV.

uncommon, and bcl6 is not always expressed; this suggests a post-germinal center immunophenotype in at least some cases.[241,255,256]

T-Cell/Histiocyte-Rich Large B-Cell Lymphoma

T-cell/histiocyte-rich large B-cell lymphoma (THRBCL), a type of diffuse large B-cell lymphoma, frequently presents with widespread disease.[258] Although it thus does not fulfill the criteria for primary hepatic lymphoma, a discussion of its pathologic features in the liver is included in this section because it often involves the liver, as well as the spleen, and many patients present with hepatosplenomegaly (also see Lymphomas of the Spleen, Chapter 6).

Pathologic Features

In the liver, THRBCL is most likely to have a predominant pattern of portal involvement rather than forming large nodules, as is characteristic of diffuse large B-cell lymphoma NOS. THRBCL has a characteristic appearance, with expansion of the portal tracts by an infiltrate of numerous reactive small lymphocytes and histiocytes and occasional large atypical neoplastic B cells, with little or no spread into sinusoids. Bile ducts within the infiltrate may be lost (Figure 5-29). Hepatic parenchyma adjacent to the lymphoma may show necrosis, steatosis, bile stasis, and sinusoidal dilatation. The large atypical neoplastic cells may be inconspicuous, and the reactive lymphohistiocytic component may be associated with damage to adjacent parenchyma in a pattern reminiscent of piecemeal necrosis; therefore, THRBCL may be mistaken for chronic active hepatitis.[259] The large B cells are CD20+, bcl6+, EMA+/−, CD15−, and CD30− and are negative for EBV (Figure 5-29, C to F).[258]

Extranodal Marginal Zone Lymphoma of Mucosa-Associated Lymphoid Tissue (MALT Lymphoma)

Clinical Features

Hepatic marginal zone lymphoma is the most common low-grade primary hepatic lymphoma. It accounts for approximately 4% to 10% of all primary hepatic lymphomas.[249,250] Hepatic marginal zone lymphoma affects adults over a wide age range, and a slight female preponderance is seen.[260] Primary hepatic marginal zone lymphoma often is an incidental finding during radiographic imaging or abdominal surgery performed for other reasons, and patients usually do not have symptoms specifically related to the lymphoma.[260-264] In one case in which the marginal zone lymphoma had undergone large cell transformation, the patient presented with abdominal pain.[265]

Among cases in which the information is available, most patients have had an inflammatory disease of the liver, including HCV, HBV, or primary biliary cirrhosis.[252,260,266,267] In cases with HBV or HCV, the disease sometimes had progressed to cirrhosis by the time the marginal zone lymphoma was

dicovered.[263,268] Two patients had *H. pylori* gastritis,[260,262] one with concurrent gastric carcinoma[262] and one with Buerger's disease.[260] Concurrent hepatocellular carcinoma has been described.[260] Other patients have had extrahepatic malignancies.[260,264] This information suggests that chronic inflammation and/or immunologic abnormalities play an important role in the pathogenesis of hepatic marginal zone lymphoma. However, because symptoms related to marginal zone lymphoma in this site often are not detectable, it is uncertain how many cases of hepatic marginal zone lymphoma arise sporadically and remain undiagnosed in patients who are otherwise well.

Pathologic Features

On gross examination, hepatic marginal zone lymphomas have the appearance of one or more well-demarcated or ill-defined, homogeneous, tan-white or yellowish nodules, ranging from less than 1 to 7.5 cm.[260,262,264,268] Hepatic marginal zone lymphomas have histologic features similar to those seen in other sites. The neoplastic infiltrate markedly expands the portal tracts, forming broad, intersecting, serpiginous bands that often entrap nodules of hepatocytes and sometimes form a diffuse, confluent infiltrate.[260,261,264,266-268] These lymphomas are composed of marginal zone cells with bland, slightly irregular nuclei and clear cytoplasm, sometimes with a component of monocytoid B cells with more abundant, clear cytoplasm and sometimes with many plasma cells (Figure 5-30). A few scattered large cells may be identified. Underlying reactive lymphoid follicles are found in some cases. Neoplastic B cells invade bile duct epithelium to form lymphoepithelial lesions.[260-264,266,268]

The neoplastic cells are CD20+, CD79a+, CD3−, CD5−, CD10−, and cyclin D1−, sometimes with co-expression of CD43. An immunostain for cytokeratin can highlight lymphoepithelial lesions. Immunostains for CD21 or CD23 highlight residual follicular dendritic meshworks (Figure 5-30, C and D). In some cases, a neoplastic plasma cell component expresses monotypic cytoplasmic immunoglobulin.[260,262-264,267,268] Genetic and cytogenetic evaluation has been performed in only a limited number of cases. However, the immunoglobulin heavy chain gene typically is clonally rearranged.[260,264,267] Cytogenetic evaluation reveals that t(14;18), resulting in *IGH/MALT1* fusion, is found in some hepatic marginal zone lymphomas.[90] In one case, a t(3;14) (q27;q32) translocation involving *BCL6* and *IGH* was identified.[264] Other translocations described in association with marginal zone lymphomas (see Table 1-1) are uncommon to absent in hepatic marginal zone lymphoma.[98,260] Trisomy 3 and trisomy 18 have been documented in a few cases.[260]

Staging, Treatment, and Outcome

In most cases, lymphoma is confined to the liver,[260,262,268] although staging occasionally has revealed lymph node and focal marrow involvement.[263]

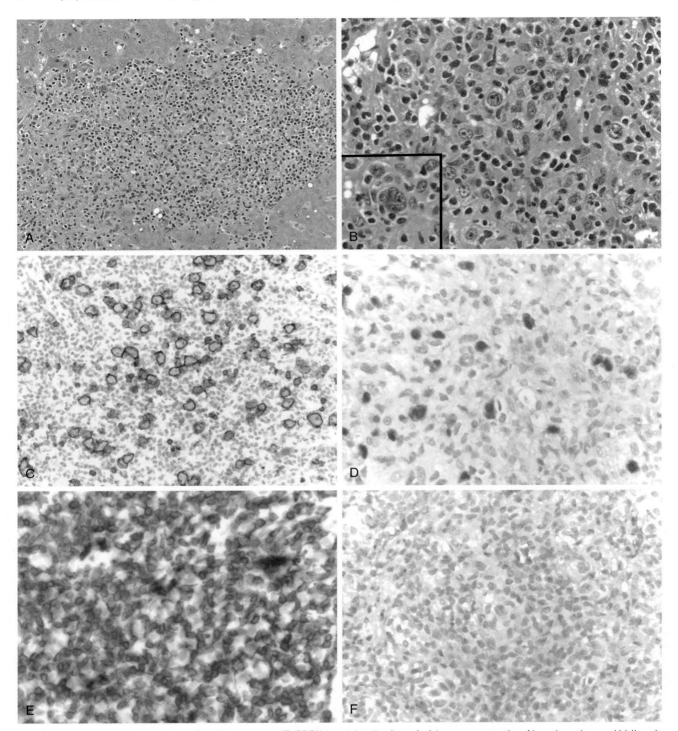

Figure 5-29   T-cell/histiocyte-rich large B-cell lymphoma (THRBCL) involving the liver. **A,** A large aggregate of lymphocytes and histiocytes, with some large atypical cells, distorts the normal hepatic architecture. **B,** High-power view shows small lymphocytes, histiocytes, and scattered large lymphoid cells, most with the appearance of centroblasts, with a very large multilobated cell shown in the inset. The large atypical cells are CD20+ B cells **(C)** that co-express bcl6 **(D)** in a background of numerous CD3+ small T cells **(E)**. There is no staining for CD30 **(F)**. (Immunoperoxidase technique on paraffin sections.)

Treatment has not been uniform. A few relapses have been documented, and follow-up sometimes has not been long. However, the behavior appears to be indolent, and patients have a very good prognosis.[252,260,264,267] A case of transformation to diffuse large B-cell lymphoma has been described[265]; in this case, the patient initially presented with hepatic diffuse large B-cell lymphoma arising in association with marginal zone lymphoma and had a local recurrence of marginal zone lymphoma 6 years later.[265]

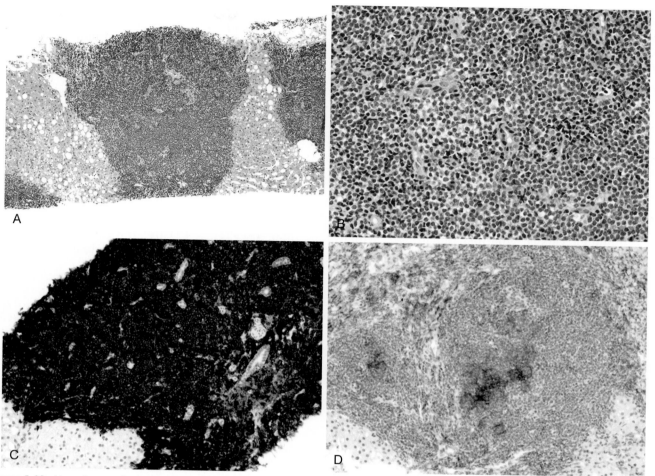

Figure 5-30 Hepatic marginal zone lymphoma. **A,** Broad bands of lymphoid cells traverse this hepatic core biopsy. **B,** Higher power view shows small, relatively uniform lymphoid cells with scant to moderate, pale cytoplasm. **C,** CD20 highlights numerous lymphoid cells; only a few T cells were present (not shown). **D,** CD23 highlights a small, distorted follicular dendritic meshwork in the lymphoma. (*C* and *D,* Immunoperoxidase technique on paraffin sections.)

Rare Primary Hepatic Lymphomas

Rare cases of follicular lymphoma,[269] Burkitt's lymphoma,[247,270,271] and peripheral T-cell lymphoma[250,252,272-277] that apparently arose in the liver have been described. Primary hepatic Burkitt's lymphoma has been reported in children,[247,270,271] in HIV-positive adults,[244] and in rare cases in immunocompetent adults.[250] Hepatic Burkitt's lymphoma among children[270,271] and HIV-positive adults[244] shows a marked male preponderance. Hepatic involvement by endemic and HIV-associated Burkitt's lymphoma in children in Africa is fairly common; hepatic involvement is more common in HIV-positive children than among HIV-negative children, but in both groups the lymphoma usually is widespread and not confined to the liver.[278] The histologic and immunophenotypic features are similar to those seen in other sites (see the earlier section, Burkitt's Lymphoma of the Gastrointestinal Tract).

The hepatic T-cell lymphomas reported sometimes have not been classified according to the WHO Classification, but most appear to be peripheral T-cell lymphoma NOS.[250,252,273-277] Anaplastic large cell lymphoma, ALK−,[272] or with ALK staining not reported[250] also has been described. Patients are mostly middle-aged or older adults, and a male preponderance is seen. As do diffuse large B-cell lymphoma and marginal zone lymphoma, the hepatic T-cell lymphomas sometimes arise in patients with HCV,[250,273] HBV,[276] or an autoimmune disease.[274,275,277] Patients with T-cell lymphoma most often present with constitutional symptoms, sometimes accompanied by abdominal pain or jaundice. The lymphomas, which may form discrete nodules or result in diffuse hepatomegaly, are composed of small, medium-sized, or large atypical T cells or of T cells of a mixture of sizes, often with an admixture of inflammatory cells.[277] Establishing a diagnosis may be difficult because of the rarity of hepatic peripheral T-cell lymphoma and because admixed inflammatory cells may obscure the neoplastic population. Careful immunophenotyping (and in challenging cases, molecular studies) to investigate the presence of a clonal population can help establish a diagnosis.

Differential Diagnosis of Primary Hepatic Lymphoma

1. **Lymphoma versus nonlymphoid tumors.** The finding of one or more hepatic lesions raises the question of hepatocellular carcinoma or metastatic carcinoma. Hepatocellular carcinoma is particularly likely to be considered in patients with previous hepatic disease that may predispose to the development of hepatocellular carcinoma, such as hepatitis B or hepatitis C.[268] The combination of a high LDH and normal CEA and AFP, particularly in an immunocompromised patient, may raise the question of lymphoma, but histologic examination is required to establish a diagnosis.[242,250,255]

2. **Lymphoma versus hepatitis.** Hepatitis C, which can be associated with prominent portal lymphoid infiltration, including invasion of biliary epithelium that mimics lymphoepithelial lesions, can enter the differential diagnosis of marginal zone lymphoma. Marginal zone lymphoma is associated with a more extensive lymphoid infiltrate and a B-cell preponderance in the infiltrate. B cells form lymphoepithelial lesions in marginal zone lymphomas, whereas in hepatitis C, the lymphocytes that infiltrate the biliary epithelium are mostly T cells. T-cell/histiocyte-rich large B-cell lymphoma (THRBCL) can be associated with changes in the adjacent hepatic tissue resembling hepatitis. Large neoplastic B cells can be inconspicuous in THRBCL, which increases the chance that THRBCL could be mistaken for hepatitis. Careful examination of well-prepared slides should reveal the large cells, which can be highlighted with immunostains for CD20 and bcl6.

3. **Marginal zone lymphoma versus hepatic pseudolymphoma.** Hepatic pseudolymphoma is a rare disorder characterized by the presence of one or (less often) two or three nodular lesions within the hepatic parenchyma. It occurs in both men and women, some of whom have autoimmune disease, carcinoma, or some other type of liver disease.[279] The lesions range from 0.5 to 5.5 cm. On microscopic examination, they consist of organized lymphoid tissue with reactive lymphoid follicles and an interfollicular area occupied by small lymphocytes, sometimes with clusters of epithelioid histiocytes and few immunoblasts and plasma cells. The lesions sometimes are partially delineated by a fibrous capsule. The lymphoid proliferation extends beyond the main lesion into adjacent parenchyma along portal tracts, but without formation of lymphoepithelial lesions. A mixture of B cells and T cells is found both within and outside follicles, and any plasma cells are polytypic. Follow-up has been uneventful.[279] The appearance could mimic that of hepatic marginal zone lymphoma. Features in favor of marginal zone lymphoma include the presence of cells with the morphology of marginal zone cells, a clear predominance of B cells outside follicles, monotypic B cells and/or plasma cells, the presence of lymphoepithelial lesions and clonal *IGH*.

4. **THRBCL versus Hodgkin's lymphoma.** The histologic picture of large tumor cells in a mixed reactive background found in THRBCL may suggest Hodgkin's lymphoma. As does THRBCL, Hodgkin's lymphoma in the liver tends to predominantly involve the portal tracts. However, it also may form solid nodules of tumor[259,280]; therefore, the pattern is little help in distinguishing THRBCL and Hodgkin's lymphoma. Immunophenotyping is helpful; THRBCL shows CD20+, CD15–, and CD30– large atypical B cells in a background composed virtually exclusively of T cells and histiocytes.[259,280,281] Classical Hodgkin's lymphoma shows large atypical cells that most often are CD15+, CD30+, and CD20– in a mixed background of T cells, B cells, histiocytes, and granulocytes.

Very few cases of nodular lymphocyte–predominant Hodgkin's lymphoma are characterized by widespread disease with hepatic involvement. In such cases, distinction from THRBCL relies on demonstration of some small B cells in the reactive background and follicular dendritic meshworks associated with the lymphoma in at least some of the involved tissues. The distinction between THRBCL and diffuse areas of nodular lymphocyte–predominant Hodgkin's lymphoma may be very difficult, particularly on a small biopsy sample. The distinction may be made more readily on a large specimen, such as an excised lymph node.

Secondary Hepatic Involvement by Lymphoma

Hepatic involvement by lymphoma in the setting of widespread disease or at relapse is more common than primary hepatic lymphoma.[280] In cases of widespread lymphoma, hepatic involvement is common.[278,282] Involvement by non-Hodgkin's lymphoma is more common than Hodgkin's lymphoma,[282] although high-stage Hodgkin's lymphoma also often involves the liver. Certain types of lymphoma have characteristic histologic patterns of hepatic involvement, even though they are not confined to the liver at presentation.[280] Diffuse large B-cell lymphoma, for example, most often involves the liver in the form of tumor nodules that obliterate normal parenchyma, but it also may predominantly involve portal tracts, with or without sinusoidal infiltration.

Follicular lymphoma most often shows portal involvement,[259,280] but it also may form tumor nodules.[280] Mantle cell lymphoma in the liver usually shows portal involvement.[280] Lymphoid leukemias, such as chronic lymphocytic leukemia, hairy cell leukemia, and B-lymphoblastic leukemia (Figure 5-31) may involve the hepatic sinusoids, although portal involvement is also common in cases of chronic lymphocytic leukemia.[280] Hepatosplenic T-cell lymphoma preferentially involves the hepatic

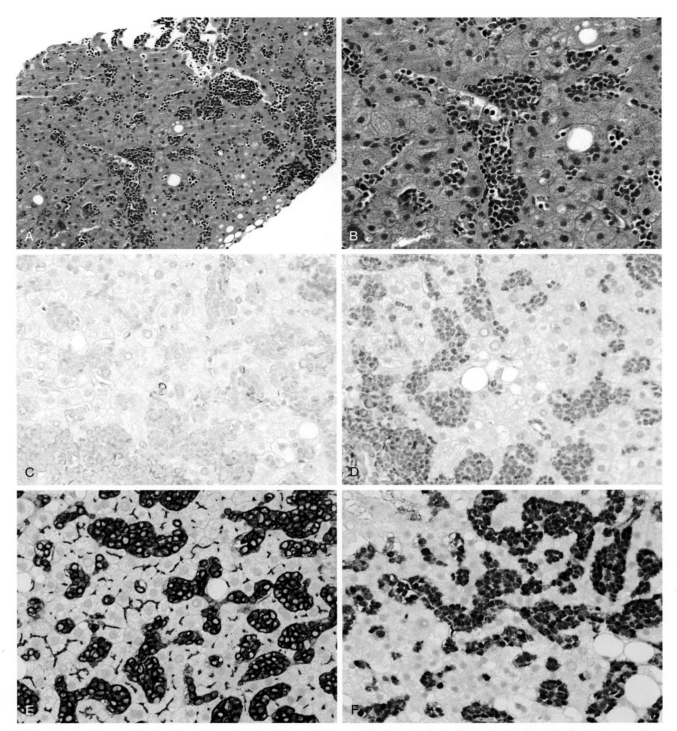

Figure 5-31   B-lymphoblastic leukemia involving the liver at relapse. **A,** Lymphoid cells fill multiple hepatic sinusoids. **B,** Lymphoid cells are small to medium-sized with oval nuclei, fine chromatin, and scant cytoplasm. The lymphoblasts are negative for CD20 **(C)** but show nuclear positivity for Pax5 (B cells, **D**), strong staining for CD10 **(E)**, and strong nuclear staining for TdT **(F)**. (Immunoperoxidase technique on paraffin sections.)

sinusoids (Figure 5-32). Pathologic features are similar for αβ and γδ variants, except that in some αβ cases, hepatic involvement is described as periportal as well as sinusoidal.[283] Hepatosplenic T-cell lymphoma is discussed in detail in Lymphomas of the Spleen, Chapter 6.

■ LYMPHOMAS OF THE GALLBLADDER

Primary Lymphomas of the Gallbladder

Primary lymphoma of the gallbladder is rare. In a series of 56,000 autopsies that evaluated tumors of the gallbladder, no cases of gallbladder lymphoma

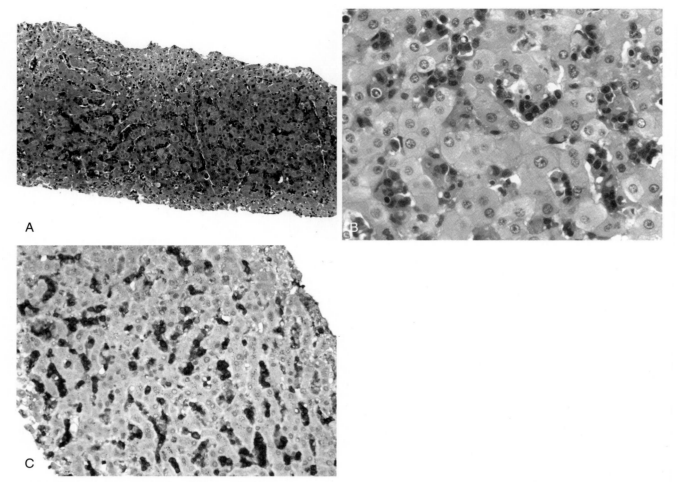

Figure 5-32 Hepatosplenic T-cell lymphoma of γδ-lineage in a renal transplant recipient with hepatosplenomegaly. **A,** Hepatic sinusoids are infiltrated by lymphoid cells throughout the needle core. **B,** The lymphoid cells have medium-sized, oval to slightly irregular nuclei; smooth chromatin; and scant to moderate, pale cytoplasm. **C,** The sinusoidal lymphoid cells are CD3+. (Immunoperoxidase technique on a paraffin section.) Immunohistochemistry together with flow cytometric analysis showed an abnormal T-cell population that was CD2+, CD3+, CD4−, CD5−, CD8−, and TCRγδ+.

were identified,[284] and only a few well-documented cases of primary lymphoma of the gallbladder have been reported.[284-296] Most patients with lymphoma primary in the gallbladder are older adults. Both men and women are affected, although a conspicuous female preponderance is seen among patients with extranodal marginal zone lymphoma of mucosa-associated lymphoid tissue (MALT lymphoma).[296,297]

Patients often present with symptoms that mimic cholecystitis, cholelithiasis, or choledocholithiasis, including right upper quadrant pain, nausea, vomiting or, in rare cases, jaundice.* Radiographic and/or gross examination often reveals thickening of the wall of the gallbladder or one or more discrete nodules; in rare cases the lymphoma forms a polypoid mass (Figure 5-33).† High-grade lymphomas tend to produce bulky masses with irregular mural thickening, whereas low-grade lymphomas may result in a more modest thickening of the gallbladder wall.[286] Most are extranodal marginal zone

lymphomas,[285,288,289,292,293] or diffuse large B-cell lymphomas.[290,298] Among the diffuse large B-cell lymphomas, bcl2 usually is positive and CD10 and bcl6 are variably expressed, although only a few cases have been studied. One lymphoma arising from the cystic duct was subclassified as a diffuse large B-cell lymphoma, anaplastic variant; this lymphoma was CD30+.[299] Several patients with large B-cell lymphomas have been HIV positive,[300] including one with a plasmablastic lymphoma and one with an HHV8+ solid variant of primary effusion lymphoma.[297] We have seen the case of an EBV+ diffuse large B-cell lymphoma (monomorphic B-lineage post-transplantation lymphoproliferative disorder) in a bone marrow transplant recipient (see Figure 5-33).

The pathologic features of the marginal zone lymphomas are similar to those observed in other sites. A dense infiltrate of marginal zone B cells with a variable admixture of small lymphocytes and plasma cells and few large cells, sometimes with interspersed reactive follicles, sometimes accompanied by the formation of lymphoepithelial lesions, involves the wall of the gallbladder, with resultant mural

---
*References 284-286, 288, 292, 293, 295, and 296.
†References 286, 287, 289, 290, 292, and 296.

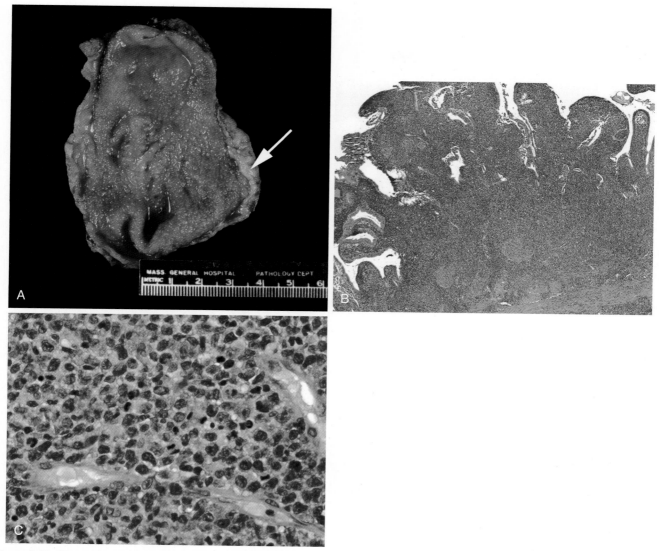

Figure 5-33 EBV+ diffuse large B-cell lymphoma involving the gallbladder in a bone marrow transplant recipient, consistent with a monomorphic post-transplantation lymphoproliferative disorder. **A,** The gallbladder wall is slightly thickened and has ill-defined nodularity. A cross section of the wall shows fleshy, light tan tissue *(arrow).* **B,** A dense lymphoid infiltrate fills the stroma of the mucosal folds and invades deep into the wall of the gallbladder. **C,** High-power view shows large lymphoid cells with oval to slightly irregular nuclei; mitoses are frequent.

thickening (Figure 5-34). Detailed immunophenotyping has been performed in a limited number of cases, but as in other sites, marginal zone lymphoma of the gallbladder is CD20+, CD5−, CD10−, CD23−, bcl6−, and bcl2+, with a low proliferation index and with markers for follicular dendritic cells highlighting residual reactive follicles.[285,292,293,295,296] In one case the presence of *API2/MALT1* fusion, indicating a t(11;18)(q21;q21), was documented using fluorescence in situ hybridization (FISH).[296]

Although only a few follicular lymphomas have been described, it is interesting that one case confined to the gallbladder was composed of lymphoid follicles lacking both bcl2 protein expression and *IGH/BCL2* gene fusion,[287] similar to certain other extranodal follicular lymphomas, whereas several other follicular lymphomas were composed of follicles that co-expressed bcl2,[286,294,297] similar to most

follicular lymphomas that arise in lymph nodes and in the tubular gut (Figure 5-35). The bcl2− follicular lymphoma occurred in a man with primary sclerosing cholangitis.[287]

Rare cases of B-lymphoblastic lymphoma and a peripheral T-cell lymphoma that was a post-transplantation lymphoproliferative disorder in a child status post cardiac transplant have been reported.[297] A case of mantle cell lymphoma with mucosal involvement, with the pattern of lymphomatous polyposis primary in the gallbladder, has been described.[297] In some cases of lymphoma of various pathologic types, concurrent chronic cholecystitis, chronic follicular cholecystitis, or cholesterolosis has been seen.[285] A number of patients with lymphomas of different types have had gallstones.[287,289,293,294,297]

On staging, the lymphoma is confined to the gallbladder in most reported cases.[284,285,287,290-292,294-297]

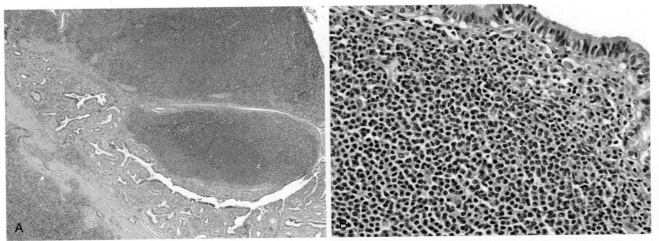

Figure 5-34 Marginal zone lymphoma arising in the gallbladder of an adult female; the lymphoma extended to the cystic duct margin. **A,** The wall of the gallbladder is thickened by a dense lymphoid infiltrate. **B,** A monotonous population of small lymphoid cells, with a few plasmacytoid cells, is present beneath an intact layer of epithelium. The immunophenotype was typical of marginal zone lymphoma.

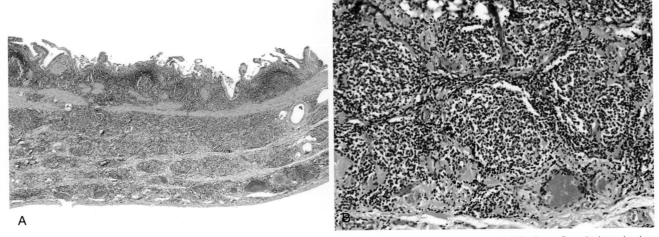

Figure 5-35 Follicular lymphoma, grade 1 of 3, arising in the gallbladder. The lymphoma was an incidental finding after cholecystectomy was performed for cholelithiasis. **A,** Low-power view shows multiple small lymphoid follicles involving the full thickness of the wall of the gallbladder. **B,** Higher power view shows several crowded, poorly delineated follicles composed of a monotonous population of small cells. The neoplastic follicles were CD20+, CD10+, bcl6+, and bcl2+, with Ki67 less than 5%.

In other cases of lymphoma interpreted as primary in the gallbladder, staging reveals involvement of lymph nodes, bone marrow, and/or other sites.[286,289,293,297]

Patients with low-grade lymphomas have a good prognosis.[286,292-296] Patients with marginal zone lymphoma usually have done well, often after surgery alone. One patient with marginal zone lymphoma treated initially with cholecystectomy alone developed a gastric relapse 5 years later but achieved remission with chemotherapy.[284] The outcome of patients with aggressive lymphomas is less favorable,[290,291] although some patients with diffuse large B-cell lymphoma treated in recent years with chemotherapy have done well.[298,299]

The etiology of lymphoma of the gallbladder is not known. However, some have suggested that these lymphomas, particularly the extranodal marginal zone type, may be related to bacterial infection and could arise from a background of cholecystitis analogous to the pathogenesis of gastric marginal zone lymphoma.[289,293,295] Given the frequency of cholecystitis and cholelithiasis in the general population, it is unclear whether this is a coincidence or whether it serves as a significant factor in the pathogenesis of the lymphomas by establishing a chronic inflammatory state in that site.

Secondary Involvement of the Gallbladder by Lymphoma

Spread to the gallbladder by lymphoma arising elsewhere and involvement of the gallbladder in cases of widespread lymphoma occasionally have been described; in some cases, gallbladder involvement was symptomatic. Some of these cases have been diffuse large B-cell lymphomas, including a case of T-cell/histiocyte-rich large B-cell lymphoma and one of EBV+ diffuse large B-cell lymphoma of the elderly.[297] Classical Hodgkin's lymphoma involving the gallbladder in the setting of widespread disease has been described.[297] The case of a man with a history of tonsillar mantle cell lymphoma that progressed to involve the gallbladder has been documented.[301] In the gallbladder, the lymphoma produced a cobblestone mucosa with the appearance of lymphomatous polyposis. On microscopic examination, a diagnosis of follicular cholecystitis initially was favored, but immunophenotyping demonstrated neoplastic mantle cells surrounding reactive follicle centers. We have seen a case of enteropathy-associated T-cell lymphoma in which the lymphoma spread to involve the gallbladder during the course of the disease.

■ LYMPHOMAS OF THE EXTRAHEPATIC BILIARY TRACT

Lymphoma is a rare cause of biliary obstruction. Approximately 1% of all cases of biliary obstruction related to malignancy are due to lymphoma.[302] In most such cases, biliary obstruction is extrinsic, related to enlarged lymph nodes in the area. Both Hodgkin's lymphoma and non-Hodgkin's lymphoma may cause extrinsic biliary obstruction. This phenomenon may occur at initial presentation or as the course of the disease progresses.[302] Lymphoma that arises primarily from the extrahepatic biliary tract is a rare phenomenon; fewer than 20 cases have been reported.[302-307] Patients with lymphoma have all been adults, and both men and women were affected. Two patients were HIV positive.

Patients with lymphoma arising from the extrahepatic biliary tract present with jaundice, fever, weight loss, right upper quadrant pain, or a combination of these findings. Cholangiography typically reveals a stricture. The clinical and radiographic features often suggest cholangiocarcinoma or sclerosing cholangitis. On gross examination, the lymphoma takes the form of mural thickening or of a nodular mass involving the bile ducts. The lymphomas sometimes have been classified using older classifications, which makes interpretation difficult; however, diffuse large B-cell lymphoma appears to be the most common type.[303-305] Rare cases of extranodal marginal zone lymphoma[306] and low-grade follicular lymphoma in which neoplastic B cells co-expressed CD20, CD10, bcl6, and bcl2[307] have been described. A case of a follicular lymphoma arising from the extrahepatic biliary tract that was grade 3A, CD20+, CD10−, bcl6+, and bcl2− has been reported; PCR showed clonal *IGH,* but FISH was negative for a translocation involving *BCL2.*[308] We also have seen a bcl2− follicular lymphoma that arose from the common bile duct (Figure 5-36); both of these bcl2− follicular lymphomas were associated with sclerosis.

■ PANCREATIC LYMPHOMAS

Primary Pancreatic Lymphomas

Introduction

A summary of the criteria proposed for a diagnosis of primary pancreatic lymphoma is as follows: (1) predominant pancreatic mass, (2) absence of lymphadenopathy except in the peripancreatic area, (3) absence of hepatic or splenic involvement, and (4) absence of peripheral blood involvement.[309] Pancreatic lymphoma is rare, accounting for fewer than 0.2% of pancreatic malignancies,[310] and fewer than 0.7% of non-Hodgkin's lymphomas.[1] Secondary involvement of the pancreas is much more common than primary lymphoma of the pancreas.[309]

Clinical Features

Primary pancreatic lymphoma affects patients over a broad age range (first to ninth decades), but almost all patients are adults, and the male to female ratio is greater than 2:1.[309,311-320] One patient was HIV positive,[312] and one lymphoma was a post-transplant lymphoproliferative disorder arising in the pancreatic allograft[321]; however, with these exceptions, patients have not had conditions predisposing to the development of lymphoma. They present with nonspecific symptoms of abdominal pain, loss of appetite, nausea, vomiting, fever, weight loss, malaise, jaundice, or a combination of these findings.[309,313-316,318,319,322] Gastrointestinal hemorrhage may result from invasion into the duodenum.[317] In rare cases the lymphoma may result in diabetes mellitus or pancreatic exocrine insufficiency.[320]

On physical examination, patients may have a palpable mass.[313,314,316,318,319] Because the signs and symptoms are so similar to those of the much more common pancreatic adenocarcinoma, patients often have undergone laparotomy and resection of tumor. Others have had a diagnosis established on an open biopsy; in some cases, computed tomography (CT)-guided percutaneous biopsy has provided diagnostic material.

The overall prognosis is difficult to assess, because most of the information is in individual case reports or is based on older reports; the lymphomas are of different types; and patients have not been treated uniformly. However, the prognosis is clearly better than for pancreatic adenocarcinoma.[309,322-324]

Pathologic Features

The lymphomas take the form of large lesions (usually larger than 6 to 8 cm in greatest dimension) that may form discrete tumors or may diffusely involve the pancreas. The head, body, or tail, or the entire pancreas, may be involved. The lesions sometimes are described as cystic or as having central necrosis. Invasion into adjacent structures such as the duodenum, retroperitoneal soft tissue, or mesentery

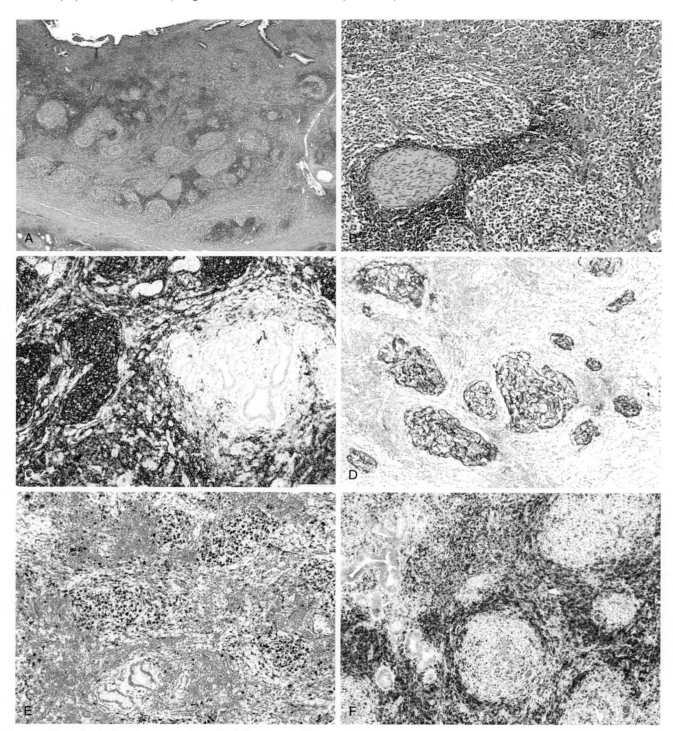

Figure 5-36   Follicular lymphoma, grade 2 of 3, follicular and diffuse pattern, arising in the common bile duct and resulting in biliary obstruction. **A,** Low-power view shows an atypical lymphoid proliferation infiltrating the full thickness of the bile duct, associated in areas with sclerosis. The lymphoma is predominantly follicular, but lymphoma in the upper right corner of the image shows a pattern that is mostly diffuse. **B,** Crowded, atypical follicles surround a nerve. **C,** B cells (CD20+) account for most of the cells in the follicles, and many scattered B cells are present outside the follicles. **D,** CD21 highlights the follicular dendritic meshworks associated with the follicles. **E** and **F,** The atypical follicles are composed of B cells that are bcl6+ and bcl2–. (*C* to *F*, Immunoperoxidase technique on paraffin sections.)

is common, and regional lymph nodes often are involved.[309,311,313-319,322,324]

The cases reported have been classified using a variety of systems, but diffuse large B-cell lymphoma appears to be most common[319,322]; a few cases have been classified as small noncleaved cell lymphoma[312] or Burkitt's lymphoma.[320] Rare cases of extranodal marginal zone lymphoma[311] and follicular lymphoma[324] have been reported. Several cases of anaplastic large cell lymphoma (two ALK+) have been described.[316-318]

Differential Diagnosis

1. **Pancreatic lymphoma versus adenocarcinoma.** Pancreatic lymphoma may mimic pancreatic adenocarcinoma clinically. Clues that may suggest lymphoma include a more gradual onset of symptoms; the presence of constitutional symptoms (e.g., fever, night sweats); a lesion that is larger than most carcinomas, which usually are smaller than 6 cm[314]; and more conspicuous lymphadenopathy.[309,323] To establish a diagnosis, tissue must be obtained for pathologic examination.

2. **Pancreatic lymphoma versus autoimmune pancreatitis.** Autoimmune pancreatitis can mimic a neoplasm clinically and radiographically. On pathologic examination, it typically is characterized by an intense periductal lymphoplasmacytic infiltrate, granulocytic epithelial lesions (periductal and ductal infiltrates of granulocytes), found in some cases, venulitis, periductal fibrosis, narrowing of ductal lumens, and an increased proportion of IgG4+ plasma cells. Lymphoid follicles often are present.[325] The lymphoplasmacytic infiltrate may suggest low-grade lymphoma, particularly on a small biopsy sample in which other characteristic features are not conspicuous. Familiarity with this entity can help prevent misdiagnosis.

REFERENCES

1. Freeman C, Berg J, Cutler S: Occurrence and prognosis of extranodal lymphomas, *Cancer* 29:252-260, 1972.
2. Gupta N, Goenka M, Jindal A et al: Primary lymphoma of the esophagus, *J Clin Gastroenterol* 23:203-206, 1996.
3. Golioto M, McGrath K: Primary lymphoma of the esophagus in a chronically immunosuppressed patient with hepatitis C infection: case report and review of the literature, *Am J Med Sci* 321:203-205, 2001.
4. Kalogeropoulos IV, Chalazonitis AN, Tsolaki S et al: A case of primary isolated non-Hodgkin's lymphoma of the esophagus in an immunocompetent patient, *World J Gastroenterol* 15:1901-1903, 2009.
5. Shim CS, Lee JS, Kim JO et al: A case of primary esophageal B-cell lymphoma of MALT type, presenting as a submucosal tumor, *J Korean Med Sci* 18:120-124, 2003.
6. George MK, Ramachandran V, Ramanan SG, Sagar TG: Primary esophageal T-cell non-Hodgkin's lymphoma, *Indian J Gastroenterol* 24:119-120, 2005.
7. Taal BG, Van Heerde P, Somers R: Isolated primary oesophageal involvement by lymphoma: a rare cause of dysphagia: two case histories and a review of other published data, *Gut* 34:994-998, 1993.
8. Zhu Q, Xu B, Xu K et al: Primary non-Hodgkin's lymphoma in the esophagus, *J Dig Dis* 9:241-244, 2008.
9. Bernal A, del Junco GW: Endoscopic and pathologic features of esophageal lymphoma: a report of four cases in patients with acquired immune deficiency syndrome, *Gastrointest Endosc* 32:96-99, 1986.
10. Tsukada T, Ohno T, Kihira H et al: Primary esophageal non-Hodgkin's lymphoma, *Intern Med* 31:569-572, 1992.
11. Sabljak P, Stojakov D, Bjelovic M et al: Primary esophageal diffuse large B-cell lymphoma: report of a case, *Surg Today* 38:647-650, 2008.
12. Koh P, Horsman J, Radstone C et al: Localised extranodal non-Hodgkin's lymphoma of the gastrointestinal tract: Sheffield Lymphoma Group experience (1989-1998), *Int J Oncol* 18:743-748, 2001.
13. Miyazaki T, Kato H, Masuda N et al: Mucosa-associated lymphoid tissue lymphoma of the esophagus: case report and review of the literature, *Hepatogastroenterology* 51:750-753, 2004.
14. Alinari L, Castellucci P, Elstrom R et al: 18F-FDG PET in mucosa-associated lymphoid tissue (MALT) lymphoma, *Leuk Lymphoma* 47:2096-2101, 2006.
15. Kitamoto Y, Hasegawa M, Ishikawa H et al: Mucosa-associated lymphoid tissue lymphoma of the esophagus: a case report, *J Clin Gastroenterol* 36:414-416, 2003.
16. Chung JJ, Kim MJ, Kie JH, Kim KW: Mucosa-associated lymphoid tissue lymphoma of the esophagus coexistent with bronchus-associated lymphoid tissue lymphoma of the lung, *Yonsei Med J* 46:562-566, 2005.
17. Fujisawa S, Motomura S, Fujimaki K et al: Primary esophageal T cell lymphoma, *Leuk Lymphoma* 33:199-202, 1999.
18. Rosenberg SA, Diamond HD, Jaslowitz B, Craver LF: Lymphosarcoma: a review of 1269 cases, *Medicine* 40:31-84, 1961.
19. Kodama T, Ohshima K, Nomura K et al: Lymphomatous polyposis of the gastrointestinal tract, including mantle cell lymphoma, follicular lymphoma and mucosa-associated lymphoid tissue lymphoma, *Histopathology* 47:467-478, 2005.
20. Michopoulos S, Petraki K, Matsouka C et al: Mantle-cell lymphoma (multiple lymphomatous polyposis) of the entire GI tract, *J Clin Oncol* 26:1555-1557, 2008.
21. Joshi A, Fields P, Simo R: Anaplastic lymphoma of the cervical esophagus presenting as a tracheoesophageal fistula, *Head Neck* 30:1264-1268, 2008.
22. Okerbloom JA, Armitage JO, Zetterman R, Linder J: Esophageal involvement by non-Hodgkin's lymphoma, *Am J Med* 77:359-361, 1984.
23. Crump M, Gospodarowicz M, Shepherd F: Lymphoma of the gastrointestinal tract, *Semin Oncol* 26:324-337, 1999.
24. Koch P, del Valle F, Berdel W et al: Primary gastrointestinal non-Hodgkin's lymphoma. I. Anatomic and histologic distribution, clinical features, and survival data of 371 patients registered in the German multicenter study GIT NHL 01/92, *J Clin Oncol* 19:3861-3873, 2001.
25. Lee J, Kim WS, Kim K et al: Intestinal lymphoma: exploration of the prognostic factors and the optimal treatment, *Leuk Lymphoma* 45:229-344, 2004.
26. Koch P, Probst A, Berdel WE et al: Treatment results in localized primary gastric lymphoma: data of patients registered within the German multicenter study (GIT NHL 02/96), *J Clin Oncol* 23:7050-7059, 2005.
27. Domizio P, Owen RA, Shepherd NA et al: Primary lymphoma of the small intestine: a clinicopathologic study of 119 cases, *Am J Surg Pathol* 17:429-442, 1993.
28. Hansen P, Vogt K, Skov R et al: Primary gastrointestinal non-Hodgkin's lymphoma in adults: a population based clinical and histopathologic study, *Int Med* 244:71-78, 1998.
29. Yoshino T, Miyake K, Ichimura K et al: Increased incidence of follicular lymphoma in the duodenum, *Am J Surg Pathol* 24:688-693, 2000.
30. Au E, Ang P, Tan P et al: Gastrointestinal lymphoma: a review of 54 patients in Singapore, *Ann Acad Med Singapore* 26:758-761, 1997.
31. Kohno S, Ohshima K, Yoneda S et al: Clinicopathological analysis of 143 primary malignant lymphomas in the small and large intestines based on the new WHO classification, *Histopathology* 43:135-143, 2003.
32. Kojima M, Nakamura S, Kurabayashi Y et al: Primary malignant lymphoma of the intestine: clinicopathologic and immunohistochemical studies of 39 cases, *Pathol Int* 45:123-130, 1995.
33. Chan J: Gastrointestinal lymphomas: an overview with emphasis on new findings and diagnostic problems, *Semin Diagn Pathol* 13:260-296, 1996.
34. Yoshida N, Nomura K, Wakabayashi N et al: Cytogenetic and clinicopathological characterization by fluorescence in situ hybridization on paraffin-embedded tissue sections of twenty-six cases with malignant lymphoma of small intestine, *Scand J Gastroenterol* 41:212-222, 2006.
35. Pickhardt P, Levy A, Rohrmann C et al: Non-Hodgkin's lymphoma of the appendix: clinical and CT findings with pathologic correlation, *Am J Roentgenol* 178:1123-1127, 2002.
36. Muller G, Dargent J, Duwel V et al: Leukemia and lymphoma of the appendix presenting as acute appendicitis or acute abdomen, *J Cancer Res Clin Oncol* 123:560-564, 1997.

37. Kitamura Y, Ohta T, Terada T: Primary T-cell non-Hodgkin's malignant lymphoma of the appendix, *Pathol Int* 50:313-317, 2000.

38. Smith D, Cataldo P: Perianal lymphoma in a heterosexual and nonimmunocompromised patient: report of a case and review of the literature, *Dis Colon Rectum* 42:952-954, 1999.

39. Nakamura S, Matsumoto T, Takeshita M et al: A clinicopathologic study of primary small intestine lymphoma: prognostic significance of mucosa-associated lymphoid tissue-derived lymphoma, *Cancer* 88:286-294, 2000.

40. Shepherd N, Hall P, Coates P, Levison D: Primary malignant lymphoma of the colon and rectum: a histopathological and immunohistochemical analysis of 45 cases with clinicopathological correlations, *Histopathology* 12:235-252, 1988.

41. Lewin K, Ranchod M, Dorfman R: Lymphomas of the gastrointestinal tract, *Cancer* 42:693-707, 1978.

42. Fan C-W, Changchien C, Wang J-Y et al: Primary colorectal lymphoma, *Dis Colon Rectum* 43:1277-1282, 2000.

43. Pasquale M, Shabahang M, Bitterman P et al: Primary lymphoma of the appendix: case report and review of the literature, *Surg Oncol* 3:243-248, 1994.

44. Powles T, Matthews G, Bower M: AIDS related systemic non-Hodgkin's lymphoma, *Sex Transm Infect* 76:335-341, 2000.

45. Beck P, Gill M, Sutherland L: HIV-associated non-Hodgkin's lymphoma of the gastrointestinal tract, *Am J Gastroenterol* 91:2377-2381, 1996.

46. Andrews CN, John Gill M, Urbanski SJ et al: Changing epidemiology and risk factors for gastrointestinal non-Hodgkin's lymphoma in a North American population: population-based study, *Am J Gastroenterol* 103:1762-1769, 2008.

47. Ferry J, Harris N: Pathology of post-transplant lymphoproliferative disorders. In Solez K, Racusen L, Billingham M, editors: *Pathology and rejection diagnosis in solid organ transplantation,* New York, 1994, Marcel Dekker.

48. Swerdlow S, Webber S, Chadburn A, Ferry J: Post-transplant lymphoproliferative disorders. In Swerdlow S, Campo E, Harris N et al, editors: *WHO classification: tumours of haematopoietic and lymphoid tissues,* ed 4, Lyon, 2008, IARC.

49. Harris N, Ferry J, Swerdlow S: Posttransplant lymphoproliferative disorders: summary of Society for Hematopathology workshop, *Semin Diagn Pathol* 14:8-14, 1997.

50. Chadburn A, Cesarman E, Knowles D: Molecular pathology of posttransplantation lymphoproliferative disorders, *Semin Diagn Pathol* 14:15-26, 1997.

51. Michael J, Greenstein S, Schechner R et al: Primary intestinal posttransplant T-cell lymphoma, *Transplantation* 75:2131-2132, 2003.

52. Ekstrom Smedby K, Vajdic CM, Falster M et al: Autoimmune disorders and risk of non-Hodgkin lymphoma subtypes: a pooled analysis within the InterLymph Consortium, *Blood* 111:4029-4038, 2008.

53. Kwon JH, Farrell RJ: The risk of lymphoma in the treatment of inflammatory bowel disease with immunosuppressive agents. *Crit Rev Oncol Hematol* 56:169-178, 2005.

54. Kandiel A, Fraser AG, Korelitz BI et al: Increased risk of lymphoma among inflammatory bowel disease patients treated with azathioprine and 6-mercaptopurine, *Gut* 54:1121-1125, 2005.

55. Loftus E, Tremaine W, Habermann T et al: Risk of lymphoma in inflammatory bowel disease, *Am J Gastroenterol* 95:2308-2312, 2000.

56. Farrell R, Ang Y, Kileen P et al: Increased incidence of non-Hodgkin's lymphoma in inflammatory bowel disease patients on immunosuppressive therapy, but overall risk is low, *Gut* 47:514-519, 2000.

57. Wong NA, Herbst H, Herrmann K et al: Epstein-Barr virus infection in colorectal neoplasms associated with inflammatory bowel disease: detection of the virus in lymphomas but not in adenocarcinomas, *J Pathol* 201:312-318, 2003.

58. Hall CH Jr, Shamma M: Primary intestinal lymphoma complicating Crohn's disease, *J Clin Gastroenterol* 36:332-336, 2003.

59. Mackey AC, Green L, Liang LC et al: Hepatosplenic T cell lymphoma associated with infliximab use in young patients treated for inflammatory bowel disease, *J Pediatr Gastroenterol Nutr* 44:265-267, 2007.

60. Buckley RH: Breakthrough in the understanding and therapy of primary immunodeficiency, *Pediatr Clin North Am* 41:665-690, 1994.

61. Harrington DS, Weisenburger DD, Purtilo DT: Malignant lymphoma in the X-linked lymphoproliferative syndrome, *Cancer* 59:1419-1429, 1987.

62. Pasic S, Vujic D, Djuricic S et al: Burkitt lymphoma–induced ileocolic intussusception in Wiskott-Aldrich syndrome, *J Pediatr Hematol Oncol* 28:48-49, 2006.

63. Dunnigan M, Yfantis H, Rapoport AP et al: Large cell lymphoma presenting as a flare of colitis in a patient with common variable immune deficiency, *Dig Dis Sci* 52:830-834, 2007.

64. Delia M, Liso V, Capalbo S et al: Common variable immunodeficiency patient with large granular lymphocytosis developing extranodal diffuse large B-cell lymphoma: a case report, *Haematologica* 91:ECR61, 2006.

65. Sneller MC, Strober W, Eisenstein E et al: New insights into common variable immunodeficiency, *Ann Intern Med* 118:720-730, 1993.

66. Castellano G, Moreno D, Galvao O et al: Malignant lymphoma of jejunum with common variable hypogammaglobulinemia and diffuse nodular hyperplasia of the small intestine, *J Clin Gastroenterol* 15:128-135, 1992.

67. Chung SJ, Kim JS, Kim H et al: Long-term clinical outcome of *Helicobacter pylori*–negative gastric mucosa–associated lymphoid tissue lymphoma is comparable to that of *H. pylori*-positive lymphoma, *J Clin Gastroenterol* 43:312-317, 2009.

68. Nakamura S, Ye H, Bacon CM et al: Clinical impact of genetic aberrations in gastric MALT lymphoma: a comprehensive analysis using interphase fluorescence in situ hybridisation, *Gut* 56:1358-1363, 2007.

69. Wang G, Auerbach A, Wei M et al: t(11;18)(q21;q21) In extranodal marginal zone B-cell lymphoma of mucosa-associated lymphoid tissue in stomach: a study of 48 cases, *Mod Pathol* 22:79-86, 2009.

70. Inagaki H, Nakamura T, Li C et al: Gastric MALT lymphomas are divided into three groups based on responsiveness to *Helicobacter pylori* eradication and detection of API2-MALT1 fusion, *Am J Surg Pathol* 28:1560-1567, 2004.

71. Montalban C, Santon A, Redondo C et al: Long-term persistence of molecular disease after histological remission in low-grade gastric MALT lymphoma treated with *H. pylori* eradication: lack of association with translocation t(11;18): a 10-year updated follow-up of a prospective study, *Ann Oncol* 16:1539-1544, 2005.

72. Fischbach W, Goebeler-Kolve M-E, Dragosics B et al: Long term outcome of patients with gastric marginal zone B cell lymphoma of mucosa associated lymphoid tissue (MALT) following exclusive *Helicobacter pylori* eradication therapy: experience from a large prospective series, *Gut* 53:34-37, 2004.

73. Hatano B, Ohshima K, Tsuchiya T et al: Clinicopathological features of gastric B-cell lymphoma: a series of 317 cases, *Pathol Int* 52:677-682, 2002.

74. de Mascarel A, Ruskone-Fourmestraux A, Lavergne-Slove A et al: Clinical, histological and molecular follow-up of 60 patients with gastric marginal zone lymphoma of mucosa-associated lymphoid tissue, *Virchows Arch* 446:219-224, 2005.

75. Ferreri A, Freschi M, Dell'Oro S et al: Prognostic significance of the histopathologic recognition of low and high-grade components in stage I-II B-cell gastric lymphomas, *Am J Surg Pathol* 25:95-102, 2001.

76. Takeshita M, Iwashita A, Kurihara K et al: Histologic and immunohistologic findings and prognosis of 40 cases of gastric large B-cell lymphoma, *Am J Surg Pathol* 24:1641-1649, 2000.

77. Yoshino T, Omonishi K, Kobayashi K et al: Clinicopathological features of gastric mucosa associated lymphoid tissue (MALT) lymphoma: high grade transformation and comparison with diffuse large B-cell lymphomas without MALT lymphoma features, *Clin Pathol* 53:187-190, 2000.

78. Ture-Ozdemir F, Gazouli M, Tzivras M et al: Association of polymorphisms of NOD2, TLR4 and CD14 genes with susceptibility to gastric mucosa–associated lymphoid tissue lymphoma, *Anticancer Res* 28:3697-3700, 2008.

79. Stathis A, Chini C, Bertoni F et al: Long-term outcome following *Helicobacter pylori* eradication in a retrospective study of 105 patients with localized gastric marginal zone B-cell lymphoma of MALT type, *Ann Oncol* 20:1086-1093, 2009.

80. Yokoi T, Nakamura T, Kasugai K et al: Primary low-grade gastric mucosa-associated lymphoid tissue (MALT) lymphoma with polypoid appearance: polypoid gastric MALT lymphoma—a clinicopathologic study of eight cases, *Pathol Int* 49:702-709, 1999.

81. Isaacson PG: Gastrointestinal lymphoma, *Hum Pathol* 25:1020-1029, 1994.

82. Zucca E, Bertoni F, Roggero E, Cavalli F: The gastric marginal zone B-cell lymphoma of MALT type, *Blood* 96:410-419, 2000.

83. Yoon SS, Coit DG, Portlock CS, Karpeh MS: The diminishing role of surgery in the treatment of gastric lymphoma, *Ann Surg* 240:28-37, 2004.

84. Fung C, Grossbard M, Linggood R et al: Mucosa-associated lymphoid tissue lymphoma of the stomach: long term outcome after local treatment, *Cancer* 85:9-17, 1999.

85. Isaacson P, Chott A, Nakamura S et al: Extranodal marginal zone lymphoma of mucosa-associated lymphoid tissue (MALT lymphoma). In Swerdlow S, Campo E, Harris N et al, editors: *WHO classification: tumours of haematopoietic and lymphoid tissues,* ed 4, Lyon, 2008, IARC.

86. Nakamura S, Yao T, Aoyagi K et al: *Helicobacter pylori* and primary gastric lymphoma: a histopathologic and immunohistochemical analysis of 237 patients, *Cancer* 79:3-11, 1997.

87. Hsi E, Singleton T, Swinnen L et al: Mucosa-associated lymphoid tissue–type lymphomas occurring in post-transplantation patients, *Am J Surg Pathol* 24:100-106, 2000.

88. Craig VJ, Arnold I, Gerke C et al: Gastric MALT lymphoma B cells express polyreactive, somatically mutated immunoglobulins, *Blood* 115:581-591, 2010.

89. Hussell T, Isaacson P, Crabtree J, Spencer J: The response of cells from low-grade B-cell gastric lymphomas of mucosa-associated lymphoid tissue to *Helicobacter pylori, Lancet* 342:571-574, 1993.

90. Raderer M, Wohrer S, Streubel B et al: Assessment of disease dissemination in gastric compared with extragastric mucosa-associated lymphoid tissue lymphoma using extensive staging: a single-center experience, *J Clin Oncol* 24:3136-3141, 2006.

91. Remstein ED, Dogan A, Einerson RR et al: The incidence and anatomic site specificity of chromosomal translocations in primary extranodal marginal zone B-cell lymphoma of mucosa-associated lymphoid tissue (MALT lymphoma) in North America, *Am J Surg Pathol* 30:1546-1553, 2006.

92. Streubel B, Seitz G, Stolte M et al: MALT lymphoma associated genetic aberrations occur at different frequencies in primary and secondary intestinal MALT lymphomas, *Gut* 55:1581-1585, 2006.

93. Liu H, Ruskon-Fourmesstraux A, Lavergne-Slove A et al: Resistance of t(11;18) positive gastric mucosa–associated lymphoid tissue lymphoma to *Helicobacter pylori* eradication therapy, *Lancet* 357:39-40, 2001.

94. Ye H, Liu H, Raderer M et al: High incidence of t(11;18)(q21;q21) in *Helicobacter pylori*-negative gastric MALT lymphoma, *Blood* 101:2547-2550, 2003.

95. Nakamura S, Ye H, Bacon CM et al: Translocations involving the immunoglobulin heavy chain gene locus predict better survival in gastric diffuse large B-cell lymphoma, *Clin Cancer Res* 14:3002-3010, 2008.

96. Hoeve M, Gisbertz I, Schouten H et al: Gastric low-grade MALT lymphoma, high-grade MALT lymphoma and diffuse large B cell lymphoma show different frequencies of trisomy, *Leukemia* 13:799-807, 1999.

97. Isaacson P: Gastrointestinal lymphomas of T- and B-cell types, *Mod Pathol* 12:151-158, 1999.

98. Ye H, Liu H, Attygalle A et al: Variable frequencies of t(11;18)(q21;q21) in MALT lymphomas of different sites: significant association with CagA strains of *H. pylori* in gastric MALT lymphoma, *Blood* 102:1012-1018, 2003.

99. Chen YW, Hu XT, Liang AC et al: High BCL6 expression predicts better prognosis, independent of BCL6 translocation status, translocation partner, or BCL6-deregulating mutations, in gastric lymphoma, *Blood* 108:2373-2383, 2006.

100. van Krieken J, Raffeld M, Raghobier S et al: Molecular genetics of gastrointestinal non-Hodgkin's lymphomas: unusual prevalence and pattern of *C-MYC* rearrangements in aggressive lymphomas, *Blood* 76:797-800, 1990.

101. de Jong D, Boot H, Taal B: Histological grading with clinical relevance in gastric mucosa–associated lymphoid tissue (MALT) lymphoma, *Cancer Res* 156:27-32, 2000.

102. Wotherspoon A, Doglioni C, Diss T et al: Regression of primary low-grade B-cell gastric lymphoma of mucosa-associated lymphoid tissue type after eradication of *Helicobacter pylori,* Lancet 342:575-577, 1993.

103. Cheng TY, Lin JT, Chen LT et al: Association of T-cell regulatory gene polymorphisms with susceptibility to gastric mucosa–associated lymphoid tissue lymphoma, *J Clin Oncol* 24:3483-3489, 2006.

104. Rollinson S, Levene A, Mensah F et al: Gastric marginal zone lymphoma is associated with polymorphisms in genes involved in inflammatory response and antioxidative capacity, *Blood* 102:1007-1011, 2003.

105. Singhal AV, Sepulveda AR: Helicobacter heilmannii gastritis: a case study with review of literature, *Am J Surg Pathol* 29:1537-1539, 2005.

106. Joo M, Kwak JE, Chang SH et al: *Helicobacter heilmannii*–associated gastritis: clinicopathologic findings and comparison with *Helicobacter pylori*–associated gastritis, *J Korean Med Sci* 22:63-69, 2007.

107. Hsi E, Eisbruch A, Greenson J et al: Classification of primary gastric lymphomas according to histologic features, *Am J Surg Pathol* 22:17-27, 1998.

108. Santon A, Garcia-Cosio M, Bellosillo B et al: Persistent monoclonality after histological remission in gastric mucosa–associated lymphoid tissue lymphoma treated with chemotherapy and/or surgery: influence of t(11;18)(q21;q21), *Leuk Lymphoma* 49:1516-1522, 2008.

109. Van Krieken J, Hoeve M: Epidemiological and prognostic aspects of gastric MALT lymphoma, *Cancer Res* 156:4-8, 2000.

110. Gobbi PG, Corbella F, Valentino F et al: Complete long-term response to radiotherapy of gastric early-stage marginal zone lymphoma resistant to both anti-*Helicobacter pylori* antibiotics and chemotherapy, *Ann Oncol* 20:465-468, 2009.

111. Thiede C, Wundisch T, Alpen B et al: Long-term persistence of monoclonal B-cells after cure of *Helicobacter pylori* infection and complete histologic remission in gastric mucosa–associated lymphoid tissue B-cell lymphoma, *J Clin Oncol* 19:1600-1609, 2001.

112. Chen LT, Lin JT, Tai JJ et al: Long-term results of anti-*Helicobacter pylori* therapy in early-stage gastric high-grade transformed MALT lymphoma, *J Natl Cancer Inst* 97:1345-1353, 2005.

113. Nakamura S, Matsumoto T, Suekane H et al: Predictive value of endoscopic ultrasonography for regression of gastric low grade and high grade MALT lymphomas after eradication of *Helicobacter pylori, Gut* 48:454-460, 2001.

114. Chen LT, Lin JT, Shyu RY et al: Prospective study of *Helicobacter pylori* eradication therapy in stage I(E) high-grade mucosa-associated lymphoid tissue lymphoma of the stomach, *J Clin Oncol* 19:4245-4251, 2001.

115. Kuo SH, Chen LT, Wu MS et al: Differential response to *H. pylori* eradication therapy of co-existing diffuse large B-cell lymphoma and MALT lymphoma of stomach: significance of tumour cell clonality and BCL10 expression, *J Pathol* 211:296-304, 2007.

116. Ang MK, Hee SW, Quek R et al: Presence of a high-grade component in gastric mucosa–associated lymphoid tissue (MALT) lymphoma is not associated with an adverse prognosis, *Ann Hematol* 88:417-424, 2009.

117. Chen ZM, Shah R, Zuckerman GR, Wang HL: Epstein-Barr virus gastritis: an underrecognized form of severe gastritis simulating gastric lymphoma, *Am J Surg Pathol* 31:1446-1451, 2007.

118. Park YH, Kim WS, Bang SM et al: Prognostic factor analysis and proposed prognostic model for conventional treatment of high-grade primary gastric lymphoma, *Eur J Haematol* 77:304-308, 2006.

119. Connor J, Ashton-Key M: Gastric and intestinal diffuse large B-cell lymphomas are clinically and immunophenotypically different: an immunohistochemical and clinical study, *Histopathology* 51:697-703, 2007.

120. Hans CP, Weisenburger DD, Greiner TC et al: Confirmation of the molecular classification of diffuse large B-cell lymphoma by immunohistochemistry using a tissue microarray, *Blood* 103:275-282, 2004.

121. McManus DT, Catherwood MA, Carey PD et al: ALK-positive diffuse large B-cell lymphoma of the stomach associated with a clathrin-ALK rearrangement, H*um Pathol* 35:1285-1288, 2004.

122. Starostik P, Greiner A, Schultz A et al: Genetic aberrations common in gastric high-grade large B-cell lymphoma, *Blood* 95:1180-1187, 2000.

123. Liang R, Chan W, Kwong Y et al: High incidence of BCL-6 gene rearrangement in diffuse large B-cell lymphoma of primary gastric origin, *Cancer Genet Cytogenet* 97:114-118, 1997.

124. Oh SY, Kwon HC, Kim WS et al: Intestinal marginal zone B-cell lymphoma of MALT type: clinical manifestation and outcome of a rare disease, *Eur J Haematol* 79:287-291, 2007.

125. Sakugawa ST, Yoshino T, Nakamura S et al: API2-MALT1 fusion gene in colorectal lymphoma, *Mod Pathol* 16:1232-1241, 2003.

126. Sinn DH, Kim YH, Lee EJ et al: Methylation and API2/MALT1 fusion in colorectal extranodal marginal zone lymphoma, *Mod Pathol* 22:314-320, 2009.

127. Kim J, Jung H, Shin K et al: Eradication of *Helicobacter pylori* infection did not lead to cure of duodenal mucosa–associated lymphoid tissue lymphoma, *Scand J Gastroenterol* 34:215-218, 1999.

128. Nagashima R, Takeda H, Maeda K et al: Regression of duodenal mucosa–associated lymphoid tissue lymphoma after eradication of *Helicobacter pylori, Gastroenterology* 111:1674-1678, 1996.

129. Nakase H, Okazaki K, Ohana M et al: The possible involvement of micro-organisms other than *Helicobacter pylori* in the development of rectal MALT lymphoma in *H. pylori*–negative patients, *Endoscopy* 34:343-346, 2002.

130. de Boer JP, Hiddink RF, Raderer M et al: Dissemination patterns in non-gastric MALT lymphoma, *Haematologica* 93:201-206, 2008.

131. Matsumoto T, Takayuki M, Iida M : Regression of mucosa-associated lymphoid tissue lymphoma of rectum after eradication of *Helicobacter pylori, Lancet* 350:115-116, 1997.

132. Azar HA: Cancer in Lebanon and the Near East, *Cancer* 15:66-78, 1962.

133. Al-Saleem T, Al-Mondhiry H: Immunoproliferative small intestinal disease (IPSID): a model for mature B-cell neoplasms, *Blood* 105:2274-2280, 2005.

134. Salem P, El-Hashimi L, Anaissie E et al: Primary small intestinal lymphoma in adults: a comparative study of IPSID versus non-IPSID in the Middle East, *Cancer* 59:1670-1676, 1987.

135. Tabbane F, Mourali N, Cammoun M, Najjar T: Results of laparotomy in immunoproliferative small intestinal disease, *Cancer* 61:1699-1706, 1988.

136. Smith WJ, Price SK, Isaacson PG: Immunoglobulin gene rearrangement in immunoproliferative small intestinal disease (IPSID), *J Clin Pathol* 40:1291-1297, 1987.

137. Lankarani KB, Masoompour SM, Masoompour MB et al: Changing epidemiology of IPSID in Southern Iran, *Gut* 54:311-312, 2005.

138. Salem PA, Estephan FF: Immunoproliferative small intestinal disease: current concepts, *Cancer J* 11:374-382, 2005.

139. Lecuit M: Immunoproliferative small intestinal disease associated with *Campylobacter jejuni, J Nat Cancer Inst* 96:571-573, 2004.

140. Lecuit M, Abachin E, Martin A et al: Immunoproliferative small intestinal disease associated with *Campylobacter jejuni, N Engl J Med* 350:239-248, 2004.

141. Economidou I, Manousos ON, Triantafillidis JK et al: Immunoproliferative small intestinal disease in Greece: presentation of 13 cases, including two from Albania, *Eur J Gastroenterol Hepatol* 18:1029-1038, 2006.

142. Fine K, Stone ML: α-Heavy chain disease, Mediterranean lymphoma, and immunoproliferative small intestinal disease, *Am J Gastroenterol* 94:1139-1152, 1999.

143. Chuang SS, Ye H, Yang SF et al: Perforation predicts poor prognosis in patients with primary intestinal diffuse large B-cell lymphoma, *Histopathology* 53:432-440, 2008.

144. Ioachim H, Antonescu C, Giancotti F et al: EBV-associated anorectal lymphomas in patients with acquired immune deficiency syndrome, *Am J Surg Pathol* 21:997-1006, 1997.

145. Chetty R, Hlatswayo N, Muc R et al: Plasmablastic lymphoma in HIV+ patients: an expanding spectrum, *Histopathology* 42:605-609, 2003.

146. Dong HY, Scadden DT, de Leval L et al: Plasmablastic lymphoma in HIV-positive patients: an aggressive Epstein-Barr virus–associated extramedullary plasmacytic neoplasm, *Am J Surg Pathol* 29:1633-1641, 2005.

147. DePond W, Said J, Tasaka T et al: Kaposi's sarcoma—associated herpesvirus and human herpesvirus 8 (KSHV/HHV8)—associated lymphoma of the bowel: report of two cases in HIV-positive men with secondary effusion lymphomas, *Am J Surg Pathol* 21:719-724, 1997.

148. Costes V, Faumont N, Cesarman E et al: Human herpesvirus-8–associated lymphoma of the bowel in human immunodeficiency virus–positive patients without history of primary effusion lymphoma, *Hum Pathol* 33:846-849, 2002.

149. Nakamura S, Jaffe E, Swerdlow S: EBV positive diffuse large B-cell lymphoma of the elderly. In Swerdlow S, Campo E, Harris N et al, editors: *WHO classification: tumours of haematopoietic and lymphoid tissues,* ed 4, Lyon, 2008, IARC.

150. Farris A, Lauwers G, Ferry J, Zukerberg L: The rectal tonsil: a reactive lymphoid proliferation that may mimic lymphoma, *Am J Surg Pathol* 32:1075-1979, 2008.

151. Shami VM, Waxman I: Lymphoid follicular proctitis mimicking rectal lymphoma: diagnosis by EMR, *Gastrointest Endosc* 60:648-652, 2004.

152. O'Briain DS, Kennedy MJ, Daly PA et al: Multiple lymphomatous polyposis of the gastrointestinal tract: a clinicopathologically distinctive form of non-Hodgkin's lymphoma of B-cell centrocytic type, *Am J Surg Pathol* 13:691-699, 1989 (review).

153. Swerdlow S, Campo E, Seto M, Muller-Hermelink H: Mantle cell lymphoma. In Swerdlow S, Campo E, Harris N et al, editors: *WHO classification: tumours of haematopoietic and lymphoid tissues,* ed 4, Lyon, 2008, IARC.

154. Cornes J: Multiple lymphomatous polyposis of the gastrointestinal tract, *Cancer* 14:249-257, 1961.

155. Salar A, Juanpere N, Bellosillo B et al: Gastrointestinal involvement in mantle cell lymphoma: a prospective clinic, endoscopic, and pathologic study, *Am J Surg Pathol* 30:1274-1280, 2006.

156. Geissmann F, Ruskone-Fourmestraux A, Hermine O et al: Homing receptor α4β7 integrin expression predicts digestive tract involvement in mantle cell lymphoma, *Am J Pathol* 153:1701-1705, 1998.

157. Isomoto H, Ohnita K, Mizuta Y et al: Clinical and endoscopic features of adult T-cell leukemia/lymphoma with duodenal involvement, *J Clin Gastroenterol* 33:241-246, 2001.

158. Hokama A, Tomoyose T, Yamamoto Y et al: Adult T-cell leukemia/lymphoma presenting multiple lymphomatous polyposis, *World J Gastroenterol* 14:6584-6588, 2008.

159. Andhavarapu S, Tolentino AM, Jha C et al: Diffuse large B-cell lymphoma presenting as multiple lymphomatous polykposis of the gastrointestinal tract, *Clin Lymphoma Myeloma* 8:179-183, 2008.

160. Harris N, Nathwani B, Swerdlow SH et al: Follicular lymphoma. In Swerdlow S, Campo E, Harris N et al, editors: *WHO classification: tumours of haematopoietic and lymphoid tissues,* ed 4, Lyon, 2008, IARC.

161. Misdraji J, Harris N, Ferry J: Follicular lymphoma of the gastrointestinal tract (abstract), *Ann Oncol* 18(s):109A, 2007.

162. Kodama M, Kitadai Y, Shishido T et al: Primary follicular lymphoma of the gastrointestinal tract: a retrospective case series, *Endoscopy* 40:343-346, 2008.

163. Huang WT, Hsu YH, Yang SF, Chuang SS: Primary gastrointestinal follicular lymphoma: a clinicopathologic study of 13 cases from Taiwan, *J Clin Gastroenterol* 42:997-1002, 2008.

164. Damaj G, Verkarre V, Delmer A et al: Primary follicular lymphoma of the gastrointestinal tract: a study of 25 cases and a literature review, *Ann Oncol* 14:623-629, 2003.

165. Shia J, Teruya-Feldstein J, Pan D et al: Primary follicular lymphoma of the gastrointestinal tract, *Am J Surg Pathol* 26:216-224, 2002.

166. Sato Y, Ichimura K, Tanaka T et al: Duodenal follicular lymphomas share common characteristics with mucosa-associated lymphoid tissue lymphomas, *J Clin Pathol* 61:377-381, 2008.

167. Misdraji J, Harris N, Hasserjian R et al: Primary follicular lymphoma of the gastrointestinal tract (in preparation).

168. Poggi MM, Cong PJ, Coleman CN, Jaffe ES: Low-grade follicular lymphoma of the small intestine, *J Clin Gastroenterol* 34:155-159, 2002.

169. Misdraji J, del Castillo C, Ferry J: Follicle center lymphoma of the ampulla of Vater presenting with jaundice, *Am J Surg Pathol* 21:484-438, 1997.

170. Takata K, Sato Y, Nakamura N et al: Duodenal and nodal follicular lymphomas are distinct: the former lacks activation-induced cytidine deaminase and follicular dendritic cells despite ongoing somatic hypermutations, *Mod Pathol* 22:940-949, 2009.

171. Chott A, Raderer M, Jager U et al: Follicular lymphoma of the duodenum: a distinct extranodal B-cell lymphoma? *Mod Pathol* 14:160A, 2001.

172. Rosty C, Briere J, Cellier C et al: Association of a duodenal follicular lymphoma and hereditary nonpolyposis colorectal cancer, *Mod Pathol* 13:586-590, 2000.

173. Bende R, Smit L, Bossenbroek J et al: Primary follicular lymphoma of the small intestine: α4β7 expression and immunoglobulin configuration suggest an origin from local antigen-experienced B cells, *Am J Pathol* 162:105-113, 2003.

174. Snuderl M, Kolman OK, Chen YB et al: B-cell lymphomas with concurrent IGH-BCL2 and MYC rearrangements are aggressive neoplasms with clinical and pathologic features distinct from Burkitt lymphoma and diffuse large B-cell lymphoma, *Am J Surg Pathol* 34:327-340, 2010.

175. Leoncini L, Raphael M, Stein H et al: Burkitt lymphoma. In Swerdlow S, Campo E, Harris N et al, editors: *WHO classification: tumours of haematopoietic and lymphoid tissues*, ed 4, Lyon, 2008, IARC.

176. Chogle A, Nguyen K, Lazare F et al: Gastric Burkitt lymphoma: a rare cause of upper gastrointestinal bleeding in a child with HIV/AIDS, *J Pediatr Gastroenterol Nutr* 48:237-239, 2009.

177. Ferry J: Burkitt's lymphoma: clinicopathologic features and differential diagnosis, *Oncologist* 11:375-383, 2006.

178. Kluin P, Harris N, Stein H et al: B-cell lymphoma, unclassifiable, with features intermediate between diffuse large B-cell lymphoma and Burkitt lymphoma. In Swerdlow S, Campo E, Harris N et al, editors: *WHO classification: tumours of haematopoietic and lymphoid tissues*, ed 4, Lyon, 2008, IARC.

179. Isaacson P: Relation between cryptic intestinal lymphoma and refractory sprue, *Lancet* 356:178-179, 2000.

180. Isaacson P, Spencer J, Connolly C et al: Malignant histiocytosis of the intestine: a T-cell lymphoma, *Lancet* ii:688-691, 1985.

181. Chott A, Vesely M, Simonitsch I et al: Classification of intestinal T-cell neoplasms and their differential diagnosis, *Am J Clin Pathol* (Pathology Patterns) 111:S68-S74, 1999.

182. Isaacson P, Chott A, Ott G, Stein H: Enteropathy-associated T-cell lymphoma. In Swerdlow S, Campo E, Harris N et al, editors: *WHO classification: tumours of haematopoietic and lymphoid tissues*, ed 4, Lyon, 2008, IARC.

183. Jaffe E, Krenacs L, Kumar S et al: Extranodal peripheral T-cell and NK-cell neoplasms, *Am J Clin Pathol* (Pathology Patterns) 111:S46-S55, 1999.

184. Harris NL, Jaffe ES, Stein H et al: A revised European-American classification of lymphoid neoplasms: a proposal from the International Lymphoma Study Group, *Blood* 84:1361-1392, 1994.

185. Smedby KE, Akerman M, Hildebrand H et al: Malignant lymphomas in coeliac disease: evidence of increased risks for lymphoma types other than enteropathy-type T cell lymphoma, *Gut* 54:54-59, 2005.

186. Verbeek WH, Van De Water JM, Al-Toma A et al: Incidence of enteropathy-associated T-cell lymphoma: a nation-wide study of a population-based registry in The Netherlands, *Scand J Gastroenterol* 43:1322-1328, 2008.

187. Gale J, Simmonds P, Mead G et al: Enteropathy-type intestinal T-cell lymphoma: clinical features and treatment of 31 patients in a single center, *J Clin Oncol* 18:795-803, 2000.

188. Chott A, Haedickle W, Mosberger I et al: Most CD56+ intestinal lymphomas are CD8+ CD5– T-cell lymphomas of monomorphic small to medium size histology, *Am J Pathol* 153:1483-1490, 1998.

189. Al-Toma A, Verbeek WH, Hadithi M et al: Survival in refractory coeliac disease and enteropathy-associated T-cell lymphoma: retrospective evaluation of single-centre experience, *Gut* 56:1373-1378, 2007.

190. Silano M, Volta U, Vincenzi AD et al: Effect of a gluten-free diet on the risk of enteropathy-associated T-cell lymphoma in celiac disease, *Dig Dis Sci* 53:972-976, 2008.

191. Holmes GKT, Prior P, Lane MR et al: Malignancy in coeliac disease: effect of a gluten free diet, *Gut* 30:333-338, 1989.

192. Cellier C, Delabesse E, Helmer C et al: Refractory sprue, coeliac disease, and enteropathy-associated T-cell lymphoma, *Lancet* 356:203-208, 2000.

193. Kluin P, Feller A, Gaulard P et al: Peripheral T/NK-cell lymphoma: a report of the Ninth Workshop of the European Association for Haematopathology, *Histopathology* 38:250-270, 2001.

194. Yuan CM, Stein S, Glick JH, Wasik MA: Natural killer–like T-cell lymphoma of the small intestine with a distinct immunophenotype and lack of association with gluten-sensitive enteropathy, *Arch Pathol Lab Med* 127:142-146, 2003.

195. Bagdi E, Diss T, Munson P, Isaacson P: Mucosal intraepithelial lymphocytes in enteropathy-associated T-cell lymphoma, ulcerative jejunitis, and refractory celiac disease constitute a neoplastic population, *Blood* 94:260-264, 1999.

196. Spencer J, Cerf-Bensussan N, Jarry A et al: Enteropathy-associated T-cell lymphoma (malignant histiocytosis of the intestine) is recognized by a monoclonal antibody (HML-1) that defines a membrane molecule on human mucosal lymphocytes, *Am J Pathol* 132:1-135, 1988.

197. Rahemtullah A, Longtine JA, Harris NL et al: CD20+ T-cell lymphoma: clinicopathologic analysis of 9 cases and a review of the literature, *Am J Surg Pathol* 32:1593-1607, 2008.

198. Obermann EC, Diss TC, Hamoudi RA et al: Loss of heterozygosity at chromosome 9p21 is a frequent finding in enteropathy-type T-cell lymphoma, *J Pathol* 202:252-262, 2004.

199. Baumgartner A, Zettl A, Chott A et al: High frequency of genetic aberrations in enteropathy-type T-cell lymphoma, *Lab Invest* 83:1509-1516, 2003.

200. Ashton-Key M, Diss T, Pan L et al: Molecular analysis of T-cell clonality in ulcerative jejunitis and enteropathy-associated T-cell lymphoma, *Am J Pathol* 151:493-498, 1997.

201. Quintanilla-Martinez L, Lome-Maldonado C, Ott G et al: Primary non-Hodgkin's lymphoma of the intestine: high prevalence of Epstein-Barr virus in Mexican lymphomas as compared with European cases, *Blood* 89:644-651, 1997.

202. Cejkova P, Zettl A, Baumgartner AK et al: Amplification of NOTCH1 and ABL1 gene loci is a frequent aberration in enteropathy-type T-cell lymphoma, *Virchows Arch* 446:416-420, 2005.

203. Holmes G: Mesenteric lymph node cavitation in celiac disease, *Gut* 27:728-733, 1986.

204. de Mascarel A, Belleannee G, Stanislas S et al: Mucosal intraepithelial T-lymphocytes in refractory celiac disease: a neoplastic population with a variable CD8 phenotype, *Am J Surg Pathol* 32:744-751, 2008.

205. Bhagat G, Naiyer AJ, Shah JG et al: Small intestinal CD8+TCRγδ+NKG2A+ intraepithelial lymphocytes have attributes of regulatory cells in patients with celiac disease, *J Clin Invest* 118:281-293, 2008.

206. Verbeek WH, von Blomberg BM, Scholten PE et al: The presence of small intestinal intraepithelial gamma/delta T-lymphocytes is inversely correlated with lymphoma development in refractory celiac disease, *Am J Gastroenterol* 103:3152-3158, 2008.

207. Carbonnel F, Grollet-Bioul L, Brouet J et al: Are complicated forms of celiac disease cryptic T-cell lymphomas? *Blood* 92:3879-3886, 1998.

208. Park YH, Kim WS, Bang SM et al: Primary gastric lymphoma of T-cell origin: clinicopathologic features and treatment outcome, *Leuk Res* 30:1253-1258, 2006.

209. Kawamoto K, Nakamura S, Iwashita A et al: Clinicopathological characteristics of primary gastric T-cell lymphoma, *Histopathology* 55:641-653, 2009.

210. Nga ME, Tan SH, Teh M et al: Lymphocytic gastritis–like T cell lymphoma: molecular evidence of an unusual recurrence, *J Clin Pathol* 57:1222-1224, 2004.

211. Hui P, Tokunaga M, Chan W et al: Epstein-Barr virus–associated gastric lymphoma in Hong Kong Chinese, *Hum Pathol* 25:947-952, 1994.

212. Chuang SS, Chang ST, Chuang WY et al: NK-cell lineage predicts poor survival in primary intestinal NK-cell and T-cell lymphomas, *Am J Surg Pathol* 33:1230-1240, 2009.

213. Svrcek M, Garderet L, Sebbagh V et al: Small intestinal CD4+ T-cell lymphoma: a rare distinctive clinicopathological entity associated with prolonged survival, *Virchows Arch* 451:1091-1093, 2007.

214. Ohshima K, Jaffe E, Kikuchi M: Adult T-cell leukaemia/lymphoma. In Swerdlow S, Campo E, Harris N et al, editors: *WHO classification: tumours of haematopoietic and lymphoid tissues*, ed 4, Lyon, 2008, IARC.

215. Tanaka K, Nakamura S, Matsumoto T et al: Long-term remission of primary gastric T cell lymphoma associated with human T lymphotropic virus type 1: a report of two cases and review of the literature, *Intern Med* 46:1783-1787, 2007.

216. Yatabe Y, Mori N, Oka K et al: Primary gastric T-cell lymphoma, *Arch Pathol Lab Med* 118:547-550, 1994.

217. Ohnita K, Isomoto H, Maeda T et al: Two cases of adult T-cell leukemia/lymphoma involving the terminal ileum, *Leuk Lymphoma* 44:973-976, 2003.

218. Isomoto H, Nishida Y, Fukuda H et al: Two cases of adult T-cell leukemia/lymphoma with oesophageal involvement, *Eur J Gastroenterol Hepatol* 14:449-452, 2002.

219. Sakata H, Fujimoto K, Iwakiri R et al: Gastric lesions in 76 patients with adult T-cell leukemia/lymphoma: endoscopic evaluation, *Cancer* 78:396-402, 1996.

220. Carey M, Medeiros L, Roepke J et al: Primary anaplastic large cell lymphoma of the small intestine, *Am J Clin Pathol* 112:696-701, 1999.

221. Morphopoulos G, Pitt M, Bisset D: Primary anaplastic large cell lymphoma of the rectum, *Histopathology* 26:190-192, 1995.

222. Kim JH, Lee JH, Lee J et al: Primary NK-/T-cell lymphoma of the gastrointestinal tract: clinical characteristics and endoscopic findings, *Endoscopy* 39:156-160, 2007.

223. Zhang YC, Sha Z, Yu JB et al: Gastric involvement of extranodal NK/T-cell lymphoma, nasal type: a report of 3 cases with literature review, *Int J Surg Pathol* 16:450-454, 2008.

224a. Mansoor A, Pittaluga S, Beck PL et al: NK-cell enteropathy: a benign NK-cell lymphoproliferative disease mimicking intestinal lymphoma: clinicopathological features and follow-up in a unique case series, *Blood* 2010, in press.

224b. Takeuchi K, Yokoyama M, Ishizawa S et al: Lymphomatoid gastropathy: a distinct clinicopathological entity of self-limited pseudomalignant NK-cell proliferation, *Blood 2010*, in press.

224c. McElroy MK, Read WL, Harmon GS, Weidner N. A unique case of an indolent CD56-positive T-cell lymphoproliferative disorder of the gastrointestinal tract: a lesion potentially misdiagnosed as natural killer/T-cell lymphoma, *Ann Diagn Pathol* 2010, in press.

225. Kumar S, Fend F, Quintanilla-Martinez L et al: Epstein-Barr virus positive primary gastrointestinal Hodgkin's disease: association with inflammatory bowel disease and immunosuppression, *Am J Surg Pathol* 24:66-73, 2000.

226. Kelly MD, Stuart M, Tschuchnigg M et al: Primary intestinal Hodgkin's disease complicating ileal Crohn's disease, *Aust N Z J Surg* 67:485-489, 1997.

227. Li S, Borowitz M: Primary Epstein-Barr virus–associated Hodgkin's disease of the ileum complicating Crohn disease, *Arch Pathol Lab Med* 125:424-427, 2001.

228. Valbuena JR, Gualco G, Espejo-Plascencia I, Medeiros LJ: Classical Hodgkin lymphoma arising in the rectum, *Ann Diagn Pathol* 9:38-42, 2005.

229. Thomas D, Huston B, Lamm K, Maia D: Primary Hodgkin's disease of the sigmoid colon, *Arch Pathol Lab Med* 121:528-532, 1997.

230. Prochorec-Sobieszek M, Majewski M, Sikorska A et al: Localized gastric diffuse large B-cell lymphoma and Hodgkin's lymphoma as secondary neoplasms in two patients with chronic lymphocytic leukemia, *Leuk Lymphoma* 47:2244-2246, 2006.

231. Grossbard M, Harris N: Case records of the Massachusetts General Hospital: case 10-1994—a 37-year-old woman with thrombocytopenia and a paragastric mass after treatment for Hodgkin's disease, *N Engl J Med* 330:698-704, 1994.

232. Horne G, Medlicott SA, Mansoor A et al: A definitive diagnosis of primary Hodgkin lymphoma on endoscopic biopsy material utilizing in-depth immunohistochemical analysis, *Can J Gastroenterol* 21:185-188, 2007.

233. Hossain FS, Koak Y, Khan FH: Primary gastric Hodgkin's lymphoma, *World J Surg Oncol* 5:119, 2007.

234. Devaney K, Jaffe E: The surgical pathology of gastrointestinal Hodgkin's disease, *Am J Clin Pathol* 95:794-801, 1991.

235. Venizelos I, Tamiolakis D, Bolioti S et al: Primary gastric Hodgkin's lymphoma: a case report and review of the literature, *Leuk Lymphoma* 46:147-150, 2005.

236. Vanbockrijck M, Cabooter M, Casselman J et al: Primary Hodgkin's disease of the ileum complicating Crohn disease, *Cancer* 72:1784-1789, 1993.

237. Dojcinov SD, Venkataraman G, Raffeld M et al: EBV positive mucocutaneous ulcer: a study of 26 cases associated with various sources of immunosuppression, *Am J Surg Pathol* 34:405-417, 2010.

238. Asano N, Yamamoto K, Tamaru J et al: Age-related Epstein-Barr virus (EBV)–associated B-cell lymphoproliferative disorders: comparison with EBV-positive classic Hodgkin lymphoma in elderly patients, *Blood* 113:2629-2636, 2009.

239. Gaulard P, Swerdlow SH, Harris N et al: Other iatrogenic immunodeficiency-associated disorders. In Swerdlow S, Campo E, Harris N et al, editors: *WHO classification: tumours of haematopoietic and lymphoid tissues,* ed 4, Lyon, 2008, IARC.

240. Krol AD, Le Cessie S, Snijder S et al: Waldeyer's ring lymphomas: a clinical study from the Comprehensive Cancer Center West population based NHL registry, *Leuk Lymphoma* 42:1005-1013, 2001.

241. Ziarkiewicz-Wroblewska B, Gornicka B, Suleiman W et al: Primary lymphoma of the liver: morphological and clinical analysis of 6 cases—success of aggressive treatment, *Neoplasma* 52:267-272, 2005.

242. Ohsawa M, Aozasa K, Horiuchi K et al: Malignant lymphoma of the liver: report of five cases and review of the literature, *Dig Sci* 37:1105-1109, 1992.

243. Memeo L, Pecorello I, Ciardi A et al: Primary non-Hodgkin's lymphoma of the liver, *Acta Oncol* 38:655-658, 1999.

244. Scerpella EG, Villareal AA, Casanova PF, Moreno JN: Primary lymphoma of the liver in AIDS: report of one new case and review of the literature, *J Clin Gastroenterol* 22:51-63, 1996.

245. Weissmann DJ, Ferry JA, Harris NL et al: Posttransplantations lymphoproliferative disorders in solid organ recipients are predominantly aggressive tumors of host origin, *Am J Clin Pathol* 103:748-755, 1995.

246. Ribas Y, Rafecas A, Figueras J et al: Post-transplant lymphoma in a liver allograft, *Transpl Int* 8:488-491, 1995.

247. Huang C-B, Eng H-L, Chuang J-H et al: Primary Burkitt's lymphoma of the liver: report of a case with long-term survival after surgical resection and combination chemotherapy, *J Pediatr Hematol Oncol* 19:135-138, 1997.

248. Osborne BM, Butler JJ, Guarda LA: Primary lymphoma of the liver: ten cases and a review of the literature, *Cancer* 56:2902-1910, 1985.

249. Page R, Romaguera J, Osborne B et al: Primary hepatic lymphoma favorable outcome after combination chemotherapy, *Cancer* 92:2023-2029, 2001.

250. Bronowicki JP, Bineau C, Feugier P et al: Primary lymphoma of the liver: clinical-pathological features and relationship with HCV infection in French patients, *Hepatology* 37:781-787, 2003.

251. Visco C, Arcaini L, Brusamolino E et al: Distinctive natural history in hepatitis C virus positive diffuse large B-cell lymphoma: analysis of 156 patients from northern Italy, *Ann Oncol* 17:1434-1440, 2006.

252. De Renzo A, Perna F, Persico M et al: Excellent prognosis and prevalence of HCV infection of primary hepatic and splenic non-Hodgkin's lymphoma, *Eur J Haematol* 81:51-57, 2008.

253. Keller BC, Nussensveig D, Dowell JE: Diffuse large B-cell lymphoma in a hepatitis C virus–infected patient presenting with lactic acidosis and hypoglycemia, *Am J Med Sci* 339:202-204, 2010.

254. Machida K, Cheng KT, Sung VM et al: Hepatitis C virus induces a mutator phenotype: enhanced mutations of immunoglobulin and protooncogenes, *Proc Natl Acad Sci USA* 101:4262-4267, 2004.

255. Scoazec J, Degott C, Brousse N et al: Non-Hodgkin's lymphoma presenting as a primary tumor of the liver: presentation, diagnosis and outcome in eight patients, *Hepatology* 13:870-875, 1991.

256. Stone VE, Bounds BC, Muse VV, Ferry JA: Case records of the Massachusetts General Hospital: case 29-2009—an 81-year-old man with weight loss, odynophagia, and failure to thrive, *N Engl J Med* 361:1189-1198, 2009.

257. Noronha V, Shafi NQ, Obando JA, Kummar S: Primary non-Hodgkin's lymphoma of the liver, *Crit Rev Oncol Hematol* 53:199-207, 2005.

258. De Wolf-Peeters C, Delabie J, Campo E et al: T-cell/histiocyte-rich large B-cell lymphoma. In Swerdlow S, Campo E, Harris N et al, editors: *WHO classification: tumours of haematopoietic and lymphoid tissues*, ed 4, Lyon, 2008, IARC.

259. Dargent J, DeWolf-Peeters C: Liver involvement by lymphoma: identification of a distinctive pattern of infiltration related to T-cell/histiocyte-rich B-cell lymphoma, *Ann Diagn Pathol* 2:363-369, 1998.

260. Koubaa Mahjoub W, Chaumette-Planckaert MT, Penas EM et al: Primary hepatic lymphoma of mucosa-associated lymphoid tissue type: a case report with cytogenetic study, *Int J Surg Pathol* 16:301-307, 2008.

261. Isaacson PG, Banks PM, Best PV et al: Primary low-grade hepatic B-cell lymphoma of mucosa-associated lymphoid tissue (MALT) type, *Am J Surg Pathol* 19:571-575, 1995.

262. Iida T, Iwahashi M, Nakamura M et al: Primary hepatic low-grade B-cell lymphoma of MALT-type associated with *Helicobacter pylori* infection, *Hepatogastroenterology* 54:1898-1901, 2007.

263. Orrego M, Guo L, Reeder C et al: Hepatic B-cell non-Hodgkin's lymphoma of MALT type in the liver explant of a patient with chronic hepatitis C infection, *Liver Transpl* 11:796-799, 2005.

264. Maes M, Depardieu J, Hermans M et al: Primary low-grade B-cell lymphoma of MALT-type occurring in the liver, *J Hepatol* 27:922-927, 1997.

265. Bouron D, Leger-Ravet MB, Gaulard P et al: [Unusual hepatic tumor], *Ann Pathol* 19:547-548, 1999.

266. Ye M, Suriawinata A, Black C et al: Primary hepatic marginal zone B-cell lymphoma of mucosa-associated lymphoid tissue type in a patient with primary biliary cirrhosis, *Arch Pathol Lab Med* 124:604-608, 2000.

267. Nakayama S, Yokote T, Kobayashi K et al: Primary hepatic MALT lymphoma associated with primary biliary cirrhosis, *Leuk Res* 34:e17-e20, 2010.

268. Nart D, Ertan Y, Yilmaz F et al: Primary hepatic marginal zone B-cell lymphoma of mucosa-associated lymphoid tissue type in a liver transplant patient with hepatitis B cirrhosis, *Transplant Proc* 37:4408-4412, 2005.

269. Gomyo H, Kagami Y, Kato H et al: Primary hepatic follicular lymphoma: a case report and discussion of chemotherapy and favorable outcomes, *J Clin Exp Hematop* 47:73-77, 2007.

270. Mantadakis E, Raissaki M, Tzardi M et al: Primary hepatic Burkitt lymphoma, *Pediatr Hematol Oncol* 25:331-338, 2008.

271. Al-Tonbary Y, Fouda A, El-Ashry R, Zalata K: Primary hepatic non-Hodgkin lymphoma presenting as acute hepatitis in a 2-year-old male, *Hematol Oncol Stem Cell Ther* 2:299-301, 2009.

272. Siebert S, Amos N, Williams BD, Lawson TM: Cytokine production by hepatic anaplastic large-cell lymphoma presenting as a rheumatic syndrome, *Semin Arthritis Rheum* 37:63-67, 2007.

273. Kim JH, Kim HY, Kang I et al: A case of primary hepatic lymphoma with hepatitis C liver cirrhosis, *Am J Gastroenterol* 95:2377-2380, 2000.

274. Tsutsumi Y, Deng YL, Uchiyama M et al: OPD4-positive T-cell lymphoma of the liver in systemic lupus erythematosus, *Acta Pathol Jpn* 41:829-833, 1991.

275. Bowman SJ, Levison DA, Cotter FE, Kingsley GH: Primary T cell lymphoma of the liver in a patient with Felty's syndrome, *Br J Rheumatol* 33:157-160, 1994.

276. Leung VK, Lin SY, Loke TK et al: Primary hepatic peripheral T-cell lymphoma in a patient with chronic hepatitis B infection, *Hong Kong Med J* 15:288-290, 2009.

277. Stancu M, Jones D, Vega F, Medeiros LJ: Peripheral T-cell lymphoma arising in the liver, *Am J Clin Pathol* 118:574-581, 2002.

278. Orem J, Maganda A, Mbidde EK, Weiderpass E: Clinical characteristics and outcome of children with Burkitt lymphoma in Uganda according to HIV infection, *Pediatr Blood Cancer* 52:455-458, 2009.

279. Zen Y, Fujii T, Nakanuma Y: Hepatic pseudolymphoma: a clinicopathologic study of five cases and review of the literature, *Mod Pathol* 23:244-250, 2010.

280. Loddenkemper C, Longerich T, Hummel M et al: Frequency and diagnostic patterns of lymphomas in liver biopsies with respect to the WHO classification, *Virchows Arch* 450:493-502, 2007.

281. Abramson JS: T-cell/histiocyte-rich B-cell lymphoma: biology, diagnosis, and management, *Oncologist* 11:384-392, 2006.

282. Salmon JS, Thompson MA, Arildsen RC, Greer JP: Non-Hodgkin's lymphoma involving the liver: clinical and therapeutic considerations, *Clin Lymphoma Myeloma* 6:273-280, 2006.

283. Macon W, Levy N, Kurtin P et al: Hepatosplenic ab T-cell lymphomas, *Am J Surg Pathol* 25:285-296, 2001.

284. Chim C, Liang R, Loong F, Lap C: Primary mucosa-associated lymphoid tissue lymphoma of the gallbladder, *Am J Med* 112:505-507, 2002.

285. Koshy M, Zhao F, Garofalo MC: Primary MALT lymphoma of the gallbladder: case report, *J Gastrointestin Liver Dis* 17:207-210, 2008.

286. Ono A, Tanoue S, Yamada Y et al: Primary malignant lymphoma of the gallbladder: a case report and literature review, *Br J Radiol* 82:e15-e19, 2009.

287. Willingham DL, Menke DM, Satyanarayana R: Gallbladder lymphoma in primary sclerosing cholangitis, *Clin Gastroenterol Hepatol* 7:A26, 2009.

288. Abe Y, Takatsuki H, Okada Y et al: Mucosa-associated lymphoid tissue lymphoma of the gallbladder associated with acute myeloid leukemia, *Intern Med* 38:442-444, 1999.

289. Bickel A, Eitan A, Tsilman B, Cohen H: Low-grade B cell lymphoma of mucosa-associated lymphoid tissue (MALT) arising in the gallbladder, *Hepatogastroenterology* 46:1643-1646, 1999.

290. Chatila R, Fiedler P, Vender R: Primary lymphoma of the gallbladder: case report and review of the literature, *Am J Gastroenterol* 91:2242-2244, 1996.

291. Friedman E, Lazda E, Grant D, Davis J: Primary lymphoma of the gallbladder, *Postgrad Med J* 69:585-587, 1993.

292. McCluggage W, Mackel E, McCusker G: Primary low grade malignant lymphoma of mucosa-associated lymphoid tissue of gallbladder, *Histopathology* 29:285-287, 1996.

293. Mosnier J, Brousse N, Sevestre C et al: Primary low-grade B-cell lymphoma of the mucosa-associated lymphoid tissue arising in the gallbladder, *Histopathology* 20:273-275, 1992.

294. Jelic TM, Barreta TM, Yu M et al: Primary, extranodal, follicular non-Hodgkin lymphoma of the gallbladder: case report and a review of the literature, *Leuk Lymphoma* 45:381-387, 2004.

295. Rajesh LS, Nada R, Yadav TD, Joshi K: Primary low-grade B-cell lymphoma of the mucosa-associated lymphoid tissue of the gallbladder, *Histopathology* 43:300-301, 2003.

296. Bisig B, Copie-Bergman C, Baia M et al: Primary mucosa-associated lymphoid tissue lymphoma of the gallbladder: report of a case harboring API2/MALT1 gene fusion, *Hum Pathol* 40:1504-1509, 2009.

297. Mani H, Climent F, Coloma L et al: Gall bladder and extrahepatic bile duct lymphomas: clinicopathological observations and biological implications, *Am J Surg Pathol* 34:1277-1286, 2010.

298. Kato H, Naganuma T, Iizawa Y et al: Primary non-Hodgkin's lymphoma of the gallbladder diagnosed by laparoscopic cholecystectomy, *J Hepatobiliary Pancreat Surg* 15:659-663, 2008.

299. Jho DH, Jho DJ, Chejfec G et al: Primary biliary B-cell lymphoma of the cystic duct causing obstructive jaundice, *Am Surg* 73:508-510, 2007.

300. O'Boyle M: Gallbladder wall mass on sonography representing large-cell non-Hodgkin's lymphoma in an AIDS patient, *J Ultrasound Med* 13:67-68, 1994.

301. Ganjifrockwala A, Jacob D, Blewitt R: Lymphomatous polyposis of the gallbladder, *Diagn Histopathol* 14:524-526, 2008.

302. Odemis B, Parlak E, Basar O et al: Biliary tract obstruction secondary to malignant lymphoma: experience at a referral center, *Dig Dis Sci* 52:2323-2332, 2007.

303. Eliason S, Grosso L: Primary biliary malignant lymphoma clinically mimicking cholangiocarcinoma, *Ann Diagn Pathol* 5:25-33, 2001.

304. Boccardo J, Khandelwal A, Ye D, Duke BE: Common bile duct MALT lymphoma: case report and review of the literature, *Am Surg* 72:85-88, 2006.

305. Das K, Fisher A, Wilson DJ et al: Primary non-Hodgkin's lymphoma of the bile ducts mimicking cholangiocarcinoma, *Surgery* 134:496-500, 2003.

306. Shito M, Kakefuda T, Omori T et al: Primary non-Hodgkin's lymphoma of the main hepatic duct junction, *J Hepatobiliary Pancreat Surg* 15:440-443, 2008.

307. Sugawara G, Nagino M, Oda K et al: Follicular lymphoma of the extrahepatic bile duct mimicking cholangiocarcinoma, *J Hepatobiliary Pancreat Surg* 15:196-199, 2008.

308. Christophides T, Samstein B, Emond J, Bhagat G: Primary follicular lymphoma of the extrahepatic bile duct mimicking a hilar cholangiocarcinoma: case report and review of the literature, *Hum Pathol* 40:1808-1812, 2009.

309. Behrns KE, Sarr MG, Strickler JG: Pancreatic lymphoma: is it a surgical disease? *Pancreas* 9:662-667, 1994.

310. Baylor S, Berg J: Cross-classification and survival characteristics of 5,000 cases of cancer of the pancreas, *Surg Oncol* 5:335-358, 1973.

311. Pecorari P, Gorji N, Melato M: Primary non-Hodgkin's lymphoma of the head of the pancreas: a case report and review of literature, *Oncol Rep* 6:1111-1115, 1999.

312. Jones W, Sheikh M, McClave S: AIDS-related non-Hodgkin's lymphoma of the pancreas, *Am J Gastroenterol* 92:335-338, 1997.

313. Borrowdale R, Strong R: Primary lymphoma of the pancreas, *Aust N Z J Surg* 64:444-446, 1994.

314. Yusuf S, Harrison J, Manhire A et al: Primary B-cell immunoblastic lymphoma of pancreas, *Eur J Surg Oncol* 17:555-557, 1991.

315. Satake K, Arimoto Y, Fujimoto Y et al: Malignant T-cell lymphoma of the pancreas, *Pancreas* 6:120-124, 1991.

316. Chim CS, Ho J, Ooi GC et al: Primary anaplastic large cell lymphoma of the pancreas, *Leuk Lymphoma* 46:457-459, 2005.

317. Cohen Y, Libster D, Amir G et al: Primary ALK positive anaplastic large cell lymphoma of the pancreas, *Leuk Lymphoma* 44:205-207, 2003.

318. Fraser CJ, Chan YF, Heath JA: Anaplastic large cell lymphoma of the pancreas: a pediatric case and literature review, *J Pediatr Hematol Oncol* 26:840-842, 2004.

319. Lin H, Li SD, Hu XG, Li ZS: Primary pancreatic lymphoma: report of six cases, *World J Gastroenterol* 12:5064-5067, 2006.

320. Meier C, Kapellen T, Trobs RB et al: Temporary diabetes mellitus secondary to a primary pancreatic Burkitt lymphoma, *Pediatr Blood Cancer* 47:94-96, 2006.

321. Dyckmans K, Lerut E, Gillard P et al: Post-transplant lymphoma of the pancreatic allograft in a kidney-pancreas transplant recipient: a misleading presentation, *Nephrol Dial Transplant* 21:3306-3310, 2006.

322. Basu A, Patil N, Mohindra P et al: Isolated non-Hodgkin's lymphoma of the pancreas: case report and review of literature, *J Cancer Res Ther* 3:236-239, 2007.

323. Qiu L, Luo Y, Peng YL: Value of ultrasound examination in differential diagnosis of pancreatic lymphoma and pancreatic cancer, *World J Gastroenterol* 14:6738-6742, 2008.

324. Sata N, Kurogochi A, Endo K et al: Follicular lymphoma of the pancreas: a case report and proposed new strategies for diagnosis and surgery of benign or low-grade malignant lesions of the head of the pancreas, *Journal of the Pancreas* [JOP] 8:44-49, 2007.

325. Kojima M, Sipos B, Klapper W et al: Autoimmune pancreatitis: frequency, IgG4 expression, and clonality of T and B cells, *Am J Surg Pathol* 31:521-528, 2007.

CHAPTER 6

Lymphomas of the Spleen

Aliyah R. Sohani•
Lawrence R. Zukerberg

■ INTRODUCTION

Accurate diagnosis and classification of lymphoma in splenectomy specimens may be challenging. Although relatively few lymphomas involve the spleen primarily, many systemic lymphomas may involve the spleen secondarily, either at presentation or at the time of disease progression. Reactive hyperplasia of the spleen may lead to splenomegaly, raising the differential diagnosis of lymphoma, and many types of B-cell lymphoma display morphologic features that overlap with those of primary splenic marginal zone lymphoma. Establishing a precise diagnosis of lymphoma on a splenectomy specimen, therefore, requires a combination of morphologic and immunophenotypic analysis, correlated with clinical features; investigation of other sites of disease involvement; and in some cases, cytogenetic studies or molecular genetic studies, including fluorescence in situ hybridization (FISH) analysis to detect recurrent genetic abnormalities or polymerase chain reaction (PCR) to detect clonal gene rearrangement.

This chapter describes the clinical and pathologic features of the major types of lymphoma that primarily and secondarily involve the spleen. Several of the types of lymphoma discussed in this chapter, including splenic marginal zone lymphoma, T-cell/histiocyte-rich large B-cell lymphoma, hairy cell leukemia, and hepatosplenic T-cell lymphoma, also typically involve the liver or bone marrow (see Lymphomas of the Bone Marrow in Chapter 13) or both at the time of initial diagnosis; they are discussed under Primary Splenic Lymphomas because they characteristically present with splenomegaly. Table 6-1 summarizes the features of various types of lymphomas involving the spleen and the various entities in their differential diagnosis.

TABLE 6-1

Pathologic Features of Lymphomas Involving the Spleen

Type of Lymphoma	Pattern of Involvement	Immunophenotype	Cytogenetic or Molecular Genetic Features	Main Entities in Differential Diagnosis
Splenic marginal zone lymphoma	Predominant WP disease with biphasic cytology and expanded pale marginal zones; RP involvement with patchy intrasinusoidal clusters or diffuse pattern	IgM+, IgD+/−, CD19+, CD20+, CD5−, CD10−, bcl6−, CD23−, cyclin D1−, CD25−, CD103−, annexin A1−	Loss of 7q21-32 seen in a subset of cases, often associated with IgD-positivity and unmutated IGH variable region	Follicular lymphoma, mantle cell lymphoma, splenic diffuse RP small B-cell lymphoma (provisional entity), chronic lymphocytic leukemia, polyclonal B-cell lymphocytosis
Diffuse large B-cell lymphoma	Predominant WP disease with macronodular or micronodular involvement; occasional cases with diffuse RP infiltration	CD20+, bcl6+, bcl2+/−, CD10+/−, cyclin D1−, high Ki67 PI, rare cases EBV+	Complex karyotype, as seen in large cell lymphoma at other sites	Micronodular T-cell–rich variant may mimic classical Hodgkin's lymphoma; cases with diffuse RP infiltration may mimic IV-LBCL with extensive splenic involvement
Hairy cell leukemia	Diffuse RP disease with formation of red blood cell lakes and WP atrophy	CD19+, CD20+ (bright), CD5−, CD10−, CD23−, CD25+, CD103+, CD11c+, DBA.44+, annexin A1+	Annexin 1 upregulation	Hairy cell leukemia variant (provisional entity, splenic diffuse RP small B-cell lymphoma (provisional entity)
Hepatosplenic T-cell lymphoma	Diffuse RP involvement by atypical medium to large cells	CD2+, CD3+, CD5−/+, CD4−, CD8−/+, CD7+/−, TCRγδ+ (more common) or TCRαβ+	Clonal TCR gene rearrangement; isochromosome 7q, trisomy 8	PTCL-NOS with splenic involvement, diffuse large B-cell lymphoma with diffuse RP infiltration
Chronic lymphocytic leukemia/small lymphocytic lymphoma	Nodular WP involvement and nodular and/or diffuse involvement of RP	CD19+, CD20+ (dim), dim surface light chain expression, FMC7−, CD5+, CD23+, CD10−, bcl6−, cyclin D1−	Trisomy 12, 17p- (TP53 loss), 11q- (ATM loss), del 13q, del 6q	Splenic marginal zone lymphoma, follicular lymphoma, mantle cell lymphoma

TABLE 6-1

Pathologic Features of Lymphomas Involving the Spleen—cont'd

Type of Lymphoma	Pattern of Involvement	Immunophenotype	Cytogenetic or Molecular Genetic Features	Main Entities in Differential Diagnosis
Follicular lymphoma	Nodular WP involvement with minimal intervening normal RP or with relative preservation of splenic architecture; minimal RP involvement	CD20+, CD10+, bcl6+, bcl2+/−; bcl2− cases typically grade 3 histology, lack t(14;18); cyclin D1−	t(14;18) (IGH-BCL2)	Splenic marginal zone lymphoma, mantle cell lymphoma, chronic lymphocytic leukemia
Lymphoplasmacytic lymphoma (Waldenström's macroglobulinemia)	Diffuse RP involvement with marked plasmacytic differentiation	CD19+, CD20+, IgM+, surface and cytoplasmic light chain expression, CD5−, CD10−, bcl6−, CD23−, cyclin D1−	Rare cases with t(9;14) (IGH-PAX5) reported	Splenic marginal zone lymphoma, splenic diffuse RP small B-cell lymphoma (provisional entity)
Mantle cell lymphoma	WP involvement with large or multiple small nodules (miliary pattern); small nodules may also be present in RP; diffuse RP involvement is seen in patients with peripheral blood leukocytosis	CD19+, CD20+ (bright), CD5+, CD10−, bcl6−, CD23−, cyclin D1+	t(11;14) (IGH-CCND1)	Follicular lymphoma, splenic marginal zone lymphoma, chronic lymphocytic leukemia
Classical Hodgkin's lymphoma	Nodular or micronodular WP involvement with scattered HRS cells	CD45−, CD30+, CD15+, CD20−/+, Pax5+ (weak), CD79a−, loss of Oct2 and/or Bob1, subset of cases EBV+	HRS cells with clonal IGH gene rearrangement and complex karyotype, as seen in Hodgkin's lymphoma at other sites	Florid immunoblastic reaction, micronodular T-cell–rich diffuse large B-cell lymphoma

EBV, Epstein-Barr virus; *HRS*, Hodgkin Reed-Sternberg cells; *IGH*, immunoglobulin heavy chain, *IV-LBCL*, intravascular large B-cell lymphoma; *PI*, proliferation index; *PTCL-NOS*, peripheral T-cell lymphoma not otherwise specified; *RP*, red pulp; *TCR*, T-cell receptor; *WP*, white pulp.

■ PRIMARY SPLENIC LYMPHOMAS

Splenic Marginal Zone Lymphoma

Clinical Features

Splenic marginal zone lymphoma is a rare, indolent B-cell lymphoma subtype with a striking propensity for involving the spleen and splenic hilar lymph nodes. Bone marrow and peripheral blood also are commonly involved; however, involvement of peripheral lymph nodes or other extranodal sites is rare. The disease affects middle-aged and older adults, typically in the sixth or seventh decades, and a slight female predominance is seen.[1,2]

Patients typically present with splenomegaly, which may be massive; anemia with or without other cytopenias; and moderate lymphocytosis with circulating villous lymphocytes.[1,3,4] An IgM paraprotein may be present but is smaller than that seen in lymphoplasmacytic lymphoma/Waldenström's macroglobulinemia, and consequent symptoms of hyperviscosity are rare.[1]

Patients commonly show autoimmune phenomena, particularly autoimmune hemolytic anemia, as well as immune thrombocytopenia purpura, IgM anticardiolipin antibodies, and lupus anticoagulants.[5-9] The autoantibodies found in affected patients may represent a direct autoimmune effect of the IgM produced by the lymphoma. An increased seroprevalence of hepatitis C virus (HCV) infection has been reported in patients with splenic marginal zone lymphoma, but this association appears to be limited to certain parts of Europe.[10,11] Patients living in malaria-endemic regions of West Africa appear to have a relatively high incidence of splenic marginal zone lymphoma.[12] In these cases, the lymphoma shares certain clinical and laboratory features with hyperreactive malarial splenomegaly caused by repeated malaria infections, and the lymphoma may be related to emergence of a B-cell clone in the setting of parasite-induced chronic antigenic stimulation.[12,13]

Splenectomy has been the mainstay of treatment and typically produces sustained partial responses, with resolution of cytopenias, paraproteinemia, and B symptoms; the median overall survival time ranges from 9 to 13 years.[1,4,14] Adverse clinical prognostic factors include autoimmune hemolytic anemia, hypoalbuminemia, an elevated serum lactate dehydrogenase, elevated serum beta$_2$-microglobulin, paraproteinemia, lymphocytosis, immune thrombocytopenia, and extranodal involvement.[4,15-19] Additional treatment options include splenic irradiation, combination chemotherapy, and monoclonal antibody therapy with rituximab.[20,21] Treatment with interferon and ribavirin would be expected to produce a response in HCV-positive patients.[10,11]

Pathologic Features

With splenic marginal zone lymphoma, the spleen is often massively enlarged (median weight, 1360 g). Gross examination of the cut surface shows a uniform multimicronodular pattern with tiny nodules,

each measuring up to 0.5 cm, dispersed throughout the splenic parenchyma; mass lesions are absent (Figure 6-1, *A*).[2] Microscopic examination characteristically shows expansion of white pulp follicles to twice or more their normal size (Figure 6-1, *B*). In some cases, the reactive germinal centers of the white pulp are reduced in size or are completely replaced by a population of small lymphocytes with irregular nuclei, condensed chromatin, and scant cytoplasm, resembling mantle zone cells, surrounded by a broad concentric zone of medium-sized cells with abundant, pale cytoplasm, resembling marginal-zone B cells (Figure 6-2).[22,23] Occasional large transformed cells may be present in the nodules (Figure 6-2, *B*), but increased numbers or sheets of large cells may indicate early transformation to diffuse large B-cell lymphoma.

The concentric growth pattern of splenic marginal zone lymphoma, with expansion of the pale marginal zones of the splenic white pulp, is the characteristic

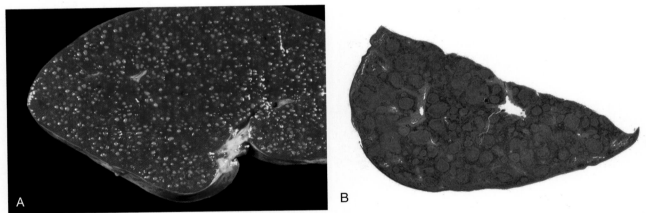

Figure 6-1   Splenic marginal zone lymphoma. **A,** This involved spleen weighed 2.4 kg. Gross examination of the cut surface shows a uniform multimicronodular pattern with small nodules throughout, representing expanded areas of the white pulp. **B,** Low-power whole mount examination shows markedly expanded white pulp nodules with a characteristic rim of pale-staining marginal zone cells at their periphery.

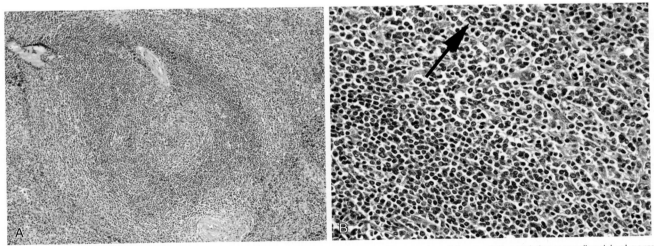

Figure 6-2   White pulp nodule replaced by splenic marginal zone lymphoma. **A,** The center of the nodule contains a small residual germinal center, which is surrounded by an inner dark concentric band, then an outer pale concentric band. **B,** The inner dark band contains small lymphocytes with condensed chromatin and scant cytoplasm, resembling mantle zone B cells *(lower left)*; these comprise part of the neoplastic clone. The outer pale band contains small to medium marginal zone–type cells with abundant, pale cytoplasm *(upper right)*. Rare large transformed cells, such as centroblasts *(arrow)*, are present.

feature from which this lymphoma derives its name. However, in our experience, recognizing the biphasic cytology may be difficult in some cases, because the marginal zone accentuation may be subtle. Many of the nodules are composed of a more uniform population of small lymphocytes with moderate, pale cytoplasm (Figure 6-3, *A*). Some cases may demonstrate plasmacytic differentiation, typically seen in the marginal zone component at the periphery of the nodules. In a minority of cases, reactive

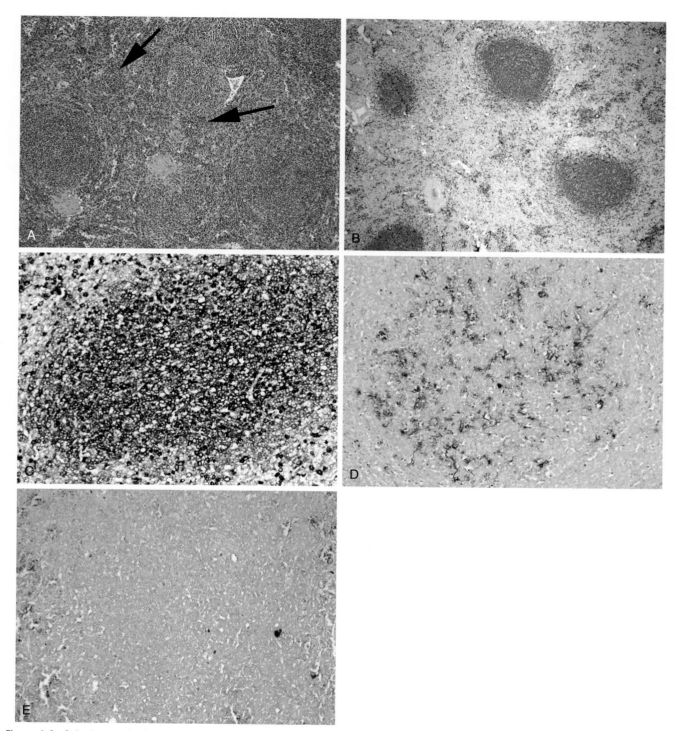

Figure 6-3 Splenic marginal zone lymphoma involving both white and red pulp. **A,** In some cases, the marginal zone accentuation is not pronounced and the white pulp nodules contain a more uniform population of small lymphocytes with moderate cytoplasm. The intervening red pulp contains small clusters of similar-appearing lymphocytes in a patchy intrasinusoidal distribution *(arrows)*. **B,** A stain for CD20 is strongly positive in the white pulp nodules and also highlights the red pulp involvement. Additional immunophenotyping shows the lymphoma cells to be strongly positive for IgM by immunohistochemistry **(C)**. A subset of the neoplastic cells demonstrates kappa immunoglobulin light chain by in situ hybridization **(D)**, with only rare lambda-positive cells **(E)**.

germinal centers at the centers of the expanded nodules are well preserved, yielding a targetoid appearance of the white pulp nodules. Red pulp infiltration is invariably present and typically is characterized by small clusters of lymphocytes present in a patchy, intrasinusoidal distribution (see Figure 6-3, *A* and *B*). Occasionally, red pulp involvement may be diffuse, without the formation of small nodules; in rare cases, the red pulp may be involved in a diffuse pattern to the extent that it obscures the nodular white pulp component, which may be apparent only on immunohistochemical staining with B-cell antigens.[22] Splenic hilar lymph nodes are enlarged and show partial effacement by an infiltrate of lymphocytes similar to those seen in the spleen; sinuses typically are patent (Figure 6-4).[22]

The lymphoma cells express mature B-cell markers (CD20, CD79a, Pax5) and IgM (see Figure 6-3, *B* and *C*). IgD is expressed in a subset of cases. Clonal surface light chain is expressed, and light chain restriction often can be demonstrated in the cytoplasm of neoplastic cells on tissue sections by immunohistochemistry or in situ hybridization (see Figure 6-3, *D* and *E*). Splenic marginal zone lymphoma typically is negative for CD5, CD10, CD23, CD25, CD43, and CD103, and cyclin D1 is not expressed. Lymphoma cells are positive for bcl2 and negative for bcl6, whereas residual small germinal centers, if present, show the opposite pattern of staining for these two antibodies. Staining with Ki67 (MIB1) shows a distinctive annular pattern of staining, with a low proliferation fraction in the neoplastic cells and a high proportion of positive nuclei in preserved reactive follicles at the centers of the nodules. Staining for follicular dendritic cell antigens (CD21, CD23) may show a dense meshwork at the centers of the white pulp nodules, as well as focal staining within the small red pulp nodules.[22,24]

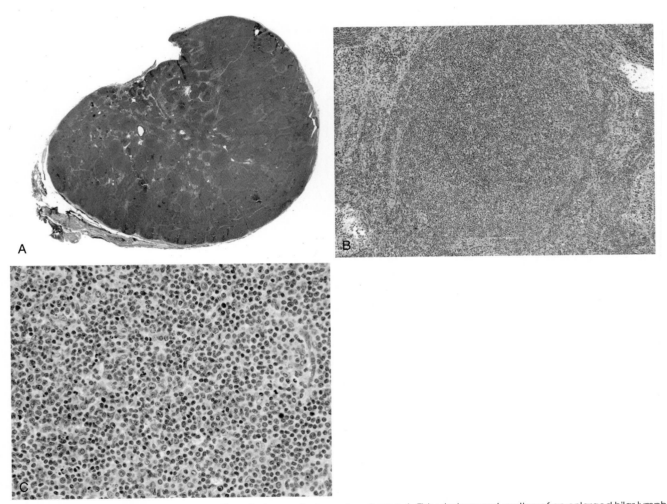

Figure 6-4   Splenic hilar lymph node involved by splenic marginal zone lymphoma. **A,** This whole mount section of an enlarged hilar lymph node from the spleen (shown in Figure 6-1) demonstrates architectural effacement by a nodular growth pattern, with relative preservation of lymph node sinuses. **B,** The enlarged nodules appear monomorphous and lack reactive-appearing germinal centers. A portion of a dilated sinusoidal space is visible in the upper right. **C,** High-power examination shows an admixture of small cells with moderate cytoplasm and larger cells with more abundant cytoplasm, resembling the small lymphocytes and marginal zone cells seen in the spleen. In the lymph nodes, the two cell types do not generally form distinct concentric bands, as is typical in the spleen. In contrast to follicular lymphoma, the cells generally are round rather than cleaved.

The cell of origin in splenic marginal zone lymphoma has been proposed to be a post-germinal center B cell of marginal zone derivation. However, recent studies suggest that this lymphoma has greater heterogeneity in terms of its cell of origin, immunophenotype, and genetics than previously inferred, and these features may predict the prognosis.[24-26] Up to half of cases have unmutated immunoglobulin heavy chain variable regions, a finding that is inconsistent with post-germinal center B-cell derivation and more supportive of origin from a naïve B cell. These cases often show allelic loss of 7q21-32, the most common cytogenetic abnormality seen in splenic marginal zone lymphoma, and patients tend to have a more aggressive clinical course. In contrast, cases with mutated immunoglobulin heavy chain variable regions often are negative for IgD and have normal cytogenetics and a more favorable clinical course. Because mutational analysis of the immunoglobulin heavy chain variable region is not routinely performed, the combination of IgD expression and FISH for 7q loss as a surrogate for somatic hypermutation status may be used to help predict the prognosis.

Differential Diagnosis

Because of the distinctive but nonspecific immunophenotype of splenic marginal zone lymphoma, the diagnosis can be made only after exclusion of other small B-cell lymphomas that may primarily or secondarily involve the spleen, as well as certain reactive conditions, such as splenic marginal zone hyperplasia and polyclonal B-cell lymphocytosis with progressive splenomegaly. In cases of splenic marginal zone hyperplasia, splenomegaly is absent or mild; white pulp nodules are only minimally expanded with accentuation of the marginal zone regions (a form of reactive hyperplasia characteristic of the splenic white pulp); and the red pulp sinusoids lack small lymphoid clusters (Figure 6-5). Flow cytometry and stains for immunoglobulin light chain confirm the polytypic nature of the lymphocytes.

Polyclonal B-cell lymphocytosis is an unusual chronic expansion of peripheral blood polyclonal B cells associated with progressive splenomegaly, which may be massive in some cases. Patients are typically adult women of varying ages, and a history of cigarette smoking is characteristic. There is an association with HLA-DR7, suggesting a genetic predisposition. Patients typically have elevated polyclonal serum IgM, a mild lymphocytosis, and circulating binucleate peripheral blood lymphocytes. Splenic histology has been described in relatively few cases, but is reported to resemble splenic marginal zone lymphoma with expansion of the white pulp marginal zone areas and a biphasic growth pattern. Bone marrow biopsies demonstrate a moderate lymphoid infiltrate with interstitial and intrasinusoidal lymphocytes. Peripheral blood and bone marrow lymphocytes are polytypic for immunoglobulin light chains and have an activated, memory B-cell phenotype by flow cytometry (CD20+, IgM+, IgD+, CD27+). Immunohistochemical stains on tissue sections of marrow and spleen characteristically show the lymphocytes to be positive for IgM, IgD and bcl2, negative for CD5, CD10, bcl6, and DBA 44, and to show polytypic light chain staining. Despite the detection of various cytogenetic abnormalities in some cases, 7q deletions and clonal *IGH* gene rearrangements are not seen and progression to lymphoma has been documented in only rare cases.[26a] Due to the degree of splenomegaly and the morphologic resemblance to splenic marginal zone lymphoma, diagnosis requires immunophenotyping by flow cytometry of peripheral blood or bone marrow or immunohistochemical analysis of tissue to support the presence of a polyclonal B-cell population. PCR to exclude a clonal *IGH* gene rearrangement may be used to further support the diagnosis.

In terms of the neoplastic differential diagnosis of splenic marginal zone lymphoma, absence of a germinal center phenotype (CD10 and bcl6) helps exclude splenic involvement by follicular lymphoma, and absence of CD5 and cyclin D1 expression excludes mantle cell lymphoma and chronic lymphocytic leukemia, all of which may show nodular involvement of the white pulp, with or without a prominent margin zone.

Cases of splenic marginal zone lymphoma with plasmacytic differentiation may raise the differential diagnosis of lymphoplasmacytic lymphoma (Waldenström's macroglobulinemia), which also lacks a specific immunophenotype and is associated with an IgM M-component. However, lymphoplasmacytic lymphoma shows predominantly red pulp disease with relative sparing of the white pulp, and plasmacytic differentiation typically is more conspicuous (Figure 6-6). Clinically, patients have more extensive disease involving the bone marrow or lymph nodes, and the spleen is secondarily involved

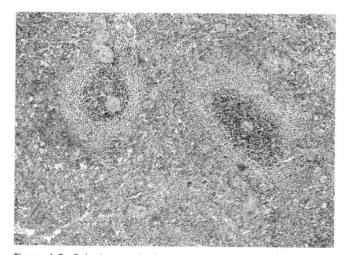

Figure 6-5 Splenic marginal zone hyperplasia. In this case, the spleen weighed less than 200 g. The white pulp nodules show prominence of the marginal zones but are only minimally expanded. Abundant intervening red pulp is present that lacks nodular aggregates of small lymphocytes.

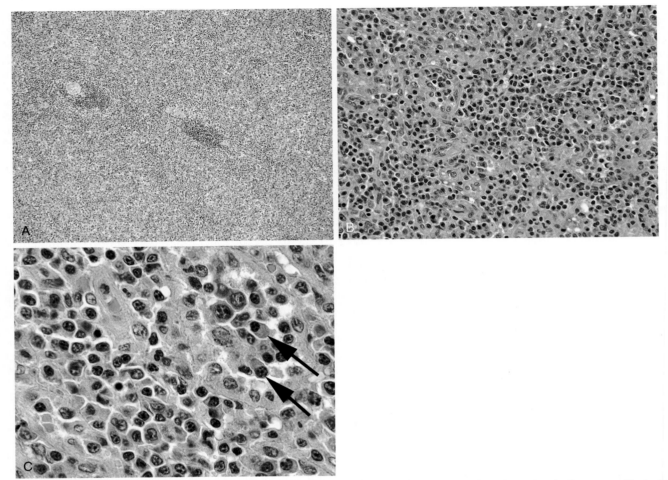

Figure 6-6 Splenic involvement by lymphoplasmacytic lymphoma. **A,** On low-power examination, the red pulp sinuses are filled with lymphocytes and plasma cells and the white pulp appears atrophic. **B,** The red pulp sinuses contain small lymphocytes and conspicuous mature plasma cells (**C,** *arrows*), as well as many intermediate forms.

with a milder degree of enlargement compared with splenic marginal zone lymphoma.

Hairy cell leukemia, another small B-cell neoplasm primarily involving the spleen, may be a differential diagnostic consideration, particularly in cases of splenic marginal zone lymphoma with circulating villous lymphocytes. However, in classic hairy cell leukemia, the pattern of splenic (and bone marrow) involvement is sufficiently different that the distinction from splenic marginal zone lymphoma is relatively straightforward. In addition, splenic marginal zone lymphoma lacks expression of CD103, CD25 and annexin A1, antigens characteristically expressed in hairy cell leukemia (see Table 6-1).[22,24]

Cases showing the nonspecific immunophenotype of splenic marginal zone lymphoma but that have diffuse red pulp involvement may be better classified as splenic diffuse red pulp small B-cell lymphoma, a provisional entity in the classification system updated in 2008 by the World Health Organization (WHO).[27,28] Cases are reported to show no expanded white pulp nodules either grossly or microscopically, but rather extensive red pulp

disease, leading to massive splenomegaly, absence of follicles, and atrophy of the white pulp, with infiltration of both the cords and sinuses by lymphoma cells (Figure 6-7, *A* and *B*). Neoplastic cells are monomorphous and small to medium with round, regular nuclei, condensed chromatin, and inconspicuous to small nucleoli with scant to moderately abundant, pale eosinophilic cytoplasm (see Figure 6-7, *B* and *C*). In extrasplenic sites, patterns of involvement may resemble splenic marginal zone lymphoma more closely: hilar lymph nodes show preservation of sinuses; bone marrow shows nonparatrabecular, interstitial, and intrasinusoidal involvement; and peripheral blood may contain circulating villous lymphocytes. The immunophenotype of the lymphoma cells is nonspecific, similar to that of splenic marginal zone lymphoma (negative for CD5, CD10, CD23 and cyclin D1), and includes the absence of expression of hairy cell leukemia-specific antigens (CD103, annexin A1). The majority of cases described to date are positive for DBA 44 and a subset are positive for CD11c. Most cases are IgG-positive and IgD-negative. Immunohistochemical staining for Ki67 shows a uniformly low proliferation index, with absence of

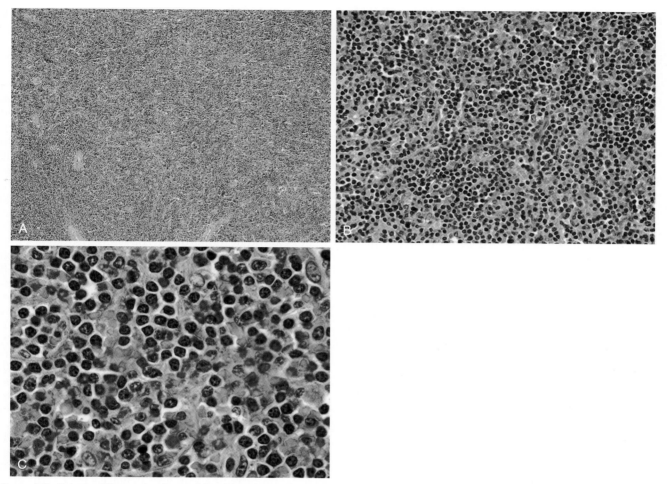

Figure 6-7 Splenic diffuse red pulp small B-cell lymphoma. **A,** Extensive red pulp disease is present with atrophy of the white pulp. **B** and **C,** Lymphoma cells are small and monomorphous, with round, regular nuclei; condensed chromatin; small, inconspicuous nucleoli; and scant cytoplasm. Plasmacytic differentiation is not evident, and large transformed cells are scarce.

the typical annular pattern seen in splenic marginal zone lymphoma.[28a]

Whether such cases represent a diffuse variant of splenic marginal zone lymphoma, as is suggested by the shared cytology, growth pattern in certain organs, and immunophenotype, or a distinct disease entity remains to be elucidated.

Diffuse Large B-Cell Lymphoma

The spleen frequently is involved by diffuse large B-cell lymphoma, the most common type of splenic lymphoma (about one half of splenic lymphoma cases). Most of the cases represent secondary involvement by diffuse large B-cell lymphoma. Primary diffuse large B-cell lymphoma of the spleen or diffuse large B-cell lymphoma presenting in the spleen is less common. In one large study, diffuse large B-cell lymphoma with initial splenic involvement represented 11% of primary splenic lymphomas.[29] The etiology of large cell lymphoma in the spleen is mostly unknown; however, one study found that HCV was associated with many cases of splenic diffuse large B-cell lymphoma.[30] The following sections

focus on large B-cell lymphomas presenting with splenic involvement.

Clinical Features

Most patients range in age from 50 to 80 years, with occasional cases occurring in younger or older patients. Splenic diffuse large B-cell lymphomas are divided into three main types based on the pattern of splenic involvement: macronodular, micronodular, and diffuse red pulp involvement. Patients with the macronodular pattern have a mean age of approximately 64 years; those with the micronodular pattern generally are younger, having a mean age of approximately 55 years. Patients with diffuse red pulp involvement have a mean age of approximately 68 years. The incidence is equal between the genders overall; however, males are more commonly reported among cases diffusely involving the red pulp.

Patients with macronodular diffuse large B-cell lymphoma mostly present with splenomegaly and abdominal pain or B symptoms. Most patients have stage I or stage II disease, and a favorable clinical outcome is expected in most cases; the remainder have a poor outcome. Patients with a micronodular or diffuse red pulp pattern of splenic involvement often have B symptoms, splenomegaly, frequent hepatic and bone marrow involvement, and an aggressive clinical course with a poor outcome in most cases. Lymphadenopathy may be absent or mild in primary splenic diffuse large B-cell lymphoma; when present, it appears to be limited to abdominal lymph nodes.[29,31-35]

Pathologic Features

Splenic Diffuse Large B-Cell Lymphoma with a Macronodular Pattern

The macronodular pattern is the most common pattern of primary splenic diffuse large B-cell lymphoma. The spleen is enlarged and partially replaced by grossly visible nodules, multiple confluent nodules, or a single large mass (Figure 6-8). These nodules, which can be larger than 10 cm, typically are composed of a relatively monomorphous population of large lymphoid cells, with numerous centroblasts and lesser numbers of admixed immunoblasts or lobated large cells (Figure 6-9). Sclerosis and necrosis are seen in some cases, and the necrosis may be extensive (see Figure 6-8 and Figure 6-9, *A* to *C*). Histiocytes are variable but can be numerous, although they typically are not as numerous as in cases of T-cell/histiocyte-rich large B-cell lymphoma (discussed later in the chapter) (see Figure 6-9, *D*). Hilar lymph nodes may be involved.[29,31-35] Splenic parenchyma away from the lymphoma usually is normal.

The lymphoma usually is positive for pan–B-cell markers, including CD20, and negative for T-cell markers, including CD3 and CD5. Most cases are bcl6 positive, and about one half are positive for CD10 or bcl2 or both. The lymphoma is negative for cyclin D1 and DBA 44. Follicular dendritic cell staining is absent. p53 overexpression is seen in approximately one third of cases and Epstein-Barr virus (EBV) positivity in only rare cases. The proliferation index,

as measured by Ki67, is high, usually greater than 70%.[29,31-35]

Splenic Diffuse Large B-Cell Lymphoma with a Micronodular Pattern

The micronodular pattern appears to be the second most common pattern of primary splenic diffuse large B-cell lymphoma. The spleen is markedly enlarged and shows a miliary pattern throughout, with coalescence of white pulp nodules that range from 0.5 to 4 cm in diameter. The nodules appear centered in the white pulp, with little or variable red pulp involvement (Figure 6-10, *A* and *B*). In some cases the nodules are predominantly composed of diffuse large B-cell lymphoma mixed with few T cells, whereas in other cases, a few large B cells are present in a background of numerous T cells and histiocytes, giving rise to the appearance of a T-cell/histiocyte-rich large B-cell lymphoma (Figure 6-10, *C*). The large B cells have the appearance of centroblasts or immunoblasts, or they may have large, pale, lobated nuclei and small nucleoli, resembling the neoplastic cells of nodular lymphocyte-predominant Hodgkin's lymphoma (LP cells). They may be difficult to identify on routine sections in the background of numerous lymphocytes and histiocytes (Figure 6-11, *A* and *B*). No residual mantle zone surrounding the neoplastic nodules is present. Some cases may have eosinophilic hyaline material or necrosis in the center of the nodules. Hilar lymph nodes may be involved.

The lymphoma cells are positive for pan–B-cell markers, including CD20 (Figure 6-11, *C*), and negative for T-cell markers, including CD3 and CD5. Most cases are bcl6 positive and negative for CD10; bcl2 may be weakly positive. The lymphoma is negative for cyclin D1 and DBA 44. Staining for follicular dendritic cell antigens is absent. Most small lymphocytes are CD3+ T cells (Figure 6-11, *D*). p53 overexpression is rare, and EBV is negative. The proliferation index, as measured by Ki67, is high, usually greater than 80% in the large neoplastic cells.

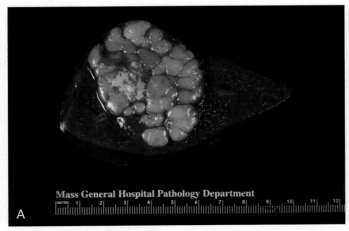
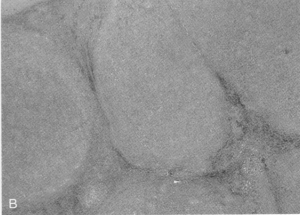

Figure 6-8   Diffuse large B-cell lymphoma of the spleen, macronodular pattern. **A,** This spleen, which weighed 360 g, contains a prominent multimacronodular mass with a tan-pink, fish-flesh cut surface and central necrosis. **B,** The large nodules with intervening fibrous bands have replaced the normal underlying splenic parenchyma.

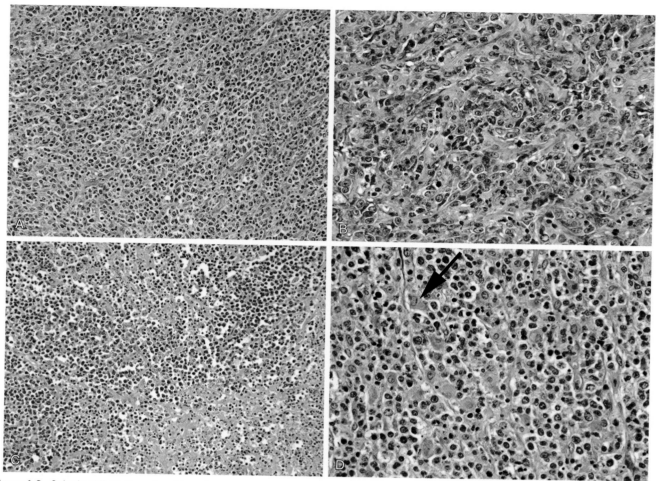

Figure 6-9 Splenic diffuse large B-cell lymphoma, microscopic features. **A** and **B,** Lymphoma cells are large with oval or irregular nuclei, vesicular chromatin, and prominent nucleoli. Fine interstitial bands of fibrosis are present. **C,** This case contains prominent cellular necrosis. **D,** In this case, scattered activated-appearing histiocytes are present admixed with large cell lymphoma cells. One of the histiocytes contains what appears to be an ingested red blood cell, suggestive of hemophagocytosis *(arrow).*

Splenic Diffuse Large B-Cell Lymphoma with Diffuse Red Pulp Infiltration

Diffuse red pulp infiltration is a rare pattern of primary splenic diffuse large B-cell lymphoma. The spleen is enlarged and has a homogeneous, beefy red appearance without discrete tumor nodules. Diffuse infiltration of the red pulp and sinusoids by large lymphoid cells with centroblastic, lobated, or pleomorphic cytology is seen (Figure 6-12). Necrosis is present in some cases. Hilar lymph nodes often are involved. Bone marrow involvement may be subtle, because the lymphoma cells may be obscured both by their resemblance to early erythroid precursors and by the predominant intrasinusoidal pattern of lymphomatous marrow infiltration. Immunohistochemistry may be necessary to detect marrow involvement and should be performed.

The differential diagnosis includes intravascular large B-cell lymphoma with splenic involvement (also see Intravascular Lymphomas in Chapter 14). In this entity, large neoplastic lymphoid cells with the appearance of centroblasts or immunoblasts are present in sinuses, small capillaries, venules, and arterioles, with involvement of numerous organs; the brain and skin are among the sites most commonly involved (Figure 6-13).

The lymphoma cells are positive for pan–B-cell markers, including CD20, and negative for T-cell markers, including CD3. The tumor cells are negative or faintly positive for CD5 by immunohistochemistry and also may be faintly CD5+ by flow cytometry. Variable expression of bcl6, bcl2, CD10, and/or DBA 44 is seen. The neoplastic cells are negative for cyclin D1. p53 overexpression is common, and EBV is negative. The proliferation index, as measured by Ki67, is high, usually greater than 75%.

T-Cell/Histiocyte-Rich Large B-Cell Lymphoma

Clinical Features

T-cell/histiocyte-rich large B-cell lymphoma is a subtype of diffuse large B-cell lymphoma with abundant, admixed reactive T cells and/or histiocytes and

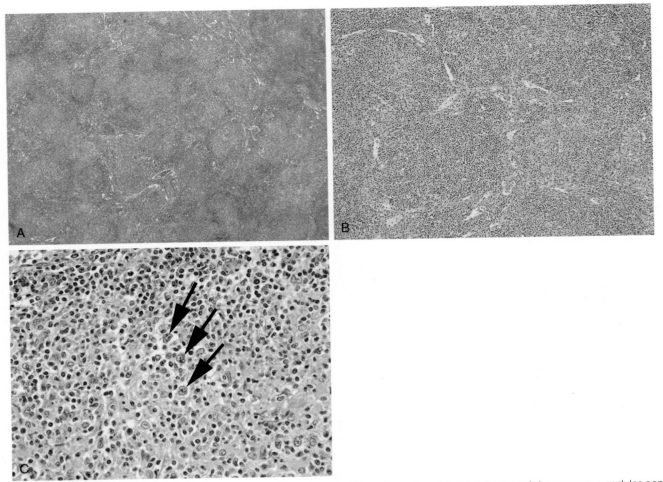

Figure 6-10 Micronodular T-cell/histiocyte-rich large B-cell lymphoma of the spleen. **A** and **B,** The spleen contains numerous nodules centered in the white pulp, with a relative paucity of intervening red pulp. The low-power features may not cause concern about high-grade lymphoma. **C,** However, high-power examination of a single white pulp nodule shows occasional large atypical cells *(arrows)* in a background rich in small lymphocytes and histiocytes.

rare to absent small B cells.[36] It has a distinct clinical presentation. It often affects middle-aged men and usually involves the lymph nodes, bone marrow, liver, and spleen. Most patients present with stage IV disease and have an aggressive course. The lymphoma often is resistant to chemotherapy regimens, especially when pathologic examination reveals a predominance of histiocytes.

Pathologic Features

Whether it involves the parenchyma of the spleen, the bone marrow, or the liver, T-cell/histiocyte-rich large B-cell lymphoma is composed of single large B cells admixed with small T cells and histiocytes. The large neoplastic cells can have a variety of appearances, ranging from centroblasts, to lymphocyte-predominant (LP) cells, to classic Hodgkin/Reed-Sternberg cells (see Figure 6-10 and Figure 6-11, *A* and *B*). Eosinophils are not commonly present among the histiocytes and lymphocytes, which helps distinguish T-cell/histiocyte-rich large B-cell lymphoma from classical Hodgkin's lymphoma. In

the spleen, a multifocal or micronodular pattern usually is found, with expansion of the white pulp, as described previously. Involvement of the liver is mainly in the form of expanded portal triads; involvement of the bone marrow is seen as small interstitial aggregates.[37]

The large neoplastic cells express pan–B-cell markers and almost always bcl6 (see Figure 6-11, *C*); bcl2 expression is variable. Some cases show staining for epithelial membrane antigen (EMA). No staining is seen with CD15, CD30, and CD138. Numerous background CD3+ T cells and CD68+, CD163+ histiocytes are present (see Figure 6-11, *D*). Lack of follicular dendritic cell staining with CD21, CD23, and CD35 and absence of IgD+ mantle zone B cells help distinguish T-cell/histiocyte-rich large B-cell lymphoma from nodular lymphocyte-predominant Hodgkin's lymphoma. Neoplastic cells are negative for EBV. Aggressive B-cell lymphomas with many reactive T cells and few neoplastic B cells that are EBV+ should not be classified as T-cell/histiocyte-rich large B-cell lymphoma, but rather considered EBV+ diffuse large B-cell lymphomas.[36]

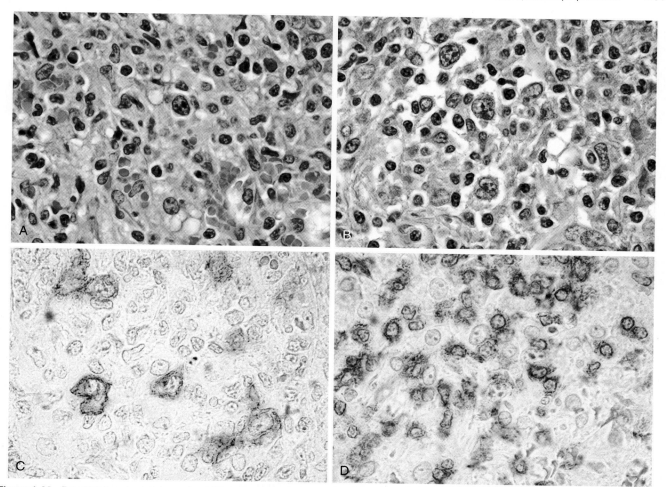

Figure 6-11 T-cell/histiocyte-rich large B-cell lymphoma. **A,** In some cases, the large atypical cells have regular, oval nuclei with multiple prominent nucleoli resembling centroblasts. **B,** In other cases, the large cells contain irregular, multilobated nuclei and are reminiscent of lymphocyte-predominant cells of nodular lymphocyte–predominant Hodgkin's lymphoma. **C,** In all cases, large cells are positive for pan–B-cell markers, such as CD20. Background small lymphocytes are negative for this antibody. **D,** The background small lymphocytes are mostly T cells and show positive staining for CD3.

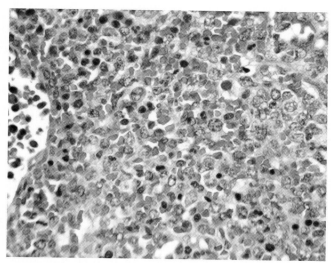

Figure 6-12 Splenic large B-cell lymphoma with diffuse red pulp infiltration. Diffuse infiltration of the red pulp by large cell lymphoma cells with oval to irregular nuclei and vesicular chromatin is present. (Photograph courtesy William G. Morice II, Mayo Clinic, Rochester, Minnesota.)

Hairy Cell Leukemia

Clinical Features

Hairy cell leukemia is a rare, chronic, mature small B-cell lymphoma/leukemia that involves the bone marrow, spleen, and peripheral blood. Its name derives from the characteristic morphology of leukemic cells containing delicate, hairlike, circumferential cytoplasmic projections, best seen on bone marrow aspirate and peripheral blood smears. The median age at presentation is 45 to 50 years, and there is a striking male predominance (the male to female ratio is 4-5:1). Unlike with other B-cell leukemic lymphomas, patients typically present with a leukopenic or sometimes a pancytopenic picture. An absolute monocytopenia is characteristic and may be a clue to the diagnosis when the number of circulating leukemic cells is small, making them difficult to identify on peripheral blood smears.

Hairy cell leukemia almost always involves the spleen, and splenomegaly is part of the typical clinical presentation.[38,39] In rare cases with an atypical

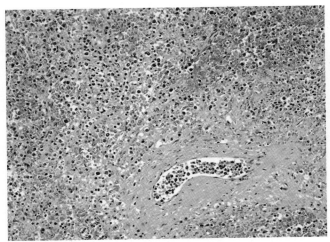

Figure 6-13 Splenic involvement by intravascular large B-cell lymphoma. In contrast to the splenic large B-cell lymphoma with diffuse red pulp infiltration in Figure 6-12, in this case the large cell lymphoma cells are present in splenic arterioles and in sinuses. This patient also had extensive intravascular lymphoma involving other organs at autopsy, including the heart, lungs, and kidneys.

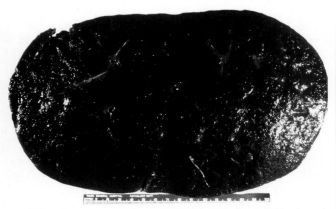

Figure 6-14 Hairy cell leukemia, gross pathology. This spleen is massively enlarged (it weighed 2 kg). It has a beefy red, cut surface, which represents extensive expansion of the red pulp. The normal pinpoint nodules of white pulp are absent.

disease distribution, splenomegaly may be mild or absent.[40] The treatment of hairy cell leukemia differs from that of other small B-cell leukemic lymphomas, which underscores the importance of diagnosing it correctly and distinguishing it from splenic marginal zone lymphoma, hairy cell leukemia variant, and other small B-cell lymphomas in leukemic phase. A single course of cladribine or 2-chlorodeoxyadenosine (2-CDA), given as a continuous intravenous infusion over 7 days, induces a durable, complete response in most patients, with resolution of splenomegaly and cytopenias.[41] Among the small proportion of patients who relapse, therapeutic options include retreatment with cladribine or rituximab monotherapy.[41,42]

Pathologic Features

In contrast to most other B-cell lymphomas involving the spleen (including splenic marginal zone lymphoma), hairy cell leukemia preferentially involves the red pulp rather than the white pulp. Grossly, the spleen is massively enlarged (median weight, 1200 g), and examination of the cut surface shows a beefy red pulp and absence of the normal pinpoint white pulp nodules (Figure 6-14).[43,44] On microscopic examination, red pulp sinuses and cords are diffusely filled with monomorphous round to oval cells with smooth nuclear contours, open chromatin, inconspicuous nucleoli, and abundant, clear cytoplasm, leading to expansion of the red pulp sinuses and atrophy of the white pulp (Figure 6-15, *A* and *B*).[45,46]

In the spleen and bone marrow, the lack of lymphoid nodules is important for distinguishing hairy cell leukemia from splenic marginal zone lymphoma and other small B-cell neoplasms. At high magnification on well-prepared cut sections, cytoplasmic projections may even occasionally be visible, and they are numerous on ultrastructural examination

(Figure 6-15, *C*).[47] Microscopic erythrocyte-filled spaces, called "pseudosinuses" or "red blood cell lakes," characteristically are present, although they are not specific to hairy cell leukemia (Figure 6-15, *B*). These may result from leukemic cell adhesion and subsequent damage to splenic sinus endothelial cells.[47,48]

Immunophenotypically, hairy cells are strongly positive for CD20 and surface light chain and usually negative for CD5, CD10, and CD23; they characteristically express DBA 44, CD103, CD25, CD11c, and CD123.[48] Expression of CD10 or CD23 may be seen in 10% to 20% of cases, and CD5 positivity has been reported in rare cases.[49-53] Up to 40% of cases express cyclin D1 (BCL1) by immunohistochemistry but lack t(11;14) by cytogenetics or FISH.[51] Annexin A1, normally present in phagocytic cells of the myeloid lineage but absent in normal B cells, has been found to be upregulated in gene expression profiling studies of hairy cell leukemia. Immunocytochemical or immunohistochemical detection of the annexin A1 protein has been shown to be highly sensitive and specific for hairy cell leukemia, distinguishing it from splenic marginal zone lymphoma and hairy cell leukemia variant.[54]

Hairy cell leukemia variant, a provisional entity in the current WHO classification system,[28] is a rare B-cell neoplasm composed of tumor cells with morphologic features intermediate between hairy cells and prolymphocytes. Cells have moderately basophilic cytoplasm with cytoplasmic projections and round to oval nuclei; however, unlike in classic hairy cell leukemia, a prominent nucleolus is present. The bone marrow, peripheral blood, and spleen are commonly involved, with preferential involvement of the splenic red pulp. Clinically, there is a leukocytosis instead of a leukopenia and absence of an absolute monocytopenia.[54] It is important to note that hairy cell leukemia variant responds poorly to drugs that are effective in hairy cell leukemia. Neoplastic cells typically are positive for CD103 and DBA 44 but lack expression of CD25 and annexin A1.[51, 54]

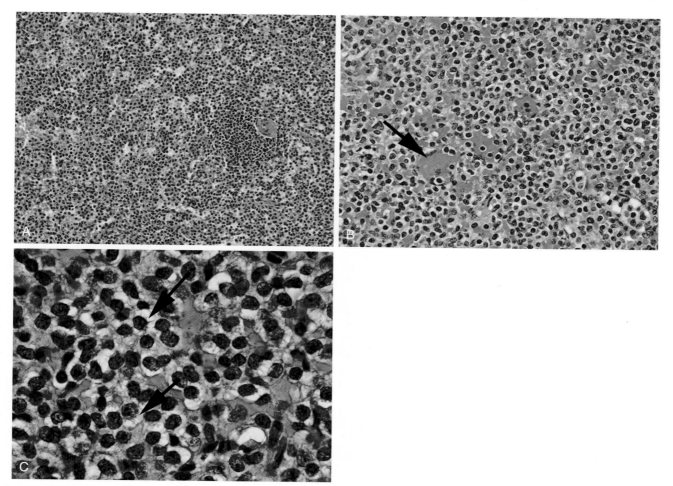

Figure 6-15 Hairy cell leukemia, microscopic features. **A,** Red pulp sinuses and cords are filled with numerous cells containing monomorphous round to oval nuclei. Adjacent white pulp appears atrophic. It is important to note that nodular lymphoid aggregates are absent. **B,** Leukemic cells contain slightly open chromatin; inconspicuous nucleoli; and abundant, pale cytoplasm. Mature erythrocytes coalesce to form pseudosinuses, or "red blood cell lakes" *(arrow).* **C,** Under high-power magnification, fine circumferential cytoplasmic projections, from which this neoplasm derives its name, may be visible *(arrows).*

The distinct clinical and immunophenotypic features of hairy cell leukemia variant have led some to suggest that it may represent a separate diagnostic entity rather than simply a morphologic variant of hairy cell leukemia.[54] The relationship, if any, between hairy cell leukemia variant and splenic diffuse red pulp small B-cell lymphoma is not known. Cases that do not fit the classic morphologic and immunophenotypic profile of hairy cell leukemia may be better placed in an unclassified category of splenic small B-cell lymphoma with diffuse red pulp involvement until more is known about the pathogenetic differences underlying such neoplasms.[55,56]

Hepatosplenic T-Cell Lymphoma

Clinical Features

Hepatosplenic T-cell lymphoma is a recently described type of lymphoma with distinctive clinical and pathologic features. Hepatosplenic T-cell lymphoma typically also involves the liver and bone marrow. Most patients are young males, and the median age is 25 years.[57] Some patients are immunosuppressed; this type of lymphoma has been reported in transplant recipients.[58] Some cases of hepatosplenic T-cell lymphoma have been described in patients with inflammatory bowel disease, particularly Crohn's disease.[59,60] Many of these patients were treated with infliximab, a chimeric monoclonal antibody to tumor necrosis factor, in combination with other immunosuppressive agents, such as azathioprine or steroids, leading to a black box warning on infliximab.[59,60] Interestingly, rare cases of hepatosplenic T-cell lymphoma also have been reported in patients with a history of *Plasmodium falciparum* malaria infection, which is associated with an expansion of γδ T cells in the peripheral blood and spleen, presumably as a result of chronic antigenic stimulation and immune dysregulation.[61,62]

The cases initially described were T-cell receptor (TCR)γδ+, TCRαβ− (hepatosplenic γδ T-cell lymphoma), but subsequently, cases expressing TCRαβ were identified. The αβ variant appears to affect patients over a wider age range, including children

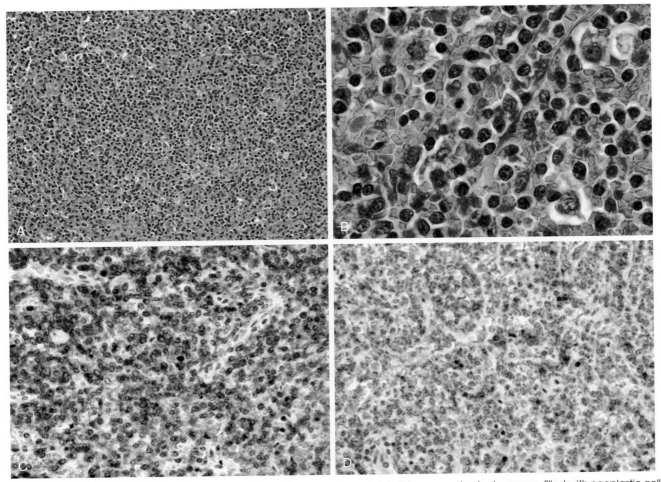

Figure 6-16 Hepatosplenic T-cell lymphoma with subtle splenic involvement. **A,** In this case, red pulp sinuses are filled with neoplastic cells with relatively mild nuclear atypia. **B,** On higher magnification, neoplastic cells are medium sized with slightly dispersed nuclear chromatin and inconspicuous or small nucleoli. **C** and **D,** Immunohistochemistry demonstrates that the sinuses are filled with numerous CD3+ T cells **(C)** that lack expression of the pan–T-cell antigen CD5 **(D)**, confirming an aberrant immunophenotype. Only rare residual CD5+ nonneoplastic T cells are present.

and older adults, to affect a higher proportion of females, and to have a slightly older median age at presentation (36 years)[57]; otherwise, the γδ and αβ variants are clinically similar.

Patients present with abdominal pain and often have fever, night sweats, or weight loss. The spleen and liver are diffusely, often strikingly enlarged, without conspicuous peripheral lymphadenopathy. Patients may have peripheral blood cytopenias, including anemia and thrombocytopenia. Circulating tumor cells may be found at presentation, but in some cases, a leukemic picture develops late in the course of the disease. Patients may respond to chemotherapy initially, but in general the disease progresses in an aggressive manner, and the lymphoma has a poor prognosis, with a median survival of less than a year.[57,63-65]

Pathologic Features

The neoplastic cells preferentially involve splenic red pulp and hepatic sinusoids (Figure 6-16, *A*, and Figure 6-17, *A*). Pathologic features are similar for γδ

and αβ variants, except that in a minority of cases, hepatic involvement in αβ cases is periportal in addition to sinusoidal.[57] Neoplastic cells in the marrow often are confined to vascular sinuses and therefore may be difficult to appreciate on routinely stained sections. Lymphoma may also infiltrate the interstitium of the marrow and in rare cases forms nodular aggregates or shows diffuse involvement. Immunohistochemical stains for T cells may be helpful in highlighting abnormal cells in an apparently normal marrow. When lymph nodes are involved, tumor cells tend to be found in sinuses. Neoplastic cells are medium-sized or occasionally large and tend to have oval nuclei with fine chromatin and abundant, pale cytoplasm (Figure 6-16, *B*, and Figure 6-17, *B*).[57, 63-65] Erythrophagocytosis in the spleen and bone marrow may be prominent.

Immunohistochemical analysis typically shows CD2+, CD3+, CD5−/+, CD4−, CD8−/+, CD7+/−, TCRγδ+ or TCRαβ+ T cells that express the cytotoxic granule–associated protein T-cell intracellular antigen 1 (TIA-1) (Figure 6-16, *C* and *D*, and Figure 6-17,

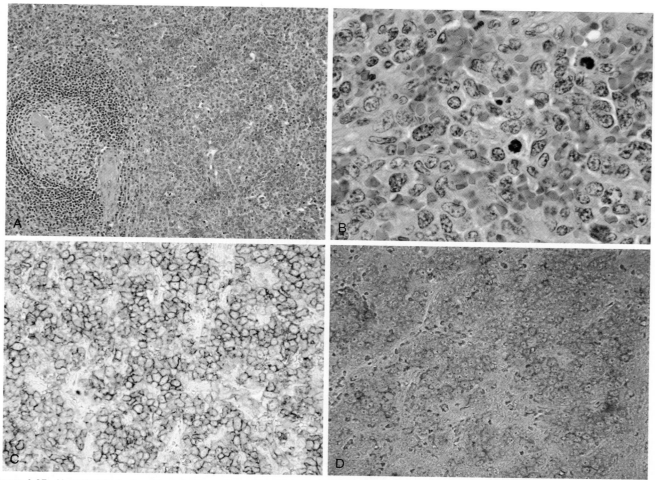

Figure 6-17 Hepatosplenic T-cell lymphoma with marked cytologic atypia. **A,** In this case, lymphomatous involvement of the spleen is more obvious than in the case in Figure 6-16, and red pulp sinuses are filled with clusters of large atypical cells. The lymphoma shows sparing of the white pulp, with a residual benign periarteriolar lymphoid follicle on the left. **B,** The neoplastic cells are large with oval to irregular nuclei and vesicular chromatin. Conspicuous mitoses are present. Neoplastic cells are positive for the pan–T-cell antigen CD5 **(C)** and weakly positive for the NK-associated antigen CD56 **(D).**

C). Other cytotoxic molecules (granzyme B and perforin) are uncommonly detected. Occasionally, natural killer (NK)-associated antigens, such as CD16 and CD56, are expressed (see Figure 6-17, *D*). Molecular genetic analysis shows clonal TCR gene rearrangement. The T cells in the γδ variant are the V-δ-1 subset.[58] The most common cytogenetic abnormalities are isochromosome 7q and trisomy 8.[58] A few cases have been positive for EBV, but most are negative.[57]

■ LYMPHOMAS SECONDARILY INVOLVING THE SPLEEN

Diffuse Large B-Cell Lymphoma

Diffuse large B-cell lymphoma is the most common lymphoid neoplasm to involve the spleen secondarily.[66] The pathologic features of secondary splenic involvement by diffuse large B-cell lymphoma are similar to those seen in the primary sites; secondary splenic involvement by diffuse large B-cell lymphoma is shown in Figures 6-8 to 6-13.

Chronic Lymphocytic Leukemia/Small Lymphocytic Lymphoma

Patients with chronic lymphocytic leukemia (CLL) frequently have splenic involvement. This may be partly related to the expression of cell surface adhesion molecules on the neoplastic B cells that allow preferential homing to the spleen over other lymphoid organs.[67,68] Although CLL is the most common of the small B-cell neoplasms to involve the spleen, the degree of splenomegaly may be less than that seen with other B-cell lymphomas.[66] The white pulp may be prominent on gross examination, and microscopically, both white and red pulp are involved (Figure 6-18 and Figure 6-19, *A*). Expanded white pulp nodules are composed of small, mature-appearing lymphocytes with scattered, admixed larger prolymphocytes and paraimmunoblasts; the latter may coalesce to form proliferation centers (Figure 6-19, *B* and *C*). Occasional residual reactive germinal centers may be present, but a marginal zone pattern is rare. Red pulp involvement may be nodular, diffuse, or a mixture of the two patterns (Figure 6-19, *D*). Hilar

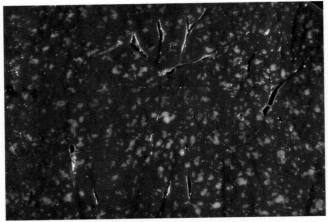

Figure 6-18 Splenic involvement by chronic lymphocytic leukemia, gross pathology. This spleen, which weighed 1 kg, shows prominent white pulp expansion by irregularly shaped nodules.

lymph node involvement is invariably present, with partial or complete architectural effacement. Lymphoma cells exhibit the typical immunophenotype of CLL, with mature B cells co-expressing CD5 and CD23. By flow cytometry, dim CD20 and surface light chain expression and absence of FMC7 help distinguish CLL from other small B-cell neoplasms. Immunohistochemistry for cyclin D1 or FISH for bcl1 rearrangement is mandatory to exclude mantle cell lymphoma.[46,69]

Follicular Lymphoma

Follicular lymphoma frequently involves the spleen, and splenectomy occasionally may be the diagnostic procedure.[70-72] Two patterns of involvement have been identified (Figure 6-20). In one pattern, the spleen shows abnormal architecture with closely packed neoplastic follicles separated by minimal red pulp. Increased numbers of interfollicular B cells

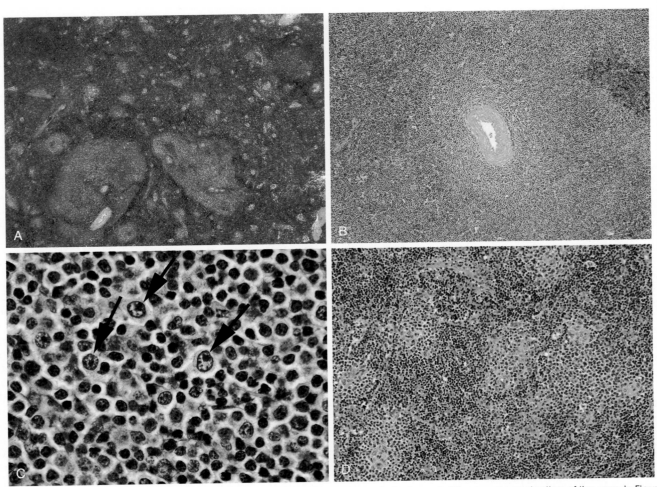

Figure 6-19 Splenic involvement by chronic lymphocytic leukemia, microscopic features. **A,** Microscopic evaluation of the case in Figure 6-18 revealed that both the white pulp and the red pulp are involved, with irregular expansions of white pulp nodules and small aggregates of lymphocytes in the red pulp. **B,** An expanded white pulp nodule contains numerous small, mature-appearing lymphocytes. Centrally, a pale-staining pseudofollicle is present, indicative of a proliferation center. **C,** Examination of the pseudofollicle under higher magnification shows a polymorphous population of small lymphocytes with condensed chromatin, slightly larger prolymphocytes with more dispersed chromatin, and large paraimmunoblasts with prominent nucleoli and vesicular chromatin (arrows). **D,** In the red pulp, involvement is diffuse and small proliferation centers are prominent.

are seen by immunohistochemistry. In the other pattern, which occurs at a similar frequency, the splenic architecture appears well preserved with only scattered neoplastic follicles preferentially involving white pulp. B cells may be present in red pulp but usually in small numbers. All cases show strong staining for B-cell and germinal center markers (CD10 and/or bcl6). bcl2 usually is overexpressed in the follicles; this finding typically correlates with a t(14;18)(q32;q21), although bcl2 expression may be weak or negative in many cases with a higher histologic grade.[72,73] The different patterns do not appear to be associated with the presence or absence of previously diagnosed follicular lymphoma, splenic weight, or clinical stage. However, bcl2− cases with a higher histologic grade are more often seen initially as a lymphoma restricted to the spleen. The cases with a purely intrafollicular growth pattern may be misdiagnosed as reactive hyperplasia, but staining for bcl2 can help with this differential. The overall survival rate for patients with follicular lymphoma

involving the spleen is about 55% at 5 years, and this does not appear to depend on bcl2 positivity or negativity.

Lymphoplasmacytic Lymphoma/ Waldenström's Macroglobulinemia

The features of splenic involvement by lymphoplasmacytic lymphoma and the differential diagnosis from splenic marginal zone lymphoma are discussed in the section on splenic marginal zone lymphoma and illustrated in Figure 6-6.

Mantle Cell Lymphoma

Mantle cell lymphoma commonly involves the spleen, and splenomegaly may be the presenting complaint.[69,74,75] Grossly, the spleen is markedly enlarged, and the white pulp appears expanded with a miliary pattern or multiple, fleshy nodules (Figure 6-21). Mantle cell lymphoma often has

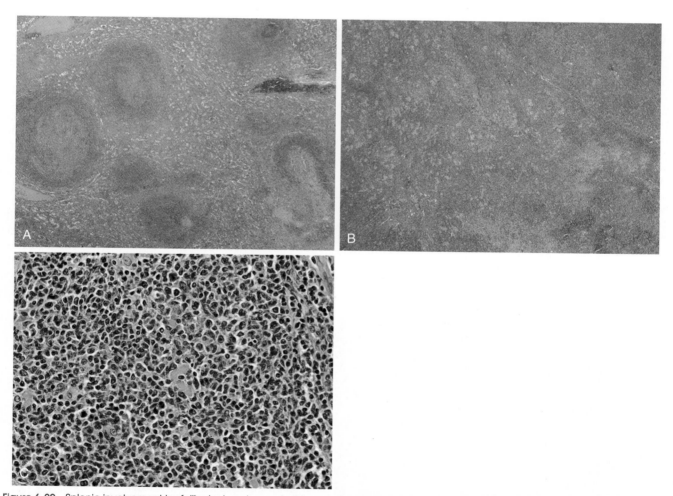

Figure 6-20 Splenic involvement by follicular lymphoma. In this case, two patterns of involvement are evident. **A,** In some areas, neoplastic follicles centered on the white pulp are spaced widely apart, with abundant intervening red pulp. **B,** In other areas, follicles are more crowded and have a confluent back-to-back arrangement; only a little intervening red pulp is visible. **C,** With both patterns, high-power examination of neoplastic follicle centers reveals a monomorphous population of centrocytes with irregular, folded nuclei and condensed chromatin. Rare centroblasts are seen in this case, reflecting a low histologic grade (grade 1-2 of 3).

larger macroscopic nodules than other small B-cell lymphomas involving the spleen (Figure 6-21, *B*). Microscopically, the white pulp is expanded by small to large nodules of lymphoma cells with typical cytologic features of mantle cell lymphoma (Figure 6-22, *A* and *B*).[46,76] Residual germinal centers usually are not seen. However, in some cases, involvement by a mantle zone growth pattern may be present, or the white pulp nodules may contain marginal zones, mimicking splenic marginal zone lymphoma.[69] Other cases may show small nodules of lymphoma cells in the red pulp, or diffuse red pulp involvement can occur in cases with a peripheral blood leukocytosis (Figure 6-22, *C*).[69] Splenic lymph nodes are almost always involved. The differential diagnosis includes splenic marginal zone lymphoma and other small B-cell lymphomas, but immunohistochemical stains, especially cyclin D1, can easily distinguish mantle cell lymphoma from other small B-cell neoplasms.

Immunohistochemical or FISH analysis for cyclin D1 is important for definitive diagnosis or exclusion of mantle cell lymphoma due to its clinically aggressive behavior in comparison to other small B cell neoplasms, and patients are typically treated with intensive chemotherapy at the time of diagnosis. Recently, however, a subset of mantle cell lymphoma patients with an indolent clinical course, prolonged time to requiring therapy and prolonged survival has been identified.[76a,76b] Such patients usually present with non-nodal disease involving the peripheral blood and often the spleen, and neoplastic cells carry a mutated immunoglobulin heavy chain variable region, in contrast to the unmutated status typically seen in conventional mantle cell lymphoma. In addition, cases of indolent mantle cell lymphoma carry a lower burden of karyotypic abnormalities and chromosomal imbalances, in comparison to conventional mantle cell lymphoma.[76a,76b] Both the conventional and indolent forms of mantle cell lymphoma appear to share a similar gene expression profile with several key differences, including expression of *SOX11*, a transcription factor that appears to be absent or underexpressed in indolent cases.[76b] SOX11 immunohistochemistry may help to identify a subset of mantle cell lymphoma patients who do well without aggressive chemotherapy and who could be managed more conservatively.[76b]

Classical Hodgkin's Lymphoma

Secondary splenic involvement by classical Hodgkin's lymphoma is relatively common. In a recent study, approximately one fourth of patients with primary refractory disease had splenic involvement, and before the advent of combination chemotherapy for the treatment of Hodgkin's lymphoma, involvement of the spleen invariably was present at the time of disease progression.[77] In contrast, primary splenic involvement by classical Hodgkin's lymphoma, with disease limited to the spleen or the spleen and abdominal lymph nodes or other organs, is relatively rare; only a few such cases have been reported.[78,79]

Once common, splenectomy as part of the staging workup for classical Hodgkin's lymphoma largely has been replaced by radiologic imaging to assess for organ involvement.[80] However, staging laparoscopy with splenectomy may be performed in selected cases in which disease otherwise appears limited so as to help determine the appropriateness of chemotherapy.[81,82]

Gross examination of the involved spleen demonstrates visibly expanded nodules centered around the white pulp (Figure 6-23). Microscopically, the normal white pulp is replaced by scattered Reed-Sternberg cells and variants, which are present in a mixed cellular background composed of small lymphocytes, histiocytes, eosinophils, and plasma cells, similar to that seen in nodal disease (see Figure 6-23, *B;* also Figure 6-24, *A* and *B*). The lymphoma initially is confined to the white pulp, with coalescence of nodules upon progression of the disease.[83] Fibrous bands may be present in the nodular sclerosis subtype. The main differential diagnosis is with a reactive process harboring immunoblasts

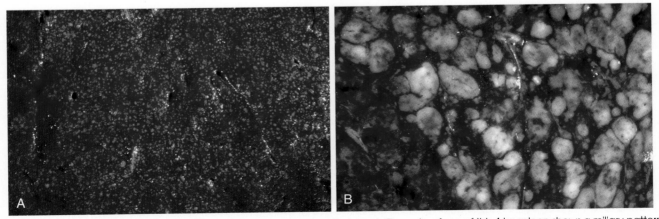

Figure 6-21   Splenic involvement by mantle cell lymphoma, gross pathology. **A,** The cut surface of this 4-kg spleen shows a miliary pattern with innumerable tiny nodules. **B,** In contrast, this case shows larger, fleshy, irregularly shaped nodules on cross section.

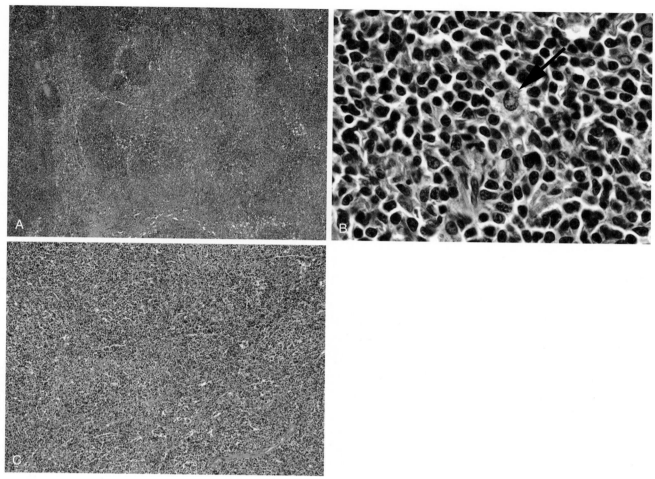

Figure 6-22 Splenic involvement by mantle cell lymphoma, microscopic features. **A,** The white pulp is markedly expanded by large, coalescent nodules. **B,** High-power examination of a white pulp nodule shows typical cytologic features of mantle cell lymphoma, with monomorphous, small to medium, centrocyte-like cells with condensed nuclear chromatin and irregular nuclear contours. Large transformed cells are absent, but occasional epithelioid histiocytes may be seen *(arrow).* **C,** Areas of involved red pulp show small nodular aggregates of lymphoma cells.

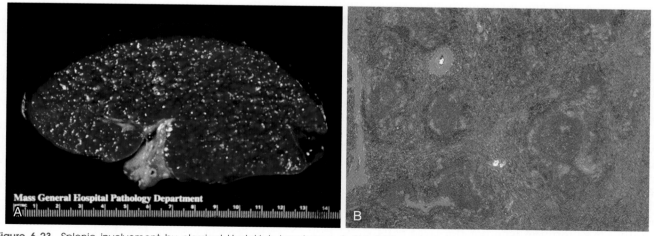

Figure 6-23 Splenic involvement by classical Hodgkin's lymphoma. **A,** This 1.7-kg spleen is grossly abnormal, showing parenchymal replacement throughout by multiple reddish brown nodules. More typically, only a few nodules are present. **B,** Microscopic examination shows that the nodules are centered on the white pulp and are composed predominantly of small lymphocytes with surrounding small clusters of histiocytes.

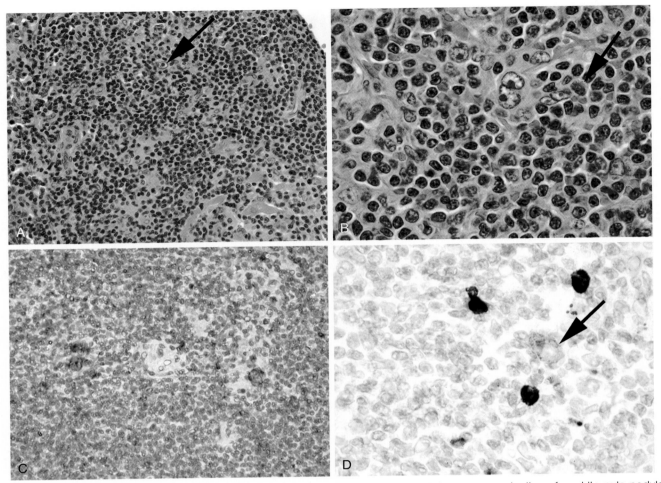

Figure 6-24 Mixed cellularity classical Hodgkin's lymphoma involving the spleen. **A,** High-power examination of a white pulp nodule reveals a mononuclear Reed-Sternberg cell variant with a large, prominent eosinophilic nucleolus *(arrow)* in a mixed cellular background composed of numerous small lymphocytes and occasional eosinophils and histiocytes. **B,** The presence of a classic binucleate Reed-Sternberg cell helps exclude a florid immunoblastic reaction or T-cell/histiocyte-rich large B-cell lymphoma. An eosinophil is to the right of the Reed-Sternberg cell *(arrow)*. Immunohistochemical staining for CD30 **(C)** and CD15 **(D,** *arrow)* shows positivity of the large, neoplastic cells, confirming the diagnosis.

that may be mistaken for mononuclear variants of Reed-Sternberg cells. Caution is necessary if no diagnostic binucleate Reed-Sternberg cells are identified and if the mononuclear cells express CD30 but not CD15. In such cases, clinical correlation is required, and additional immunohistochemistry should be undertaken to support a diagnosis of Hodgkin's lymphoma (e.g., Pax5 to look for weak Pax5 expression; Oct2 and Bob1 to look for loss of one or both of these antigens). Cases of Hodgkin's lymphoma with a monotonous lymphohistiocytic background involving the spleen may mimic the micronodular T-cell/histiocyte-rich variant of large B-cell lymphoma. The latter entity typically lacks classic Reed-Sternberg cells, fibrosis, and eosinophilia; however, appropriate immunohistochemical staining to determine whether the large cells show or lack a normal expression profile of mature B cells is necessary to resolve this differential diagnosis (Figure 6-24, *C* and *D*).

REFERENCES

1. Berger F, Felman P, Thieblemont C et al: Non-MALT marginal zone B-cell lymphomas: a description of clinical presentation and outcome in 124 patients, *Blood* 95:1950-1956, 2000.
2. Diebold J, Le Tourneau A, Comperat E et al: Primary splenic and nodal marginal zone lymphoma, *J Clin Exp Hematopathol* 45:1-14, 2005.
3. Dogan A, Isaacson PG: Splenic marginal zone lymphoma, *Semin Diagn Pathol* 20:121-127, 2003.
4. Thieblemont C, Felman P, Callet-Bauchu E et al: Splenic marginal-zone lymphoma: a distinct clinical and pathological entity, *Lancet Oncol* 4:95-103, 2003.
5. Ciaudo M, Horellou MH, Audouin J et al: Lupus anticoagulant associated with primary malignant lymphoplasmacytic lymphoma of the spleen: a report of four patients, *Am J Hematol* 38:271-276, 1991.
6. Martin SE, Abel RF: Splenic marginal zone lymphoma, iliac vein thrombosis, and monoclonal immunoglobulin M-kappa antiphospholipid antibody with Annexin A5 interaction, *Leuk Lymphoma* 47:1994-1996, 2006.

7. Murakami H, Irisawa H, Saitoh T et al: Immunological abnormalities in splenic marginal zone cell lymphoma, *Am J Hematol* 56:173-178, 1997.

8. Sawamura M, Yamaguchi S, Murakami H et al: Multiple autoantibody production in a patient with splenic lymphoma, *Ann Hematol* 68:251-254, 1994.

9. Ziakas PD, Giannouli S, Tasidou A et al: Multiple autoimmune phenomena in splenic marginal zone lymphoma, *Leuk Lymphoma* 47:772-775, 2006.

10. De Renzo A, Perna F, Persico M et al: Excellent prognosis and prevalence of HCV infection of primary hepatic and splenic non-Hodgkin's lymphoma, *Eur J Haematol* 81:51-57, 2008.

11. Saadoun D, Suarez F, Lefrere F et al: Splenic lymphoma with villous lymphocytes associated with type II cryoglobulinemia and HCV infection: a new entity? *Blood* 105:74-76, 2005.

12. Bates I, Bedu-Addo G, Rutherford T et al: Splenic lymphoma with villous lymphocytes in tropical West Africa, *Lancet* 340:575-577, 1992.

13. Bates I, Bedu-Addo G, Rutherford TR et al: Circulating villous lymphocytes: a link between hyperreactive malarial splenomegaly and splenic lymphoma, *Trans R Soc Trop Med Hyg* 91:171-174, 1997.

14. Oscier D, Owen R, Johnson S: Splenic marginal zone lymphoma, *Blood Rev* 19:39-51, 2005.

15. Arcaini L, Zibellini S, Passamonti F et al: Splenic marginal zone lymphoma: clinical clustering of immunoglobulin heavy chain repertoires, *Blood Cells Mol Dis* 42:286-291, 2009.

16. Chacon JI, Mollejo M, Munoz E et al: Splenic marginal zone lymphoma: clinical characteristics and prognostic factors in a series of 60 patients, *Blood* 100:1648-1654, 2002.

17. Fodor A, Molnar MZ, Krenacs L et al: Autoimmune hemolytic anemia as a risk factor of poor outcome in patients with splenic marginal zone lymphoma, *Pathol Oncol Res* 15:597-603, 2009.

18. Parry-Jones N, Matutes E, Gruszka-Westwood AM et al: Prognostic features of splenic lymphoma with villous lymphocytes: a report on 129 patients, *Br J Haematol* 120:759-764, 2003.

19. Thieblemont C, Felman P, Berger F et al: Treatment of splenic marginal zone B-cell lymphoma: an analysis of 81 patients, *Clin Lymphoma* 3:41-47, 2002.

20. Abramson JS, Chatterji M, Rahemtullah A: Case records of the Massachusetts General Hospital: case 39-2008—a 51-year-old woman with splenomegaly and anemia, *N Engl J Med* 359:2707-2718, 2008.

21. Kalpadakis C, Pangalis GA, Dimopoulou MN et al: Rituximab monotherapy is highly effective in splenic marginal zone lymphoma, *Hematol Oncol* 25:127-131, 2007.

22. Isaacson PG, Matutes E, Burke M et al: The histopathology of splenic lymphoma with villous lymphocytes, *Blood* 84:3828-3834, 1994.

23. Van Huyen JP, Molina T, Delmer A et al: Splenic marginal zone lymphoma with or without plasmacytic differentiation, *Am J Surg Pathol* 24:1581-1592, 2000.

24. Papadaki T, Stamatopoulos K, Belessi C et al: Splenic marginal-zone lymphoma: one or more entities? A histologic, immunohistochemical, and molecular study of 42 cases, *Am J Surg Pathol* 31:438-446, 2007.

25. Algara P, Mateo MS, Sanchez-Beato M et al: Analysis of the IgV(H) somatic mutations in splenic marginal zone lymphoma defines a group of unmutated cases with frequent 7q deletion and adverse clinical course, *Blood* 99:1299-1304, 2002.

26. Stamatopoulos K, Belessi C, Papadaki T et al: Immunoglobulin heavy- and light-chain repertoire in splenic marginal zone lymphoma, *Mol Med* 10:89-95, 2004.

26a. Del Giudice I, Pileri SA, Rossi M et al: Histopathological and molecular features of persistent polyclonal B-cell lymphocytosis (PPBL) with progressive splenomegaly, *Br J Haematol* 144:726-731, 2009.

27. Mollejo M, Algara P, Mateo MS et al: Splenic small B-cell lymphoma with predominant red pulp involvement: a diffuse variant of splenic marginal zone lymphoma? *Histopathology* 40:22-30, 2002.

28. Piris MA, Foucar K, Mollejo M et al: Splenic B-cell lymphoma/leukemia, unclassifiable. In Swerdlow S, Campo E, Harris N et al, editors: *WHO classification: tumours of haematopoietic and lymphoid tissues*, ed 4, Lyon, 2008, IARC.

28a. Kanellis G, Mollejo M, Montes-Moreno S et al: Splenic diffuse red pulp small B-cell lymphoma: revision of a series of cases reveals characteristic clinico-pathological features, *Haematologica* 95:1122-1129, 2010.

29. Mollejo M, Algara P, Mateo MS et al: Large B-cell lymphoma presenting in the spleen: identification of different clinico-pathologic conditions, *Am J Surg Pathol* 27:895-902, 2003.

30. Takeshita M, Sakai H, Okamura S et al: Prevalence of hepatitis C virus infection in cases of B-cell lymphoma in Japan, *Histopathology* 48:189-198, 2006.

31. Dogan A, Burke JS, Goteri G et al: Micronodular T-cell/histiocyte-rich large B-cell lymphoma of the spleen: histology, immunophenotype, and differential diagnosis, *Am J Surg Pathol* 27:903-911, 2003.

32. Harris NL, Aisenberg AC, Meyer JE et al: Diffuse large cell (histiocytic) lymphoma of the spleen: clinical and pathologic characteristics of ten cases, *Cancer* 54:2460-2467, 1984.

33. Kan E, Levy I, Benharroch D: Splenic micronodular T-cell/histiocyte-rich large B-cell lymphoma, *Ann Diagn Pathol* 12:290-292, 2008.

34. Kashimura M, Noro M, Akikusa B et al: Primary splenic diffuse large B-cell lymphoma manifesting in red pulp, *Virchows Arch* 453:501-509, 2008.

35. Morice WG, Rodriguez FJ, Hoyer JD et al: Diffuse large B-cell lymphoma with distinctive patterns of splenic and bone marrow involvement: clinicopathologic features of two cases, *Mod Pathol* 18:495-502, 2005.

36. De Wolf-Peeters C, Delabie J, Campo E et al: T-cell/histiocyte-rich large B-cell lymphoma. In Swerdlow S, Campo E, Harris N et al, editors: *WHO classification: tumours of haematopoietic and lymphoid tissues*, ed 4, Lyon, 2008, IARC.

37. Delabie J, Vandenberghe E, Kennes C et al: Histiocyte-rich B-cell lymphoma: a distinct clinicopathologic entity possibly related to lymphocyte predominant Hodgkin's disease, paragranuloma subtype, *Am J Surg Pathol* 16:37-48, 1992.

38. Cannon T, Mobarek D, Wegge J et al: Hairy cell leukemia: current concepts, *Cancer Invest* 26:860-865, 2008.

39. Fanta PT, Saven A: Hairy cell leukemia, *Cancer Treat Res* 142:193-209, 2009.

40. Farkash EA, Ferry JA, Harris NL et al: Rare lymphoid malignancies of the breast: a report of two cases illustrating potential diagnostic pitfalls, *J Hematopathol* 2:237-244, 2009.

41. Tallman MS, Hakimian D, Rademaker AW et al: Relapse of hairy cell leukemia after 2-chlorodeoxyadenosine: long-term follow-up of the Northwestern University experience, *Blood* 88:1954-1959, 1996.

42. Angelopoulou MK, Pangalis GA, Sachanas S et al: Outcome and toxicity in relapsed hairy cell leukemia patients treated with rituximab, *Leuk Lymphoma* 49:1817-1820, 2008.

43. Golomb HM, Vardiman JW: Response to splenectomy in 65 patients with hairy cell leukemia: an evaluation of spleen weight and bone marrow involvement, *Blood* 61:349-352, 1983.

44. Mintz U, Golomb HM: Splenectomy as initial therapy in twenty-six patients with leukemic reticuloendotheliosis (hairy cell leukemia), *Cancer Res* 39:2366-2370, 1979.

45. Burke JS, Byrne GE Jr, Rappaport H: Hairy cell leukemia (leukemic reticuloendotheliosis). I. A clinical pathologic study of 21 patients, *Cancer* 33:1399-1410, 1974.

46. van Krieken JH, Feller AC, te Velde J: The distribution of non-Hodgkin's lymphoma in the lymphoid compartments of the human spleen, *Am J Surg Pathol* 13:757-765, 1989.

47. Pilon VA, Davey FR, Gordon GB et al: Splenic alterations in hairy-cell leukemia. II. An electron microscopic study, *Cancer* 49:1617-1623, 1982.

48. Del Giudice I, Matutes E, Morilla R et al: The diagnostic value of CD123 in B-cell disorders with hairy or villous lymphocytes, *Haematologica* 89:303-308, 2004.

49. Chen D, Morice DG, Viswanatha DS et al: CD5-positive hairy cell leukemia: a rare but distinct variant, *Mod Pathol* 22:258A, 2009 (abstract).

50. Chen YH, Tallman MS, Goolsby C et al: Immunophenotypic variations in hairy cell leukemia, *Am J Clin Pathol* 125:251-259, 2006.

51. Dong HY, Weisberger J, Liu Z et al: Immunophenotypic analysis of CD103+ B-lymphoproliferative disorders: hairy cell leukemia and its mimics, *Am J Clin Pathol* 131:586-595, 2009.

52. Jasionowski TM, Hartung L, Greenwood JH et al: Analysis of CD10+ hairy cell leukemia, *Am J Clin Pathol* 120:228-235, 2003.

53. Rahemtullah A, Rezk S, Wang SA et al: Aberrant expression of CD5 and CD10 in hairy cell leukemia: correlation with clinical presentation and outcome, *Mod Pathol* 19:242A-243A, 2006 (abstract).

54. Falini B, Tiacci E, Liso A et al: Simple diagnostic assay for hairy cell leukaemia by immunocytochemical detection of annexin A1 (ANXA1), *Lancet* 363:1869-1870, 2004.

55. Chuang SS, Chang ST, Huang WT et al: Variant hairy cell leukemia without distinct nucleoli, *Leuk Lymphoma* 48:1050-1052, 2007.

56. Traverse-Glehen A, Baseggio L, Bauchu EC et al: Splenic red pulp lymphoma with numerous basophilic villous lymphocytes: a distinct clinicopathologic and molecular entity? *Blood* 111:2253-2260, 2008.

57. Macon WR, Levy NB, Kurtin PJ et al: Hepatosplenic alpha-beta T-cell lymphomas: a report of 14 cases and comparison with hepatosplenic gamma-delta T-cell lymphomas, *Am J Surg Pathol* 25:285-296, 2001.

58. Wu H, Wasik MA, Przybylski G et al: Hepatosplenic gamma-delta T-cell lymphoma as a late-onset posttransplant lymphoproliferative disorder in renal transplant recipients, *Am J Clin Pathol* 113:487-496, 2000.

59. Mackey AC, Green L, Liang LC et al: Hepatosplenic T cell lymphoma associated with infliximab use in young patients treated for inflammatory bowel disease, *J Pediatr Gastroenterol Nutr* 44:265-267, 2007.

60. Rosh JR, Gross T, Mamula P et al: Hepatosplenic T-cell lymphoma in adolescents and young adults with Crohn's disease: a cautionary tale? *Inflamm Bowel Dis* 13:1024-1030, 2007.

61. Belhadj K, Reyes F, Farcet JP et al: Hepatosplenic gamma-delta T-cell lymphoma is a rare clinicopathologic entity with poor outcome: report on a series of 21 patients, *Blood* 102:4261-4269, 2003.

62. Hassan R, Franco SA, Stefanoff CG et al: Hepatosplenic gamma-delta T-cell lymphoma following seven malaria infections, *Pathol Int* 56:668-673, 2006.

63. Farcet JP, Gaulard P, Marolleau JP et al: Hepatosplenic T-cell lymphoma: sinusal/sinusoidal localization of malignant cells expressing the T-cell receptor gamma delta, *Blood* 75:2213-2219, 1990.

64. Pouderoux P, Gris JC, Pignodel C et al: Primary sinusoidal lymphoma of the liver revealed by autoimmune hemolytic anemia, *Gastroenterol Clin Biol* 21:514-518, 1997.

65. Wong KF, Chan JK, Matutes E et al: Hepatosplenic gamma delta T-cell lymphoma: a distinctive aggressive lymphoma type, *Am J Surg Pathol* 19:718-726, 1995.

66. Arber DA, Rappaport H, Weiss LM: Non-Hodgkin's lymphoproliferative disorders involving the spleen, *Mod Pathol* 10:18-32, 1997.

67. Bairey O, Zimra Y, Rabizadeh E et al: Expression of adhesion molecules on leukemic B cells from chronic lymphocytic leukemia patients with predominantly splenic manifestations, *Isr Med Assoc J* 6:147-151, 2004.

68. Hartmann TN, Grabovsky V, Wang W et al: Circulating B-cell chronic lymphocytic leukemia cells display impaired migration to lymph nodes and bone marrow, *Cancer Res* 69:3121-3130, 2009.

69. Kansal R, Ross CW, Singleton TP et al: Histopathologic features of splenic small B-cell lymphomas: a study of 42 cases with a definitive diagnosis by the World Health Organization classification, *Am J Clin Pathol* 120:335-347, 2003.

70. Bende RJ, Smit LA, van Noesel CJ: Molecular pathways in follicular lymphoma, *Leukemia* 21:18-29, 2007.

71. Gandhi MK, Marcus RE: Follicular lymphoma: time for a rethink? *Blood Rev* 19:165-178, 2005.

72. Howard MT, Dufresne S, Swerdlow SH et al: Follicular lymphoma of the spleen: multiparameter analysis of 16 cases, *Am J Clin Pathol* 131:656-662, 2009.

73. Mollejo M, Rodriguez-Pinilla MS, Montes-Moreno S et al: Splenic follicular lymphoma: clinicopathologic characteristics of a series of 32 cases, *Am J Surg Pathol* 33:730-738, 2009.

74. Narang S, Wolf BC, Neiman RS: Malignant lymphoma presenting with prominent splenomegaly: a clinicopathologic study with special reference to intermediate cell lymphoma, *Cancer* 55:1948-1957, 1985.

75. Pittaluga S, Verhoef G, Criel A et al: "Small" B-cell non-Hodgkin's lymphomas with splenomegaly at presentation are either mantle cell lymphoma or marginal zone cell lymphoma: a study based on histology, cytology, immuno-histochemistry, and cytogenetic analysis, *Am J Surg Pathol* 20:211-223, 1996.

76. van Krieken JH: Histopathology of the spleen in non-Hodgkin's lymphoma, *Histol Histopathol* 5:113-122, 1990.

76a. Orchard J, Garand R, Davis Z et al: A subset of t(11;14) lymphoma with mantle cell features displays mutated IgVH genes and includes patients with good prognosis, nonnodal disease, *Blood* 101:4975-4981, 2003.

76b. Fernandez V, Salamero O, Espinet B et al: Genomic and gene expression profiling defines indolent forms of mantle cell lymphoma, *Cancer Res* 70:1408-1418, 2010.

77. Akhtar S, El Weshi A, Abdelsalam M et al: Primary refractory Hodgkin's lymphoma: outcome after high-dose chemotherapy and autologous SCT and impact of various prognostic factors on overall and event-free survival—a single institution result of 66 patients, *Bone Marrow Transplant* 40:651-658, 2007.

78. Gupta R, Jain P, Bakshi S et al: Primary Hodgkin's disease of spleen: a case report, *Indian J Pathol Microbiol* 49:435-437, 2006.

79. Midorikawa Y, Kubota K, Mori M et al: Advanced primary Hodgkin's disease of the spleen cured by surgical resection: report of a case, *Surg Today* 29:367-370, 1999.

80. Picardi M, Soricelli A, Pane F et al: Contrast-enhanced harmonic compound US of the spleen to increase staging accuracy in patients with Hodgkin lymphoma: a prospective study, *Radiology* 251:574-582, 2009.

81. Rueffer U, Sieber M, Stemberg M et al: Spleen involvement in Hodgkin's lymphoma: assessment and risk profile, *Ann Hematol* 82:390-396, 2003.

82. Lefor AT: Laparoscopic interventions in lymphoma management, *Semin Laparosc Surg* 7:129-139, 2000.

83. Falk S, Muller H, Stutte HJ: Hodgkin's disease in the spleen: a morphological study of 140 biopsy cases, *Virchows Arch A Pathol Anat Histopathol* 411:359-364, 1987.

CHAPTER 7

Adrenal Lymphomas

Judith A. Ferry

PRIMARY ADRENAL LYMPHOMAS

SECONDARY ADRENAL INVOLVEMENT
BY LYMPHOMA

■ PRIMARY ADRENAL LYMPHOMAS

Clinical Features

Primary adrenal lymphoma is defined as lymphoma that arises in the adrenal gland. Some authorities require that the lymphoma be confined to the adrenal glands, whereas others consider cases to be acceptable as primary adrenal lymphoma even if other sites of disease are present, so long as the dominant site of disease is the adrenals.[1,2]

Primary adrenal lymphoma is a rare disease; Freeman's series of 1467 extranodal lymphomas makes no mention of adrenal lymphoma.[3] Affected patients are adults in the third to ninth decades of life, and the median age is in the seventh decade.[2,4,5] A male to female ratio of 2-3:1 is seen.[4-6] A disproportionate number of cases are reported from Asia, but whether primary adrenal lymphoma actually is more prevalent among Asians is not clear. Rare patients are HIV positive,[7] and several have had autoimmune disorders[8,9]; however, the disease has no known specific predisposing factors.

Patients present with abdominal pain, fever, night sweats, or weight loss.[2,5-7,9,10] Review of the literature reveals that approximately half of all patients have had manifestations of adrenal insufficiency (including hyperpigmentation, weakness, hyponatremia, and hyperkalemia) and that nearly all such patients have bilateral adrenal involvement.[6,8,10] In a more recent series of 10 adrenal lymphomas, however, only one patient had adrenal insufficiency,[2] which suggests that this manifestation of adrenal lymphoma may not be as common as previously thought.

A variety of radiographic techniques, including ultrasound, computed tomography (CT), and magnetic resonance imaging (MRI), can be used to detect these tumors, which have a tendency to show hemorrhage, necrosis, and/or calcification and also can appear cystic radiographically.[11]

Pathologic Features

Primary adrenal lymphoma characteristically produces bulky masses,[1,2,12] which are larger than 10 cm in greatest dimension in most cases.[2] Almost all well-documented cases have been diffuse large B-cell lymphomas, although rare cases of peripheral T-cell lymphoma also have been reported.[1,4-8,10-12] Individual cases of EBV+ plasmablastic lymphoma,[2] Burkitt's lymphoma,[1] and follicular lymphoma, grade 2, with diffuse areas[1] have been described. Rare cases of rapidly fatal extranodal natural killer (NK)/T-cell lymphoma, nasal type, have been reported.[2,13] We have seen an unusual case of adrenal low-grade B-cell lymphoma with prominent plasmacytic differentiation in an elderly woman who presented with systemic symptoms and an adrenal mass (Figure 7-1). Adrenal diffuse large B-cell lymphomas typically have a non-germinal center B-cell immunophenotype (CD10−, bcl6+/−, MUM1/IRF4+).[2] In one study, approximately 38% of diffuse large B-cell lymphomas

were positive for Epstein-Barr virus by in situ hybridization.[7] In another study, however, only one of eight cases of diffuse large B-cell lymphoma not otherwise specified (NOS) was clearly EBV+.[2] Additional study is required to determine the significance and prevalence of EBV in adrenal lymphomas. When fluorescence in situ hybridization (FISH) is used, rearrangements of the *BCL6* gene appear to be common, whereas translocations involving immunoglobulin heavy chain (*IGH*) are found in only a minority of cases. Rearrangements of *MYC* and *BCL2* have not been documented,[2] although few cases have been studied. Mutations of the genes for p53 and c-kit are common, which suggests that they may be involved in the pathogenesis of adrenal lymphoma.[4]

Staging, Treatment, and Outcome

In up to approximately 75% of cases, both adrenals are involved, often without detectable disease outside the adrenals.[5,7,8] When staging reveals other sites of involvement, these sites often are extranodal; they include abdominal and retroperitoneal structures, such as the kidneys, liver, and pancreas, as well as the central nervous system and bone marrow in occasional cases.[1] The adrenal tumors may invade directly into surrounding structures.[14]

The prognosis traditionally is considered poor, and in some cases the diagnosis is not even established until autopsy.[8,12] The best outcome appears to be associated with combination chemotherapy, with possible benefit from the addition of rituximab, and, with bilateral adrenalectomy, corticosteroid replacement therapy.[5,6,9,10]

Even with modern therapy, the prognosis is guarded. In one series of 15 cases treated with combination chemotherapy, five patients were free of disease at last follow-up and 10 had died. Eight of the 10 who succumbed to lymphoma did so within 2 years of diagnosis.[1] In another series that included eight cases of diffuse large B-cell lymphoma NOS and one case of plasmablastic lymphoma, at last follow-up one patient was alive and well, one was alive with lymphoma, one had died of other causes, and six had died of lymphoma within 1 year of diagnosis.[2] A number of patients have had progression or relapse in the central nervous system.[1,2,11]

Differential Diagnosis

Diagnosis can be challenging, particularly on a small biopsy specimen. Other neoplasms that may involve the adrenals include metastatic carcinoma, metastatic melanoma, and primary adrenal cortical and medullary neoplasms. Primary adrenal cortical neoplasms and pheochromocytomas are composed of cells that typically are larger than lymphoma cells and that have abundant cytoplasm. For other neoplasms in the differential diagnosis, as in other sites, an accurate clinical history and careful evaluation of routinely stained slides, in addition to immunohistochemistry, can establish a diagnosis.

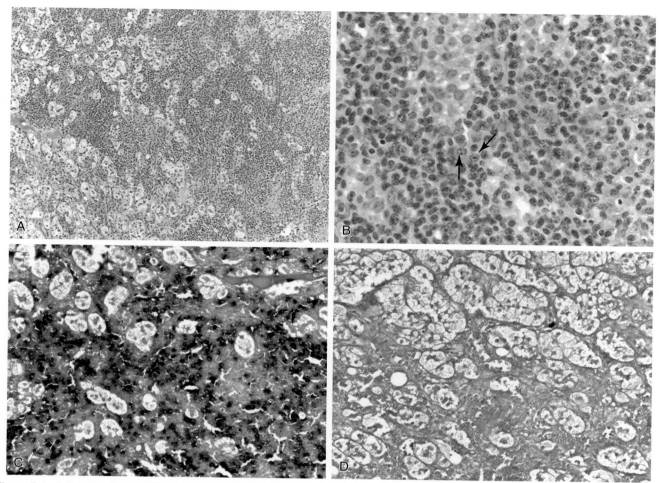

Figure 7-1   B-cell lymphoma with plasmacytic differentiation. **A,** Low-power view shows a dense infiltrate of lymphoid cells with scattered islands of residual pale adrenal cortical cells. **B,** High-power view shows a predominance of small lymphocytes with occasional plasma cells *(arrows)* and a few large cells. **C** and **D,** In situ hybridization for kappa and lambda shows monotypic staining of plasma cells for kappa **(C),** with only rare lambda-positive cells **(D).** (In situ hybridization on paraffin sections.) Most of the lymphocytes were B cells; a minority were T cells (not shown).

■ SECONDARY ADRENAL INVOLVEMENT BY LYMPHOMA

Secondary involvement of the adrenal gland by lymphoma is much more common than primary adrenal lymphoma. Up to 25% of patients with non-Hodgkin's lymphoma who die of lymphoma have adrenal involvement at autopsy.[5] Adrenal involvement can be found at presentation with widespread disease[12] or at relapse of lymphoma arising in a variety of sites. The adrenal gland can be directly invaded by lymphoma that arises in the kidney (see

Figure 8-2, *D*). Diffuse large B-cell lymphoma is a common type in the setting of secondary adrenal involvement.[12,15,16] We have recently seen a case of lymphomatoid granulomatosis that presented with lung nodules and an adrenal mass; the diagnosis was established on the basis of an adrenalectomy specimen (Figure 7-2). (Lymphomatoid granulomatosis is discussed in detail in Pulmonary Lymphomas in Chapter 4.) As is true of primary adrenal lymphoma, extensive bilateral involvement in the setting of disseminated lymphoma can be associated with adrenal insufficiency.[16]

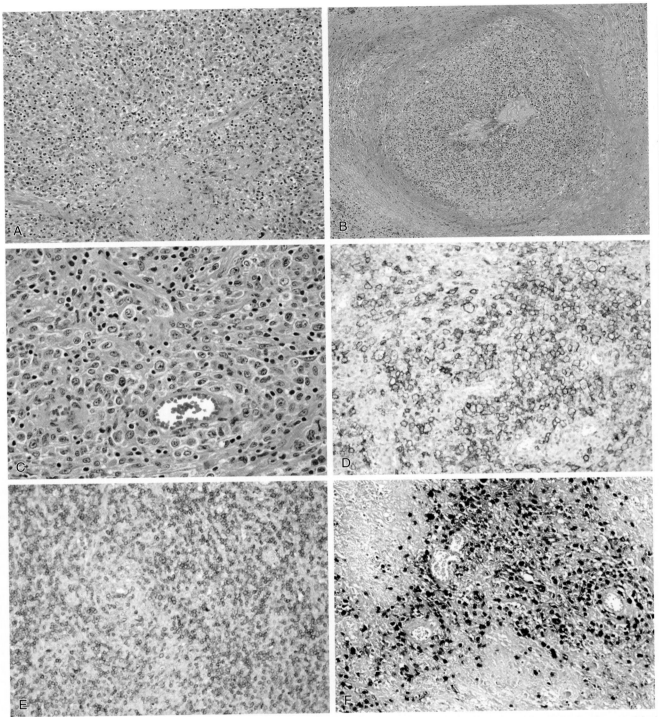

Figure 7-2   Lymphomatoid granulomatosis, grade 3. **A,** The adrenal has been replaced by an infiltrate of small lymphocytes, immunoblasts, and histiocytes surrounding an area of necrosis; the appearance is vaguely granulomatous. **B,** This large blood vessel has been extensively infiltrated by lymphoid cells. **C,** A small blood vessel is surrounded by lymphoid cells; numerous large lymphoid cells are present. **D,** CD20 highlights many B cells, which range in size but often are large. **E,** CD3 stains many small T cells. (*D* and *E,* immunoperoxidase technique on paraffin sections.) **F,** In situ hybridization for Epstein-Barr virus (Epstein-Barr–encoded RNA (EBER) probe) shows staining of numerous B cells, which tend to cluster around blood vessels. (In situ hybridization on a paraffin section.)

REFERENCES

1. Grigg A, Connors J: Primary adrenal lymphoma, *Clin Lymphoma* 4:154-160, 2003.
2. Mozos A, Ye H, Chuang WY et al: Most primary adrenal lymphomas are diffuse large B-cell lymphomas with non-germinal center B-cell phenotype, BCL6 gene rearrangement and poor prognosis, *Mod Pathol* 22:1210-1217, 2009.
3. Freeman C, Berg J, Cutler S: Occurrence and prognosis of extranodal lymphomas, *Cancer* 29:252-260, 1972.
4. Nakatsuka S, Hongyo T, Syaifudin M et al: Mutations of p53, c-kit, K-ras, and β-catenin in non-Hodgkin's lymphoma of adrenal gland, *Jpn J Cancer Res* 93:267-274, 2002.
5. Wu H, Shih L, Chen T et al: A patient with bilateral primary adrenal lymphoma, presenting with fever of unknown origin and achieving long-term disease-free survival after resection and chemotherapy, *Ann Hematol* 78:289-292, 1999.
6. Kim KM, Yoon DH, Lee SG et al: A case of primary adrenal diffuse large B-cell lymphoma achieving complete remission with rituximab-CHOP chemotherapy, *J Korean Med Sci* 24:525-528, 2009.
7. Ohsawa M, Tomita Y, Hashimoto M et al: Malignant lymphoma of the adrenal gland: its possible correlation with the Epstein-Barr virus, *Mod Pathol* 9:534-543, 1996.
8. Al-Fiar FZ, Pantalony D, Shepherd F: Primary bilateral adrenal lymphoma, *Leuk Lymphoma* 27:543-549, 1997.
9. Yamamoto E, Ozaki N, Nakagawa M, Kimoto M: Primary bilateral adrenal lymphoma associated with idiopathic thrombocytopenic purpura, *Leuk Lymphoma* 35:403-408, 1999.
10. Fujiwara T, Kawamura M, Sasaki A et al: Transient spontaneous regression of aggressive non-Hodgkin's lymphoma confined to the adrenal glands, *Ann Hematol* 80:561-564, 2001.
11. Hahn JS, Choi HS, Suh CO, Lee WJ: A case of primary bilateral adrenal lymphoma (PAL) with central nervous system (CNS) involvement, *Yonsei Med J* 43:385-390, 2002.
12. Singh D, Kumar L, Sharma A et al: Adrenal involvement in non-Hodgkin's lymphoma: four cases and review of literature, *Leuk Lymphoma* 45:789-794, 2004.
13. Thompson MA, Habra MA, Routbort MJ et al: Primary adrenal natural killer/T-cell nasal type lymphoma: first case report in adults, *Am J Hematol* 82:299-303, 2007.
14. Zhang L, Talwalkar SS, Shaheen SP II: A case of primary unilateral adrenal Burkitt-like large cell lymphoma presenting as adrenal insufficiency, *Ann Diagn Pathol* 11:127-131, 2007.
15. Park CK, Miller C, Lawrence G: Addison's disease from non-Hodgkin's lymphoma with normal-size adrenal glands, *J Clin Oncol* 25:2322-2324, 2007.
16. Levy N, Young WJ, Habermann T et al: Adrenal insufficiency as a manifestation of disseminated non-Hodgkin's lymphoma, *Mayo Clin Proc* 72:818-822, 1997.

CHAPTER 8

Lymphomas of the Urinary Tract

Judith A. Ferry

■ LYMPHOMAS OF THE KIDNEY

Primary Renal Lymphomas

Introduction

Renal involvement by lymphoma in the setting of widespread disease is common,[1] but lymphoma confined to one or both kidneys is rare.[2] Many cases reported in the literature as primary renal lymphoma are lymphomas that present primarily with renal involvement, even though the disease is not always limited to the kidney. Renal lymphoma accounts for approximately 0.7% of all extranodal lymphomas.[3]

Clinical Features

Patients mostly are middle-aged or older adults, and the mean age is in the sixth decade. A slight male preponderance is seen.[4-15] A few cases also have been described in children, and a few patients have been HIV positive.[7] A number of cases of post-transplantation lymphoproliferative disorders that affect the allograft in iatrogenically immunosuppressed renal allograft recipients have been reported.[16] In some cases, patients with renal lymphoma also have had other malignancies, autoimmune diseases, or other disorders[4,5,7,8,17]; however, the renal lymphomas have been a variety of different types, and the associated conditions could have occurred by chance. Except for the tendency of post-transplantation lymphoproliferative disorders to involve the renal allograft, predisposing conditions specific for renal lymphoma have not been defined.

Patients present with flank pain, loss of appetite, nausea, hematuria, fever, weight loss, or fatigue. They also may have renal insufficiency, particularly with bilateral renal involvement.[6-8,10,14,15,18-20] Cases with diffuse interstitial bilateral renal involvement are most likely to be associated with acute renal failure.[20] In contrast, intravascular large B-cell lymphoma with prominent glomerular involvement causes acute renal failure somewhat less often but may result in proteinuria that may be sufficient to cause nephrotic syndrome (see also Intravascular Large B-Cell Lymphoma in Chapter 14).[20,21] Most transplant recipients with post-transplantation lymphoproliferative disorders that involve the allograft present with fever and graft dysfunction.[16] In rare cases, renal lymphoma is an incidental finding.[8,22]

Pathologic Features and Clinicopathologic Correlation

Most patients (approximately three fourths) have unilateral renal lymphoma.[4,6-8,10] Nephrectomy specimens reveal one or more lesions ranging from less than 5 cm to massive. Lymphoma may be associated with discrete lesions or with diffuse enlargement of the kidney and obliteration of the renal parenchyma. A minority appear to arise from the renal pelvis (Figure 8-1). The lesions may be fleshy or firm and yellow, gray, or tan. Frequently the tumors invade adjacent tissues, including perinephric fat, the psoas muscle, and even the pancreas and duodenum. Vascular or ureteral encasement and sometimes compression by the lymphoma may occur. Extension into the renal vein and even the inferior vena cava has been described, analogous to renal cell carcinoma.[6-8,12,22,23]

The most common renal lymphoma is the diffuse large B-cell type, which accounts for slightly more than half of the cases.* The remainder are a variety of low- and high-grade types that are nearly always of B-lineage; they include extranodal marginal zone lymphoma of mucosa-associated lymphoid tissue (MALT lymphoma) (see Figure 8-1 and Figure 8-2)[10,19,25-27]; follicular lymphoma, sometimes with diffuse areas[8,23]; and lymphoplasmacytic, lymphoblastic, and Burkitt's lymphomas.[4,6-8,11,13,27] A case of ALK+ anaplastic large cell lymphoma confined to one kidney has been described.[12] Lymphomas in HIV-positive patients have been diffuse large B-cell or Burkitt's lymphomas.[7] Children with renal lymphoma usually have Burkitt's lymphoma, B-lymphoblastic lymphoma or, less often, T-lymphoblastic lymphoma.[2,7,28]

Post-transplantation lymphoproliferative disorders (PTLDs) that involve the renal allograft most often are monomorphic B-lineage PTLDs consistent with diffuse large B-cell lymphoma. Polymorphic B-lineage PTLDs also have been described.[16] We recently encountered a case of an EBV+ polymorphic PTLD with the features of a diffuse large B-cell lymphoma that involved an allograft and other sites. It developed 3 months after transplantation and resulted in the patient's death after only 2 months (Figure 8-3) (also see Table 5-1, Post-Transplantation Lymphoproliferative Disorders).

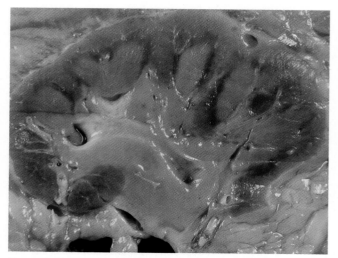

Figure 8-1 Extranodal marginal zone lymphoma of mucosa-associated lymphoid tissue (MALT lymphoma) arising in the kidney. Fleshy, light tan tumor fills the renal pelvis, distorting the calyces. Much of the cortex is spared.

*References 2, 6, 8, 14, 15, and 24.

Patients with renal diffuse large B-cell lymphoma occasionally have had other malignancies before, at the same time as, or after the diagnosis of lymphoma. One patient with hepatitis C virus infection[24] and one with a previous diagnosis of multicentric Castleman's disease[17] each developed renal diffuse large B-cell lymphoma. Bilateral renal diffuse large B-cell lymphoma has been reported in a patient with systemic lupus erythematosus who was treated with methotrexate.[29] The large B-cell lymphomas have

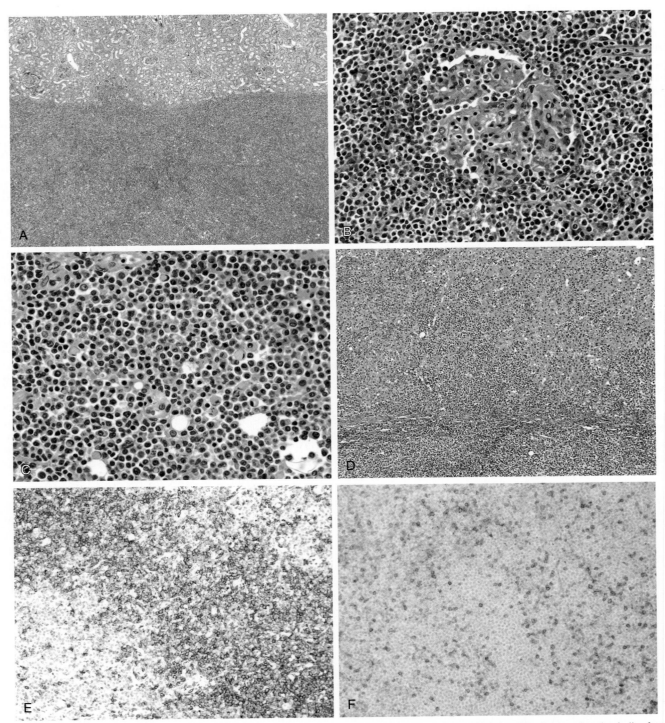

Figure 8-2 Extranodal marginal zone lymphoma arising in the kidney. **A,** In this case, lymphoma mainly involves the renal cortex in the form of a dense, diffuse infiltrate of lymphoid cells. **B,** The lymphoma is composed of small lymphoid cells and many plasma cells, in this field surrounding and invading a glomerulus. **C,** Plasmacytic differentiation is prominent. Numerous plasma cells are present, including many with Dutcher bodies (intranuclear protrusions of cytoplasm containing immunoglobulin) and large cytoplasmic immunoglobulin inclusions. **D,** The lymphoma invaded perinephric fat as well as the adrenal gland; residual adrenal parenchyma is present in the upper part of this image. The lymphoma is composed predominantly of CD20+ B cells **(E),** with scattered admixed small CD3+ T cells **(F).**

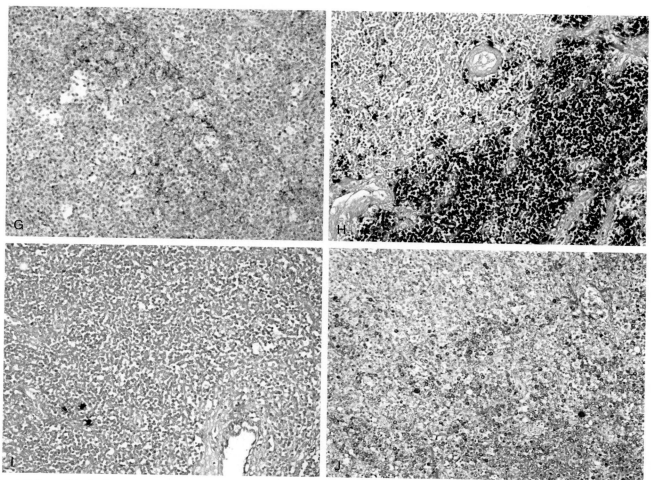

Figure 8-2, cont'd   G, Occasional remnants of CD21+ dendritic meshworks are present, consistent with the presence of underlying lymphoid follicles. The plasmacytic component expresses monotypic kappa immunoglobulin light chain **(H)**, with only rare lambda-positive cells **(I)** (in situ hybridization on paraffin sections). **J,** Plasma cells co-express mu heavy chain, shown here. Thus, this lymphoma expresses monotypic IgMκ. This lymphoma was associated with an IgM paraprotein, raising the question of lymphoplasmacytic lymphoma. Presentation as a localized extranodal lesion and the presence of follicular dendritic meshworks favored extranodal marginal zone lymphoma over lymphoplasmacytic lymphoma. (*E* to *G* and *J*, Immunoperoxidase technique on paraffin sections.)

an appearance similar to that of diffuse large B-cell lymphoma that arises elsewhere. They may be composed of centroblasts, although in rare cases they have a spindle cell morphology or an admixture of large bizarre cells. Tumor cells are CD20+.[8,15]

Patients with extranodal marginal zone lymphoma occasionally have had an autoimmune disease or some other source of chronic inflammation, including Sjögren's syndrome,[30] sarcoidosis,[22] another malignancy,[26] previous nephrotic syndrome,[31] and others; however, many patients have had no other concurrent illness that would predispose to the development of lymphoma.[25]

As in other sites, marginal zone lymphoma in the kidney is composed of marginal zone cells with slightly irregular nuclei and clear cytoplasm, sometimes with a component of plasma cells, plasmacytoid cells, or monocytoid B cells (see Figure 8-2). Reactive lymphoid follicles may be interspersed. Neoplastic B cells may infiltrate the renal tubules to form lymphoepithelial lesions. Neoplastic cells

are CD20+, CD5−, CD10−, CD23−, bcl6−, and cyclin D1−, with monotypic surface immunoglobulin (best detected if fresh tissue is available for evaluation) and with monotypic cytoplasmic immunoglobulin in cases with plasmacytic differentiation (see Figure 8-2, *H* to *J*).[22,25,31] Large cell transformation has been reported.[30]

Staging, Treatment, and Outcome

Only a minority of patients presenting with lymphoma primarily involving the kidney have Ann Arbor stage I disease. Staging reveals disseminated disease in most patients.[6-10] The renal insufficiency found in some cases of bilateral renal lymphoma usually responds promptly to chemotherapy, but patients with bilateral disease tend to have a worse prognosis than those with unilateral renal lymphoma, and some patients eventually succumb to the lymphoma despite a good initial response to therapy.[7,9,20,32] Historically, renal diffuse large B-cell

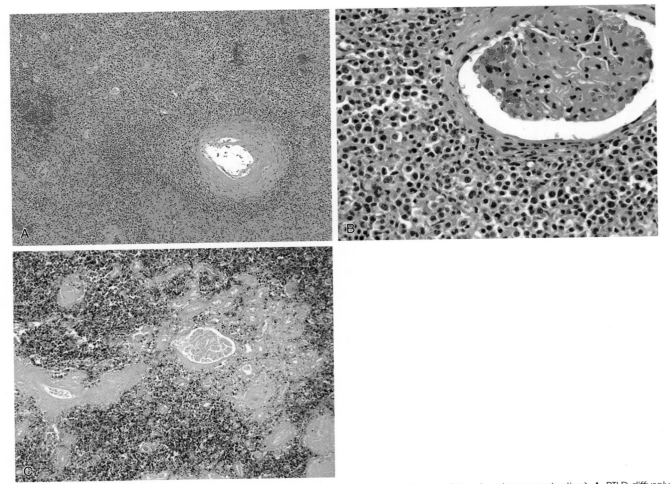

Figure 8-3 Post-transplantation lymphoproliferative disorder (PTLD) involving a renal allograft (postmortem examination). **A,** PTLD diffusely involves the renal parenchyma. **B,** The PTLD, shown here surrounding a glomerulus, comprises a polymorphous population of lymphoid cells with prominent plasmacytic differentiation. **C,** The cells of the PTLD are diffusely positive for Epstein-Barr virus. (In situ hybridization on a paraffin section, Epstein-Barr–encoded RNA (EBER) probe).

lymphoma has often behaved in an aggressive manner, but the prognosis may be improved with optimal therapy.*

As for other renal lymphomas, some marginal zone lymphomas have been localized to the kidney at presentation, but others have shown involvement of lymph nodes or other extranodal sites. Among the small number of patients with marginal zone lymphoma who have had follow-up, the outcome has varied. Some are alive and disease free at last follow-up; some are alive with disease; and a few have died of lymphoma.[10,22,26,30,31] In one remarkable case, the patient experienced a total of eight relapses in a wide variety of extranodal sites over 13 years. The relapses were treated with radiation, and the patient was well at last follow-up.[25] Allograft recipients with lymphoma confined to the transplanted kidney appear to have a favorable prognosis.[16] Too few cases of other types of renal lymphoma have occurred to draw definite conclusions about the prognosis.

Differential Diagnosis

Renal lymphomas, particularly when unilateral, may be mistaken clinically and radiographically for renal cell carcinomas* or transitional cell carcinomas.[31,33] Less often, they may mimic metastases, polycystic kidney disease,[7] soft tissue tumors,[34] or inflammatory lesions,[34] including unusual infectious diseases.[33] Lymphoma is more likely than renal cell carcinoma to be bilateral; therefore, bilateral disease may suggest lymphoma preoperatively.[8] The distinction is important, because other renal neoplasms often are treated with nephrectomy, which is not required as therapy for lymphoma. Diffuse bilateral renal involvement that presents with renal insufficiency can mimic medical renal disease clinically.[20] Lymphoma generally can be readily distinguished from the entities in the clinical differential diagnosis on microscopic examination.

---

*References 6, 8, 15, 17, 24, 29, and 32.

*References 5, 7, 8, 15, 17-19, and 31.

Secondary Renal Involvement by Lymphoma

Secondary involvement of the kidneys by lymphoma, including renal involvement in the setting of wide-spread disease[1] and relapse in the kidney, is more common than primary renal lymphoma. Among individuals who die of lymphoma, renal involvement is even more prevalent. Disease more often is bilateral than unilateral, often with multiple nodules in each kidney. Lymphoma less often secondarily involves the kidney by direct extension from retroperitoneal sites of involvement. The lymphoma may be asymptomatic, or it may extensively involve the kidney and perinephric tissues, resulting in renal insufficiency or vascular or ureteral compression.[35,36] The lymphomas are a variety of types.[36,37]

■ URETERAL LYMPHOMAS

One or both ureters occasionally are involved by lymphoma. Patients present with abdominal pain, nausea and vomiting, dysuria, hematuria, and/or fever. Ureteral obstruction may develop, with hydroureter, hydronephrosis, and renal insufficiency.[7,38-43] Primary ureteral lymphoma is exceedingly unusual, but rare unilateral and bilateral cases have been described[39-41]; cases have been subclassified as diffuse large B-cell lymphoma[27,40] and follicular lymphoma with diffuse areas.[41]

Ureteral involvement by lymphoma usually is found in the setting of widespread disease or retroperitoneal lymphoma with compression or invasion of the ureters, and the involvement can be unilateral or bilateral.[44] Lymphoma that involves retroperitoneal lymph nodes or arises from the kidney or the genital tract,[38,42,43,45] especially the uterine cervix (see Uterine Lymphomas in Chapter 10) may be associated with ureteral obstruction. Lymphoma that arises in the kidney also can extend to involve the ureter (Figure 8-4).

Diffuse large B-cell lymphoma is the most common lymphoma to secondarily involve the ureters, although other types, including Burkitt's lymphoma,[43] have been described. The differential diagnosis of lymphoma that affects the ureter includes other malignancies and nonneoplastic processes, particularly retroperitoneal fibrosis.[46] Retroperitoneal fibrosis is characterized by a chronic inflammatory cell infiltrate, often including reactive lymphoid follicles and plasma cells, with sclerosis. A subset of cases of retroperitoneal fibrosis appears to be part of the spectrum of IgG4-associated sclerosing disease; these cases have increased numbers of IgG4+ plasma cells and are likely to show eosinophils and obliterative phlebitis.[46] Lymphomas in the retroperitoneum can be associated with marked sclerosis, and crush artifact may obscure cytologic detail, making differentiation of lymphoma and retroperitoneal fibrosis difficult. A dense, diffuse lymphoid infiltrate, cytologic atypia of lymphoid cells, and the presence of many B cells outside lymphoid follicles suggest lymphoma.

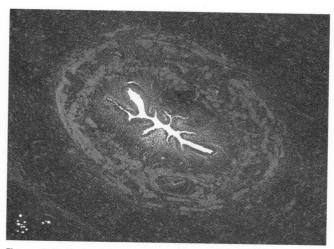

Figure 8-4 Ureteral involvement by renal lymphoma. The lymphoma has invaded from the renal pelvis, surrounding and infiltrating the wall of the ureter (same case as shown in Figure 8-1).

■ LYMPHOMAS OF THE URINARY BLADDER

Primary Lymphoma of the Urinary Bladder

Primary lymphoma of the urinary bladder may be defined as lymphoma that arises in the urinary bladder, with presenting symptoms related to the bladder and the bulk of the disease within the bladder, without direct extension from lymphoma involving adjacent organs. Primary non-Hodgkin's lymphoma of the bladder accounts for fewer than 1% of neoplasms in this site and for 0.2% of all extranodal lymphomas.[47,48] Among lymphomas that involve the bladder, an estimated 17% are primary and the remainder involve the bladder at the time of presentation in the setting of widespread disease or at the time of relapse.[49]

Clinical Features

In contrast to most lymphomas, primary bladder lymphoma predominantly affects women. Most patients are older adults; the age range is 22 to 85 years, and the mean age is in the sixties.[7,47,49-51] Patients present with hematuria, urinary frequency, and dysuria. Some have ureteral outlet obstruction. Analogous to the pathogenesis of extranodal marginal zone lymphomas in other sites, marginal zone lymphomas in the bladder may be related to previous inflammatory disease, because a number of patients have a history of chronic cystitis or bacteriuria.[7,47-49,52]

Pathologic Features

Cystoscopic or gross pathologic examination reveals single, occasionally multiple, submucosal, exophytic, sessile nodules that range from less than 1 cm to 15 cm. Diffuse mucosal thickening also has been described. Sectioning usually reveals pale, firm tissue, although some tumors are soft and vary in color.[7,49,53] Invasion of the muscularis is common, but the lymphoma does not usually invade beyond the bladder.[7,54] Infiltration of surrounding structures typically is minor, compared with that expected in a carcinoma of comparable size.[55] In a few cases, lymphoma obstructs the ureteral outlet.[7]

Most cases are extranodal marginal zone lymphomas of mucosa-associated lymphoid tissue (MALT lymphomas).[7,49,51,52,56] The histologic features are similar to those seen in other sites: a diffuse or vaguely nodular proliferation of marginal zone cells with oval to slightly irregular nuclei and pale cytoplasm, as well as small lymphocytes, often with admixed reactive lymphoid follicles and sometimes with follicular colonization and numerous plasma cells. As in other sites, the lymphomas are composed of CD20+ B cells that lack CD5 and CD10 expression and have a low proliferation index (Figure 8-5).

Lymphoepithelial lesions may form in association with cystitis cystica,[57] cystitis glandularis,[47,49,51] and transitional surface epithelium.[50] Associated follicular cystitis sometimes is seen. A minority of cases are diffuse large B-cell lymphomas; some of them may represent large cell transformation of an underlying marginal zone lymphoma.[27,50,54,56,58] Other types of lymphoma are rare. Burkitt's lymphoma in an HIV-positive man has been described,[59] and a case of primary follicular lymphoma also has been reported.[27] Peripheral T-cell lymphoma in a patient with long-standing schistosomiasis has been reported.[60]

Staging, Treatment, and Outcome

Nearly all patients have Ann Arbor stage I disease at presentation,[7,49,51,57] which indicates that bladder lymphoma has a tendency to remain localized for a long time. Treatment has changed over time. Earlier cases often were treated with surgical excision, sometimes involving radical cystectomy, or even anterior pelvic exenteration, with or without radiation.[7] More recent cases have managed with biopsy or limited resection followed by chemotherapy, with or without radiation.[7,51] Rare marginal zone lymphomas have been treated successfully with antibiotics.[52,61]

The prognosis is favorable, because bladder lymphoma tends to be localized, and it frequently is low grade and responsive to therapy.[7,49-51] The outlook for patients with marginal zone lymphoma is very good. The diffuse large B-cell lymphomas may behave in a more aggressive manner.

Differential Diagnosis

The main entities in the differential diagnosis of lymphoma of the bladder are marked chronic inflammation and carcinoma,[7] including small cell carcinoma, lymphoepithelioma-like carcinoma, and poorly differentiated transitional cell carcinoma. The distinction is critical because of differences in treatment and prognosis; in general, lymphoma that arises in the bladder has a better prognosis than carcinoma.[58]

1. **Small cell carcinoma versus lymphoma.** Small cell carcinoma rarely arises in the bladder; its frequency is similar to that of lymphoma, and it mainly affects older adults. In contrast to lymphoma, small cell carcinoma shows a male preponderance. Careful attention to histologic features should reveal at least some areas with cohesive growth and nuclear molding, providing evidence against lymphoma.

2. **Lymphoepithelioma-like carcinoma versus lymphoma.** Lymphoepithelioma-like carcinoma is rare in the bladder. Microscopic examination reveals syncytial aggregates of large cells in a background of small lymphocytes.[58] Immunostains using antibody to cytokeratin can help establish a diagnosis by highlighting the malignant epithelial cells. Occasional transitional cell carcinomas are associated with a marked lymphoid infiltrate that is not as striking as that of lymphoepithelioma-like carcinoma but that can still partially obscure the carcinoma.[62]

3. **Poorly differentiated transitional cell carcinoma, including plasmacytoid transitional cell carcinoma, versus lymphoma.** Infrequently, transitional cell carcinomas grow in a diffuse pattern with little intervening stroma, an appearance that could suggest lymphoma.[62] In the rare variant known as *plasmacytoid transitional cell carcinoma,* neoplastic cells have eccentric nuclei, which may mimic plasma cells or plasmacytoid lymphoid cells.[62-64] Plasmacytoid transitional cell carcinomas typically are associated with high-stage disease, high-grade histologic features, and a poor prognosis.

   Factors that favor a diagnosis of carcinoma are: at least some areas of cohesive growth, the presence of carcinoma in situ, and cytokeratin staining of the neoplastic cells. Like normal and neoplastic plasma cells, plasmacytoid transitional cell carcinoma often is CD138+[63,64]; if a broader panel of immunostains, including cytokeratin, is not performed, the CD138 positivity could lead to a misdiagnosis of plasmacytic neoplasm.

4. **Low-grade lymphomas versus chronic cystitis.** Low-grade lymphomas may be mistaken for chronic inflammatory disorders.[7,51] The presence of a mass lesion composed mainly of B cells suggests lymphoma; plasma cells that express monotypic immunoglobulin confirm the diagnosis. Histologically, chronic inflammation (including the lymphoid infiltrate associated with carcinomas)[62] usually is marked by the presence mainly of T cells, often with a component of polytypic plasma cells.

5. **Lymphoma versus spindle cell neoplasms.** Some lymphomas, including occasional diffuse large B-cell lymphomas and rare anaplastic large cell lymphomas, have a spindle cell morphology, which raises the question of sarcoma, sarcomatoid

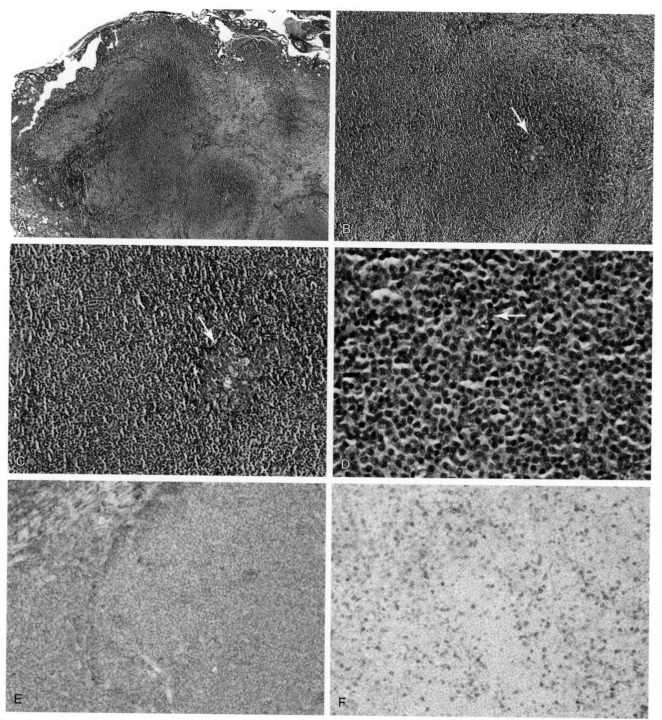

Figure 8-5 Extranodal marginal zone lymphoma arising in the urinary bladder. **A,** Low-power view shows a vaguely nodular proliferation of lymphoid cells replacing this portion of the bladder wall. **B,** Slightly higher power view shows ill-defined zones of cells with an increased amount of clear cytoplasm. The arrow indicates a small reactive follicle center. **C,** Higher power view shows that the reactive follicle center (arrow) is composed of cells that overall are larger and more variable in size than the surrounding smaller marginal zone cells. Tingible body macrophages are admixed with the follicle center cells. **D,** The marginal zone cells are small, oval to minimally irregular, uniform cells with pale cytoplasm. Only rare large cells with vesicular nuclei and prominent nucleoli (arrow) are present. **E,** Numerous cells are CD20+. **F,** Scattered admixed T cells are CD5+; the neoplastic B cells are negative for CD5.

Continued

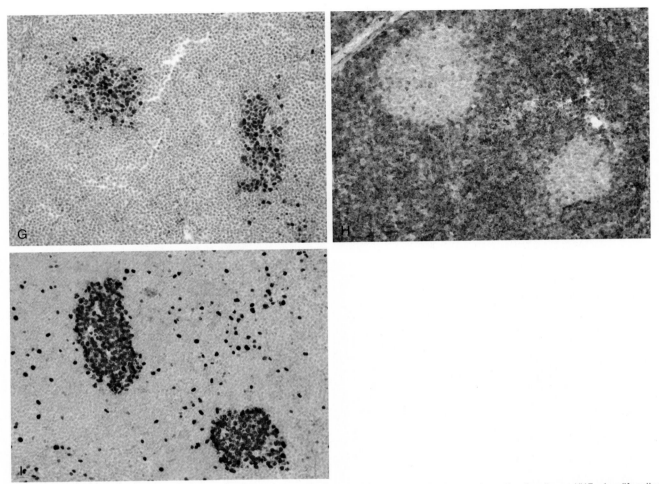

Figure 8-5, cont,d   G to I, The interspersed reactive follicle centers are bcl6+ **(G)** and bcl2– **(H),** and nearly all cells are Ki67+ (proliferation **(I)).** The neoplastic marginal zone cells are bcl6– and bcl2+; they have a low proliferation index. (*E* to *I,* Immunoperoxidase technique on paraffin sections.)

carcinoma, or inflammatory myofibroblastic tumor. Sarcomatoid carcinomas may be accompanied by carcinoma in situ of the intact urothelium and may show cohesive growth of tumor cells at least in some areas.

Inflammatory myofibroblastic tumor poses special problems in the differential diagnosis. It is composed of a variably cellular proliferation of stellate cells or spindle cells, sometimes with an admixture of lymphocytes, plasma cells, and eosinophils. Mitoses may be present. It can involve a wide variety of sites, but one of the more frequently involved sites is the urinary tract.[65] Inflammatory myofibroblastic tumors present with a variety of symptoms, including fever, weight loss, mass effect, and, in the urinary tract, hematuria. In the bladder, inflammatory myofibroblastic tumor often takes the form of a polypoid lesion, for which a cut surface shows pale, firm tissue. A subset of cases is positive for ALK protein (typically cytoplasmic). Lymphomas with a spindle cell pattern show more striking cytologic atypia and express lymphoid-associated antigens. ALK+ anaplastic large cell lymphoma expresses

CD30 diffusely and strongly, and ALK usually is nuclear and cytoplasmic. Familiarity with the entity of inflammatory myofibroblastic tumor helps prevent its misdiagnosis as lymphoma. A carefully chosen panel of immunostains can help establish a diagnosis.

Secondary Involvement of the Urinary Bladder by Lymphoma

The bladder can be involved secondarily by lymphoma that arises in lymph nodes[49] or other extranodal sites[49] in the setting of disseminated disease, by direct extension from adjacent structures, or at relapse. Secondary involvement is much more common than primary bladder lymphoma, and in contrast to primary bladder lymphoma, a male predominance is seen.[49] In this setting, non-Hodgkin's lymphomas of various types can affect the bladder. Diffuse large B-cell lymphoma is most common, followed by follicular lymphoma (Figure 8-6) and then by marginal zone lymphoma; other types are uncommon. The prognosis is much less favorable than for primary lymphoma of the bladder.[49,50]

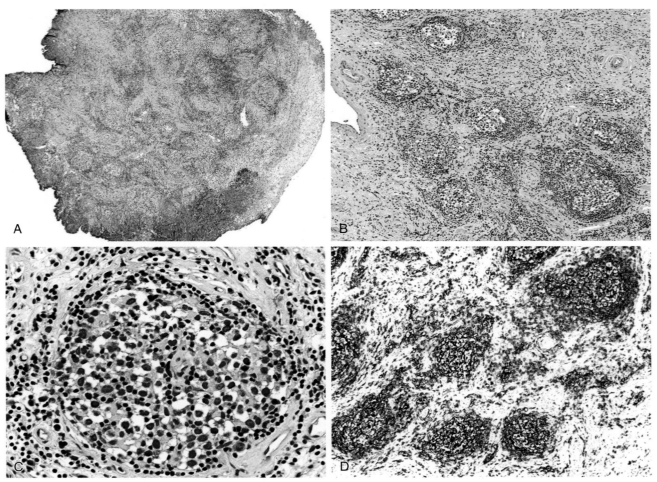

Figure 8-6 Urinary bladder involvement by follicular lymphoma, grade 3B. The patient had a large pelvic mass associated with invasion of the bladder, with urinary obstruction and renal failure. **A,** Biopsy sample of the bladder shows a mottled lymphoid infiltrate involving the bladder wall. **B,** Higher power view shows that the infiltrate is composed of poorly formed, ill-defined lymphoid follicles with attenuated mantles; the infiltrate is associated with sclerosis. **C,** The follicles are composed of solid aggregates of large cells, consistent with follicular lymphoma, grade 3B. **D,** An immunostain for CD20 highlights the follicular pattern of the lymphoma. (Immunoperoxidase technique on a paraffin section.)

Rare cases of widespread ALK+ anaplastic large cell lymphoma that presents with bladder involvement,[66,67] including a case with sarcomatoid features,[68] have been described. Hodgkin's lymphoma involving the bladder is rare; however, a well-documented case of Epstein-Barr virus–positive, classical Hodgkin's lymphoma in an elderly woman who presented with symptoms related to bladder involvement has been described. The bladder contained a large ulcerated tumor; however, the patient also had lymphadenopathy, and the bladder involvement likely was secondary.[69]

■ URETHRAL LYMPHOMAS

Lymphoma rarely arises in the urethra, the portion of the lower urinary tract least often involved by lymphoma. Despite its rarity, primary urethral lymphoma shows distinctive clinical and pathologic features. As does lymphoma of the bladder, urethral lymphoma tends to affect older patients, and

a female preponderance is seen.[7,70-74] Rare patients have been HIV positive or have had an autoimmune disease, but most have no predisposing conditions for the development of lymphoma.[7,75] Patients present with hematuria, dysuria, obstructive symptoms, or a mass. The lesions range from 1.5 to 7 cm in greatest dimension. The neoplasm often is a polypoid mass, although occasional tumors are infiltrative. In women the mass often protrudes from the urethral meatus, mimicking a caruncle.[7,54,72,76]

Diffuse large B-cell lymphoma accounts for about half of cases[*]; in one case, the lymphoma was positive for Epstein-Barr virus.[77] Other cases have been diagnosed as extranodal marginal zone lymphoma.[76] A number of urethral lymphomas have been reported using older classification systems, but the descriptions suggest that some are marginal zone lymphoma.[7,72,73] Nearly all lymphomas have been localized at presentation (Ann Arbor stage I or occasionally stage II).[73,77]

---

[*]References 70, 71, 74, 75, 77, and 78.

Based on the small number of reported cases, localized urethral lymphoma appears to have a good prognosis, particularly in cases of marginal zone lymphoma,[7,70,71,73] although some large cell lymphomas have resulted in the patient's death.[75] Suspecting urethral lymphoma before biopsy is difficult, but the diagnosis usually is straightforward when adequate tissue is obtained. The differential diagnosis is similar to that of lymphoma of the urinary bladder. Polypoid lymphomas with surface erosion and admixed inflammatory cells could mimic a caruncle pathologically as well as clinically.[79]

The urethra also may be involved in the setting of widespread disease.[78] Urethral relapse of lymphoma that arose outside the urinary tract has been reported.[80]

REFERENCES

1. Yunus SA, Usmani SZ, Ahmad S, Shahid Z: Renal involvement in non-Hodgkin's lymphoma: the Shaukat Khanum experience, *Asian Pac J Cancer Prev* 8:249-252, 2007.
2. Stallone G, Infante B, Manno C et al: Primary renal lymphoma does exist: case report and review of the literature, *J Nephrol* 13:367-372, 2000.
3. Freeman C, Berg J, Cutler S: Occurrence and prognosis of extranodal lymphomas, *Cancer* 29:252-260.
4. Abbas Z, Johnston DA, Murray FE: Renal lymphoma: an unusual cause of extrahepatic biliary obstruction, *Postgraduate Med J* 72:617-618, 1996.
5. Ahmad AH, Maclennan GT, Listinsky C: Primary renal lymphoma: a rare neoplasm that may present as a primary renal mass, *J Urol* 173:239, 2005.
6. Dimopoulos MA, Moulopoulos LA, Constantinides C et al: Primary renal lymphoma: a clinical and radiological study, *J Urol* 155:1865-1867, 1996.
7. Ferry J, Young R: Malignant lymphoma of the genitourinary tract, *Curr Diagn Pathol* 4:145-169, 1997.
8. Ferry JA, Harris NL, Papanicolaou N, Young RH: Lymphoma of the kidney: a report of 11 cases, *Am J Surg Pathol* 19:134-144, 1995.
9. Okuno SH, Hoyer JD, Ristow K, Witzig TE: Primary renal non-Hodgkin's lymphoma: an unusual extranodal site, *Cancer* 75:2258-2261, 1995.
10. Parveen T, Navarro-Roman L, Medeiros L et al: Low-grade B-cell lymphoma of mucosa-associated lymphoid tissue arising in the kidney, *Arch Pathol Lab Med* 117:780-783, 1993.
11. Porcaro A, D'Amico A, Novella G et al: Primary lymphoma of the kidney: report of a case and update of the literature, *Arch Ital Urol Androl* 74:44-47, 2002.
12. Venizelos I, Rombis V, Tulupidis S, Garipidou V: Primary anaplastic large cell lymphoma of the kidney, *Leuk Lymphoma* 44:353-355, 2003.
13. Yasunaga Y, Hoshida H, Hashimoto M et al: Malignant lymphoma of the kidney, *J Surg Oncol* 64:207-211, 1997.
14. James TC, Shaikh H, Escuadro L, Villano JL: Bilateral primary renal lymphoma, *Br J Haematol* 143:1, 2008.
15. Kose F, Sakalli H, Mertsoylu H et al: Primary renal lymphoma: report of four cases, *Onkologie* 32:200-202, 2009.
16. Cobo F, Garcia C, Talavera P et al: Diffuse large B-cell lymphoma in a renal allograft associated with Epstein-Barr virus in the recipient: a case report and a review of lymphomas presenting in a transplanted kidney, *Clin Transplant* 22:512-519, 2008.
17. Onishi T, Yonemura S, Sakata Y, Sugimura Y: Renal lymphoma associated with Castleman's disease, *Scand J Urol Nephrol* 38:90-91, 2004.
18. Osborne BM, Brenner M, Weitzner S, Butler JJ: Malignant lymphoma presenting as a renal mass: four cases, *Am J Surg Pathol* 11:375-382, 1987.
19. Tuzel E, Mungan MU, Yorukoglu K et al: Primary renal lymphoma of mucosa-associated lymphoid tissue, *Urology* 61:463, 2003.
20. Tornroth T, Heiro M, Marcussen N, Franssila K: Lymphomas diagnosed by percutaneous kidney biopsy, *Am J Kidney Dis* 42:960-971, 2003.
21. Kameoka Y, Takahashi N, Komatsuda A et al: Kidney-limited intravascular large B cell lymphoma: a distinct variant of IVL-BCL? *Int J Hematol* 89:533-537, 2009.
22. Qiu L, Unger PD, Dillon RW, Strauchen JA: Low-grade mucosa-associated lymphoid tissue lymphoma involving the kidney: report of 3 cases and review of the literature, *Arch Pathol Lab Med* 130:86-89, 2006.
23. Bozas G, Tassidou A, Moulopoulos LA et al: Non-Hodgkin's lymphoma of the renal pelvis, *Clin Lymphoma Myeloma* 6:404-406, 2006.
24. Kaya A, Kanbay M, Bayrak O et al: Primary renal lymphoma associated with hepatitis C virus infection, *Leuk Lymphoma* 47:1976-1978, 2006.
25. Jindal B, Sharma SC, Das A, Banerjee AK: Indolent behaviour of low-grade B cell lymphoma of mucosa-associated lymphoid tissue arising in the kidney, *Urol Int* 67:91-93, 2001.
26. Mita K, Ohnishi Y, Edahiro T et al: Primary mucosa-associated lymphoid tissue lymphoma in the renal pelvis, *Urol Int* 69:241-243, 2002.
27. Schniederjan SD, Osunkoya AO: Lymphoid neoplasms of the urinary tract and male genital organs: a clinicopathological study of 40 cases, *Mod Pathol* 22:1057-1065, 2009.
28. Olowu WA, Adelusola KA, Badmos KB, Aina OJ: Autopsy diagnosis of endemic Burkitt lymphoma as the primary etiology of acute renal failure in children, *Pediatr Hematol Oncol* 22:315-321, 2005.
29. Nasr SH, Alobeid B, Jacobs JM et al: Methotrexate-associated B-cell lymphoma presenting with acute renal failure and bilateral nephromegaly, *Kidney Int* 71:272-275, 2007.
30. Pelstring RJ, Essell JH, Kurtin PJ et al: Diversity of organ site involvement among malignant lymphomas of mucosa-associated tissues, *Am J Clin Pathol* 96:738-745, 1991.
31. Kato Y, Hasegawa M, Numasato S et al: Primary mucosa-associated lymphoid tissue–type lymphoma arising in the kidney, *Int J Urol* 15:90-92, 2008.
32. Morel P, Dupriez B, Herbrecht R et al: Aggressive lymphomas with renal involvement: a study of 48 patients treated with the LNH-84 and LNH-87 regimens, *Br J Cancer* 70:154-159, 1994.
33. Sheth S, Ali S, Fishman E: Imaging of renal lymphoma: patterns of disease with pathologic correlation, *Radiographics* 26:1151-1168, 2006.
34. Matsushima H, Fujita K, Kunitake T et al: Renal lymphoma: report of 2 cases and review of the literature, *Nippon Hinyokika Gakkai Zasshi* 83:1521-1524, 1992.
35. Eyre RC, Huberman MS, Balogh K: Non-Hodgkin's lymphoma of the kidney with inferior vena caval extension, *Urol Int* 51:43-45, 1993.
36. Davies J, Healey DA, Wood KM et al: Acute renal failure due to mantle cell lymphoma: a case report and discussion of the literature, *Clin Nephrol* 67:394-396, 2007.
37. Miyake O, Namiki M, Sonoda T, Kitamura H: Secondary involvement of genitourinary organs in malignant lymphoma, *Urol Int* 42:360-362, 1987.
38. Bhattachary V, Gammall MM: Case report: bilateral non-Hodgkin's intrinsic lymphoma of ureters, *Br J Urol* 75:673-674, 1995.
39. Lebowitz JA, Rofsky NM, Weinreb JC, Friedmann P: Ureteral lymphoma: MRI demonstration, *Abdom Imaging* 20:173-175, 1995.
40. Hashimoto H, Tsugawa M, Nasu Y et al: Primary non-Hodgkin lymphoma of the ureter, *BJU Int* 83:148-149, 1999.
41. Kubota Y, Kawai A, Tsuchiya T et al: Bilateral primary malignant lymphoma of the ureter, *Int J Clin Oncol* 12:482-484, 2007.
42. Buck DS, Peterson MS, Borochovitz D, Bloom EJ: Non-Hodgkin lymphoma of the ureter: CT demonstration with pathologic correlation, *Urol Radiol* 14:183-187, 1992.
43. Comiter S, Glasser J, Al-Askari S: Ureteral obstruction in a patient with Burkitt's lymphoma and AIDS, *Urology* 39:277-280, 1992.
44. Scharifker D, Chalasani A: Ureteral involvement by malignant lymphoma, *Arch Pathol Metab Med* 102:541-542, 1978.

45. Stein A, Aghai E, Cohen O et al: Kidney conservation by delayed contralateral autotransplantation in a case of retroperitoneal lymphoma involving the ureter, *Urol Int* 55:167-168, 1995.

46. Zen Y, Onodera M, Inoue D et al: Retroperitoneal fibrosis: a clinicopathologic study with respect to immunoglobulin G4, *Am J Surg Pathol* 33:1833-1839, 2009.

47. Al-Maghrabi J, Kamel-Reid S, Jewett M et al: Primary low-grade B-cell lymphoma of mucosa-associated lymphoid tissue type arising in the urinary bladder: report of 4 cases with molecular genetic analysis, *Arch Pathol Lab Med* 125: 332-336, 2001.

48. Riccioni R, Carulli G, de Maria M et al: Primary lymphoma of the bladder: case report, *Am J Hematol* 81:77-78, 2001.

49. Kempton C, Kurtin P, Inwards D et al: Malignant lymphoma of the bladder: evidence from 36 cases that low-grade lymphoma of the MALT-type is the most common primary bladder lymphoma, *Am J Surg Pathol* 21:1324-1333, 1997.

50. Bates A, Norton A, Baithun S: Malignant lymphoma of the urinary bladder: a clinicopathological study of 11 cases, *J Clin Pathol* 53:458-461, 2000.

51. Pawade J, Banerjee SS, Harris M et al: Lymphomas of mucosa-associated lymphoid tissue arising in the urinary bladder, *Histopathology* 23:147-151, 1993.

52. Oscier D, Bramble J, Hodges E, Wright D: Regression of mucosa-associated lymphoid tissue lymphoma of the bladder after antibiotic therapy, *J Clin Oncol* 20:882, 2002.

53. Siegel RJ, Napoli VM: Malignant lymphoma of the urinary bladder: a case with signet-ring cells simulating urachal adenocarcinoma, *Arch Pathol Lab Med* 115:635-637, 1991.

54. Simpson RHW, Bridger JE, Anthony PP et al: Malignant lymphoma of the lower urinary tract: a clinicopathologic study with review of the literature, *Br J Urol* 65:254-260, 1990.

55. Bhansali SK: Primary malignant lymphoma of the bladder, *Br J Urol* 32:440-454, 1960.

56. Isaacson PG: Critical commentary to "Primary malignant lymphoma of the bladder," *Pathol Res Pract* 192:164-165, 1996.

57. Kuhara H, Tamura Z, Suchi T et al: Primary malignant lymphoma of the urinary bladder: a case report, *Acta Pathol Jpn* 40:764-769, 1990.

58. Leite K, Bruschini H, Camara-Lopes L: Primary lymphoma of the bladder, *Int Braz J Urol* 30:37-39, 2004.

59. Mearini L, Mearini E, Costantini E et al: Primary Burkitt's lymphoma of bladder in patient with AIDS, *Urol Int* 68:91-94, 2002.

60. Mourad W, Khalil S, Radwi A et al: Primary T-cell lymphoma of the urinary bladder, *Am J Surg Pathol* 22:373-377, 1993.

61. van den Bosch J, Kropman R, Blok P, Wijermans P: Disappearance of a mucosa-associated lymphoid tissue (MALT) lymphoma of the urinary bladder after treatment for *Helicobacter pylori*, *Eur J Haematol* 68:187-188, 2002.

62. Zukerberg LR, Harris NL, Young RH: Carcinomas of the urinary bladder simulating malignant lymphoma: a report of five cases, *Am J Surg Pathol* 15:569-576, 1991.

63. Nigwekar P, Tamboli P, Amin MB et al: Plasmacytoid urothelial carcinoma: detailed analysis of morphology with clinicopathologic correlation in 17 cases, *Am J Surg Pathol* 33:417-424, 2009.

64. Ro JY, Shen SS, Lee HI et al: Plasmacytoid transitional cell carcinoma of urinary bladder: a clinicopathologic study of 9 cases, *Am J Surg Pathol* 32:752-757, 2008.

65. Freeman A, Geddes N, Munson P et al: Anaplastic lymphoma kinase (ALK 1) staining and molecular analysis in inflammatory myofibroblastic tumours of the bladder: a preliminary clinicopathological study of nine cases and review of the literature, *Mod Pathol* 17:765-771, 2004.

66. Murphy AJ, O'Neill P, O'Brien F et al: Anaplastic large cell lymphoma: a unique presentation with urinary bladder involvement—a case report, *Int J Surg Pathol* 13:369-373, 2005.

67. Pai SA, Naresh KN, Patil PU: Systemic anaplastic large cell lymphoma presenting as a bladder neoplasm, *Leuk Lymphoma* 45:841-843, 2004.

68. Allory Y, Merabet Z, Copie-Bergman C et al: Sarcomatoid variant of anaplastic large cell lymphoma mimics ALK-1–positive inflammatory myofibroblastic tumor in bladder, *Am J Surg Pathol* 29:838-839, 2005.

69. de Leval L, Jardon-Jeghers C, Gennigens C, Boniver J: Hodgkin's lymphoma presenting as a bladder tumour, *Haematologica* 91:ECR03, 2006.

70. Hatcher PA, Wilson DD: Primary lymphoma of the male urethra, *Urology* 49:142-144, 1997.

71. Hofmockel G, Dammrich J, Manzanilla Garcia H et al: Primary non-Hodgkin's lymphoma of the male urethra: a case report and review of the literature, *Urol Int* 55:177-180, 1995.

72. Kakizaki H, Nakada T, Sugano O et al: Malignant lymphoma in the female urethra, *Int J Urol* 1:281-282, 1994.

73. Kitamura H, Umehara T, Miyake M et al: Non-Hodgkin's lymphoma arising in the urethra of a man, *J Urol* 156:175-176, 1996.

74. Richter LA, Hegde P, Taylor JA III: Primary non-Hodgkin's B-cell lymphoma of the male urethra presenting as stricture disease, *Urology* 70:1008.e11-1008.e12, 2007.

75. Lopez AE, Latiff GA, Ciancio G, Antun R: Lymphoma of the urethra in a man with acquired immune deficiency syndrome, *Urology* 42:596-598, 1993.

76. Masuda A, Tsujii T, Kojima M et al: Primary mucosa-associated lymphoid tissue (MALT) lymphoma arising from the male urethra: a case report and review of the literature, *Pathol Res Pract* 198:571-575, 2002.

77. Ohsawa M, Mishima K, Suzuki A et al: Malignant lymphoma of the urethra: report of a case with detection of Epstein-Barr virus genome in the tumour cells, *Histopathology* 24:525-529, 1994.

78. Vapnek JM, Turzan CW: Primary malignant lymphoma of the female urethra: report of a case and review of the literature, *J Urol* 147:701-703, 1992.

79. Young RH, Oliva E, Saenz Garcia JA et al: Urethral caruncle with atypical stromal cells simulating lymphoma or sarcoma—a distinctive pseudoneoplastic lesion of females: a report of six cases, *Am J Surg Pathol* 20:1190-1195, 1996.

80. Melicow MM, Lattes R, Pierre-Louis C: Lymphoma of the urethra masquerading as a caruncle, *J Urol* 108:748-749, 1972.

CHAPTER 9

Lymphomas of the Male Genital Tract

Judith A. Ferry

■ TESTICULAR LYMPHOMAS

Primary Testicular Lymphomas

Introduction

In 1877, Malassez, a French physician, described the case of a man who presented with a left testicular mass. Pathologic examination after surgery revealed a tumor of "lymphadénome type, à réticulum fin, à petites cellules."[1] Within a few weeks, the patient developed progressive disease; he died 7 months after diagnosis with widespread disease, which included involvement of the skin and opposite testicle. Malassez's report is the first published description of primary testicular lymphoma.

Lymphoma that arises in the testis accounts for 1% to 2% of all lymphomas, for 4% of extranodal lymphomas, and for 5% of testicular neoplasms.[2,3] Although uncommon, it is the most frequent testicular neoplasm in men older than 50 years of age.[3] Children are only rarely affected.[4-8] Eighty percent to 90% of primary testicular lymphomas are the diffuse large B-cell type; other types are rare (Table 9-1).[2,9,10]

Diffuse Large B-Cell Lymphoma

Clinical Features

Testicular diffuse large B-cell lymphoma is predominantly a disease of older adults, although in rare cases young adults and even teenagers are affected (Figures 9-1 and 9-2). In most large series, the mean or median age is in the sixties.[2,3,6,9-16] Recent epidemiologic analysis suggests that testicular diffuse large B-cell lymphoma is more prevalent among white men than among black men.[16]

Nearly all testicular lymphomas arise sporadically with no specific predisposing factors, although a few patients have been infected with the human immunodeficiency virus (HIV).[9,11,17] One case report describes a rapidly fatal testicular diffuse large B-cell lymphoma in a man who was iatrogenically immunosuppressed, having received steroids and then azathioprine.[18] We have seen a plasmablastic lymphoma that occurred as a post-transplantation lymphoproliferative disorder in a patient status post cardiac transplantation (Figure 9-3; see also Lymphomas of the Oral Cavity in Chapter 3).

TABLE 9-1

Primary Testicular Lymphomas			
Parameter	Diffuse Large B-Cell Lymphoma	Follicular Lymphoma	Extranodal NK/T-Cell Lymphoma, Nasal Type
Frequency	80% to 90% of testicular lymphomas	Rare	Rare
Patients usually affected	Older men	Boys, young adults	Young, middle-aged, and older men
Histology	Diffuse infiltrate of large lymphoid cells; some intertubular spread at periphery of tumor; tubular invasion common; sclerosis common	Crowded, ill-defined neoplastic follicles, often with many large cells (follicular lymphoma, grade 3 of 3)	Diffuse infiltrate of small, medium-sized, and/or large atypical lymphoid cells; zonal necrosis common
Usual immunophenotype	CD20+, CD10−/+, bcl6+, bcl2+, MUM1/IRF4+, TdT−	CD20+, CD5−, CD10+/−, bcl6+, bcl2−, p53−, mib1/Ki67 high	CD2+, sCD3−, cCD3+, CD56+, TIA-1+, granzyme B+, perforin+, CD16−, CD57−, TdT−
Usual Epstein-Barr virus status of tumor	EBER−	EBER− in the rare cases tested	EBER+
Usual genetic features	Clonal IGH; absence of BCL2 rearrangement	Clonal IGH; absence of BCL2 rearrangement	Absence of clonal IGH and TCR rearrangement
Relapses	Common, often in extranodal sites, especially CNS and opposite testis; nodal relapses also common; relapses may occur many years after presentation	Not reported	Present in all reported cases, almost always to extranodal sites, especially GI tract, CNS, upper respiratory tract, and skin
Prognosis	Relatively poor; worse than for DLBCL arising in most other sites	Excellent, although few cases have long follow-up	Dismal; almost all patients die of the lymphoma in less than 1 year

CNS, Central nervous system; DLBCL, diffuse large B-cell lymphoma; EBER, Epstein-Barr–encoded RNA; GI, gastrointestinal; TCR, T-cell receptor; +, positive in the vast majority of cases; +/−, positive in most cases; −/+, positive in a minority of cases; −, negative in the vast majority of cases.

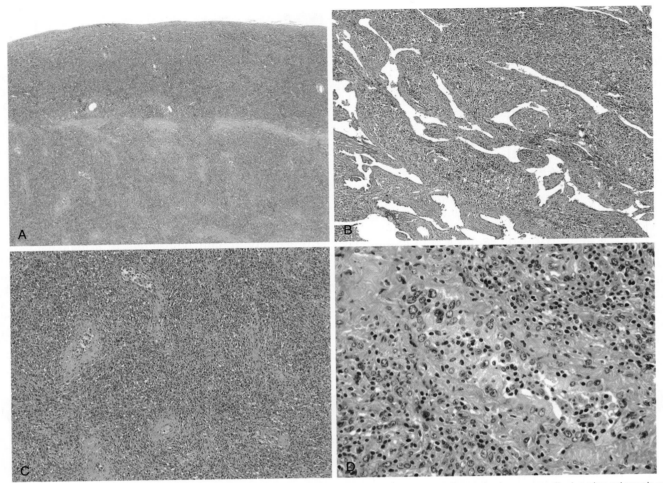

Figure 9-1   Testicular diffuse large B-cell lymphoma in a 65-year-old man. **A,** The lymphoma formed a large mass that replaced much of the testis and invaded the tunica albuginea *(top).* Scattered residual sclerotic seminiferous tubules are present. **B,** The lymphoma infiltrates the rete testis. **C,** The lymphoma in this area has an intertubular pattern; seminiferous tubules are atrophic with thickened, hyalinized walls. **D,** This tubule has been surrounded and invaded by large atypical lymphoid cells; a few cytologically bland Sertoli cells remain. Small lymphocytes are admixed with the large neoplastic lymphoid cells.

Patients typically present with a hard, painless, scrotal mass that usually is unilateral but may be bilateral. Lymphoma is thought to be the most common bilateral primary testicular tumor, although the frequency varies widely among different series; on average, approximately 10% to 15% of cases are bilateral.* In a minority of cases, patients present with constitutional symptoms (fever, weight loss, weakness, or anorexia)[3,4,13] or, in some patients with distant spread, with symptoms related to extratesticular disease (e.g., abnormal neurologic or ophthalmologic findings).[5] Ultrasound examination reveals a hypoechoic mass in the normally highly echogenic parenchyma of the testis.[17]

Pathologic Features

The diagnosis is almost always established on an orchiectomy specimen. Gross examination reveals a circumscribed, fleshy or firm, tan, pink, gray, or white tumor ranging in size from a few millimeters to 16 cm in greatest dimension (median, approximately 6 cm), which often has replaced most of the testis and invaded into or through the tunica albuginea (see Figure 9-1).[5,17] The epididymis is involved in most cases. In up to 40% of cases, the spermatic cord may be involved.[5]

On microscopic examination, the lymphomas typically obliterate the seminiferous tubules in at least some areas, with peripheral areas that may show intertubular spread of the tumor. In most cases, neoplastic cells invade some seminiferous tubules, occupying the periphery of the tubules and displacing germ cells and Sertoli cells centrally or filling the tubules completely. In one third of cases, the tumor is associated with sclerosis.[5] Most tumors are composed of centroblasts (large noncleaved cells), but some show a predominance of immunoblasts, large centrocytes (large cleaved cells), or multilobated lymphoid cells (see Figure 9-1). A few cases may show minor foci with neoplastic follicle formation.[5]

_____
*References 2, 3, 5, 12, 13, and 17.

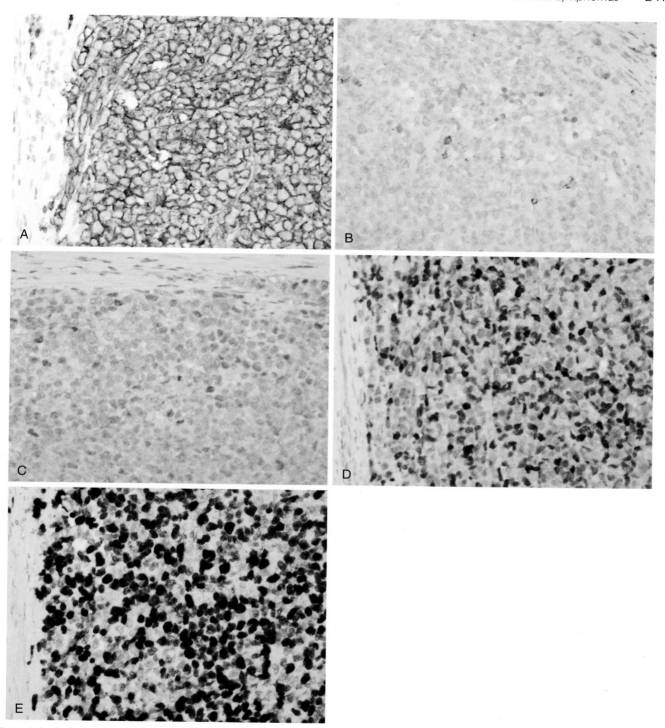

Figure 9-2 Testicular diffuse large B-cell lymphoma, usual immunophenotype. The large atypical lymphoid cells are CD20+ **(A)**, with a few admixed small T cells (CD2+ **(B)**). The large B cells are bcl6+/− **(C)** and MUM1/IRF4+ **(D)**, with approximately 80% Ki67+ **(E)** (immunoperoxidase technique on paraffin sections). In situ hybridization showed no evidence of Epstein-Barr virus in the neoplastic cells.

Immunohistochemical analysis reveals features that overlap with those of diffuse large B-cell lymphoma in other sites.[4-6] Leukocyte common antigen (CD45) and pan–B-cell markers (e.g., CD20) are diffusely strongly expressed. The proportion of cases expressing bcl6 in different series has been variable. bcl2 and MUM1/IRF4 each are detected by immunohistochemistry in 80% or more of cases; a minority of cases (17% in one series,[12] 6% in another[9]) are CD10+ (see Figure 9-2). Therefore, only a minority of primary testicular diffuse large B-cell lymphomas have a germinal center B-cell–like phenotype. Although the bcl2 protein usually is expressed, a translocation involving the *BCL2* gene typically is absent.[19]

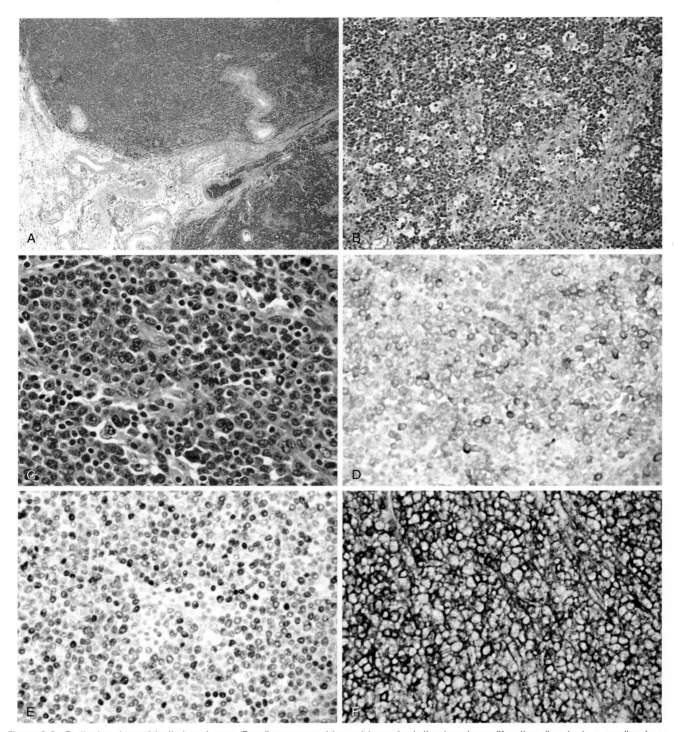

Figure 9-3 Testicular plasmablastic lymphoma /B-cell monomorphic post-transplantation lymphoproliferative disorder in a cardiac transplant recipient. This lymphoma initially was misdiagnosed as seminoma because of the appearance of the tumor cell nuclei and the lack of CD20 expression by tumor cells. **A,** Much of the testis is obliterated by a densely cellular infiltrate. A few seminiferous tubules remain within the lymphoma and around its periphery. **B,** Higher power view shows many scattered, pale histiocytes with apoptotic debris, imparting a starry sky pattern. **C,** Neoplastic cells are large and discohesive, with round to oval nuclei, prominent central nucleoli, and a scant to moderate amount of eosinophilic cytoplasm. Rare binucleated and multinucleated tumor cells are present. The neoplastic cells are CD79a+ **(D),** MUM1/IRF4+ **(E),** and CD138+ **(F).** They were negative for CD20 (not shown).

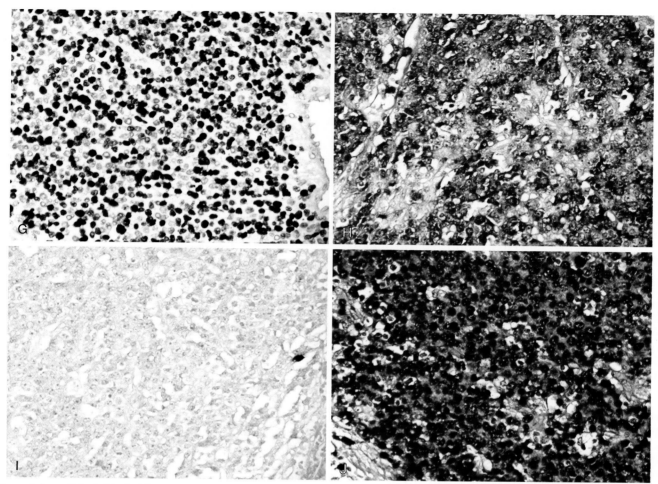

Figure 9-3, cont'd   G, Most of the tumor cells are Ki67+; a high proliferation fraction is characteristic of plasmablastic lymphoma. (*D* to *G*, Immunoperoxidase technique on paraffin sections.) Neoplastic cells express monotypic kappa immunoglobulin light chain **(H),** with only rare mature plasma cells expressing lambda light chain **(I)** (in situ hybridization on paraffin sections). **J,** Neoplastic cells harbor EBV, as is the case in most plasmablastic lymphomas and most post-transplantation lymphoproliferative disorders. (In situ hybridization for Epstein-Barr–encoded RNA (EBER) on a paraffin section.)

Plasmablastic lymphoma that presents in the testis has histologic and immunophenotypic features very similar to those in the oral cavity: large cells with the appearance of immunoblasts, plasmacytoid immunoblasts, or plasmablasts that are negative for CD20 and typically positive for markers expressed at a plasma cell stage of differentiation, such as MUM1/IRF4 and CD138. Most cases are positive for Epstein-Barr virus, as demonstrated by in situ hybridization for Epstein-Barr virus–encoded RNA (EBER).[20] The lack of CD20 may lead to failure to consider a diagnosis of lymphoma (see Figure 9-3).

Some have hypothesized that because testicular diffuse large B-cell lymphoma is a lymphoma that arises in an immunologically privileged site, it may have genetic features that distinguish it from diffuse large B-cell lymphomas that arise elsewhere.[21] In contrast to nodal diffuse large B-cell lymphoma, testicular diffuse large B-cell lymphoma commonly shows loss of chromosomal material on 6p, in the region of the human leukocyte antigen (HLA) genes, potentially leading to ineffective immune response to the tumor.[21] Often, testicular lymphoma also shows gains in the region of chromosome 19q13, although this change is uncommon in nodal diffuse large B-cell lymphoma.[21] Multiple genes reside on 19q13 that may play a role in the pathogenesis of testicular diffuse large B-cell lymphoma; for example, expression of high levels of *LILRA3*, a member of the leukocyte immunoglobulin–like receptor (*LILR*) gene family, could interfere with activation of tumor-infiltrating lymphocytes. *BCL2L12*, *PPP5C* and *PAK4* are thought to play a role in the inhibition of apoptosis. *SPIB*, the direct target of the B-cell transcription factor BOB1, also resides in this region.[21] Abnormalities affecting the p53 pathway likewise are common in testicular diffuse large B-cell lymphoma, although p53 pathway aberrations also are found, albeit somewhat less frequently, in nodal diffuse large B-cell lymphomas.[21]

Staging, Treatment, and Outcome

In approximately half of cases, patients have Ann Arbor stage I disease (lymphoma confined to the testis with or without involvement of adjacent structures). Approximately one fourth of patients have stage II disease (with involvement of lymph nodes below the diaphragm), and almost all of the remainder have stage IV disease (with involvement of other extranodal sites). Only a few have stage III disease.* In patients with stage IV disease, sites of disease found on staging include the bone marrow, bone, central nervous system (CNS), skin, orbit, gastrointestinal tract, and a variety of others.[3,5] In some series, bilateral testicular involvement was seen only at presentation in patients with widespread disease,[5,12] although other series identified some cases of bilateral testicular lymphoma in patients with limited stage disease.[2,3] Most patients have a low or low-intermediate risk according to the International Prognostic Index (IPI).[3,11,12,22]

Testicular diffuse large B-cell lymphoma has a relatively poor prognosis. Currently, therapy most often consists of orchiectomy followed by combination chemotherapy, with or without radiation to the opposite testis or other sites, sometimes combined with intrathecal therapy.[3,12] Approximately 80% of patients achieve complete remission; most of these are patients with limited stage disease. Patients with advanced stage disease achieve complete remission less often.† Most of those who do not attain complete remission die of lymphoma within 1 year.[3,6,10,12,13]

Even when the lymphoma is treated aggressively and the patient appears free of disease, relapses are relatively common and may continue to occur for many years after initial diagnosis; therefore, whether a patient is ever truly cured of the lymphoma is difficult to determine.[3,12,22] When relapses occur, they often involve extranodal sites, most often the central nervous system[3,6,14,23] but also the opposite testis, bone, lung, skin, Waldeyer's ring, liver, kidney, and other sites; relapses also may involve lymph nodes.[3,5,6,17] When spread to the CNS occurs, it more often is parenchymal than meningeal, in contrast to most other lymphomas with secondary involvement of the CNS.[3,12] Most relapses cannot be salvaged.[5,12] Although median survival as long as 96 months has been reported for patients with stage I disease,[9] in recent series, the median overall survival time for all patients is less than 5 years, and for patients presenting with advanced stage disease, it is only about 1 year.[3,6,12-14]

The prognosis for testicular diffuse large B-cell lymphoma usually is considered worse than for diffuse large B-cell lymphoma that arises in lymph nodes and in other extranodal sites, except for primary CNS diffuse large B-cell lymphoma (see Primary Central Nervous System Lymphomas in Chapter 2).[24] In one recent study, patients with testicular diffuse large B-cell lymphoma had better survival than patients with comparable lymph node lymphomas in the early years of follow-up. However, on longer follow-up, the tendency of testicular lymphoma patients to continue to experience relapses eliminated their apparent survival advantage.[16]

A number of clinical and pathologic features affect the prognosis of patients with large B-cell lymphoma. Advanced age, decreased serum albumin, and high lactate dehydrogenase (LDH) levels are associated with a poor prognosis.[3,16,22] Surprisingly, patients with stage I disease with right-sided tumors have been reported to have a better prognosis than those with left-sided tumors.[5,16] A favorable IPI score also is associated with a better prognosis.[3,12] Patients who present with localized disease have a significantly better outcome than those with widespread disease.[3,5,13,16,23] Sclerosis is associated with a favorable prognosis. In one study, patients who had lymphomas with sclerosis had a much better outcome than those who had lymphomas without sclerosis (72% and 16%, respectively, for the 5-year disease-free survival rate for all patients; 90% and 34%, respectively, for the 5-year disease-free survival rate for stage I patients).[5]

Optimal therapy remains controversial,[6,14] but an improved outcome has been associated with anthracycline-based chemotherapy. Administration of intrathecal chemotherapy or high-dose intravenous methotrexate appears to reduce the risk of CNS relapse, and scrotal irradiation appears to reduce the risk of relapse in the opposite testis.*

Follicular Lymphoma

In the rare cases in which boys develop primary testicular lymphoma, it most often is follicular lymphoma. Follicular lymphoma has been reported in adults but is far less common than diffuse large B-cell lymphoma in that age group.[2,25] Primary testicular follicular lymphoma that occurs in children and adults is a distinctive clinicopathologic entity. Based on the small number of cases reported, adult patients are mostly younger (under 35 years of age).[25] The children usually are in the first decade of life. Most have no other medical problems, although several have had hydroceles,[8,26] and in one case, there was hypospadias.[27] They present with unilateral testicular enlargement.

On gross examination most tumors are 2 to 4 cm, quite a bit smaller than the average testicular diffuse large B-cell lymphoma. The tumors form tan-gray or yellow-tan, firm to fleshy lesions that replace all or part of the testis.[8,26-30]

Microscopic examination shows poorly delineated follicles composed of large centrocytes, centroblasts, and/or multilobated lymphoid cells lacking mantles that displace or infiltrate between seminiferous tubules, sometimes associated with sclerosis within or around neoplastic follicles (Figure 9-4). In most cases, large cells are sufficiently numerous for a diagnosis of follicular lymphoma, grade 3 of 3. Some cases show focal diffuse areas. The tumor may be confined to the testis or may extend to involve the epididymis

---

*References 2, 3, 5, 6, 11-14, and 22.
†References 2, 3, 5, 6, 11-14, and 22.

*References 2, 3, 10, 12, 22, and 23.

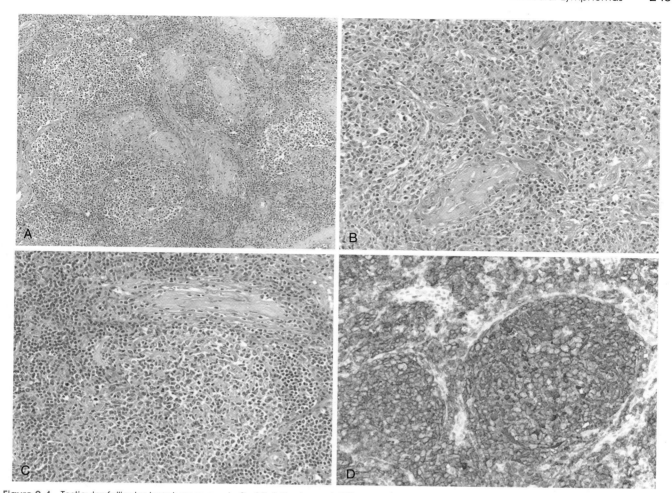

Figure 9-4   Testicular follicular lymphoma, grade 2 of 3, follicular and diffuse pattern. **A,** Ill-defined follicles have replaced much of the testicular parenchyma. The remaining seminiferous tubules are hyalinized. **B,** In some areas, the lymphoma has a diffuse pattern. **C,** Individual follicles are composed of irregular centrocytes and scattered, large centroblasts. This follicle is surrounded by small lymphocytes. **D,** An immunostain for CD20 highlights the follicular architecture of the lymphoma.

Continued

or, infrequently, the spermatic cord. In some cases many small lymphocytes are present between neoplastic follicles or around the periphery of the tumor.

Neoplastic cells are positive for CD20, usually express bcl6, and often express CD10; small T cells typically are present in an interfollicular pattern (see Figure 9-4, *D* to *F*).[8,25-30] Tumor cells lack bcl2 expression (see Figure 9-4, *G*) and, when tested, also lack p53 protein expression.[25-27,29,30] Proliferation, as assessed by mib1, is high.[26,30] *BCL2* rearrangement has been absent, although clonal rearrangement of the immunoglobulin heavy chain gene (*IGH*) usually can be demonstrated. Rearrangement of the *BCL6* gene was demonstrated in one case,[26] and mutations of *BCL6* were found in another.[30]

Patients almost always have localized disease (stage IE). They usually have been treated with orchiectomy combined with chemotherapy[8,25,26,28] or in rare cases with surgery alone.[27] Based on the small number of cases reported, the prognosis appears excellent, although follow-up sometimes is of limited duration, and no follow-up beyond 5 years has been reported.[8,25,28]

In contrast to nodal follicular lymphoma, therefore, testicular follicular lymphoma preferentially affects children and young adults, presents with localized disease, is typically grade 3, lacks expression of the bcl2 protein, lacks *BCL2* rearrangement, and may be curable with the currently available therapy. The cases with *BCL6* rearrangement and mutation raise the question of the role of the *BCL6* gene (rather than *BCL2*) in the pathogenesis of at least a subset of cases.

Extranodal NK/T-Cell Lymphoma, Nasal Type

A rare but distinctive type of testicular lymphoma that has an exceedingly poor prognosis is extranodal natural killer (NK)/T-cell lymphoma, nasal type.[31-34] Also, a case has been reported in which the closely related, aggressive NK-cell lymphoma/leukemia presented as a testicular tumor.[35] These neoplasms affect adults over a broad age range and have a predilection to affect Asians.

Patients present with unilateral or, in rare cases, bilateral[31] testicular enlargement, which is

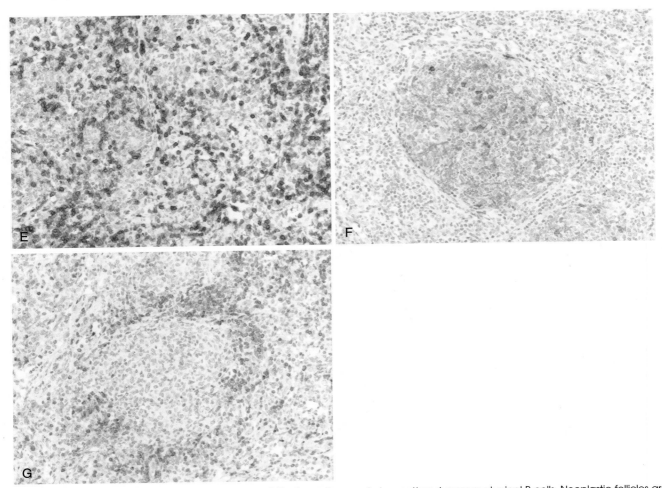

Figure 9-4, cont'd   E, CD3 stains small T cells in an interfollicular pattern and also scattered among atypical B cells. Neoplastic follicles are CD10+ **(F)** and bcl2– **(G).** (*D* to *G,* Immunoperoxidase technique on paraffin sections.)

accompanied in some cases by fever and weight loss. The pathologic features are similar to those of extranodal NK/T-cell lymphoma, nasal type, that occurs in other anatomic sites (see Extranodal NK/T-Cell Lymphoma, Nasal-Type, in Chapter 3). Orchiectomy reveals lymphoma composed of medium-sized to large (less often, small to medium-sized) atypical cells with irregular nuclei, granular chromatin, distinct nucleoli, and pale cytoplasm. Infiltration of seminiferous tubules, associated with reduplication of the basement membrane, may be seen. The tumors are associated with coagulative necrosis and may show angioinvasion and perineural invasion.

Immunophenotyping typically shows expression of CD3 on paraffin sections but not on frozen sections. The lymphomas also express CD2, CD56, and cytotoxic granule proteins (e.g., TIA-1, granzyme B, and perforin) but not B-cell antigens. In situ hybridization demonstrates Epstein-Barr virus (EBV) in tumor cells. The few cases studied have shown no clonal rearrangement of *IGH*. A small minority have clonal rearrangement of T-cell receptor genes (*TCR*); in conjunction with the results of immunophenotyping, this suggests a cytotoxic T-cell origin.[34] However, no clonal T-cell population has been detected

in most cases, consistent with an NK-cell origin (see Table 9-1).[31-33,35,36] Extranodal NK/T-cell lymphoma, nasal type, and aggressive NK-cell lymphoma/leukemia cannot be distinguished based on findings in the testis.

Staging sometimes shows disease confined to the testis[31,33-36] but may reveal involvement of other sites, particularly the nasal area[32]; this raises the question of whether some testicular NK/T-cell lymphomas actually represent spread from a primary in the upper aerodigestive tract.

Patients have been treated with surgery, radiation and/or chemotherapy. Most of these aggressive lymphomas have relapsed within 6 months of diagnosis with some even progressing during initial therapy. Nearly all patients are dead within a year. The extranodal NK/T-cell lymphomas, nasal type, spread to the CNS, gastrointestinal tract, skin and other extranodal sites.[31-33] The aggressive NK-cell lymphoma/leukemia spread to the spleen, marrow, and peripheral blood, a pattern typical of that entity.[35] Because CD56 is expressed in normal testis as well as in the skin, gastrointestinal tract, and spleen[33] and because CD56 has the capacity for homophilic binding, CD56 expression could play a role in the

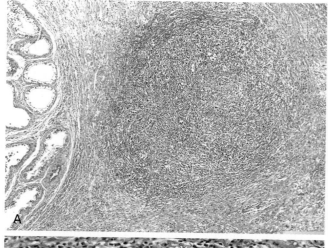

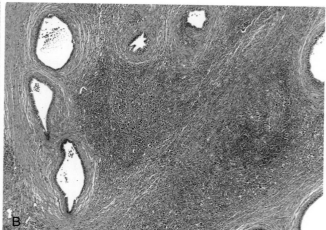

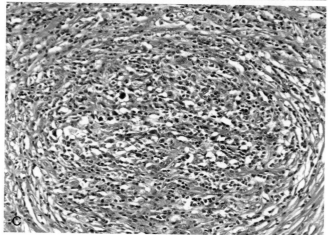

Figure 9-5 Nodular sclerosis classical Hodgkin's lymphoma involving the testis and epididymis. **A,** A cellular nodule surrounded by sclerosis is present adjacent to the epididymis. **B,** Poorly delineated aggregates of lymphocytes with scattered, large, dark atypical cells infiltrate the epididymis. **C,** Higher power view of a nodule shows lymphocytes, occasional eosinophils, and scattered large atypical cells. Tumor cells were CD30+ and rarely CD15+; they were negative for CD45, CD20, CD79a, CD3, CD5, and epithelial markers.

testicular presentation and pattern of spread of these lymphomas.[32,37]

Patients with testicular NK/T-cell lymphoma should have a careful otorhinolaryngeal examination, even in the absence of symptoms related to this site, to exclude an occult primary in the upper respiratory tract.[32]

Miscellaneous Primary Testicular Lymphomas

B-cell lymphomas that arise primary in the testis, other than those described previously, are exceptional, although rare cases of Burkitt's lymphoma[7] and B-lymphoblastic lymphoma[15] that presented with testicular involvement have been described. Only a few cases of T-lineage lymphoma have been described; these have included peripheral T-cell lymphoma not otherwise specified,[12,38] anaplastic large cell lymphoma,[39,40] and T-lymphoblastic lymphoma.[41] Convincing cases of testicular Hodgkin's lymphoma are vanishingly rare. We have seen one case of a patient who presented with a testicular mass that proved to be nodular sclerosis classical Hodgkin's lymphoma on examination of an orchiectomy specimen (Figure 9-5). The patient later was found to have ipsilateral inguinal and iliac lymphadenopathy; therefore, the Hodgkin's lymphoma

may have arisen in lymph nodes and involved the testis secondarily.[42]

Differential Diagnosis

1. **Lymphoma versus seminoma.** Misdiagnosis of testicular lymphoma is relatively common.[5,9] The most important entity in the differential diagnosis of testicular lymphoma is germ cell tumors, especially seminoma.[5] Misdiagnosis is especially likely for younger patients with testicular lymphoma (i.e., those in the age range typical for germ cell tumors).[9] Compared with seminoma, lymphoma is more often bilateral, is more likely to involve the epididymis and spermatic cord, and is more likely to metastasize to extranodal sites, such as the CNS.[5] Seminomas are composed of nests of neoplastic cells with abundant, pale, glycogen-rich cytoplasm and uniform oval, euchromatic nuclei that are often flattened along one side and have prominent nucleoli (Figure 9-6). Nests of neoplastic cells are delineated by fibrous septa that contain small lymphocytes and sometimes granulomas. Seminomas express Oct4 and placental alkaline phosphatase (PLAP).

2. **Lymphoma versus orchitis.** Testicular lymphomas, both diffuse large B-cell lymphoma

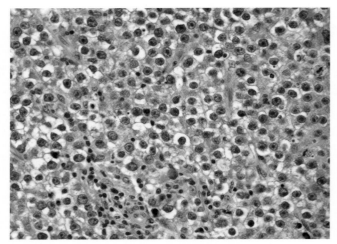

Figure 9-6 In this seminoma, neoplastic cells are large, with oval nuclei with finely stippled to smooth chromatin, large central nucleoli, and abundant, clear cytoplasm.

and follicular lymphoma, particularly those with prominent sclerosis and large numbers of admixed nonneoplastic lymphocytes, may suggest a diagnosis of orchitis, including bacterial or viral infection or granulomatous orchitis. Acute inflammation with abscess formation and well-formed granulomas tends to exclude lymphoma. The presence of atypical lymphoid cells, even if interspersed among small lymphocytes, indicates that lymphoma should be included in the differential diagnosis. Distinguishing testicular follicular lymphoma from orchitis may be difficult, but the presence of crowded follicles, non-polarized follicle centers, B-cell predominance, atypical B cells outside follicles, light chain restriction, and clonal *IGH* supports a diagnosis of lymphoma.

A distinctive type of orchitis has histologic features that resemble those of mumps orchitis, but it does not have a proven viral etiology; this entity has been designated *viral-type orchitis*. Viral-type orchitis is characterized by patchy inflammation, an intratubular infiltrate composed predominantly of histiocytes, and an intertubular infiltrate composed of small T cells and histiocytes with few admixed B cells. Variably conspicuous interstitial hemorrhage usually is seen. The parenchymal architecture is at most slightly distorted by the inflammation (Figure 9-7). The architectural preservation, predominant intratubular distribution of inflammation, cytologic features of the infiltrate, and immunophenotype readily exclude lymphoma.[43]

3. **Lymphoma versus plasmacytoma.** Testicular plasmacytomas are rare, and when they do occur, patients usually have or develop plasma cell myeloma (Figure 9-8).[44] Plasmacytoma occasionally can enter the differential diagnosis of lymphoma, but clinical and histologic features, augmented by immunophenotyping, establish a diagnosis. The neoplastic plasma cells typically

have a lower nuclear to cytoplasmic ratio than do the neoplastic cells of diffuse large B-cell lymphoma. They have eccentric nuclei, sometimes with clock face chromatin, and a recognizable paranuclear hof. Plasma cells typically are CD20−, CD138+, and cIg+, in contrast to neoplastic B cells (Figure 9-9). Plasmablastic lymphoma may be in the differential diagnosis of plasmacytoma in the testis, as well as other sites. Plasmablastic lymphoma typically occurs in individuals who are immunocompromised, usually because of HIV infection, and who do not have associated plasma cell myeloma. Plasmablastic lymphoma is composed predominantly of large lymphoid cells with a high proliferation fraction. Immunophenotypic overlap with plasmacytoma/plasma cell myeloma is seen, but plasmablastic lymphoma usually is EBV+, in contrast to plasmacytoma/plasma cell myeloma (compare Figures 9-3 and 9-9).

4. **Lymphoma versus myeloid sarcoma.** In rare cases the testis is involved by myeloid or monocytic sarcoma. When this occurs in a patient without a history of acute myeloid leukemia, myelodysplasia, or other myeloproliferative disorder, misdiagnosis as lymphoma is common. Myeloid sarcoma is composed of cells that overall are slightly smaller than those of diffuse large B-cell lymphoma and that have finer chromatin; in some cases, the cytoplasm has a pink blush, indicating the presence of myeloid granules. Immunophenotyping readily distinguishes between the two possibilities (Figure 9-10).[45-47]

Secondary Testicular Involvement by Lymphoma

Testicular involvement is infrequently found on staging in adult or pediatric patients with lymphoma arising in other sites. The testis occasionally is involved during relapse or progression of lymphoma arising in another site; this has been reported to be more common than primary testicular lymphoma.[17] The primary site may be in lymph nodes but often is an extranodal site, such as the sinonasal tract, skin, thyroid, or central nervous system.[4,5,48] The testis is among the most common sites for relapse of primary CNS lymphoma (Figure 9-11).[49]

Among adults, a variety of types of lymphoma may be encountered. The diffuse large B-cell type is the most common (Figure 9-12). Rare cases of involvement by follicular lymphoma have been reported.[50] We have seen a case of testicular involvement by lymphoplasmacytic lymphoma (Figure 9-13). In one case, the testis was the site of large cell transformation of a follicular lymphoma that arose in the tonsil.[51] Testicular involvement has been described during disease progression of an EBV+ plasmablastic lymphoma arising in an HIV-positive male.[52]

Up to approximately 5% of boys with non-Hodgkin's lymphoma have testicular involvement either at presentation or at relapse,[53] although the number of boys who develop relapses has declined substantially in recent years because of improvements in

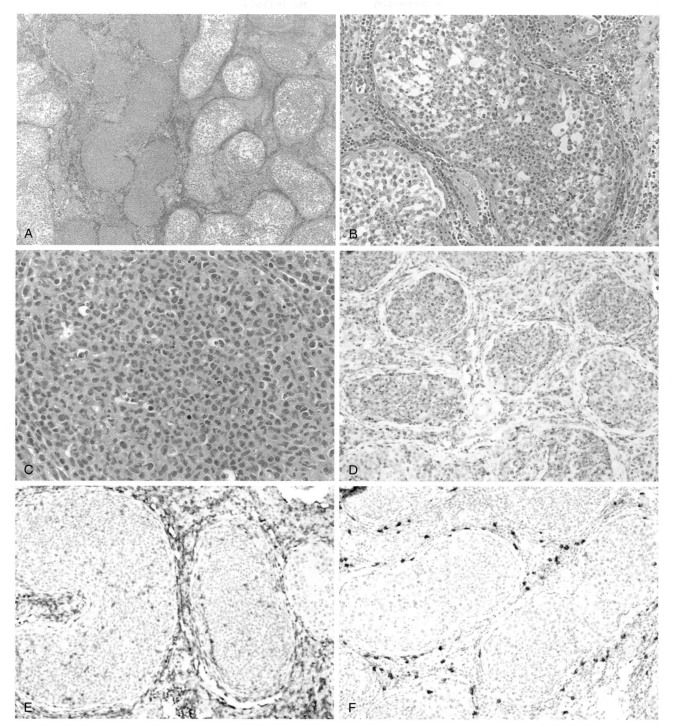

Figure 9-7 Viral-type orchitis. **A,** Low-power view of this orchiectomy specimen shows a zone of tubules heavily infiltrated by inflammatory cells alternating with tubules containing smaller numbers of inflammatory cells. Sparse interstitial hemorrhage also is present. The architecture is preserved. **B,** These tubules contain residual germ cells with many admixed inflammatory cells. The interstitium contains a sparse infiltrate of small lymphocytes and a small amount of extravasated blood. **C,** High-power view of a tubule shows numerous histiocytes with indented and folded nuclei and fine chromatin, along with scattered neutrophils and a few eosinophils. **D,** Most of the cells in the tubules are histiocytes (CD68+); CD68 also highlights intertubular histiocytes. Most of the lymphocytes are T cells (CD3+ **(E)**), present mainly in the interstitium. A few interstitial small B cells are present (CD20+ **(F)**). B cells are virtually absent in the tubules. (*D* to *F,* Immunoperoxidase technique on paraffin sections.)

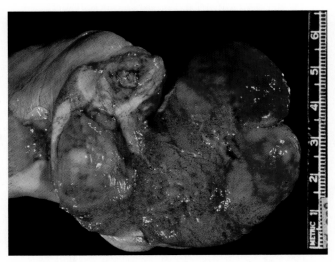

Figure 9-8 These testicular plasmacytomas were found at postmortem examination in a patient with plasma cell myeloma. Several white-tan and red nodules of tumor are present within the testis.

therapy. When lymphoma involves the testis at presentation, it typically is in the setting of widespread disease, and the testis is only rarely considered the primary site.[7,53] Whether found on initial staging or at relapse, the lymphoma usually is diffuse high-grade lymphoma, usually B-lineage, including Burkitt's lymphoma, diffuse large B-cell lymphoma and B or T lymphoblastic leukemia/lymphoma[7,53]; with currently available chemotherapy, lymphoma involving the testis often can be eliminated without orchiectomy. The testis is a fairly common site of involvement by endemic Burkitt's lymphoma; involvement was bilateral in one third of such cases in the experience of Dr. Burkitt.[54]

In general, the lymphomas have pathologic features similar to those of lymphomas in extratesticular sites. One report described that, in contrast to primary testicular lymphoma, lymphomas secondarily involving the testis were unlikely to invade the seminiferous tubules.[41]

■ EPIDIDYMAL LYMPHOMAS

Lymphoma that arises in the epididymis is rare. Only a few cases have been reported, all in adult men.[5,55-60] Patients with primary epididymal lymphoma present with a unilateral mass (although in one case the mass was bilateral).[57] Several of the younger patients (under 40 years of age) had lymphomas with sclerosis that were entirely or partially follicular (Figure 9-14).[4,5,25,57] One patient was reported to have a marginal zone lymphoma.[56] The remaining patients had diffuse large cell lymphoma (B-lineage when immunophenotyped).[4,55,58-60]

Staging in these cases usually has shown no disease spread beyond the epididymis. The number of cases reported is too small to allow definite conclusions to be drawn about behavior, but rare

epididymal lymphomas that occur in younger men appear to have a follicular component and relatively indolent behavior, analogous to testicular follicular lymphoma. The clinical and pathologic features of the remaining cases may be more akin to testicular diffuse large B-cell lymphoma. Direct extension into the epididymis by testicular lymphoma is much more common than primary epididymal lymphoma.[5] In rare cases, the epididymis is involved by disseminated lymphoma that arises in other sites.[57]

■ LYMPHOMAS OF THE SPERMATIC CORD

Lymphoma that arises in the spermatic cord is rare. Only 0.04% of non-Hodgkin's lymphomas present with involvement of the spermatic cord.[60-62] Patients' ages have ranged from 21 to 89 years; the mean age is in the 50s. The usual presentation is a hard, painless mass in the upper scrotum or the inguinal canal. The most common lymphoma is the diffuse large cell type (B-lineage when immunophenotyped)[60-62]; two cases have been intravascular lymphoma.[5,63]

One case of human herpes virus type 8 (HHV8+) immunoblastic lymphoma with plasmacytic differentiation that arose in the spermatic cord has been described in an HIV-positive male with multicentric Castleman's disease.[64] It may be pertinent that the spermatic cord is a mesothelial-covered structure and that primary effusion lymphoma, an HHV8+ lymphoma, arises in mesothelial-lined cavities (see Lymphomas of the Pleura and Pleural Cavity in Chapter 4 for a discussion of primary effusion lymphoma).

Most patients have been treated with orchiectomy with or without radiation or chemotherapy, and most developed distant relapses within a few months of diagnosis. Relapses tend to be widespread or to involve the CNS, and the outcome has been poor.[61,62] Based on the small number of reported cases, lymphomas presenting with spermatic cord involvement appear to behave in a manner similar to that of testicular lymphoma.[61,62] As with the epididymis, the spermatic cord most often is involved by lymphoma secondary to spread from testicular lymphoma.[5]

■ PROSTATIC LYMPHOMAS

Primary Prostatic Lymphomas

Introduction

Prostatic lymphoma is rare. Only about 100 cases, including both primary and secondary prostatic lymphomas, have been reported. Primary lymphoma of the prostate accounts for 0.1% of all non-Hodgkin's lymphomas and for 0.09% of prostatic neoplasms.[65] In a large series of prostatic biopsies, transurethral resection specimens, and prostatectomies, 0.17% of cases harbored primary prostatic lymphoma.[66]

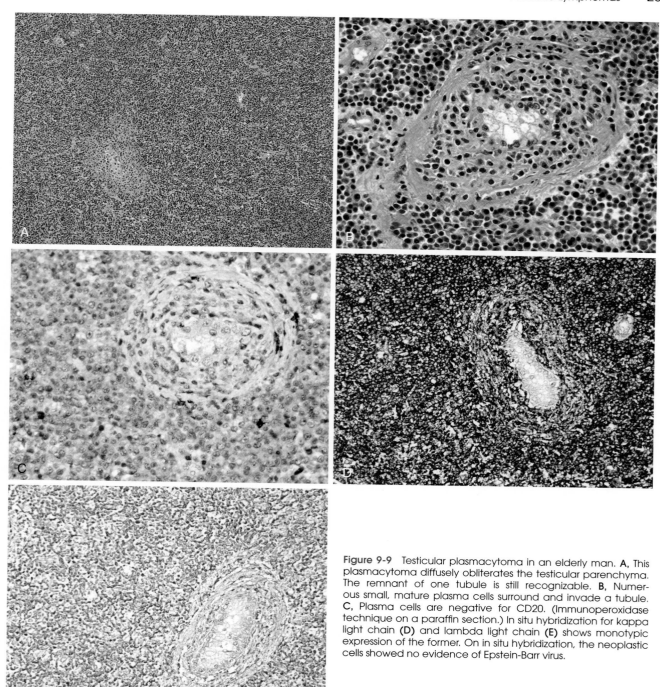

Figure 9-9 Testicular plasmacytoma in an elderly man. **A,** This plasmacytoma diffusely obliterates the testicular parenchyma. The remnant of one tubule is still recognizable. **B,** Numerous small, mature plasma cells surround and invade a tubule. **C,** Plasma cells are negative for CD20. (Immunoperoxidase technique on a paraffin section.) In situ hybridization for kappa light chain **(D)** and lambda light chain **(E)** shows monotypic expression of the former. On in situ hybridization, the neoplastic cells showed no evidence of Epstein-Barr virus.

Clinical Features

Patients' ages have ranged from 18 to 86, and the mean age has been approximately 60 years.[4,65,67-69] Most patients present with symptoms of bladder outlet obstruction, occasionally with acute urinary retention, and sometimes with hematuria.[66,67,69-72] A few patients have hydronephrosis,[69] sometimes with renal failure.[65,73,74] In some cases, prostatic lymphoma is an incidental finding on a routine physical examination.[72,75]

On physical examination, the prostate usually is enlarged, nontender, and typically without nodularity. The gland may have normal consistency or may be firm, but it is not as hard as in cases of carcinoma.[68] The median furrow may be obliterated. Cystoscopic examination sometimes reveals

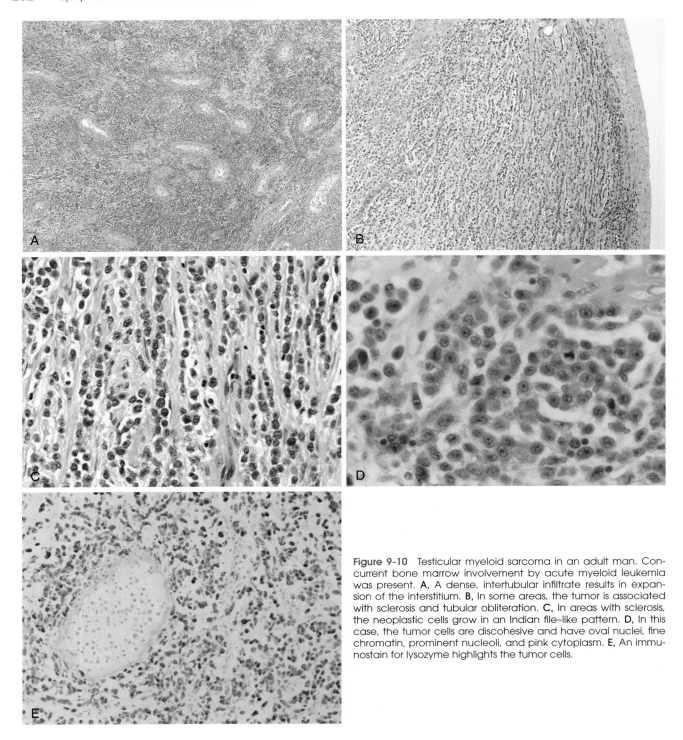

Figure 9-10 Testicular myeloid sarcoma in an adult man. Concurrent bone marrow involvement by acute myeloid leukemia was present. **A,** A dense, intertubular infiltrate results in expansion of the interstitium. **B,** In some areas, the tumor is associated with sclerosis and tubular obliteration. **C,** In areas with sclerosis, the neoplastic cells grow in an Indian file–like pattern. **D,** In this case, the tumor cells are discohesive and have oval nuclei, fine chromatin, prominent nucleoli, and pink cytoplasm. **E,** An immunostain for lysozyme highlights the tumor cells.

urethral narrowing and bladder trabeculation.[76] Serum prostatic specific antigen levels usually are normal.[76,77]

Based on the clinical features, patients often are thought to have benign prostatic hyperplasia,[4] and the diagnosis of lymphoma is only rarely suspected prospectively. In those cases with rapid onset of symptoms, the pace of evolution of the disease makes benign prostatic hyperplasia less likely.[76]

Pathologic Features

The lymphomas are a variety of types, but the most common appears to be diffuse large B-cell lymphoma.[*] Other cases have almost always been B-cell lymphomas; reported cases have included follicular lymphoma,[67,68] Burkitt's lymphoma,[65] and a few cases of marginal zone lymphoma.[70,71,78]

---

*References 15, 67, 68, 72-74, 76, and 77.

Microscopic examination reveals an atypical lymphoid infiltrate that usually is patchy but may be unifocal, extensive and obliterative, or perivascular. The lymphoma infiltrates among fibromuscular bundles and occasionally infiltrates glandular epithelium (Figure 9-15).[68]

Staging, Treatment, and Outcome

Staging has shown the extent of disease to be Ann Arbor stage I in most cases. In rare cases concurrent involvement of the bladder and prostate is seen.[76] Cases with involvement of lymph nodes and of other extranodal sites have been reported, although in such cases it may be difficult to determine with certainty whether the lymphoma truly arose from the prostate. The marginal zone lymphomas are associated with an indolent course and a good prognosis. The aggressive lymphomas, as in other sites, often respond to therapy, although treatment may lead to complications, particularly among elderly patients. Overall survival has improved over time with improvements in therapy[65]; a number of cases with a good outcome have been described.[76,77]

Differential Diagnosis

The differential diagnosis of prostatic lymphoma includes poorly differentiated carcinoma and prostatitis. However, even in poorly differentiated carcinoma, neoplastic cells at least focally form cords, cohesive sheets, and sometimes glandular lumens. In the differential diagnosis with prostatitis, the presence of a dense, monomorphous, cytologically atypical lymphoid infiltrate favors lymphoma. Immunophenotyping can be helpful for distinguishing a low-grade lymphoma from marked chronic inflammation; a dense infiltrate composed predominantly of B cells suggests lymphoma.

Secondary Involvement of the Prostate by Lymphoma

Secondary involvement of the prostate by lymphoma is more common than primary prostatic lymphoma; primary sites have been nodal and extranodal. Symptoms are similar to those seen in patients with primary prostatic lymphoma. The lymphomas have been a variety of low- and high-grade types; the most common have been chronic lymphocytic leukemia and diffuse large B-cell lymphoma.[67,68,79] Rare cases of secondary involvement by peripheral T-cell lymphoma also have been reported.[67]

■ LYMPHOMAS OF THE PENIS

The penis is the least common site in the male genital tract to give rise to lymphoma. Most lymphomas involving the penis are cutaneous lymphomas

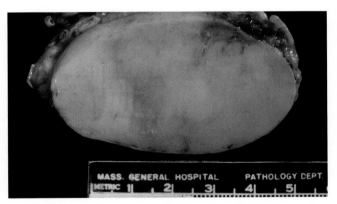

Figure 9-11 Diffuse large B-cell lymphoma involving the testis in a patient with a history of primary central nervous system diffuse large B-cell lymphoma. Yellow-tan tumor has replaced the testis.

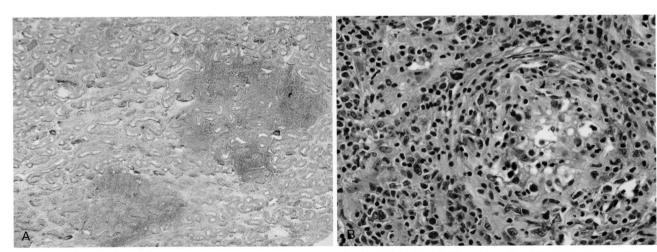

Figure 9-12 Diffuse large B-cell lymphoma involving the testis in a patient with a history of diffuse large B-cell lymphoma presenting with lymph node involvement. **A,** The testis contains multiple small foci of lymphoma; this pattern is uncommon for primary testicular lymphoma. **B,** Higher power view shows large atypical lymphoid cells, many with irregular nuclei, surrounding and invading this tubule. Interspersed small, nonneoplastic lymphocytes also are present.

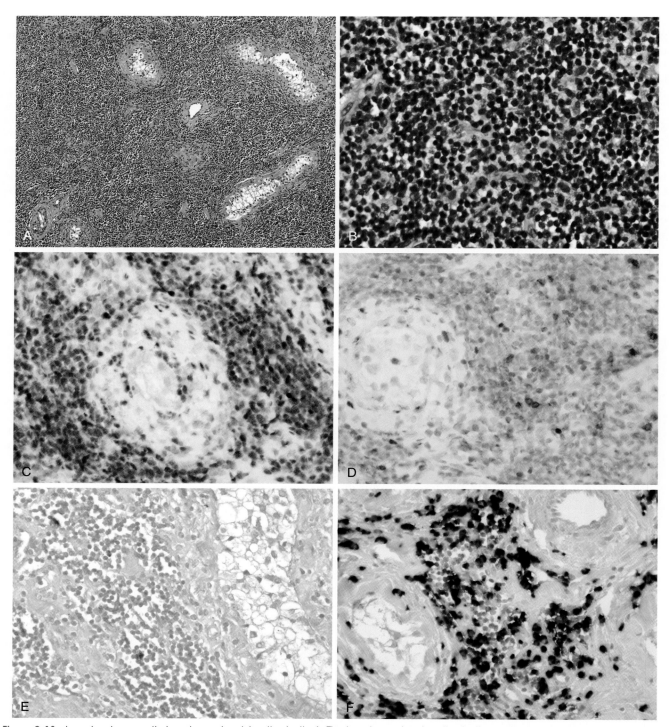

Figure 9-13   Lymphoplasmacytic lymphoma involving the testis. **A,** The lymphoma involves the testis predominantly in an intertubular pattern. **B,** High-power view shows small lymphocytes and occasional single scattered and clustered plasmacytoid lymphocytes and plasma cells *(arrow)*. Most of the infiltrate consists of B cells (Pax5+ **(C)**) with scattered T cells (CD2+ **(D)**) (immunoperoxidase technique on paraffin sections). **E** and **F,** In situ hybridization shows absence of staining for kappa light chain **(E)**, as well as numerous plasma cells and plasmacytoid cells with monotypic staining for lambda light chain **(F)**.

(see Cutaneous Lymphomas in Chapter 11). In rare cases, cutaneous lymphoma is confined to the penis.[80] Lymphomas involving the penis, other than those that arise in the skin, occur in adults[81-85] and rarely in children.[86] The penile lymphoma may be the presenting site of widespread lymphoma,[83] but a few cases of primary penile lymphoma have been reported.[81,82,84-86] One patient had a history of venereal disease before the development of lymphoma.[85] In one intriguing case, primary penile lymphoma arose at the site of injections for erectile dysfunction.[82]

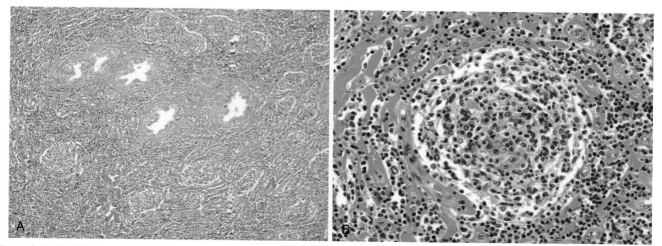

Figure 9-14 Epididymal follicular lymphoma. **A,** The epididymis has been mostly replaced by a proliferation of atypical, small, poorly delineated follicles that lack mantles and are associated with prominent sclerosis. **B,** High-power view of a follicle shows that it is composed predominantly of centrocytes.

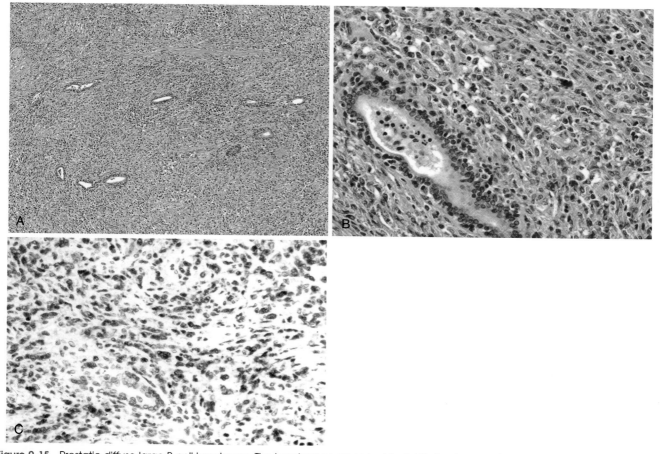

Figure 9-15 Prostatic diffuse large B-cell lymphoma. The lymphoma was an incidental finding in a prostatectomy performed for adenocarcinoma. **A,** A cellular proliferation infiltrates between prostatic glandular structures. **B,** High-power view shows atypical, discohesive cells with irregular, lobated, sometimes elongated nuclei and scant cytoplasm. **C,** The atypical lymphoid cells are Pax5+ (immunoperoxidase technique on a paraffin section); they also were CD20+ and bcl6+ and negative for CD5, CD10, and bcl2.

Patients present with a firm, usually painless mass or swelling, sometimes accompanied by urinary symptoms. The shaft is involved more often than the glans. The lesions are associated with ulceration in some cases. The lymphomas have not always been classified precisely, but diffuse large B-cell lymphoma appears to be the most common type (Figure 9-16).[82,84,85]

Therapy has varied, as has the outcome. Chemotherapy, with or without radiation, has been

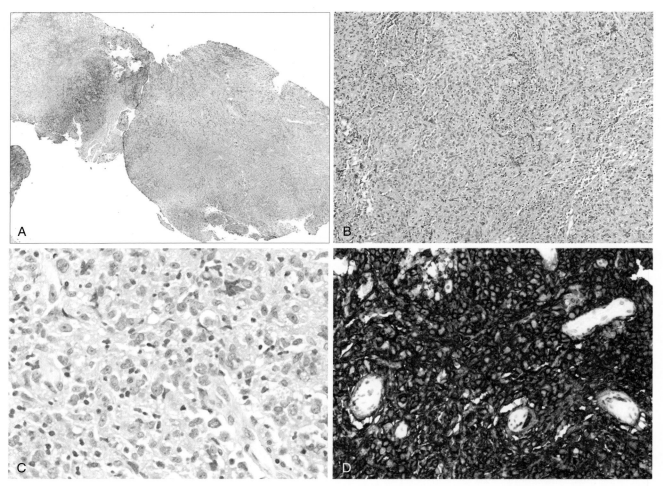

Figure 9-16   Diffuse large B-cell lymphoma of the penis in an adult man. **A,** Low power examination shows fragments of soft tissue replaced by lymphoma. **B,** Large atypical lymphoid cells diffusely infiltrate the biopsy specimen. **C,** The neoplastic cells are large and have oval, irregular, or lobated nuclei; distinct nucleoli; and scant cytoplasm. The diameter of their nuclei is more than twice that of the few interspersed small lymphocytes. **D,** Tumor cells are strongly positive for CD20. (Immunoperoxidase technique on a paraffin section.)

recommended as the optimal therapy.[84,85] The addition of rituximab to chemotherapy may be beneficial.[85] Some patients have been well after therapy,[85,86] whereas others have developed distant spread and died of lymphoma.[82,84]

REFERENCES

1. Malassez M: Lymphadenome du testicule, *Bull Soc Anat Paris* 52:176-178, 1877.
2. Darby S, Hancock BW: Localised non-Hodgkin lymphoma of the testis: the Sheffield Lymphoma Group experience, *Int J Oncol* 26:1093-1099, 2005.
3. Zucca E, Conconi A, Mughal TI et al: Patterns of outcome and prognostic factors in primary large-cell lymphoma of the testis in a survey by the International Extranodal Lymphoma Study Group, *J Clin Oncol* 21:20-27, 2003.
4. Ferry J, Young R: Malignant lymphoma of the genitourinary tract, *Curr Diagn Pathol* 4:145-169, 1997.
5. Ferry JA, Harris NL, Young RH et al: Malignant lymphoma of the testis, epididymis, and spermatic cord: a clinicopathologic study of 69 cases with immunophenotypic analysis, *Am J Surg Pathol* 18:376-390, 1994.
6. Fonseca R, Habermann T, Colgan J et al: Testicular lymphoma is associated with a high incidence of extranodal recurrence, *Cancer* 88:154-161, 2000.
7. Dalle J, Mechinaud F, Michon J et al: Testicular disease in childhood B-cell non-Hodgkin's lymphoma: the French Society of Pediatric Oncology experience, *J Clin Oncol* 19:2397-2403, 2001.
8. Pakzad K, MacLennan GT, Elder JS et al: Follicular large cell lymphoma localized to the testis in children, *J Urol* 168:225-228, 2002.
9. Al-Abbadi MA, Hattab EM, Tarawneh MS et al: Primary testicular diffuse large B-cell lymphoma belongs to the nongerminal center B-cell–like subgroup: a study of 18 cases, *Mod Pathol* 19:1521-1527, 2006.
10. Gupta D, Sharma A, Raina V et al: Primary testicular non-Hodgkin lymphoma: a single institution experience from India, *Indian J Cancer* 46:46-49, 2009.
11. Aviles A, Neri N, Huerta-Guzman J et al: Testicular lymphoma: organ-specific treatment did not improve outcome, *Oncology* 67:211-214, 2004.
12. Hasselblom S, Ridell B, Wedel H et al: Testicular lymphoma: a retrospective, population-based, clinical and immunohistochemical study, *Acta Oncol* 43:758-765, 2004.
13. Pectasides D, Economopoulos T, Kouvatseas G et al: Anthracycline-based chemotherapy of primary non-Hodgkin's lymphoma of the testis: the Hellenic Cooperative Oncology Group experience, *Oncology* 58:286-292, 2000.
14. Lagrange JL, Ramaioli A, Theodore CH et al: Non-Hodgkin's lymphoma of the testis: a retrospective study of 84 patients treated in the French anticancer centres, *Ann Oncol* 12:1313-1319, 2001.

15. Schniederjan SD, Osunkoya AO: Lymphoid neoplasms of the urinary tract and male genital organs: a clinicopathological study of 40 cases, *Mod Pathol* 22:1057-1065, 2009.

16. Gundrum JD, Mathiason MA, Moore DB, Go RS: Primary testicular diffuse large B-cell lymphoma: a population-based study on the incidence, natural history, and survival comparison with primary nodal counterpart before and after the introduction of rituximab, *J Clin Oncol* 27:5227-5232, 2009.

17. Shahab N, Doll D: Testicular lymphoma, *Semin Oncol* 26:259-269, 1999.

18. Barthelmes L, Thomas KJ, Seale JR: Prostatic involvement of a testicular lymphoma in a patient with myasthenia gravis on long-term azathioprine, *Leuk Lymphoma* 43:2425-2426, 2002.

19. Lambrechts AC, Looijenga LHJ, vant's Veer MB et al: Lymphomas with testicular localisation show a consistent BCL-2 expression without a translocation (14,18): a molecular and immunohistochemical study, *Br J Cancer* 71:73-77, 1995.

20. Stein H, Harris N, Campo E: Plasmablastic lymphoma. In Swerdlow S, Campo E, Harris N et al, editors: *WHO classification: tumours of haematopoietic and lymphoid tissues*, ed 4, Lyon, 2008, IARC.

21. Booman M, Szuhai K, Rosenwald A et al: Genomic alterations and gene expression in primary diffuse large B-cell lymphomas of immune-privileged sites: the importance of apoptosis and immunomodulatory pathways, *J Pathol* 216:209-217, 2008.

22. Seymour J, Solomon B, Wolf M et al: Primary large-cell non-Hodgkin's lymphoma of the testis: a retrospective analysis of patterns of failure and prognostic factors, *Clin Lymphoma* 2:109-115, 2001.

23. Zouhair A, Weber D, Belkacemi Y et al: Outcome and patterns of failure in testicular lymphoma: a multicenter Rare Cancer Network study, *Int J Radiat Oncol Biol* 52:652-656, 2002.

24. Moller MB, Pedersen NT, Christensen BE: Diffuse large B-cell lymphoma: clinical implications of extranodal versus nodal presentation: a population-based study of 1575 cases, *Br J Haematol* 124:151-159, 2004.

25. Bacon C, Ye H, Diss T et al: Primary follicular lymphoma of the testis and epididymis in adults, *Am J Surg Pathol* 31:1050-1058, 2007.

26. Finn L, Viswanatha D, Belasco J et al: Primary follicular lymphoma of the testis in childhood, *Cancer* 85:1626-1635, 1999.

27. Heller KN, Teruya-Feldstein J, La Quaglia MP, Wexler LH: Primary follicular lymphoma of the testis: excellent outcome following surgical resection without adjuvant chemotherapy, *J Pediatr Hematol Oncol* 26:104-107, 2004.

28. Moertel CL, Watterson J, McCormick SR, Simonton SC: Follicular large cell lymphoma of the testis in a child, *Cancer* 75:1182-1186, 1995.

29. Lu D, Medeiros L, Eskenazi A, Abruzzo L: Primary follicular large cell lymphoma of the testis in a child, *Arch Pathol Lab Med* 125:551-554, 2001.

30. Pileri S, Sabattini E, Rosito P et al: Primary follicular lymphoma of the testis in childhood: an entity with peculiar clinical and molecular characteristics, *J Clin Pathol* 55:684-688, 2002.

31. Ballereau C, Leroy X, Morschhauser F et al: Testicular natural killer T-cell lymphoma, *Int J Urol* 12:223-224, 2005.

32. Chan JKC, Tsang WYW, Lau W-H et al: Aggressive T/natural killer cell lymphoma presenting as testicular tumor, *Cancer* 77:1198-1205, 1996.

33. Kim Y, Chang S, Yang W-I et al: Primary NK/T cell lymphoma of the testis, *Acta Haematol* 109:95-100, 2003.

34. Ornstein DL, Bifulco CB, Braddock DT, Howe JG: Histopathologic and molecular aspects of CD56+ natural killer/T-cell lymphoma of the testis, *Int J Surg Pathol* 16:291-300, 2008.

35. Sun T, Brody J, Susin M et al: Aggressive natural killer cell lymphoma/leukemia: a recently recognized clinicopathologic entity, *Am J Surg Pathol* 17:1289-1299, 1993.

36. Totonchi K, Engel G, Weisenberg E et al: Testicular natural killer/T-cell lymphoma, nasal type, of true natural killer–cell origin, *Arch Pathol Lab Med* 126:1527-1529, 2002.

37. Chan J, Sin V, Wong K et al: Nonnasal lymphoma expressing the natural killer cell marker CD56: a clinicopathologic study of 49 cases of an uncommon aggressive neoplasm, *Blood* 89:4501-4513, 1997.

38. Froberg M, Hamati H, Kant J et al: Primary low-grade T-helper cell testicular lymphoma, *Arch Pathol Lab Med* 121:1096-1099, 1997.

39. Akhtar M, Al-Dayel F, Siegrist K, Ezzat SIA: Neutrophil-rich Ki-1–positive anaplastic large cell lymphoma presenting as a testicular mass, *Mod Pathol* 9:812-815, 1996.

40. Azua-Romeo J, Alvarez-Alegret R, Serrano P, Mayayo E: Primary anaplastic large cell lymphoma of the testis, *Int Urol Nephrol* 36:393-396, 2004.

41. Wilkins BS, Williamson JMS, O'Brien CJ: Morphological and immunohistochemical study of testicular lymphomas, *Histopathology* 15:147-156, 1989.

42. Seliem R, Chikwava K, Swerdlow S et al: Classical Hodgkin's lymphoma presenting as a testicular mass: report of a case, *Int J Surg Pathol* 15:207-212, 2007.

43. Braaten KM, Young RH, Ferry JA: Viral-type orchitis: a potential mimic of testicular neoplasia, *Am J Surg Pathol* 33:1477-1484, 2009.

44. Ferry JA, Young RH, Scully RE: Plasmacytoma of the testis: a report of 7 cases, including 3 that were the initial manifestation of plasma cell myeloma, *Am J Surg Pathol* 21:590-598, 1997.

45. Ferry JA, Srigley JR, Young RH: Granulocytic sarcoma of the testis: a report of two cases of a neoplasm prone to misinterpretation, *Mod Pathol* 10:320-325, 1997.

46. Hull D, Alexander H, Markey G et al: Histiocytic lymphoma presenting as a testicular tumour and terminating in acute monoblastic leukaemia, *J Clin Pathol* 53:788-790, 2000.

47. Valbuena JR, Admirand JH, Lin P, Medeiros LJ: Myeloid sarcoma involving the testis, *Am J Clin Pathol* 124:445-452, 2005.

48. Abbondanzo S, Wenig B: Non-Hodgkin's lymphoma of the sinonasal tract: a clinicopathologic and immunophenotypic study of 120 cases, *Cancer* 75:1281-1291, 1995.

49. Jahnke K, Thiel E, Martus P et al: Relapse of primary central nervous system lymphoma: clinical features, outcome and prognostic factors, *J Neurooncol* 80:159-165, 2006.

50. Jacobsen E, Lomo L, Briccetti F et al: Follicular lymphoma with bilateral testicular and epididymal involvement: case report and review of the literature, *Leuk Lymphoma* 46:1663-1666, 2005.

51. Dolken MT, Schuler F, Hirt C et al: Multiple osteolytic lesions and testicular involvement at first relapse of follicular lymphoma grade 1 in transformation, *Leuk Lymphoma* 47:369-371, 2006.

52. Schichman S, McClure R, Schaefer R, Mehta P: HIV and plasmablastic lymphoma manifesting in sinus, testicles and bones: a further expansion of the disease spectrum, *Am J Hematol* 77:291-295, 2004.

53. Kellie SJ, Pui C-H, Murphy SB: Childhood non-Hodgkin's lymphoma involving the testis: clinical features and treatment outcome, *J Clin Oncol* 7:1066-1070, 1989.

54. Burkitt D, Wright D: *Burkitt's lymphoma*, Edinburgh, 1970, E & S Livingstone.

55. Ginaldi L, De Pasquale A, De Martinis M et al: Epididymal lymphoma: a case report, *Tumori* 79:147-149, 1993.

56. Kausch I, Doehn C, Buttner H et al: Primary lymphoma of the epididymis, *J Urol* 160:1801-1802, 1998.

57. McDermott MB, O'Briain DS, Shiels OM, Daly PA: Malignant lymphoma of the epididymis: a case report of bilateral involvement by a follicular large cell lymphoma, *Cancer* 75:2174-2179, 1995.

58. Novella G, Porcaro A, Righetti R et al: Primary lymphoma of the epididymis: case report and review of the literature, *Urol Int* 67:97-99, 2001.

59. Okabe M, Kurosawa M, Suzuki S et al: Primary lymphoma of spermatic cord, *Leuk Lymphoma* 40:663-666, 2001.

60. Vega F, Medeiros L, Abruzzo L: Primary paratesticular lymphoma: a report of 2 cases and review of literature, *Arch Pathol Lab Med* 125:428-432, 2001.

61. Moller MB: Non-Hodgkin's lymphoma of the spermatic cord, *Acta Haematol* 91:70-72, 1994.

62. Lands RH: Non-Hodgkin's lymphoma originating in the spermatic cord, *South Med J* 89:352-353, 1996.

63. Tranchida P, Bayerl M, Voelpel MJ, Palutke M: Testicular ischemia due to intravascular large B-cell lymphoma: a novel presentation in an immunosuppressed individual, *Int J Surg Pathol* 11:319-324, 2003.

64. Boulanger E, Gerard L, Gabarre J et al: Prognostic factors and outcome of human herpesvirus 8–associated primary effusion lymphoma in patients with AIDS, *J Clin Oncol* 23:4372-4380, 2005.

65. Sarris A, Dimopoulos M, Pugh W, Cabanillas F: Primary lymphoma of the prostate: good outcome with doxorubicin-based combination chemotherapy, *J Urol* 153:1852-1854, 1995.

66. Chu P, Huang Q, Weiss L: Incidental and concurrent malignant lymphomas discovered at the time of prostatectomy and prostate biopsy, *Am J Surg Pathol* 29:693-699, 2005.

67. Bostwick D, Iczkowski K, Amin M et al: Malignant lymphoma involving the prostate, *Cancer* 83:732-738, 1998.

68. Bostwick DG, Mann RB: Malignant lymphomas involving the prostate: a study of 13 cases, *Cancer* 56:2932-2938, 1985.

69. Ghose A, Baxter-Smith DC, Eeles H et al: Lymphoma of the prostate treated with radiotherapy, *Clin Oncol (Royal Coll Radiol)* 7:134, 1995.

70. Tomaru U, Ishikura H, Kon S et al: Primary lymphoma of the prostate with features of low grade B-cell lymphoma of mucosa associated lymphoid tissue: a rare cause of urinary obstruction, *J Urol* 162:496-497, 1999.

71. Jhavar S, Agarwal J, Naresh K, Dinshaw K: Primary extranodal mucosa associated lymphoid tissue (MALT) lymphoma of the prostate, *Leuk Lymphoma* 41:445-449, 2001.

72. Mermershtain W, Benharroch D, Lavrenkov K et al: Primary malignant lymphoma of the prostate: a report of three cases, *Leuk Lymphoma* 42:809-811, 2001.

73. Appu S, Pham T, Costello AJ: Primary lymphoma of the prostate, *ANZ J Surg* 71:329-330, 2001.

74. Antunes AA, Dall'Oglio M, Srougi M: Primary lymphoma of the prostate: a rare cause of urinary obstruction, *Int Braz J Urol* 30:410-412, 2004.

75. Bouet R, Thwaites D, Harris SB et al: Asymptomatic follicular lymphoma of the prostate discovered by abnormal digital rectal examination, *J Urol* 171:795-796, 2004.

76. Choi WW, Yap RL, Ozer O et al: Lymphoma of the prostate and bladder presenting as acute urinary obstruction, *J Urol* 169:1082-1083, 2003.

77. Alvarez CA, Rodriguez BI, Perez LA: Primary diffuse large B-cell lymphoma of the prostate in a young patient, *Int Braz J Urol* 32:64-65, 2006.

78. Tissier F, Badoual C, Saporta F et al: Prostatic lymphoma of mucosa-associated lymphoid tissue: an uncommon location, *Histopathology* 40:111-113, 2002.

79. Yavuz S, Paydas S, Disel U et al: Prostatic hypertrophy and prostatic infiltration in small lymphocytic lymphoma, *Leuk Lymphoma* 45:201-202, 2004.

80. Pomara G, Cuttano MG, Tripodo C et al: Primary T-cell rich B-cell lymphoma of the penis: a first case, *BJU Int* 91:889, 2003.

81. Arena F, di Stefano C, Peracchia G et al: Primary lymphoma of the penis: diagnosis and treatment, *Eur Urol* 39:232-235, 2001.

82. Beal K, Mears JG: Short report: penile lymphoma following local injections for erectile dysfunction, *Leuk Lymphoma* 42:247-249, 2001.

83. Gallardo F, Pujol RM, Barranco C, Salar A: Progressive painless swelling of glans penis: uncommon clinical manifestation of systemic non-Hodgkin's lymphoma, *Urology* 73:929, e3-e5, 2009.

84. el-Sharkawi A, Murphy J: Primary penile lymphoma: the case for combined modality therapy, *Clin Oncol (R Coll Radiol)* 8:334-335, 1996.

85. Kim HY, Oh SY, Lee S et al: Primary penile diffuse large B cell lymphoma treated by local excision followed by rituximab-containing chemotherapy, *Acta Haematol* 120:150-152, 2008.

86. Wei CC, Peng CT, Chiang IP, Wu KH: Primary B cell non-Hodgkin lymphoma of the penis in a child, *J Pediatr Hematol Oncol* 28:479-480, 2006.

CHAPTER 10

Lymphomas of the Female Genital Tract

Judith A. Ferry

■ INTRODUCTION

Lymphoma only rarely presents with female genital tract involvement. The ovaries are most commonly affected, followed by the uterine cervix, the uterine corpus, the vagina, the vulva, and the fallopian tube. Nearly all cases are B-cell lymphoma; diffuse large B-cell lymphoma is the most common type throughout the female genital tract. T-cell lymphoma is infrequent; natural killer (NK)-cell lymphoma is uncommon; and Hodgkin's lymphoma is vanishingly rare.[1,2] Except in rare cases of lymphoma that arises in the setting of human immunodeficiency virus (HIV) infection or iatrogenic immunosuppression,[3-5] or in the case of endemic Burkitt's lymphoma, there are no known predisposing factors for the development of female genital tract lymphoma.

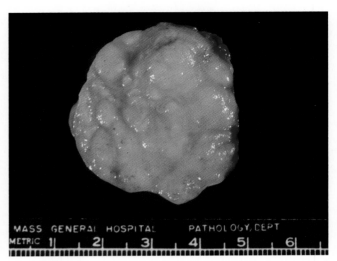

Figure 10-1 Ovarian diffuse large B-cell lymphoma. Cross section reveals ovary replaced by poorly delineated, sometimes confluent nodules of homogeneous light tan tissue.

■ OVARIAN LYMPHOMAS

Primary Ovarian Lymphomas

Introduction

The precise criteria for accepting a case as primary ovarian lymphoma have been debated in the literature; however, most series on ovarian lymphoma consist of cases in which patients present with predominant ovarian involvement but also may have extraovarian disease.[6] In general, fewer than 1% of lymphomas present with ovarian involvement,[1,7,8] and fewer than 1.5% of neoplasms that arise in the ovary are lymphomas. In striking contrast, however, in countries where Burkitt's lymphoma is endemic, approximately 50% of malignant ovarian tumors in childhood are Burkitt's lymphoma.[9]

Clinical Features

Ovarian lymphoma affects patients over a wide age range, from early childhood to advanced age[1]; the peak incidence is in the fourth or fifth decade.[1,7,10] Occasional cases have been recognized during pregnancy.[1,11] Rare patients have been HIV positive.[5]

The most common presenting complaints are abdominal pain and increasing abdominal girth.[7,10,12] A minority of patients have weight loss, fatigue, fever, or abnormal vaginal bleeding.[7] The lymphoma has been an incidental finding in a few cases.[10]

Pathologic Features

On gross examination, ovarian lymphomas range from microscopic, representing incidental findings,[10] to 25 cm in diameter; the average diameter is 11 to 14 cm.[1,10] These lymphomas typically have an intact external surface that may be smooth or nodular. The consistency ranges from soft and fleshy to firm and rubbery, depending on the degree of associated sclerosis. On sectioning, the tumors usually are white, tan, or gray-pink (Figure 10-1). A minority

have cystic degeneration, hemorrhage, or necrosis.[1] Rare cases of lymphoma involving the ovary in association with, and possibly arising from, a teratoma have been described.[13]

The most common type of lymphoma is diffuse large B-cell lymphoma, followed by Burkitt's lymphoma and follicular lymphoma.[7] Adolescents and children almost always have diffuse, aggressive lymphomas, including Burkitt's lymphoma, B-lymphoblastic lymphoma, and diffuse large B-cell lymphoma.[2] Ovarian lymphoma may spare the corpora lutea, corpora albicantia, developing follicles, and a peripheral rim of cortical tissue, but it otherwise typically obliterates the normal ovarian parenchyma.

Diffuse Large B-Cell Lymphoma

The histologic appearance of lymphoma in the ovary is similar to that in extraovarian sites (Figure 10-2). However, in the ovary, associated sclerosis often is seen, and tumor cells may appear to grow in cords and nests and simulate carcinoma[9]; or, they may have an elongate shape, grow in a storiform pattern, and mimic a spindle cell sarcoma (Figure 10-3). A few diffuse large B-cell lymphomas have a component of follicular lymphoma.[10,12] They are CD20+, and in the few cases studied, expression of bcl6, CD10, and bcl2 is common.[10]

Burkitt's Lymphoma

Burkitt's lymphoma appears to be most common among children and adolescents,[2] although adults occasionally are affected. Both sporadic and endemic Burkitt's lymphoma may present with ovarian involvement. In contrast to other types of ovarian lymphoma, Burkitt's lymphoma almost always is bilateral.[14] Burkitt's lymphoma that occurs in pregnancy is thought to have a tendency to involve hormonally stimulated organs, including the ovary.[11]

The histologic features are the same as those in other sites (Figure 10-4); and, as in other sites, the

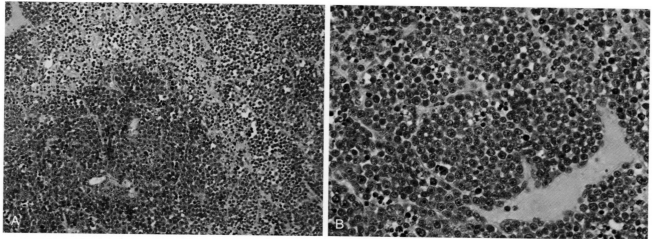

Figure 10-2 Ovarian diffuse large B-cell lymphoma composed of immunoblasts. **A,** Ovarian parenchyma is obliterated by a dense proliferation of atypical lymphoid cells with foci of necrosis but without intervening fibrous stroma. **B,** High-power view shows that nearly all cells are immunoblasts with large oval nuclei and prominent central nucleoli.

characteristic immunophenotype is CD20+, CD10+, CD5−, bcl6+, and bcl2−; Ki67 is about 100%, and the neoplastic cells harbor a translocation involving MYC[2,15,16] (see Burkitt's Lymphoma of the Gastrointestinal Tract, Chapter 5).

Follicular Lymphoma

Ovarian follicular lymphoma mainly affects older patients. Follicular lymphomas of all three grades occur in the ovary. The follicular lymphomas may have conspicuous diffuse areas.[14] Detailed information on immunophenotyping is only occasionally available, but two cases in one series were CD10+, bcl6+, and bcl2−[10]; the lack of bcl2 in these cases is in contrast to most lymph node follicular lymphomas, which typically are bcl2+.

Miscellaneous Rare Lymphomas

Rare cases of anaplastic large cell lymphoma and B- and T-lymphoblastic lymphoma presenting with ovarian involvement have been reported.[2,10,17] A well-documented case of ALK+ anaplastic large cell lymphoma in a 14-year-old girl presenting primarily with an ovarian mass has been reported, although extraovarian involvement by lymphoma also was found on staging.[18]

Staging, Treatment, and Outcome

Laparotomy shows involvement of one or both ovaries with approximately equal frequency. Extraovarian spread is found in most cases, most commonly to pelvic or paraaortic lymph nodes and occasionally to the peritoneum, other portions of the female genital tract, or more distant sites.[1,7] Ovarian lymphoma traditionally has been considered an aggressive tumor with a poor outcome; however, in more recent reports, with combination chemotherapy the prognosis appears similar to that for nodal lymphomas of comparable stage and histologic type.[6,7,10]

Secondary Ovarian Involvement by Lymphoma

Among patients with disseminated lymphoma, the ovary is a relatively common site of involvement, although the disease may not be clinically apparent. Seven percent to 25% of women who die with lymphoma have involvement of the ovaries.[1] The ovary is the most common site in the female genital tract to be involved by lymphoma at autopsy.[19] Any type of lymphoma may spread to the ovary, but primary mediastinal large B-cell lymphoma (see also Lymphomas of the Thymus in Chapter 4) has a distinct tendency to involve certain extranodal sites, including the ovary, on progression or at the time of relapse.[20,21]

In a case presented in the Case Records of the Massachusetts General Hospital, a woman with mediastinal large B-cell lymphoma presented during pregnancy with dyspnea and a lymphomatous breast mass; she was found to have ovarian involvement by lymphoma during successful delivery of the infant by cesarean section (Figure 10-5).[22] We have seen the unusual case of a patient with a history of follicular lymphoma who had a mature cystic teratoma that was involved by the follicular lymphoma (Figure 10-6).

Differential Diagnosis of Ovarian Lymphoma

The differential diagnosis of ovarian lymphoma is broad; it includes dysgerminoma; metastatic carcinoma; primary ovarian small cell carcinoma of hypercalcemic type, as well as pulmonary type; adult granulosa cell tumor[12]; spindle cell sarcoma; undifferentiated carcinoma; and myeloid sarcoma.[1] Attention to cytologic detail and familiarity with the spectrum of histologic features of ovarian lymphoma are helpful in establishing a diagnosis.

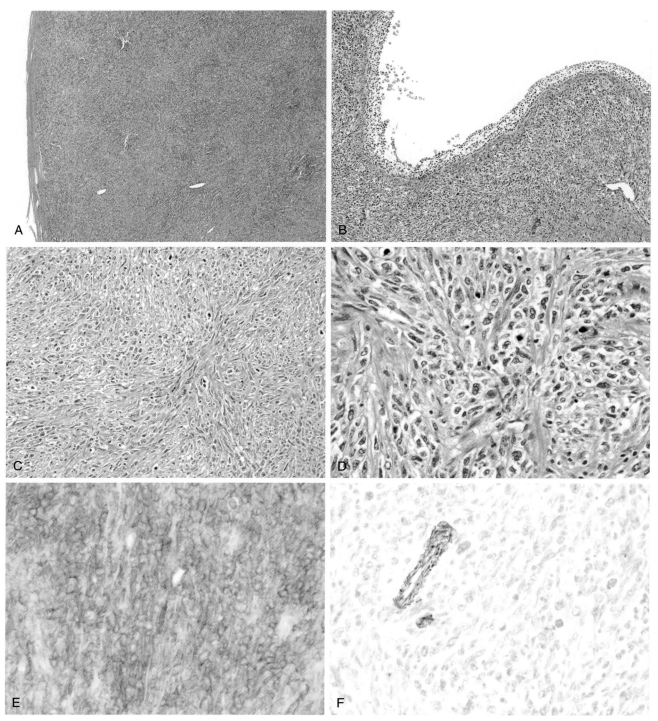

Figure 10-3 Ovarian diffuse large B-cell lymphoma composed of spindle cells. **A,** Except for a very narrow band of collagenized tissue beneath the ovarian surface, the ovary has been replaced by a cellular neoplasm. **B,** The lymphoma has spared this developing follicle. **C,** In some areas, the lymphoma has a storiform pattern. Neoplastic cells are often elongate, and interstitial sclerosis is present. **D,** High-power view shows elongate tumor cells with blunt-ended nuclei, as well as tumor cells with lobated nuclei, associated with sclerosis. Neoplastic cells are diffusely CD20+ **(E)**, indicating B-lineage, and negative for vimentin **(F)**. A small blood vessel stains for vimentin. (Immunoperoxidase technique on paraffin sections.)

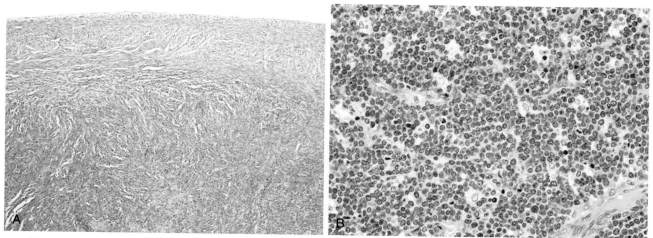

Figure 10-4 Ovarian Burkitt's lymphoma. **A,** The lymphoma has spared the superficial portion of the ovarian cortex. **B,** The lymphoma is composed of closely packed, medium-sized, round, dark blue cells with frequent mitoses, scattered pale tingible body macrophages, and little or no intervening stroma.

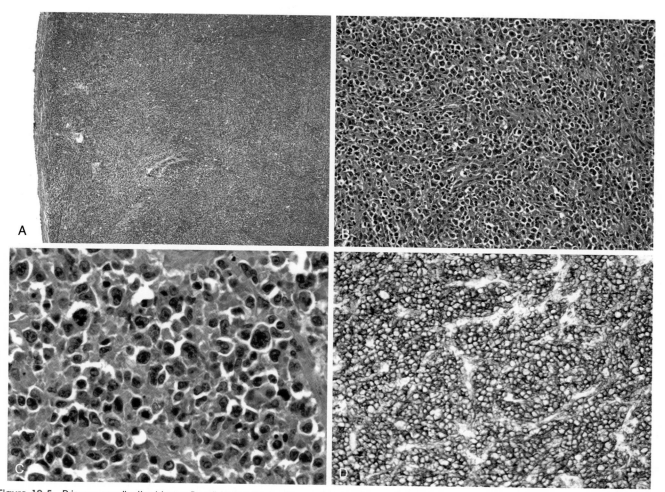

Figure 10-5 Primary mediastinal large B-cell lymphoma with ovarian involvement. **A,** Microscopic examination shows a cellular tumor replacing the ovarian parenchyma. **B,** Slightly higher power view shows discohesive, dark cells associated with sclerosis. **C,** High-power view shows medium to large atypical lymphoid cells with irregular, sometimes lobated, nuclei. Neoplastic cells are diffusely positive for CD20, indicating B-lineage **(D).**

Continued

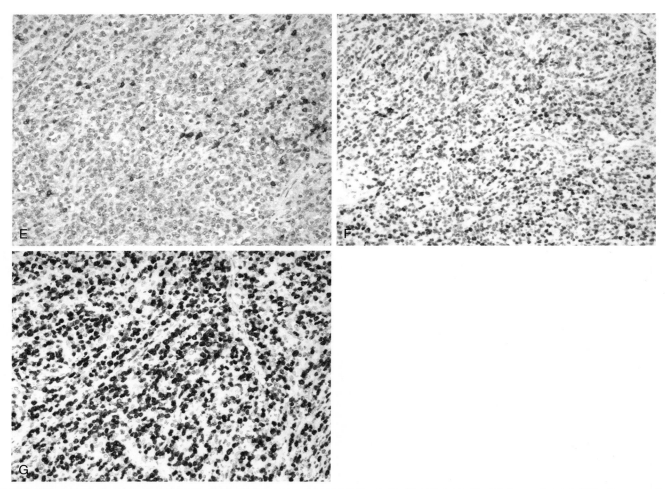

Figure 10-5, cont'd   Scattered small T cells (CD3+ **(E)**) also are present. Most neoplastic cells are bcl6+ **(F)**. Approximately 80% of tumor cells are Ki67+ (proliferation **(G)**). (Immunoperoxidase technique on paraffin sections.)

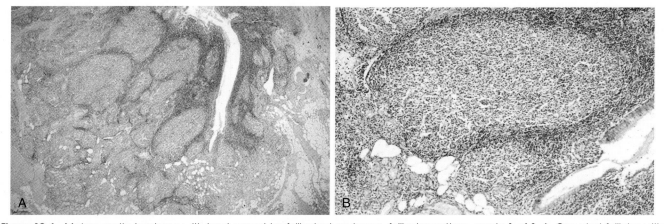

Figure 10-6   Mature cystic teratoma with involvement by follicular lymphoma, follicular pattern, grade 1 of 3. **A,** Crowded follicles with attenuated mantles preferentially occupy stroma adjacent to an epithelial-lined structure, reminiscent of the distribution of normal and acquired mucosa-associated lymphoid tissue in sites such as the gastrointestinal tract or bronchial tree. **B,** This neoplastic follicle is composed of a monotonous population of centrocytes with only rare large centroblasts, consistent with a low-grade follicular lymphoma (grade 1 of 3).

Immunohistochemical studies readily confirm or exclude lymphoma. Selected problems in differential diagnosis are discussed in the following list.

1. **Dysgerminoma versus lymphoma.** The large, oval nuclei and prominent central nucleoli of the neoplastic cells of dysgerminoma may raise the question of a large cell lymphoma. However, dysgerminomas are composed of cells with abundant, pale, glycogen-rich cytoplasm and distinct cell membranes. Tumor cells grow in cohesive sheets, nests, or trabeculae. The tumor may have fibrous bands containing lymphocytes and sometimes lymphoid follicles. An associated granulomatous reaction may be seen as well. Although dysgerminoma and lymphoma should be readily distinguished on the basis of routinely stained sections, some of the characteristic features of dysgerminoma may be difficult to appreciate if the tumor is not well fixed. In contrast to lymphoma, dysgerminoma has PAS+ cytoplasm, with immunoreactivity for placental alkaline phosphatase (PLAP) and Oct4.

2. **Carcinoma versus lymphoma.** When lymphoma is associated with sclerosis, it can have cordlike or nested growth that can mimic carcinoma. The appearance can be reminiscent of the "Indian file" pattern of breast carcinoma, raising the question of metastasis. Familiarity with this growth pattern of lymphoma, reinforced by a basic panel of immunostains, should readily establish a diagnosis.

3. **Adult granulosa cell tumor versus lymphoma.** Adult granulosa cell tumors are composed of cells with large, oval nuclei and usually scant cytoplasm that sometimes grow in a haphazard pattern, potentially mimicking lymphoma. Examination of granulosa cell tumors often reveals areas with growth in trabecular, insular, microfollicular, and/or macrofollicular patterns, sometimes with formation of Call-Exner bodies, which excludes lymphoma. The nuclear chromatin in granulosa cells usually is paler and more evenly dispersed than in lymphoma, and in contrast to lymphoma, a subset of neoplastic granulosa cells often shows nuclear grooves.

■ FALLOPIAN TUBE LYMPHOMAS

Primary malignant lymphoma of the fallopian tube is rare. A case of primary tubal marginal zone lymphoma associated with salpingitis,[23] two cases of primary tubal follicular lymphoma (Figure 10-7),[1,24] and a bilateral primary tubal peripheral T-cell lymphoma[25] have been reported. One follicular lymphoma was low grade (see Figure 10-7).[1] The other

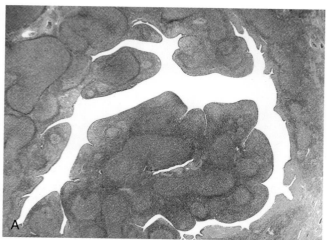

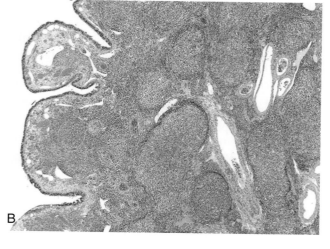

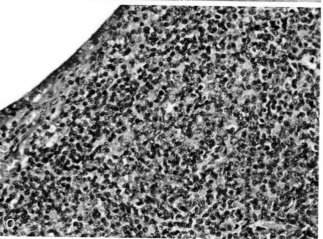

Figure 10-7 Follicular lymphoma, follicular pattern, grade 1 of 3, presenting with isolated involvement of the fallopian tube. **A,** Low-power view shows circumferential mural involvement by a proliferation of lymphoid follicles that fill and expand the plicae. **B,** The follicles are crowded and poorly delineated, with attenuated or absent mantles. **C,** High-power view shows an atypical follicle composed almost entirely of centrocytes with only rare centroblasts, consistent with a low-grade follicular lymphoma (grade 1 of 3).

was a grade 3B follicular lymphoma with a minor component of diffuse large B-cell lymphoma that expressed CD10 and bcl6 but not bcl2, without detectable *BCL2* translocation by polymerase chain reaction (PCR); this patient was alive and well 18 months after surgical excision alone.[24]

Among patients with lymphoma of the ovaries, secondary tubal involvement is common. Secondary spread to the tube also may occur from other sites in the absence of ovarian involvement.[12] Diffuse large B-cell lymphoma and Burkitt's lymphoma are most common[26]; follicular lymphoma also has been described.[12]

■ UTERINE LYMPHOMAS

Primary Uterine Lymphomas

Introduction

Malignant lymphoma that arises in the uterus is rare; fewer than 1% of extranodal lymphomas arise in this site.[8] Lymphoma arises more often in the cervix than in the corpus; one series showed a 10:1 ratio,[27] although other series have not shown such a striking excess of cervical lymphomas.[2]

Clinical Features

The patients range in age from 20 to 80 years,[28] and the mean and median ages are in the 40s.[28-31] The most common presenting symptom is abnormal vaginal bleeding.[1,26,28,30,32-35] Less common complaints are dyspareunia or perineal, pelvic, or abdominal pain. Only a small minority of patients have systemic symptoms, such as fever or weight loss.[1,29,31] Because the lymphomas typically are not associated with ulceration, only occasionally can uterine lymphoma be detected on a Papanicolaou smear.

Pathologic Features

Cervical lymphomas usually produce bulky lesions readily identifiable on pelvic examination. The classic appearance is diffuse, circumferential enlargement of the cervix ("barrel-shaped" cervix) (Figure 10-8). The lymphoma also may form a discrete submucosal tumor (Figure 10-9),[28,32] a polypoid or multinodular lesion,[28,35,36] or a fungating, exophytic mass; ulceration is unusual.[28] The tumors have been variously described as fleshy, rubbery, or firm. They usually are white-tan or yellow (Figure 10-10).[28] Extensive local spread to sites such as the vagina, parametria, or even the pelvic side walls is common (Figure 10-8)[28,33,35]; invasion into the urinary bladder has been described.[37] Ureteral obstruction with hydronephrosis is common.[1,28,33] Lymphomas of the uterine corpus usually are fleshy or soft, pale gray, yellow, or cream colored. They may form a polypoid mass or diffusely infiltrate the endometrium, sometimes with deep invasion of the myometrium.[1,28]

The microscopic appearance of the lymphomas is similar to that of nodal and other extranodal sites, although there are some distinctive features. In the cervix, a band of uninvolved normal tissue often is present just beneath the surface epithelium, and the overlying epithelium usually is intact. A large biopsy or hysterectomy specimen usually shows

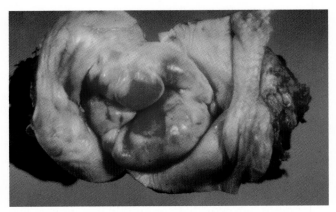

Figure 10-8 Uterine cervix with circumferential involvement by lymphoma, so-called barrel-shaped cervix. The cervical mucosa sometimes is congested but shows no obvious ulceration. The subepithelial stroma expands and distorts the cervix and extends into the adjacent vaginal stroma and adjacent paracervical soft tissue.

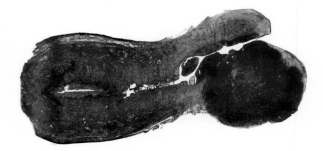

Figure 10-9 Lymphoma of the uterine cervix. Whole mount view of this uterus reveals a relatively discrete lesion forming a large mass in the wall of the cervix.

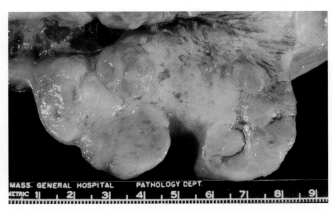

Figure 10-10 Lymphoma of the uterine cervix. Cross section shows multiple infiltrative light yellow–tan or white nodules replacing much of the cervix.

deep invasion of the cervical wall. In small biopsy specimens, squeeze artifact often is prominent.

Diffuse Large B-Cell Lymphoma

By far, the most common type of primary uterine lymphoma in both the corpus and the cervix is diffuse large B-cell lymphoma (Figure 10-11),[26,27,34-37] which accounts for about 70% of such cases.[26,29] The cervical lymphomas, but not the endometrial lymphomas, frequently are associated with prominent sclerosis,[14,26,36] which may be associated with a cord-like arrangement of tumor cells or spindle-shaped tumor cells.[28] The spindle cell pattern may be sufficiently prominent to mimic a sarcoma; the terms "spindle cell variant"[38] and "sarcomatoid variant"[39] have been suggested to describe such cases. In one case, a lymphoma has been described as an Epstein-Barr virus–positive endometrial T-cell-rich large B-cell lymphoma[40]; this disease arose in the uterus of a woman who had had an intrauterine device

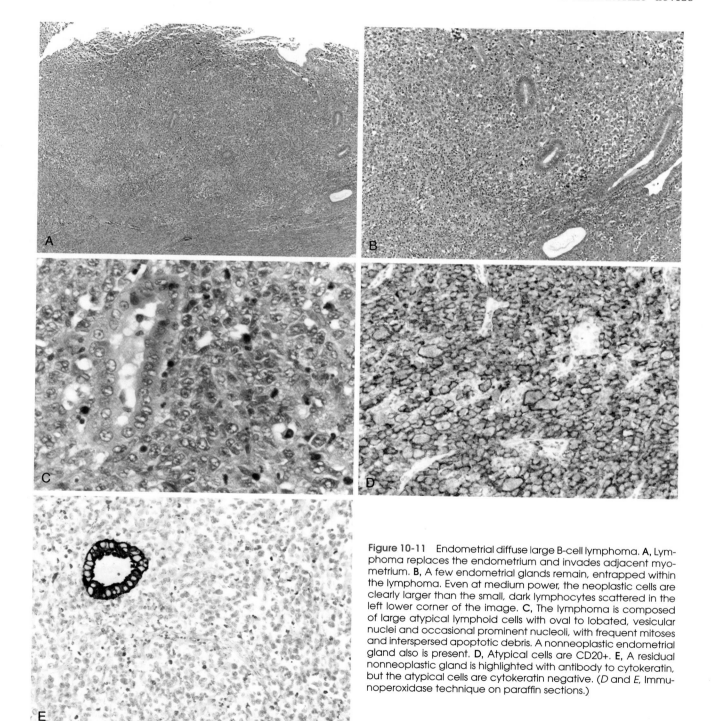

Figure 10-11 Endometrial diffuse large B-cell lymphoma. **A,** Lymphoma replaces the endometrium and invades adjacent myometrium. **B,** A few endometrial glands remain, entrapped within the lymphoma. Even at medium power, the neoplastic cells are clearly larger than the small, dark lymphocytes scattered in the left lower corner of the image. **C,** The lymphoma is composed of large atypical lymphoid cells with oval to lobated, vesicular nuclei and occasional prominent nucleoli, with frequent mitoses and interspersed apoptotic debris. A nonneoplastic endometrial gland also is present. **D,** Atypical cells are CD20+. **E,** A residual nonneoplastic gland is highlighted with antibody to cytokeratin, but the atypical cells are cytokeratin negative. (*D* and *E,* Immunoperoxidase technique on paraffin sections.)

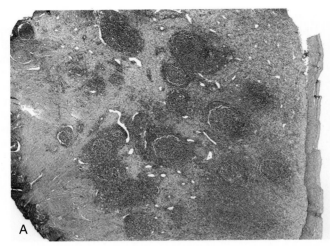

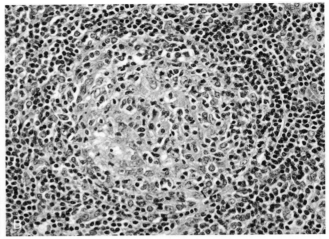

Figure 10-12 Follicular lymphoma, follicular pattern, arising in the uterine cervix. **A,** The squamous epithelium is intact, and a thin layer of subepithelial stroma appears largely spared by the lymphoma. A proliferation of atypical, poorly delineated follicles invades deep into the cervical wall. **B,** This follicle has a monotonous cellular composition and lacks the polarization and tingible body macrophages typically found in reactive follicles.

(IUD) in place for more than 20 years. As currently defined, T-cell/histiocyte rich large B-cell lymphoma does not contain EBV (see Chapter 6, Lymphomas of the Spleen) and precise subclassification in this case using updated criteria is uncertain.

Follicular Lymphoma

Follicular lymphoma is the second most common type of uterine lymphoma, and follicular lymphomas of all three grades have been reported.[2] As is diffuse large B-cell lymphoma, cervical follicular lymphoma often is associated with sclerosis. Neoplastic follicles often are found in a perivascular location as they invade the wall of the cervix (Figures 10-12 and 10-13).[28]

Extranodal Marginal Zone Lymphoma of Mucosa-Associated Lymphoid Tissue

Several cases of endometrial marginal zone lymphoma and rare cervical marginal zone lymphomas* have been reported. Given the frequency of follicular cervicitis and the concept that marginal zone lymphomas arise in a background of acquired mucosa-associated lymphoid tissue (MALT), the rarity of cervical marginal zone lymphomas is surprising.

In 1997, three cases of a distinctive type of low-grade endometrial B-cell lymphoma were described.[42] The lymphomas all affected women in their 60s and were all incidental findings; the lymphoma was confined to the uterus and did not form a grossly apparent mass. These lymphomas shared common histologic and immunohistologic features. Microscopic examination showed that they were made up of large nodules composed of a monotonous population of small lymphoid cells with slightly irregular nuclei and scant, pale cytoplasm adjacent to and sometimes surrounding endometrial glands. Immunohistochemical analysis showed B

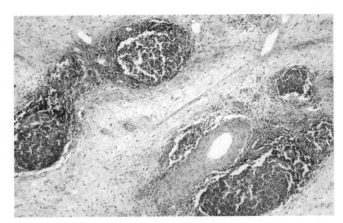

Figure 10-13 Perivascular spread of neoplastic follicles deep into the cervical wall.

cells with aberrant co-expression of CD43. Clonality was confirmed with evaluation of the immunoglobulin heavy chain gene *(IGH)* by PCR. Follow-up, when available, was uneventful.

The authors of this study were reluctant to subclassify their lymphomas as the marginal zone type for a number of reasons: lymphoepithelial lesions were inconspicuous; a marginal zone pattern and reactive follicle centers were absent; and only limited immunophenotyping could be performed.

Subsequently, other investigators have described two cases with identical histologic features, also in women in their 60s with lymphoma confined to the uterus. The neoplastic cells were CD20+, bcl2+, and CD79a+, without expression of CD5, CD10, bcl6, or cyclin D1 (all markers were not tested in both cases). The cellular nodules were associated with altered follicular dendritic cell meshworks that were positive for CD21[17] or for CD23.[43] Clonal rearrangement of *IGH* was demonstrated in one case.[43] These cases were interpreted as endometrial marginal zone lymphomas.

---

*References 1, 2, 26, 27, 41, and 42.

We have seen two cases with features virtually identical to those of the published cases. These cases are best classified as endometrial marginal zone lymphomas of mucosa-associated lymphoid tissue (MALT lymphomas), albeit with distinctive clinical and pathologic features (Figure 10-14).

Miscellaneous Rare Lymphomas

A few cases of Burkitt's lymphoma[2,44] and rare cases of B-lymphoblastic lymphoma,[2] peripheral T-cell lymphoma,[45,46] and cervical extranodal NK/T-cell lymphoma, nasal type,[26] have been reported. One of the peripheral T-cell lymphomas appeared to arise in a leiomyoma and involved endometrial glands in a pattern reminiscent of enteropathy-type T-cell lymphoma; this epitheliotropic lymphoma had a cytotoxic phenotype (CD8+, TIA-1+). A monomorphic B-cell post-transplantation lymphoproliferative disorder confined to the cervix and lower uterine segment has been described.[3] A case of lymphocyte-depleted classical Hodgkin's lymphoma has been reported in which the diagnosis was confirmed with immunophenotyping that showed CD15 and CD30 expression by the neoplastic cells.[2]

Staging, Treatment, and Outcome

Although most uterine lymphomas have reached a large size by the time of diagnosis, most are localized (Ann Arbor stage I or stage II) at presentation; stage I is more frequent than stage II.[27,32] Uterine lymphoma has a relatively good prognosis.[1,26,35,47] Patients have been treated with surgery, radiation, chemotherapy, or a combination of these modalities; optimal therapy for this disease has not been determined precisely. In a few cases, young women have been successfully treated with combination chemotherapy and some of them have maintained fertility.[1,36] Only a few recently diagnosed cases have been treated with rituxan; therefore, its role in the treatment of this disease is unclear.[33]

In reviews of this topic, approximately 70% to 90% of patients were alive and free of disease at last follow-up.[29,32] The 5-year survival rate for cervical lymphoma is approximately 80%.[27,30] Most

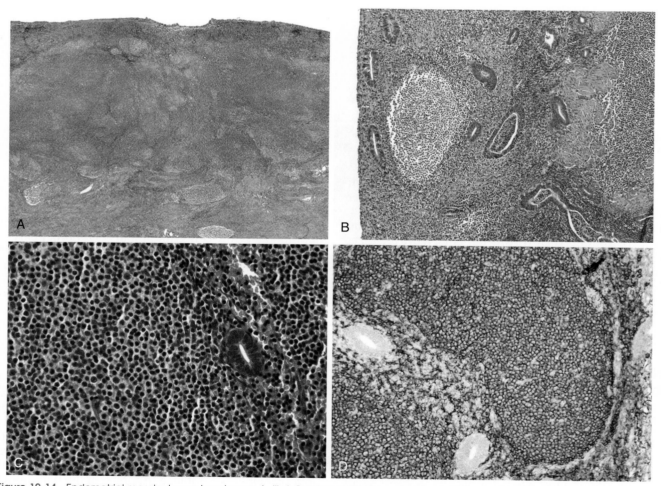

Figure 10-14 Endometrial marginal zone lymphoma. **A,** Ill-defined nodules of lymphoid cells fill the endometrium and invade subjacent myometrium. **B,** Higher power view shows monotonous nodules of lymphoid cells displacing endometrial glands. **C,** High-power view shows monotonous small lymphoid cells with moderately abundant, pale cytoplasm adjacent to an endometrial gland. **D,** Nodules of small lymphoid cells are composed of CD20+ B cells.

Continued

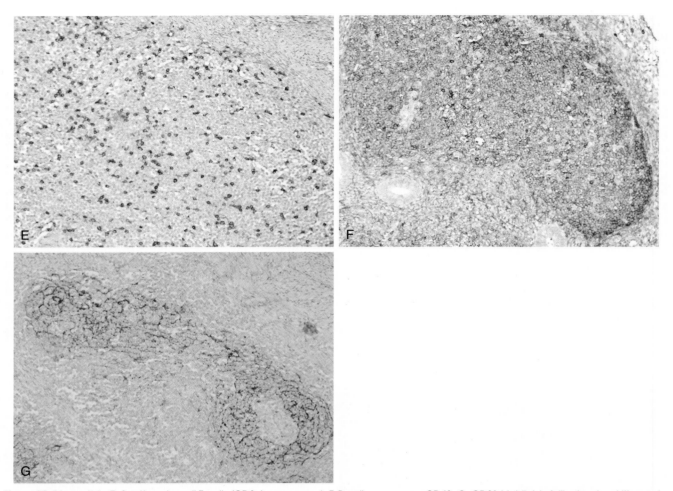

Figure 10-14, cont'd   E, Scattered small T cells (CD3+) are present. **F,** B cells co-express CD43. **G,** CD21 highlights follicular dendritic meshworks associated with nodules of lymphoid cells. (*D* to *G,* Immunoperoxidase technique on paraffin sections.)

information on uterine lymphoma is related to lymphoma that arises in the cervix. Not enough information is available to allow definite conclusions to be drawn about the prognosis of the rare endometrial lymphomas. However, patients with localized disease tend to do well, including those with endometrial marginal zone lymphomas,[42] the epitheliotropic T-cell lymphoma noted previously,[46] and one well-documented endometrial peripheral T-cell lymphoma.[45] Patients with advanced disease that presents with endometrial involvement tend to fare poorly.[28]

Secondary Uterine Involvement by Lymphoma

Secondary involvement of the uterus in cases of disseminated lymphoma is not unusual. Secondary involvement of the female genital tract may be asymptomatic or may be accompanied by vaginal bleeding or discharge.[1,2,26] In contrast to primary uterine lymphoma, when the uterus is secondarily involved by lymphoma, the corpus is involved at least as often as the cervix. The types of lymphomas encountered also vary more than in primary cases,

with a less pronounced predominance of diffuse large B-cell lymphoma. They include diffuse large B-cell lymphoma, follicular lymphoma, chronic lymphocytic leukemia, lymphoblastic lymphoma[1,2,26] and extranodal NK/T-cell lymphoma.[48] The prognosis is much worse than for primary uterine lymphoma.[27,48] We have seen the case of a patient with a history of chronic lymphocytic leukemia in which a diffuse large B-cell lymphoma developed (Richter's transformation) and involved the uterus (Figure 10-15).

■ PLACENTAL INVOLVEMENT BY LYMPHOMA

Approximately 0.1% of women have a malignancy during pregnancy, a subset of which is lymphoma. In rare cases, lymphoma during pregnancy spreads to involve the placenta.[49-52] Some patients have been treated successfully for the lymphoma, and others have succumbed to the disease. Most often, placental involvement does not lead to spread of the lymphoma to the fetus, although in rare cases this does occur.[51,52] The fetal immune system, or the placenta itself, may serve as a barrier to fetal involvement by lymphoma.

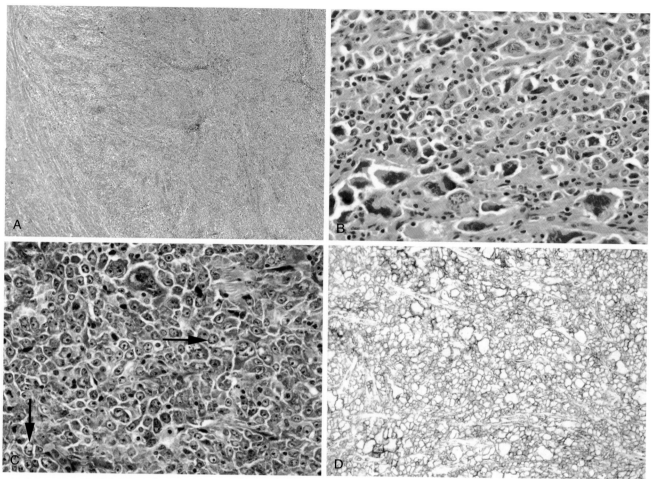

Figure 10-15   Richter's transformation of chronic lymphocytic leukemia, presenting with uterine involvement as a polypoid lesion of the endocervix. **A,** A cellular tumor involves the stroma. **B,** High-power view shows many large lymphoid cells with oval nuclei and prominent nucleoli, a few binucleated cells, and many bizarre giant cells *(bottom of image).* **C,** A Giemsa stain illustrates the vesicular chromatin, prominent nucleoli, and deeply basophilic cytoplasm of the large cells in this lymphoma. Most cells are immunoblasts, with single, prominent, central nucleoli. A few are centroblasts with several peripherally located nucleoli *(arrows).* A few very large bizarre cells are also seen. **D,** Neoplastic cells are CD45+ (immunoperoxidase technique on a paraffin section). They also were diffusely positive for CD20 (not illustrated).

On gross examination, the involved placenta may show white nodules, white granular areas, or infarcts.[49,50] Microscopic examination shows a variably dense infiltrate of neoplastic cells in the intervillous space (maternal circulation). In rare cases, neoplastic cells also are found within the chorionic villi involving blood vessels (fetal circulation)[51,52]; involvement of chorionic villi may be associated with spread of the malignancy to the fetus, resulting in death within a few months of delivery (Figure 10-16). This underscores the importance of careful gross and microscopic examination of the placenta in the setting of maternal malignancy.

Lymphomas that involve the placenta have been aggressive lymphomas of B- and T-lineage.[49] Single cases of mediastinal large B-cell lymphoma[50] and ALK+ anaplastic large cell lymphoma[49] have been reported. We have seen an EBV+ aggressive NK-cell leukemia/lymphoma[51] that presented in the third trimester of pregnancy in a young woman; EBV+

neoplastic cells were identified in the placenta and were transmitted to the fetus (see Figure 10-16). Both the mother and infant succumbed to the lymphoid malignancy.

■ VAGINAL LYMPHOMAS

Primary Vaginal Lymphomas

Clinical Features

Lymphoma rarely arises in the vagina.[1,31,53,54] Patients with primary vaginal lymphoma have ranged in age from 19 to 79 years; the mean age is in the 40s. They present with vaginal bleeding, discharge, pain or discomfort, dyspareunia, urinary frequency, or a mass. The lesion may compress the urethra and cause anuria[55] or bladder distension.[53] On physical examination, the tumors typically result in ill-defined thickening or induration of the vaginal

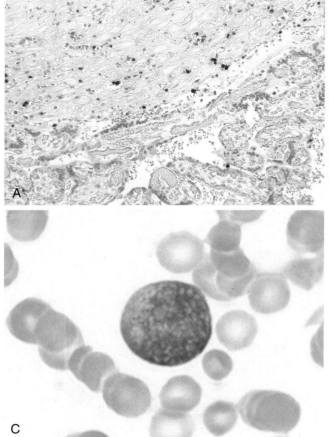

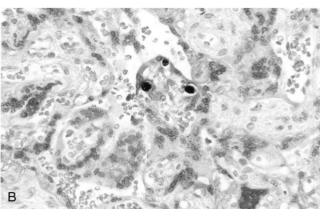

Figure 10-16 Aggressive NK cell leukemia involving the placenta. **A,** Scattered EBV+ cells are present in the decidua, and a few also are in the intervillous space. **B,** Rare EBV+ cells are present in a villus in the fetal circulation. **C,** Large atypical lymphoid cells were found in the infant's blood shortly after birth, and the child died at 2 months of age. (*A* and *B,* In situ hybridization with an Epstein-Barr virus–encoded RNA (*E,* Probe on paraffin sections.)

wall, often with invasion of adjacent structures such as the cervix and the rectovaginal septum[53]; extension to the parametrium and even to the pelvic side walls has been described.[54] In rare cases a firm, bulky vaginal lymphoma may mimic a leiomyoma on physical examination.[56] Because the surface epithelium usually is intact, Papanicolaou smears generally are negative.[57]

Pathologic Features

The pathologic features are very similar to those of cervical lymphoma. Nearly all the lymphomas are the diffuse large B-cell type (Figure 10-17),[1,2,53,54,56] but rare cases of follicular lymphoma,[2,28,33] Burkitt's lymphoma, lymphoplasmacytic lymphoma,[2] T-cell lymphoma,[1,57] and one well-documented marginal zone lymphoma[55] have been reported. As in the cervix, vaginal diffuse large B-cell lymphomas often are associated with marked sclerosis, and some are composed of neoplastic cells with spindle cell morphology (Figure 10-18), sometimes accompanied by a storiform pattern of growth. In the very small number of spindle cell diffuse large B-cell lymphomas studied, the lymphomas have been CD20+, CD5−, CD10−, bcl6+, MUM1/IRF4−, CD138−, Epstein-Barr virus negative (EBV−), and human herpes virus type 8 negative (HHV8−) with somatic mutation of both

immunoglobulin and *BCL6* genes. These features suggest that the so-called "spindle cell variant" of diffuse large B-cell lymphoma corresponds to a germinal center stage of B-cell maturation.[38] Isolated cases of EBV+ primary vaginal lymphoma have been reported.[58] We have seen a case of B-lymphoblastic lymphoma that presented with vaginal involvement. The surface of the lesion had a papillary configuration, and the clinical impression had been condyloma acuminatum (Figure 10-19).

Staging, Treatment, and Outcome

Cases classified as primary vaginal lymphoma present with localized disease (stage IE or IIE). Treatment has not been uniform, but vaginal lymphoma appears to have a favorable prognosis.[31,33,53-55,57,58] For example, in one series of eight cases of diffuse large B-cell lymphoma, only one patient died of lymphoma.[53]

Secondary Vaginal Involvement by Lymphoma

Secondary involvement of the vagina by malignant lymphoma is more common than primary vaginal lymphoma.[1] In contrast to primary vaginal lymphoma, cases of widespread lymphoma that present with vaginal involvement do not have a favorable prognosis.[53,57]

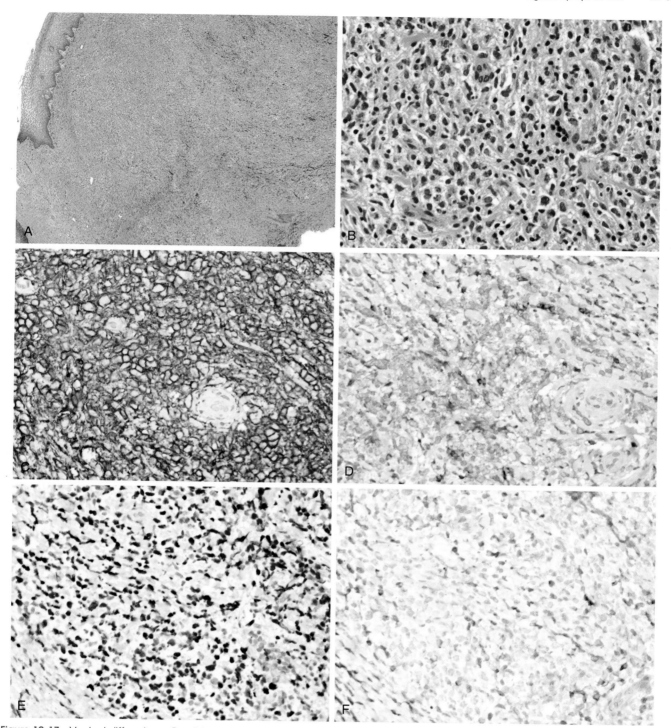

Figure 10-17 Vaginal diffuse large B-cell lymphoma. **A,** Biopsy sample shows a densely cellular infiltrate extending deep into the vaginal wall. The overlying squamous epithelium is intact. **B,** High-power view shows large atypical cells with oval, irregular and lobated nuclei, and associated delicate interstitial sclerosis. Scattered small, dark, reactive lymphocytes also are present. The atypical cells are diffusely positive for CD20 **(C),** faintly positive for CD10 **(D),** positive for bcl6 **(E),** and negative for bcl2 **(F).** The few bcl2+ cells are reactive T cells (immunoperoxidase technique on paraffin sections).

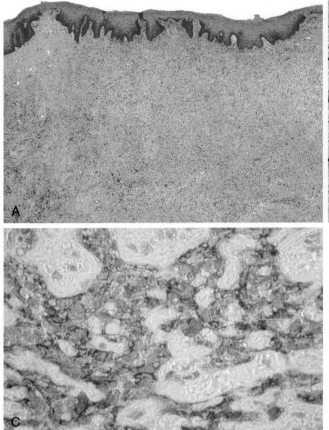

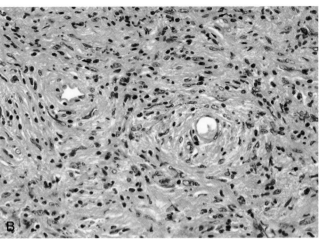

Figure 10-18 Vaginal diffuse large B-cell lymphoma composed of spindle cells, with prominent sclerosis. **A,** A cellular proliferation diffusely involves the vaginal stroma. The surface epithelium is intact. **B,** High-power view shows atypical cells with elongate, sometimes twisted, occasionally oval or lobated nuclei and scant cytoplasm associated with coarse sclerosis. The atypical cells are CD20+ **(C).** (Immunoperoxidase technique on a paraffin section.)

■ VULVAR LYMPHOMAS

Primary Vulvar Lymphomas

Primary vulvar lymphoma is rare. Patients are adults who present with a nodule, swelling, or induration of the vulva.[1,59] Rare patients have presented with a mass of Bartholin's gland[60] or with a clitoral mass.[2] Based on the small number of reported cases, patients on average appear to be older than those with lymphoma that arises in other parts of the female genital tract.[2] Rare patients are HIV positive or iatrogenically immunosuppressed (Figure 10-20).[1,4,59,61] Diffuse large B-cell lymphoma is the most common type.[1,59,60,62] Several cases of lymphoplasmacytic lymphoma have been reported[2]; other types are rare. We have seen an example of peripheral T-cell lymphoma that occurred in a renal allograft recipient (Figure 10-20).[4] Vulvar lymphoma is overall relatively aggressive, but occasional patients have long disease-free survival times.

Secondary Vulvar Involvement by Lymphoma

Secondary involvement of the vulva by lymphoma is rare but has been reported.[19] The lymphomas have been of various types.[2] Mycosis fungoides may involve the vulva, but typically skin elsewhere also

is involved.[26] In rare cases patients with widespread lymphoma have symptoms related to vulvar involvement at initial presentation.[1] A case of MUM1/IRF4+, CD138+, CD20–, EBV+ plasmablastic lymphoma in a young HIV-positive child who presented initially with vulvar involvement has been reported; staging revealed widespread disease.[63] This case is especially unusual, because plasmablastic lymphoma is rare in children and also because vulvar involvement by plasmablastic lymphoma had not been documented previously. (Plasmablastic lymphoma is discussed in more detail in Lymphomas of the Oral Cavity in Chapter 3.)

A case of classical Hodgkin's lymphoma that presented with a vulvar mass has been described in a patient with long-standing Crohn's disease.[64] The patient had had recurring anovaginal fistulas before the lymphoma developed. The histologic features and the immunophenotype of the neoplastic cells (CD15+, CD30+, CD45–, CD20–) were typical of classical Hodgkin's lymphoma. Staging revealed widespread disease. The findings in this case may be analogous to the rare but well-documented phenomenon of classical Hodgkin's lymphoma that arises in the gastrointestinal tract of patients with Crohn's disease with preferential involvement of areas of the bowel involved by Crohn's disease (see Hodgkin's Lymphoma of the Gastrointestinal Tract in Chapter 5).

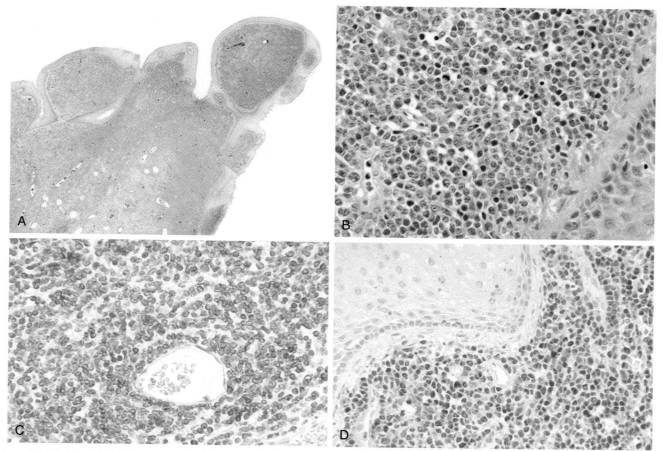

Figure 10-19 B-lymphoblastic lymphoma presenting with vaginal involvement. **A,** The lymphoma forms an exophytic lesion with a papillary surface; clinically it was thought to be a condyloma. **B,** High-power view shows a proliferation of slightly enlarged lymphoid cells with oval to slightly irregular nuclei, fine chromatin, pinpoint nucleoli, and scant cytoplasm. Mitoses are frequent. Atypical cells are CD79a+ **(C)** and TdT+ **(D)** (immunoperoxidase technique on paraffin sections). They were also CD10+, CD43+, CD45 dim+, and negative for CD3 and for myeloperoxidase (not illustrated), which confirmed a diagnosis of B-lymphoblastic lymphoma.

Differential Diagnosis of Lymphoma of the Lower Female Genital Tract

The differential diagnosis of lymphoma of the lower female genital tract includes chronic inflammatory processes, carcinoma, sarcomas, undifferentiated malignant tumors, and other conditions. Some of the entities in the differential diagnosis are more common than lymphoma in this site, which compounds the difficulty of reaching the correct diagnosis.

1. **Lymphoma of the lower female genital tract versus reactive lymphoid infiltrates.**
   a. *Nonspecific chronic inflammation.* Lymphoma tends not to involve the most superficial part of the cervical or vaginal wall and is easily distorted by crush artifact; therefore, unless a deep biopsy specimen is obtained and the specimen is handled carefully, it may be nondiagnostic or mistaken for a reactive lymphoid infiltrate.
   b. *Marked chronic inflammation.* Inflammatory processes are much more common than lymphoma in the female genital tract, but severe chronic cervicitis can potentially mimic a low-grade lymphoma. Follicular cervicitis accompanied by a dense infiltrate of small lymphocytes and plasma cells may suggest the possibility of a marginal zone lymphoma with admixed reactive follicles. A superficially located infiltrate with a mixed composition focally involving the cervix favors an inflammatory process. In difficult cases, immunophenotyping can be performed; a mixture of B and T cells and polytypic plasma cells favors a reactive process.
   c. *Lymphoma-like lesion.* The uterine cervix, and less often the endometrium and vulva, can be involved by a prominent reactive lymphoid infiltrate often with a conspicuous component of large lymphoid cells; these lymphoid infiltrates have been referred to as "lymphoma-like lesions."[65-67] The atypical appearance often raises the possibility of lymphoma, although a number of clues can help the pathologist arrive at the correct diagnosis. Lymphoma-like lesions almost all occur in patients of reproductive age and only rarely affect postmenopausal patients. Abnormal uterine bleeding is common. A few patients have developed

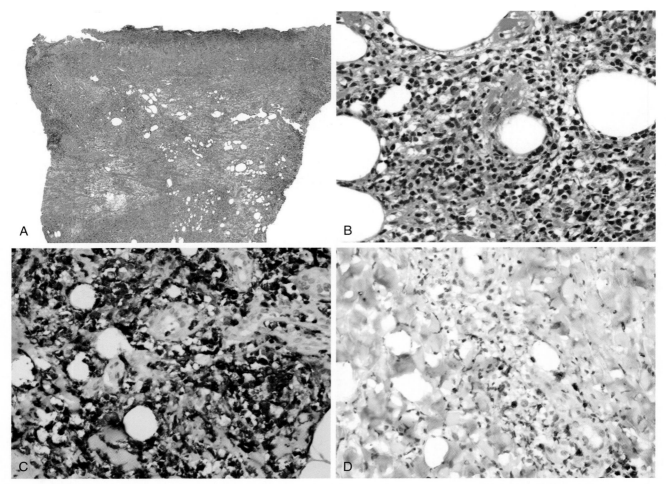

Figure 10-20   Peripheral T-cell lymphoma involving the vulva in a renal allograft recipient. **A,** Punch biopsy specimen of skin shows extensive necrosis and a patchy, lymphoid infiltrate. **B,** Needle biopsy also was performed; this specimen showed areas with a denser lymphoid infiltrate. The atypical cells are a range of sizes and have dark, irregular nuclei and scant cytoplasm. Immunostains show that the lymphoid cells are CD3+ **(C)** and CD5– **(D)**; they also were negative for CD4 and CD8, an abnormal immunophenotype.

lymphoma-like lesions in the setting of pelvic inflammatory disease or infectious mononucleosis. A lymphoma-like lesion occasionally may be an incidental finding in a patient biopsied for investigation of an abnormal Papanicolaou smear.

Colposcopic examination of cervical lesions reveals polyps and eroded, friable mucosa or small nodules confined to the cervix. Large masses are uncommon. The rare vulvar lesions may be small ulcers. Microscopic examination reveals a mixture of large lymphoid cells, small lymphocytes, plasma cells, and neutrophils in a diffuse pattern, occasionally with interspersed lymphoid follicles. Large cells may form small or large collections. The infiltrate typically is superficially located and associated with erosion. Within the wall of the cervix, the infiltrate generally is no more than 3 mm deep, and it only infrequently extends deeper than the endocervical glands (Figure 10-21). A background of chronic endometritis in endometrial lesions and of nonspecific acute and chronic

cervicitis in cervical lesions often is seen. Sclerosis is not associated with lymphoma-like lesions. Immunohistochemical studies show that large cells are B cells (CD20+, CD79a+) without aberrant antigen expression. Large cells in follicles are CD10+, bcl6+, and bcl2–.[66] Plasma cells are polytypic. In occasional cases of lymphoma-like lesion, PCR reveals a clonal B-cell population, which may heighten the suspicion of lymphoma.[67] However, lymphoma-like lesions with and without clonal B cells otherwise are indistinguishable from one another, and the clonal B cells may represent a focused response to antigen, perhaps the infection or other process responsible for the development of the lymphoma-like lesion. Establishing a diagnosis requires careful correlation of the clinical, histologic, and immunophenotypic data. In this setting, the finding of clonal B cells is not considered sufficient for a diagnosis of lymphoma. Because lymphoma-like lesions may resolve spontaneously, rebiopsy may be helpful in difficult cases.

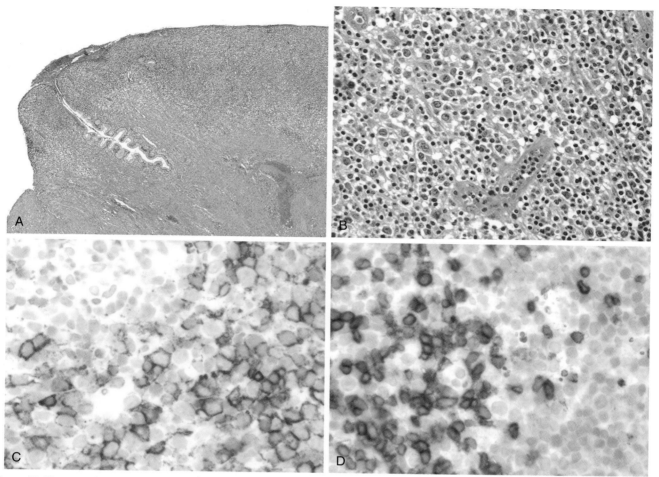

Figure 10-21   Lymphoma-like lesion of the uterine cervix. **A,** Low-power view shows a prominent but superficially located infiltrate in a bandlike pattern. The infiltrate involves the surface epithelium. Sclerosis is not conspicuous. **B,** The infiltrate consists of scattered and loosely clustered large lymphoid cells in a mixed background of small lymphocytes, plasma cells, and a few neutrophils. **C,** Large cells and a few small cells are CD20+ B cells. **D,** CD3 highlights many small T cells. (*C* and *D,* Immunoperoxidase technique on paraffin sections.)

In contrast, lymphomas typically produce large, deeply invasive masses that often invade adjacent structures (see Figures 10-8 through 10-10). Surface involvement and ulceration are unusual. The neoplastic population is more monomorphous and often is associated with sclerosis.

   d. *Leiomyoma with lymphoid infiltration.* Leiomyoma with lymphoid infiltration is a rare condition in which uterine leiomyomas harbor a variably dense infiltrate of small lymphocytes with scattered larger lymphoid cells, occasionally with germinal centers, plasma cells and, in rare cases, eosinophils. The inflammatory cells usually are confined to the leiomyoma. The polymorphous nature of the infiltrate and its confinement to the leiomyoma help distinguish it from lymphoma. The etiology is unknown, but possibilities include inflammation related to an intrauterine contraceptive device,[68] autoimmune disease, and use of gonadotropin-releasing hormone (GnRH) agonists.[69] In all reported cases of leiomyoma with lymphoid infiltration, follow-up has been uneventful.[68]

2. **Lymphoma of the lower female genital tract versus carcinoma.** Poorly differentiated carcinoma, especially lymphoepithelial carcinoma and small cell carcinoma, may enter the differential diagnosis of lymphoma. Some poorly differentiated carcinomas or poorly fixed carcinomas may be composed of cells that appear discohesive. Careful examination of the best preserved areas may reveal definite cohesive growth, which excludes lymphoma. Carcinoma tends to invade and obliterate normal structures; lymphoma tends to infiltrate around these structures, with relative preservation of endometrial and endocervical glands and sparing of the most superficial subepithelial stroma. Adjacent in situ squamous or adenocarcinoma favors carcinoma.

3. **Lymphoma of the lower female genital tract versus sarcoma.**

   a. *Spindle cell sarcoma.* The tendency of some cervical and vaginal lymphomas to assume a spindle cell or sarcomatoid pattern may

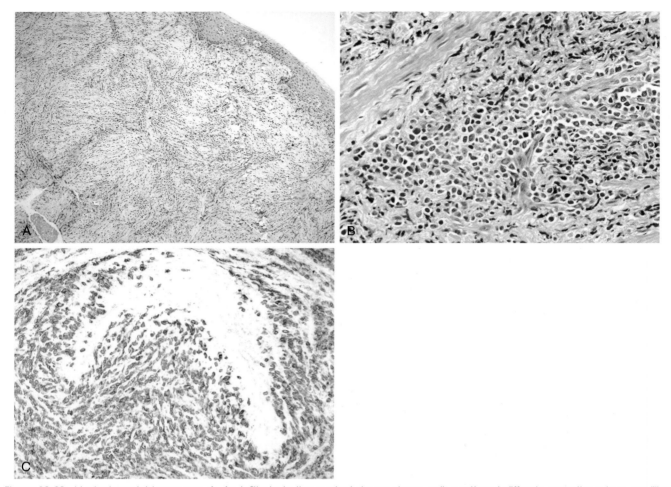

Figure 10-22 Vaginal myeloid sarcoma. **A,** An infiltrate in the vaginal stroma shows cells scattered diffusely, sometimes in a cordlike pattern. **B,** The neoplasm consists of medium-sized, discohesive, primitive cells with fine chromatin, small nucleoli, and scant cytoplasm. **C,** Tumor cells are positive for myeloperoxidase. (Immunoperoxidase technique on a paraffin section.)

raise the question of a spindle cell sarcoma. Awareness of this histologic pattern and a basic panel of immunostains can help establish a diagnosis.

b. *Low-grade endometrial stromal sarcoma.* The relatively small, dark nuclei and high nuclear to cytoplasmic ratio characteristic of endometrial stromal cells may bring low-grade endometrial stromal sarcoma into the differential diagnosis of lymphoma. Endometrial stromal sarcoma often invades in the form of a nodular or wormlike protrusion into the myometrium and/or blood vessels. Endometrial stromal cells tend to be less closely packed than lymphoid cells. Small arterioles are characteristically interspersed among neoplastic stromal cells, a finding not associated with most lymphomas.

c. *Embryonal rhabdomyosarcoma.* Embryonal rhabdomyosarcoma may be considered in the differential diagnosis, but this neoplasm is more common in children and more likely to have a myxoid background and alternating hypocellular and hypercellular areas.

4. **Lymphoma of the lower female genital tract versus extramedullary hematopoiesis.** The uterus is rarely involved by extramedullary hematopoiesis,[70] which could be mistaken for an abnormal lymphoid infiltrate, particularly if erythroid elements predominate. In roughly half of reported cases, an underlying hematologic disorder has been found. The endometrial stroma is the most common site of involvement, although in rare cases extramedullary hematopoiesis is seen in the myometrium or in uterine malignancies.[70]

5. **Lymphoma of the lower female genital tract versus Langerhans' cell histiocytosis.** The vulva, and less often other portions of the lower female genital tract, may be affected by Langerhans' cell histiocytosis (histiocytosis X, eosinophilic granuloma).[71] Female genital tract involvement can occur in isolation or in association with disease in other anatomic sites. Vulvar Langerhans' cell histiocytosis produces one or more pruritic lesions, often with ulceration. As in other sites, the neoplastic cells have large oval, folded, or twisted nuclei, which may show longitudinal

grooves, and abundant pale pink cytoplasm. In contrast, large lymphoid cells have oval, irregular, lobated, or elongate nuclei that often are vesicular; coarse chromatin along the nuclear membrane; frequently prominent nucleoli; and scant cytoplasm. Interspersed eosinophils may provide a clue to the diagnosis of Langerhans' cell histiocytosis. The immunophenotype of Langerhans' cells (S100+, CD1a+, Langerin+) differs from that of lymphoid cells.

6. **Lymphoma of the lower female genital tract versus myeloid sarcoma.** Myeloid sarcoma rarely involves the female genital tract[72]; when it does, it may cause problems in the differential diagnosis with lymphoma. Features helpful in distinguishing female genital tract myeloid sarcoma from lymphoma are similar to those in other sites. Primitive myeloid cells, on average, are slightly smaller and have more finely dispersed chromatin and smaller nucleoli than large lymphoid cells (Figure 10-22). If some maturation of the neoplastic myeloid cells has occurred, some cells may have a variable amount of pink cytoplasm consistent with the presence of myeloid granules. Immunophenotyping establishes the diagnosis (also see Differential Diagnosis of Testicular Lymphoma in Chapter 9 and Table 12-2, Lymphomas of Bone and Their Differential Diagnosis, in Chapter 12).

REFERENCES

1. Ferry J, Young R: Malignant lymphoma of the genitourinary tract, *Curr Diagn Pathol* 4:145-169, 1997.
2. Kosari F, Daneshbod Y, Parwaresch R et al: Lymphomas of the female genital tract: a study of 186 cases and review of the literature, *Am J Surg Pathol* 29:1512-1520, 2005.
3. Nagarsheth NP, Kalir T, Rahaman J: Post-transplant lymphoproliferative disorder of the cervix, *Gynecol Oncol* 97:271-275, 2005.
4. Kaplan MA, Jacobson JO, Ferry JA, Harris NL: T cell lymphoma of the vulva with erythrophagocytosis in a renal allograft recipient, *Am J Surg Pathol* 17:842-849, 1993.
5. Lanjewar D, Dongaonkar D: HIV-associated primary non-Hodgkin's lymphoma of ovary: a case report, *Gynecol Oncol* 102:590-592, 2006.
6. Mansouri H, Sifat H, Gaye M et al: Primary malignant lymphoma of the ovary: an unusual presentation of a rare disease, *Eur J Gynaec Oncol* 21:616-618, 2000.
7. Dimopoulos MA, Daliani D, Pugh W et al: Primary ovarian non-Hodgkin's lymphoma: outcome after treatment with combination chemotherapy, *Gynecol Oncol* 64:446-450, 1997.
8. Freeman C, Berg J, Cutler S: Occurrence and prognosis of extranodal lymphomas, *Cancer* 29:252-260, 1972.
9. Scully RE: Tumors of the ovary and maldeveloped gonads. In *Atlas of tumor pathology*, Second series, Fascicle 16, pp 117-127, Washington, DC, 1979, Armed Forces Institute of Pathology.
10. Vang R, Medeiros L, Warnke R et al: Ovarian non-Hodgkin's lymphoma: a clinicopathologic study of eight primary cases, *Mod Pathol* 14:1093-1099, 2001.
11. Magloire LK, Pettker CM, Buhimschi CS, Funai EF: Burkitt's lymphoma of the ovary in pregnancy, *Obstet Gynecol* 108:743-745, 2006.
12. Neuhauser TS, Tavassoli FA, Abbondanzo SL: Follicle center lymphoma involving the female genital tract: a morphologic and molecular genetic study of three cases, *Ann Diagn Pathol* 4:293-299, 2000.
13. McKelvey A, McKenna D, McManus D, Joyce M: A case of lymphoma occurring in an ovarian teratoma, *Gynecol Oncol* 90:474-477, 2003.
14. Lagoo AS, Robboy SJ: Lymphoma of the female genital tract: current status, *Int J Gynecol Pathol* 25:1-21, 2006.
15. Leoncini L, Raphael M, Stein H et al: Burkitt lymphoma. In Swerdlow S, Campo E, Harris N et al, editors: *WHO classification: tumours of haematopoietic and lymphoid tissues*, ed 4, pp 262-264, Lyon, 2008, IARC.
16. Chishima F, Hayakawa S, Ohta Y et al: Ovarian Burkitt's lymphoma diagnosed by a combination of clinical features, morphology, immunophenotype, and molecular findings and successfully managed with surgery and chemotherapy, *Int J Gynecol Cancer* 16(suppl 1):337-343, 2006.
17. Iyengar P, Deodhare S: Primary extranodal marginal zone B-cell lymphoma of MALT type of the endometrium, *Gynecol Oncol* 93:238-241, 2004.
18. Chong AL, Ngan BY, Weitzman S, Abla O: Anaplastic large cell lymphoma of the ovary in a pediatric patient, *J Pediatr Hematol Oncol* 31:702-704, 2009.
19. Lathrop JC: Malignant pelvic lymphomas, *Obstet Gynecol* 30:137-145, 1967.
20. de Leval L, Ferry J, Falini B et al: Expression of bcl-6 and CD10 in primary mediastinal large cell lymphoma: evidence for derivation from germinal center B cells? *Am J Surg Pathol* 25:1277-1282, 2001.
21. Zinzani P, Martelli M, Bertini M et al: Induction chemotherapy strategies for primary mediastinal large B-cell lymphoma with sclerosis: a retrospective multinational study on 426 previously untreated patients, *Haematologica* 87:1258-1264, 2002.
22. Shulman LN, Hitt RA, Ferry JA: Case records of the Massachusetts General Hospital: case 4-2008—a 33-year-old pregnant woman with swelling of the left breast and shortness of breath, *N Engl J Med* 358:513-523, 2008.
23. Noack F, Lange K, Lehmann V et al: Primary extranodal marginal zone B-cell lymphoma of the fallopian tube, *Gynecol Oncol* 86:384-386, 2002.
24. Goodlad JR, MacPherson S, Jackson R et al: Extranodal follicular lymphoma: a clinicopathological and genetic analysis of 15 cases arising at non-cutaneous extranodal sites, *Histopathology* 44:268-276, 2004.
25. Gaffan J, Herbertson R, Davis P et al: Bilateral peripheral T-cell lymphoma of the fallopian tubes, *Gynecol Oncol* 95:736-738, 2004.
26. Vang R, Medeiros LJ, Fuller GN et al: Non-Hodgkin's lymphoma involving the gynecologic tract: a review of 88 cases, *Adv Anat Pathol* 8:200-217, 2001.
27. Vang R, Medeiros LJ, Ha CS, Deavers M: Non-Hodgkin's lymphomas involving the uterus: a clinicopathologic analysis of 26 cases, *Mod Pathol* 13:19-28, 2000.
28. Harris NL, Scully RE: Malignant lymphoma and granulocytic sarcoma of the uterus and vagina: a clinicopathologic analysis of 27 cases, *Cancer* 53:2530-2545, 1984.
29. Dursun P, Gultekin M, Bozdag G et al: Primary cervical lymphoma: report of two cases and review of the literature, *Gynecol Oncol* 98:484-489, 2005.
30. Makarewicz R, Kuzminska A: Non-Hodgkin's lymphoma of the uterine cervix: a report of three patients, *Clin Oncol (R Coll Radiol)* 7:198-199, 1995.
31. Perren T, Farrant M, McCarthy K et al: Lymphomas of the cervix and upper vagina: a report of five cases and a review of the literature, *Gynecol Oncol* 44:87-95, 1992.
32. Chan JK, Loizzi V, Magistris A et al: Clinicopathologic features of six cases of primary cervical lymphoma, *Am J Obstet Gynecol* 193:866-872, 2005.
33. Cohn DE, Resnick KE, Eaton LA et al: Non-Hodgkin's lymphoma mimicking gynecological malignancies of the vagina and cervix: a report of four cases, *Int J Gynecol Cancer* 17:274-279, 2007.
34. Alvarez A, Ortiz J, Sacristan F: Large B-cell lymphoma of the uterine corpus: case report with immunohistochemical and molecular study, *Gynecol Oncol* 65:534-538, 1997.
35. Chandy L, Kumar L, Dawar R: Non-Hodgkin's lymphoma presenting as a primary lesion in uterine cervix: case report, *J Obstet Gynaecol Res* 24:183-187, 1998.

36. Garavaglia E, Taccagni G, Montoli S et al: Primary stage I-IIE non-Hodgkin's lymphoma of uterine cervix and upper vagina: evidence for a conservative approach in a study on three patients, *Gynecol Oncol* 97:214-218, 2005.

37. Kawauchi S, Fukuma F, Morioka H et al: Malignant lymphoma arising as a primary tumor of the uterine corpus, *Pathol Int* 52:423-424, 2002.

38. Carbone A, Gloghini A, Libra M et al: A spindle cell variant of diffuse large B-cell lymphoma possesses genotypic and phenotypic markers characteristic of a germinal center B-cell origin, *Mod Pathol* 19:299-306, 2006.

39. Kahlifa M, Buckstein R, Perez-Ordonez B: Sarcomatoid variant of B-cell lymphoma of the uterine cervix, *Int J Gynecol Pathol* 22:289-293, 2003.

40. Gutman PD, Williams JP, Dveksler GS et al: T-cell-rich B-cell lymphoma and Epstein-Barr virus infection of the uterus in a patient with an intrauterine contraceptive device in place for over 20 years, *Gynecol Oncol* 68:288-292, 1998.

41. Ballesteros E, Osborne BM, Matsushima AY: CD5+ low-grade marginal zone B-cell lymphomas with localized presentation, *Am J Surg Pathol* 22:201-207, 1998.

42. van de Rijn M, Kamel O, Chang P et al: Primary low grade endometrial B-cell lymphoma, *Am J Surg Pathol* 21:187-194, 1997.

43. Heeren JH, Croonen AM, Pijnenborg JM: Primary extranodal marginal zone B-cell lymphoma of the female genital tract: a case report and literature review, *Int J Gynecol Pathol* 27:243-246, 2008.

44. Nomura S, Ishii K, Shimamoto Y et al: Burkitt lymphoma of the uterus in a human T lymphotropic virus type-1 carrier, *Intern Med* 45:215-217, 2006.

45. Kirk CM, Naumann RW, Hartmann CJ et al: Primary endometrial T-cell lymphoma: a case report, *Am J Clin Pathol* 115:561-566, 2001.

46. Merz H, Lange K, Koch B et al: Primary extranodal CD8 positive epitheliotropic T-cell lymphoma arising in a leiomyoma of the uterus, *BJOG* 110:527-529, 2003.

47. Nasu K, Yoshimatsu J, Urata K, Miyakawa I: A case of primary non-Hodgkin's lymphoma of the uterine cervix treated by combination chemotherapy (THP-COP), *J Obstet Gynaecol Res* 24:157-160, 1998.

48. Murase T, Inagaki H, Takagi N et al: Nasal NK-cell lymphoma followed by relapse in the uterine cervix, *Leuk Lymphoma* 43:203-206, 2002.

49. Meguerian-Bedoyan Z, Lamant L, Hopfner C et al: Anaplastic large cell lymphoma of maternal origin involving the placenta: case report and literature survey, *Am J Surg Pathol* 21:1236-1241, 1997.

50. Nishi Y, Suzuki S, Otsubo Y et al: B-cell–type malignant lymphoma with placental involvement, *J Obstet Gynaecol Res* 26:39-43, 2000.

51. Catlin EA, Roberts JD Jr, Erana R et al: Transplacental transmission of natural killer–cell lymphoma, *N Engl J Med* 341:85-91, 1999.

52. Maruko K, Maeda T, Kamitomo M et al: Transplacental transmission of maternal B-cell lymphoma, *Am J Obstet Gynecol* 191:380-381, 2004.

53. Vang R, Medeiros L, Silva E et al: Non-Hodgkin's lymphoma involving the vagina: a clinicopathologic analysis of 14 patients, *Am J Surg Pathol* 24:719-725, 2000.

54. Akbayir O, Gungorduk K, Gulkilik A et al: Successful treatment of primary vaginal diffuse large B-cell lymphoma using chemotherapy, *Taiwan J Obstet Gynecol* 47:334-337, 2008.

55. Yoshinaga K, Akahira J, Niikura H et al: A case of primary mucosa-associated lymphoid tissue lymphoma of the vagina, *Hum Pathol* 35:1164-1166, 2004.

56. Mahendran SM: Primary non-Hodgkin's lymphoma of the vagina masquerading as a uterine fibroid in pregnancy, *J Obstet Gynaecol* 28:456-458, 2008.

57. Prevot S, Hugol D, Audouin J, Diebold J: Primary non Hodgkin's malignant lymphoma of the vagina: report of 3 cases with review of the literature, *Pathol Res Pract* 188:78-85, 1992.

58. Domingo S, Perales A, Torres V et al: Epstein-Barr virus positivity in primary vaginal lymphoma, *Gynecol Oncol* 95:719-721, 2004.

59. Vang R, Medeiros L, Malpica A et al: Non-Hodgkin's lymphoma involving the vulva, *Int J Gynecol Pathol* 19:236-242, 2000.

60. Tjalma W, Van de Velde A, Schroyens W: Primary non-Hodgkin's lymphoma in Bartholin's gland, *Gynecol Oncol* 87:308-309, 2002.

61. Kaplan EJ, Chadburn A, Caputo TA: Case report: HIV-related primary non-Hodgkin's lymphoma of the vulva, *Gynecol Oncol* 61:131-138, 1996.

62. Macleod C, Palmer A, Findlay M: Primary non-Hodgkin's lymphoma of the vulva: a case report, *Int J Gynecol Cancer* 8:504-508, 1998.

63. Chabay P, De Matteo E, Lorenzetti M et al: Vulvar plasmablastic lymphoma in a HIV-positive child: a novel extraoral localisation, *J Clin Pathol* 62:644-646, 2009.

64. Winnicki M, Gariepy G, Sauthier PG, Funaro D: Hodgkin lymphoma presenting as a vulvar mass in a patient with Crohn disease: a case report and literature review, *J Low Genit Tract Dis* 13:110-114, 2009.

65. Young RH, Harris NL, Scully RE: Lymphoma-like lesions of the lower female genital tract: a report of 16 cases, *Int J Gynecol Pathol* 4:289-299, 1985.

66. Ma J, Shi Q, Zhou X et al: Lymphoma-like lesion of the uterine cervix: report of 12 cases of a rare entity, *Int J Gynecol Pathol* 26:194-198, 2007.

67. Geyer J, Ferry J, Harris N et al: Florid reactive lymphoid hyperplasia of the lower female genital tract (lymphoma-like lesion): a benign condition that frequently harbors clonal immunoglobulin heavy chain gene rearrangements, *Am J Surg Pathol* 34:161-168, 2010.

68. Ferry JA, Harris NL, Scully RE: Leiomyomas with lymphoid infiltration simulating lymphoma: a report of 7 cases, *Int J Gynecol Pathol* 8:263-270, 1989.

69. Saglam A, Guler G, Taskin M et al: Uterine leiomyoma with prominent lymphoid infiltrate, *Int J Gynecol Cancer* 15:167-170, 2005.

70. Valeri RM, Ibrahim N, Sheaff MT: Extramedullary hematopoiesis in the endometrium, *Int J Gynecol Pathol* 21:178-181, 2002.

71. Axiotis C, Merino M, Duray P: Langerhans' cell histiocytosis of the female genital tract, *Cancer* 67:1650-1660, 1991.

72. Oliva E, Ferry JA, Young RH et al: Granulocytic sarcoma of the female genital tract: a clinicopathologic study of 11 cases, *Am J Surg Pathol* 21:1156-1165, 1997.

CHAPTER 11

Cutaneous Lymphomas

Lyn M. Duncan • Johanna L. Baran • Judith A. Ferry

■ INTRODUCTION

Classification of Cutaneous Lymphomas

Evolving technologies, including immunohisto-chemical and molecular genetic analysis, have allowed for a better understanding of the types of lymphoma that occur in the skin. The practice of dermatopathology requires an understanding of the lymphoma classification schemes and the reactive processes that mimic lymphoma in the skin. Lymphomas that occur as primary tumors of the skin are listed in Table 11-1; although many are indolent, some may be lethal.

In 1994 the Revised European-American Classification of Lymphoid Neoplasms (REAL), a proposal from the International Lymphoma Study Group, laid the groundwork for the development of a World Health Organization (WHO) classification scheme for lymphomas.[1] These classifications are based on the identification of distinct clinical entities that may be recognized by pathologists using available techniques.[2,3] Morphology, immunophenotype, genetic features, and clinical features are all used to define the diseases. The tumors are classified predominantly by lineage with a normal counterpart postulated for each neoplasm.

Shortly after publication of the REAL classification, the European Organization for Research and Treatment of Cancer (EORTC) Cutaneous Lymphoma Program Project Group devised a classification scheme specifically for primary cutaneous lymphoma (see Table 11-1).[4] The EORTC scheme incorporated the clinical presentation and biologic behavior of these cutaneous tumors and presented definitions of primary cutaneous lymphoma. It paid particular attention to lymphomas manifesting clinical behaviors that could not be predicted using classification schemes designed for nodal lymphomas.

In 2005 a consensus EORTC-WHO classification scheme for cutaneous lymphomas was published.[3,5] The most recent WHO Classification of Haematopoietic and Lymphoid Tissues and the EORTC Classification for Cutaneous Lymphomas recognize the same diseases.

An understanding of how the terms "primary" and "secondary" have been applied to cutaneous lymphomas is critical to an understanding the classification schemes. *Primary cutaneous lymphoma* is defined as lymphoma that arises in the skin without evidence of extracutaneous lymphoma on staging studies at the time of the diagnosis. The term *secondary cutaneous lymphoma* is used to describe lymphoma that develops in the skin as a secondary manifestation of a primary extracutaneous lymphoma.[6] The term "secondary cutaneous lymphoma" occasionally has also been used to describe cutaneous lymphoma that develops as a high-grade transformation of a low-grade cutaneous lymphoma.[7,8] However, these transformed tumors are not considered "secondary" cutaneous lymphomas in the EORTC or WHO classification schemes.

General Features

In contrast to lymphomas that arise in many other sites, most primary cutaneous lymphomas are T-cell lymphomas (more than 70% of cases). B-cell lymphomas account for fewer than 30% of cases.[9] Most cutaneous T-cell lymphomas have distinctive clinical presentations that help differentiate them from histologically similar processes. Cutaneous T-cell lymphoma may present as a solitary erythematous or violaceous nodule, as solitary or multiple patches and infiltrated erythematous plaques, or as a markedly pruritic erythroderma. In contrast, most cutaneous B-cell lymphomas appear clinically similar to one another.[10] These tumors usually occur as solitary or multiple erythematous papules or nodules that may coalesce to form plaques. Ulceration rarely occurs in cutaneous B-cell lymphomas. Some regional predilection is seen. For example, follicle center lymphoma more commonly arises on the scalp; extranodal marginal zone lymphoma usually occurs on the trunk or extremities; and the aggressive diffuse large B-cell lymphoma, leg type, usually arises on the lower leg. Nevertheless, all types of cutaneous B-cell lymphoma

TABLE 11-1

WHO-EORTC Classification of Cutaneous Lymphomas with Primary Cutaneous Manifestations

Cutaneous T-Cell and NK-Cell Lymphomas
Mycosis fungoides (MF)
MF variants and subtypes
   Folliculotropic MF
   Pagetoid reticulosis
   Granulomatous slack skin
Sézary syndrome
Primary cutaneous CD30+ lymphoproliferative disorders
   Primary cutaneous anaplastic large cell lymphoma
   Lymphomatoid papulosis
Subcutaneous panniculitis-like T-cell lymphoma
Extranodal NK/T-cell lymphoma, nasal type
Primary cutaneous peripheral T-cell lymphoma, rare subtypes
   Primary cutaneous gamma-delta T-cell lymphoma
   Primary cutaneous CD8+ aggressive epidermotropic cytotoxic T-cell lymphoma (provisional entity)
   Primary cutaneous CD4+ small/medium T-cell lymphoma (provisional entity)

Cutaneous B-Cell Lymphomas
Extranodal marginal zone lymphoma of mucosa-associated lymphoid tissue (MALT)
Primary cutaneous follicle center lymphoma
Primary cutaneous diffuse large B-cell lymphoma, leg type
Intravascular large B-cell lymphoma

Modified from Swerdlow SH, Campo E, Harris NL et al, editors: *WHO classification of tumours of haematopoietic and lymphoid tissues,* ed 4, Lyon, 2008, IARC; and Willemze R, Jaffe ES, Burg G et al: WHO-EORTC classification for cutaneous lymphomas, *Blood* 105:3768-3785, 2005.
WHO, World Health Organization; *EORTC,* European Organization for Research and Treatment of Cancer.

can occur at any cutaneous site; consequently, the clinical findings are not particularly useful in differential diagnosis for an individual patient.

Several types of cutaneous T-cell lymphoma are characterized by epidermotropism, in contrast to B-cell lymphomas, in which the tumor cells spare the epidermis and usually are separated from it by a grenz zone of papillary dermis free of tumor. Two features historically used by pathologists to support a diagnosis of cutaneous lymphoid hyperplasia are no longer valid; a "top heavy" infiltrate and the presence of reactive lymphoid follicles both are commonly observed in primary cutaneous B-cell lymphomas, although these findings historically were considered to favor a reactive infiltrate.

An aberrant T-cell immunophenotype, particularly the loss of pan–T-cell antigens (CD2, CD3, or CD5), or loss of both CD4 and CD8 supports a diagnosis of cutaneous T-cell lymphoma. Expression of CD7, a marker found on many but not all normal T cells, often is undetectable in cutaneous T-cell lymphoma. However, it also may be absent in CD4+ T cells of nonneoplastic T-cell infiltrates, which likely reflects expansion of a normal CD4+, CD7– T-cell population. Decreased expression of CD7, therefore, is not as definitive a predictor of neoplasia as is loss of true pan–T-cell antigens. As with T-cell lymphomas, an aberrant B-cell immunophenotype (e.g., co-expression of CD43 or CD5 or expression of germinal center markers [CD10, BCL6] in interfollicular areas) may suggest a diagnosis of B-cell lymphoma. In addition, a monotypic proliferation of B lymphocytes may be demonstrated using immunohistochemical stains or in situ hybridization for kappa and lambda light chains on paraffin sections in some cases; this is successful mainly in lymphomas with plasmacytic differentiation. The usual responder cells in cutaneous inflammation are T cells; therefore, a diffuse cutaneous infiltrate composed of more than 75% B lymphocytes is worrisome for B-cell lymphoma. On the other hand, dense reactive T-cell infiltrates frequently are seen in cutaneous B-cell lymphomas; this should be kept in mind when immunohistochemical stains are interpreted, because neoplastic B cells may account for only a minority of the infiltrate.

Polymerase chain reaction (PCR)–based techniques for identifying T-cell receptor and immunoglobulin gene rearrangements are quite sensitive; they can detect as few as 0.001% to 1% clonal cells. Clonal populations are detected in most cases of cutaneous T-cell lymphoma and in approximately 50% of cases of cutaneous B-cell lymphoma.[11,12] Unfortunately, PCR-based techniques also may detect small clonal B- or T-cell populations in reactive processes. As with any diagnostic tool, the genetic results must be interpreted in the context of the clinical, histologic, and immunophenotypic findings.[13]

With the exception of mycosis fungoides, for which many therapeutic options exist, most cutaneous lymphomas have a similar treatment algorithm. Solitary or localized tumors usually are treated with excision or radiation therapy or both; solitary low-grade lymphomas also may be treated with injection of corticosteroids or interferon. Multifocal or disseminated cutaneous lymphoma usually is treated with chemotherapy. Single-agent chemotherapy is used for more indolent tumors, whereas multiagent chemotherapy is instituted for biologically aggressive lymphomas.

■ CUTANEOUS T-CELL AND NK-CELL LYMPHOMAS

Mycosis Fungoides

Mycosis fungoides is a cutaneous T-cell lymphoma characterized by an epidermotropic proliferation of small to medium neoplastic T lymphocytes with cerebriform nuclear features (Figure 11-1).[14] The term *mycosis fungoides* is used for lymphomas characterized by the classical evolution of patch, plaque, and tumor stage and for variants with a similar course.

Clinical Features

Mycosis fungoides is the most common form of cutaneous T-cell lymphoma. It occurs in adults, and the peak incidence is seen in the sixth and seventh decades of life. The skin lesions present as erythematous, round, oval or arciform patches or plaques. Mycosis fungoides is a usually indolent T-cell lymphoma that primarily involves the skin; however, it may spread to involve the lymph nodes, blood, and viscera (usually the liver, lungs, and spleen). Progression from patches to plaques and ultimately to tumors occurs over several decades. Occasionally patients present with an erythroderma that is not associated with the diagnostic criteria for Sézary syndrome.

In rare cases mycosis fungoides may evolve into a CD30+ large cell lymphoma that may resemble primary cutaneous anaplastic large cell lymphoma; this large cell transformation is associated with a poor prognosis.[15,16] Mycosis fungoides also has been described in advanced stages of chronic actinic dermatitis (actinic reticuloid),[17] although some consider that this disease may have represented lymphoma from the outset. In rare cases mycosis fungoides has been found in association with lymphomatoid papulosis and Hodgkin's lymphoma.[18]

Pathologic Features

The histologic hallmark of mycosis fungoides is epidermotropism.[19] Epidermotropism is defined as the presence of atypical T cells within the epidermis, often in a pagetoid growth pattern or in a linear distribution along the dermal-epidermal junction.[20,21] Epidermal spongiosis usually is absent. The neoplastic T cells are small to medium sized but larger than normal lymphocytes. The neoplastic T-cell nuclei characteristically display dense nuclear chromatin with extensive convolutions of the nuclear membrane. The irregular nuclear shape is most commonly termed *cerebriform,* and sharp angulations of

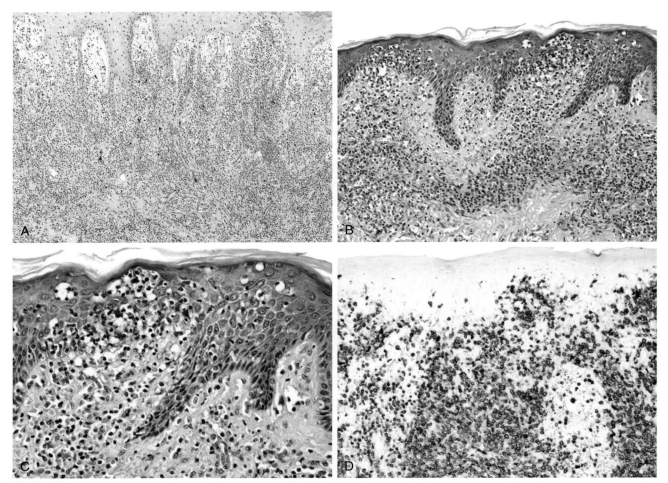

Figure 11-1 Mycosis fungoides is characterized by an epidermotropic proliferation of cytologically atypical lymphocytes. Epidermal hyperplasia **(A)** or epidermal atrophy **(B)** may be seen. The tumor cells form intraepidermal Pautrier collections **(C)** and stain positively for CD3 **(D)**.

the nuclei, termed *inscisorum*, may be seen. A clear space or halo around the atypical lymphocytes also may be observed.

A particularly useful histologic finding is the presence of Pautrier collections, intraepidermal aggregates of three or more cytologically atypical T cells (see Figure 11-1). The dermal lymphoid infiltrate in mycosis fungoides often is superficial and bandlike (lichenoid). In the tumor stage, it may extend deep into the subcutaneous fat as a dense dermal nodule of neoplastic T cells. In the tumor stage of mycosis fungoides, scattered large atypical cells that express CD30 may be seen. Histologic progression (large cell or "blast" transformation) is defined as a proportion greater than 25% of large lymphoid cells (which may or may not express CD30).

Although epidermotropism, Pautrier collections, and cerebriform nuclear changes are the diagnostic features of mycosis fungoides, these findings may not be present in the early stages of the disease. Several biopsies may have to be done over time before a definitive diagnosis is established histologically. Because the cytologic appearance of activated T cells may be similar to the early cerebriform changes of

mycosis fungoides, distinguishing epidermotropism of neoplastic T cells from a reactive exocytosis may be difficult. In the late tumor stage of mycosis fungoides, the disease's distinctive epidermotropism may be absent. In these diagnostically difficult cases, clinical correlation combined with immunohistochemical and molecular genetic studies may be helpful for arriving at the diagnosis of mycosis fungoides.

Mycosis fungoides usually is a neoplastic proliferation of CD4+, CD8− T cells that also express CD2, CD3, CD5, and the alpha-beta T-cell receptor (TCR). In rare cases (usually in pediatric patients), the tumors have a CD8+ immunophenotype; the prognosis is similar to that for CD4+ mycosis fungoides.[22] The diagnosis of lymphoma is supported by the presence of an aberrant immunophenotype (e.g., T cells that lack one or more of the pan–T-cell antigens). Neoplastic cells often lack CD7. Loss of CD5, CD2, and CD3 occurs less often.[23,24] Loss of one or more pan–T-cell antigens in addition to loss of CD7 is particularly supportive of a diagnosis of T-cell lymphoma. The immunophenotypic features are not specific for mycosis fungoides and may be seen in other peripheral T-cell lymphomas.[25] In the

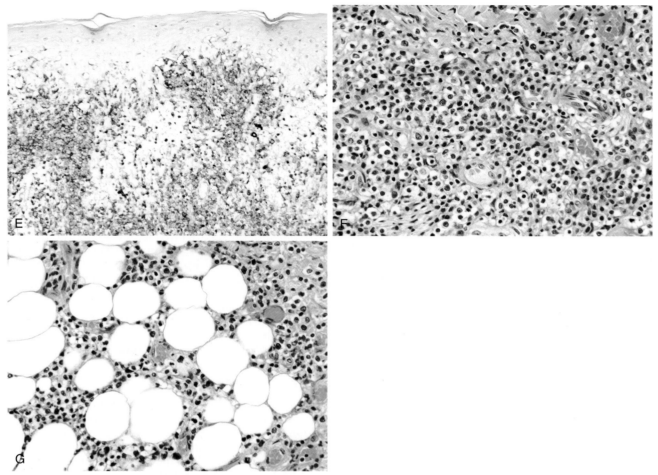

Figure 11-1, cont'd   The tumor cells also stain positively for CD4 **(E)**. In the tumor stage, the tumor cells diffusely infiltrate the dermis **(F)** and subcutaneous fat **(G)**.

interpretation of the immunohistochemical results, it is important to remember that apparent loss of only CD7 by T cells may represent expansion of a normal CD4+, CD7– T-cell population; this may be observed in some reactive processes. Scattered CD30+ large cells are observed in many cases of mycosis fungoides, particularly with progression to the tumor stage[26]; this finding is not specific, however, because occasional CD30+ cells also may be seen in reactive processes and in other T-cell and B-cell lymphomas.

Clonal rearrangement of the T-cell receptor genes typically is found in mycosis fungoides; however, this should not by itself be interpreted as proof of lymphoma, because PCR-based techniques may detect lymphocyte populations with clonally rearranged T-cell receptor genes in some reactive processes.[13] Correlation of the genetic results with the clinical, histologic, and immunophenotypic findings is imperative before a definitive diagnosis of lymphoma is rendered. TCR gene rearrangement results from PCR-based techniques have been suggested as possible predictors of the prognosis in patients with mycosis fungoides when a clone is identified in a lymph node or peripheral blood.[27-29]

Staging, Treatment, and Outcome

The stage of the disease is the most important prognostic factor for patients with mycosis fungoides. The prognosis is excellent for patients with limited, patch-stage disease. Patients who develop the cutaneous tumor stage or extracutaneous dissemination have a poor prognosis.[30] Other markers of a poor prognosis include large cell transformation (more than 25% large cells), an elevated lactate dehydrogenase (LDH) level, and age over 60 years. Patients commonly are treated with psoralen and ultraviolet light (PUVA) and occasionally with topical nitrogen mustard, interferon, electron beam therapy, photopheresis, or radiotherapy. Disseminated disease may be treated with combination chemotherapy.

Differential Diagnosis

The early lesions of mycosis fungoides with minimal cytologic atypia and the late tumors without epidermotropism are the most diagnostically challenging. In early cases, repeated skin biopsies and immunophenotypic and molecular genetic studies aid determination of the appropriate diagnosis. In early lesions, the presence of an infiltrate composed entirely of CD4+ cells with epidermotropism in the absence of spongiosis, dyskeratosis, or parakeratosis supports the diagnosis of mycosis fungoides. In later lesions, the presence of cytologically atypical CD4+ cells with an aberrant T-cell immunophenotype supports a diagnosis of T-cell lymphoma; identification of areas of epidermotropism and clinical information about the evolution of the disease over time help with subclassification as mycosis fungoides.

The differential diagnosis of an atypical cutaneous lymphoid infiltrate with epidermotropism includes a hypersensitivity reaction to a drug,[31] adult T-cell leukemia/lymphoma (human T-cell leukemia virus type 1 [HTLV-1] positive), and primary cutaneous CD8+ aggressive epidermotropic cytotoxic T-cell lymphoma. The presence of Pautrier collections of CD4+ medium-sized lymphocytes with cerebriform nuclei supports the diagnosis of mycosis fungoides. Cutaneous mycosis fungoides–like drug reactions often display epidermal keratinocyte dyskeratosis, intraepidermal Langerhans' cell collections, and papillary dermal pigment–laden macrophages. Immunohistochemical stains may also be helpful. Mycosis fungoides usually displays a relatively uniform proliferation of CD4+ T cells with rare scattered CD8+ cells; drug reactions usually display a pattern of CD8+ cells in the epidermis and CD4+ cells in the dermis. Serologic studies for HTLV-1 are useful for evaluating the possibility of adult T-cell leukemia/lymphoma.

Mycosis Fungoides Variants

Significant variability in the clinical and pathologic features of mycosis fungoides has led to the identification of a number of mycosis fungoides variants, three of which are specified in the WHO classification: pagetoid reticulosis, granulomatous slack skin, and folliculotropic mycosis fungoides.

Pagetoid reticulosis is a localized variant of mycosis fungoides that usually occurs on the distal extremities. It is characterized clinically by patches or plaques and histologically by marked, or pagetoid, epidermotropism with little underlying dermal infiltration (Woringer-Kolopp disease).[14,32-34] The neoplastic cells may be CD8+ or CD4+ and may co-express CD30. The prognosis for patients with this condition is excellent. It is important that this disorder not be confused with the so-called "Ketron-Goodman" type of pagetoid reticulosis, which presents as disseminated disease and now is believed in most cases to represent CD8+ aggressive epidermotropic cytotoxic T-cell lymphoma or gamma-delta T-cell lymphoma.[35,36]

Granulomatous slack skin presents with the gradual appearance of lax folds of skin in the axillae and groin. The disease is characterized histologically by a granulomatous infiltrate with histiocytes, multinucleated giant cells, elastolysis, and a clonal proliferation of CD4+ T cells.[37] The clinical course for most patients is indolent.[38]

Folliculotropic mycosis fungoides is characterized by infiltration of the hair follicle epithelium by neoplastic T cells. This folliculotropism may be associated with the formation of intrafollicular Pautrier collections. The lesions usually involve the head and neck and may be associated with alopecia. Other distinctive findings that may be seen in benign processes include follicular mucinosis (hyaluronic acid deposition in the hair follicle epithelium), syringotropism, and eccrine gland hyperplasia (Figure 11-2).[39-41] Whether idiopathic follicular mucinosis and follicular mucinosis in mycosis fungoides are ends of a spectrum or two distinct diseases remains unclear.[42] Clear-cut clinical, histologic, and/or molecular genetic criteria for distinguishing between idiopathic and mycosis fungoides–associated follicular mucinosis are elusive.[42] With extracutaneous spread, the T cells retain their cerebriform morphology and may show epitheliotropism.[43] Patients with folliculotropic mycosis fungoides have a 5-year survival rate of approximately 70%, much worse than that for the patch or plaque stage of mycosis fungoides. In a recent study of folliculotropic mycosis fungoides, 24% of patients had distant lymph node involvement and 30% had circulating Sézary cells.[41]

Sézary Syndrome

Sézary syndrome is a T-cell lymphoma defined by the presence of erythroderma, generalized lymphadenopathy, and the presence of Sézary cells in the skin, lymph node, and peripheral blood.[44,45] At least one of the following criteria must be met: an expanded CD4+ population with a CD4:CD8 ratio greater than 10; loss of one or more pan–T-cell antigens; or an absolute Sézary cell count greater than 1000 cells/mm.[3,46]

Clinical Features

Pruritic erythroderma is the characteristic dermatologic finding in Sézary syndrome. Palmar plantar hyperkeratosis, onychodystrophy, and alopecia also may be present. Generalized lymphadenopathy is present in the early stages; in advanced stages, any of a variety of organs may be involved. The bone marrow often is spared.

Pathologic Features

Sézary cells have the cytologic features of the CD4+ neoplastic T cells in mycosis fungoides. Although the histologic features of skin biopsies in Sézary syndrome may be identical to those seen in mycosis fungoides, the infiltrate often is composed nearly entirely of neoplastic cells with few reactive small lymphocytes. Also, epidermotropism may be absent. In nearly 30% of cases of Sézary syndrome, the cutaneous biopsy is not diagnostic.[47] The nuclear convolutions of Sézary cells are most clearly visible on peripheral blood smears or 1-μm plastic sections (Figure 11-3).

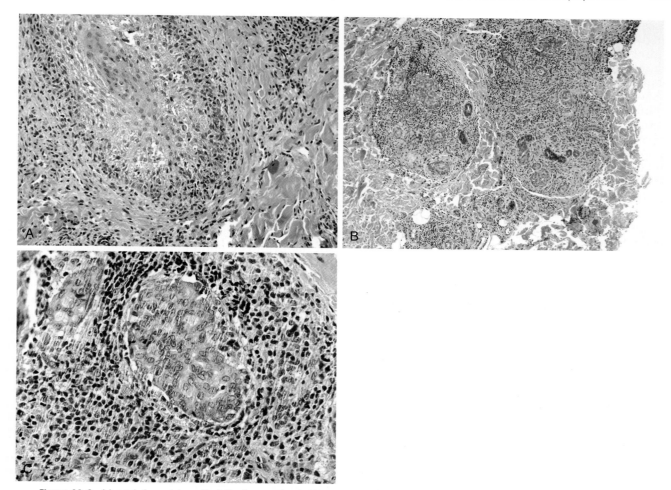

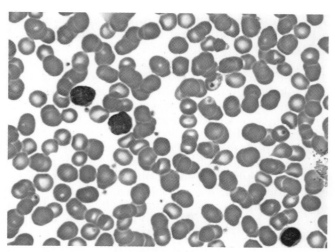

Figure 11-2 Mycosis fungoides with follicular mucinosis **(A)** and syringotropism and eccrine epithelial hyperplasia **(B and C)**.

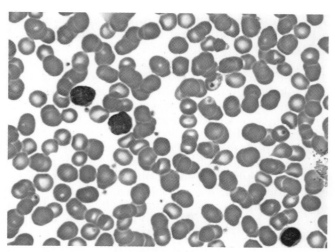

Figure 11-3 Sézary syndrome. The nuclear hyperconvolutions are best appreciated on a peripheral blood smear.

The tumor cells of Sézary syndrome are immunophenotypically similar to the cells of mycosis fungoides: CD2, CD3, CD5, TCRαβ, CLA, and CCR4+ T cells, usually with a CD4+ phenotype.[48] CD7 and CD26 characteristically are absent.[49] Recent investigation suggests that Sézary syndrome is a malignancy of central memory T cells, whereas mycosis fungoides is a malignancy of skin-resident effector memory T cells.[50] Clonal rearrangement of the T-cell receptor genes and complex karyotypes is seen, along with numeric and structural abnormalities and a high rate of unbalanced translocations and associated chromosomal deletions.

Staging, Treatment, and Outcome

As noted previously, bone marrow involvement is rare in Sézary syndrome. The extent of lymph node and peripheral blood involvement is the most reliable prognostic factor.[51] The 5-year overall survival rate for patients with Sézary syndrome is less than 15%, and opportunistic infections cause the most morbidity and mortality.[3]

Primary Cutaneous CD30+ Lymphoproliferative Disorders

Primary cutaneous CD30+ lymphoproliferative disorders are characterized by the presence of CD30+ large cells. These disorders represent a spectrum of disease, ranging from small lesions with only scattered CD30+ cells to large tumors composed almost entirely of CD30+ large cells.[52] These diseases constitute the second most common form of primary cutaneous lymphoma, after mycosis fungoides; they account for about 30% of primary cutaneous T-cell lymphomas. The term "borderline," when applied to these tumors, indicates failure to define whether the process represents anaplastic large cell lymphoma or lymphomatoid papulosis; however, the clinical follow-up usually reveals the true nature of the CD30+ lymphoproliferative disorder, allowing for appropriate diagnosis.

Primary Cutaneous Anaplastic Large Cell Lymphoma

Primary cutaneous anaplastic large cell lymphoma (ALCL) is composed of large cells with an anaplastic, pleomorphic, or immunoblastic cytomorphology that express the CD30 antigen in more than 75% of the tumor cells. Patients do not have clinical evidence or a history of mycosis fungoides. This disease must be distinguished from systemic ALCL (ALK+ and ALK−), which has different clinical and pathologic features.

Clinical Features

Primary cutaneous ALCL usually presents as a solitary cutaneous nodule in patients in the seventh or eighth decade of life.[53] (It occurs only rarely in children[54,55].) Multiple tumor nodules or papules may be present, but they usually are localized to one cutaneous region. In rare cases primary cutaneous ALCLs regress spontaneously; frequently they relapse in the skin. Dissemination to extracutaneous sites occurs in fewer than 15% of patients and even then usually is limited to the regional lymph nodes and is associated with a 4-year disease-specific survival rate exceeding 90%.[56,57]

Primary cutaneous ALCL has a much more favorable prognosis than does cutaneous involvement by systemic ALCL.[7,58] Therefore, these two types of ALCL must be differentiated. If the patient has a history of mycosis fungoides, a diagnosis of large cell transformation of mycosis fungoides (in which the large atypical cells may express CD30) is much more likely than the more prognostically favorable primary cutaneous ALCL.

Pathologic Features

The tumors of primary cutaneous ALCL are characterized by dermal sheets of CD30+ large neoplastic lymphoid cells that extend into the subcutaneous fat. These CD30+ cells comprise more than 75% of the infiltrating cells. They have oval, indented, or irregularly shaped nuclei, prominent eosinophilic macronucleoli, and abundant cytoplasm (Figure 11-4, A-D). Binucleated and multinucleated forms occasionally are seen. Numerous mitoses are present, as is a moderately dense reactive inflammatory infiltrate at the periphery of the tumor. The epidermis may be hyperplastic, but epidermotropism is rare. Ulcerated lesions may show an inflammatory background rich in eosinophils, histiocytes, and neutrophils. The neutrophil-rich variant shows numerous neutrophils, which sometimes obscure the CD30+ neoplastic large cell population (see Figure 11-4).

The tumor cells of cutaneous ALCL are strongly positive for CD30 and show a characteristic punctate accentuation of staining in the perinuclear Golgi region (see Figure 11-4, E-G). Staining for the pan–T-cell antigens CD2, CD3, and CD5 is inconsistent or weak. The tumor cells usually are positive for CLA, HLA-DR, CD25, and CD45RO but do not express EMA or ALK. The CD30+ cells characteristically are activated CD4+ cells with frequent expression of the cytotoxic granule proteins granzyme B, TIA, and perforin. In fewer than 5% of cases, a CD8+, CD30+ phenotype is observed. Even more uncommon is CD56 expression. Neither CD8 nor CD56 expression is associated with a worse prognosis. Clonal rearrangement of the T-cell receptor genes usually is seen.[59] In contrast to ALCL, ALK+, the t(2;5)(p23;q35) translocation and the resultant p80 NPM-ALK protein by definition are not present in cutaneous ALCL.[60-63]

Staging, Treatment, and Outcome

When confined to the skin, CD30+ ALCL has a good prognosis and has even been known to regress spontaneously.[64] The overall 10-year survival rate exceeds 90%, and the extent of disease and degree of cytologic anaplasia do not seem to affect the prognosis.

Differential Diagnosis

The histologic differential diagnosis of cutaneous ALCL includes transformed mycosis fungoides and a variety of reactive processes that can be associated with a remarkably dense infiltrate of CD30+ large activated T cells.[65-67] Viral infections, particularly molluscum contagiosum and herpes infection of the hair follicle epithelium, can lead to the production of dermal reactive infiltrates composed predominantly of CD30+ large cells.[66] In these cases, sections at additional levels may be required to identify the virally infected epithelium. Arthropod bites may yield a similar histologic picture; however, neutrophils or eosinophils usually are present, and the surface of the specimen may show epidermal and superficial dermal changes of lichen simplex chronicus (Figure 11-5). These findings are not specific, however, and the clinical history is helpful for arriving at the correct diagnosis. An abnormal T-cell immunophenotype supports a neoplastic process.

Lymphomatoid Papulosis

Lymphomatoid papulosis is a chronic, recurring, self-healing cutaneous eruption characterized by a dermal lymphoid infiltrate that contains large atypical immunoblastic, anaplastic, or Hodgkin-like CD30+ cells scattered in an inflammatory background. In 1968 Macaulay described lymphomatoid papulosis as a continuing, self-healing eruption that was clinically benign but histologically malignant.[68] In the 1970s and 1980s, lymphomatoid papulosis was described as a variant of pityriasis lichenoides et varioliformis acuta (PLEVA) because of the clinical and histologic resemblance of these two disorders. Since then, immunophenotyping has shown that these are distinct entities.

Clinical Features

Lymphomatoid papulosis is a skin-limited disease that usually occurs in adults but in rare cases may be seen in children. Women are affected more often than men. It presents clinically as recurrent crops of erythematous papules and nodules on the proximal extremities and trunk. The skin lesions may develop as small, ulcerated papules that heal with scarring. Lymphomatoid papulosis may be self-limited, lasting only a few months, or may persist for decades.

Pathologic Features

The histologic appearance of lymphomatoid papulosis is quite varied. Most biopsies show epidermal changes, including parakeratosis, acanthosis, spongiosis, basal layer vacuolization, and occasionally a focus of epidermal erosion. Often endothelial cell swelling with erythrocyte extravasation is seen (Figure 11-6). The perivascular lymphoid infiltrate frequently is quite dense and may have a wedge-shaped appearance on scanning magnification. The infiltrate is composed of small banal lymphocytes and large atypical cells.

Three types of lymphomatoid papulosis have been described. In type A, scattered CD30+ cells, occasionally clustered, are seen in a background of inflammatory cells. Type B is characterized by an epidermotropic infiltrate of atypical lymphocytes, similar to that seen in mycosis fungoides, without a CD30+ cell population but with the clinical features of lymphomatoid papulosis. Type C shows a monotonous population of CD30+ cells with few admixed inflammatory cells. Recently a group of investigators identified cases with

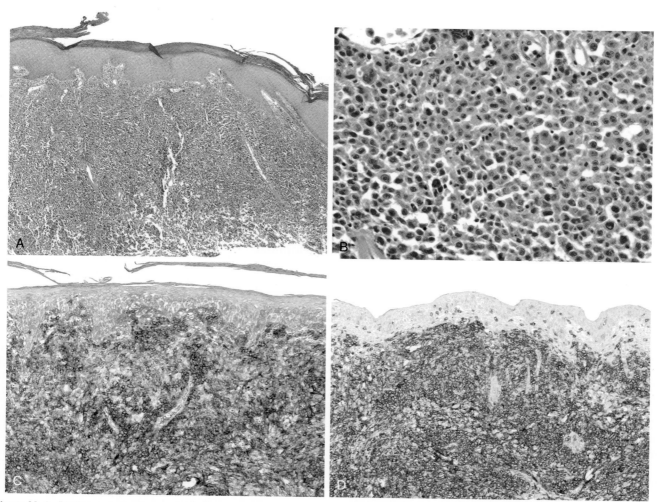

Figure 11-4 Primary cutaneous anaplastic large cell lymphoma. **A,** The tumor cells diffusely infiltrate the dermis and may abut the epidermis. The nuclei, which are large and vesicular and have eosinophilic macronucleoli **(B),** stain positively for CD30 **(C)** and CD4 **(D).**

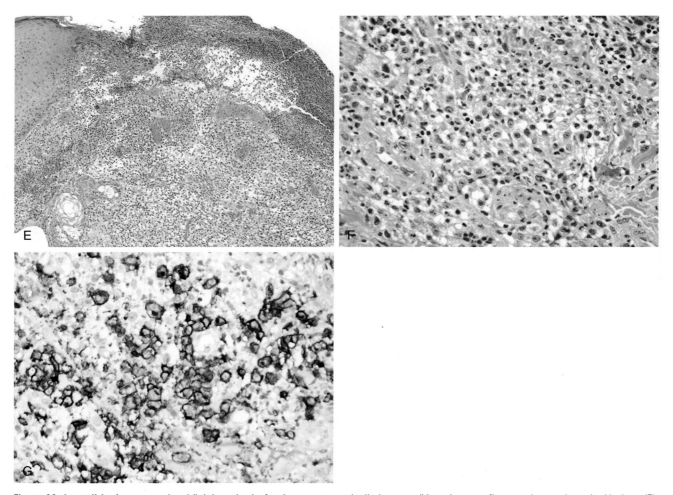

Figure 11-4, cont'd A rare, neutrophil-rich variant of cutaneous anaplastic large cell lymphoma often produces ulcerated lesions **(E)** and is characterized by a dense infiltrate of neutrophils and scattered clusters of large anaplastic T cells **(F)** that stain positively for CD30 **(G)**; large cells were also CD3+, CD5+, CD2+/–, CD4–/+, CD7–, CD8– (not illustrated) consistent with abnormal T-cell immunophenotype.

the clinical behavior of lymphomatoid papulosis but with histologic and immunophenotypic features closely resembling those of primary cutaneous CD8+ aggressive epidermotropic cytotoxic T-cell lymphoma; a designation of lymphomatoid papulosis, type D, has been proposed for such cases.[69]

Most of the cells in the infiltrate have a CD4+ phenotype. The large lymphocytes may show loss of some pan–T-cell antigens.[16] The CD30+ Reed-Sternberg–like cells observed in the type A and type C forms of lymphomatoid papulosis usually are CD15–, CD45R+, although a recent report described CD15+ cells in some cases of lymphomatoid papulosis (see Figure 11-6).[7] Rare cases of lymphomatoid papulosis expressing CD8 and CD56 have been reported. Type B tumor cells have a CD3+, CD4+, CD8– immunophenotype; the type B form is rare, accounting for fewer than 10% of cases of lymphomatoid papulosis.

Clonal rearrangement of T-cell receptor genes has been reported in more than 50% of cases of lymphomatoid papulosis. However, the presence of clonal rearrangements is not correlated with a poor prognosis. As with primary cutaneous ALCL, the t(2;5)(p23;q35) characteristic of ALCL, ALK+ is not detected in lymphomatoid papulosis.[7]

Staging, Treatment, and Outcome

Lymphomatoid papulosis is believed to represent the indolent end of the spectrum of CD30+ lympho-proliferative disorders.[58,70] It may be preceded by, associated with, or progress to lymphoma in approximately 20% of cases, usually mycosis fungoides,[71] anaplastic large cell lymphoma[16,72,73] or, in rare cases, Hodgkin's lymphoma.[74] In some of these cases, similar immunophenotypes and T-cell receptor gene rearrangements have been observed in the cells of the lymphomatoid papulosis and the subsequent lymphoma. No genetic or phenotypic pattern predicts which patients will develop lymphoma.[7,61,75-77] The clinical signs of lymphoma development in patients with lymphomatoid papulosis include skin lesions that persist or enlarge, lymphadenopathy, and circulating atypical cells.[16] The overall 5-year survival rate for lymphomatoid papulosis exceeds 98%; however, careful follow-up is recommended because of the patient's risk of developing associated lymphoma.

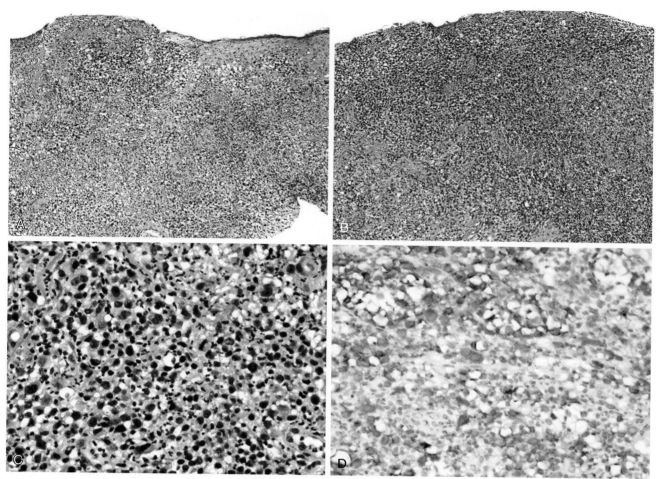

Figure 11-5 Reaction to an arthropod (spider) bite. Note the ulceration of the epidermis with overlying scale crust and a dense dermal inflammatory infiltrate (**A**). Scattered small lymphocytes are accompanied by a proliferation of large cells (**B**) with pleomorphic nuclei and ample cytoplasm (**C**) that stain positively for CD30 (**D**).

Differential Diagnosis

The most common process in the histologic differential is *pityriasis lichenoides et varioliformis acuta (PLEVA)* because of the clinical and histologic resemblance of these two disorders (see Figure 11-6). Both may show a papulonecrotic eruption that heals with superficial scarring and a dense dermal mixed inflammatory infiltrate with distinctive epidermal changes. However, few, if any, CD30+ large cells are present in PLEVA, whereas clustered and an increased density of CD30+ large cells are required for a diagnosis of lymphomatoid papulosis. Also, erythrocyte extravasation with erythrocytic exocytosis in the epidermis and occasional vasculitis are more characteristically observed in PLEVA than in lymphomatoid papulosis.

Significant overlap occurs among the three forms of lymphomatoid papulosis and also between lymphomatoid papulosis and cutaneous ALCL. Clinical findings and the density of the CD30+ large cells may be helpful for differentiating these processes. In contrast to lymphomatoid papulosis, CD30+ ALCL usually presents as a solitary nodule predominantly composed of CD30+ large cells.

The differential diagnosis of lymphomatoid papulosis includes a broad range of inflammatory dermatoses that may manifest scattered CD30+ large cells. Most notably, reactions to arthropod bites (see Figure 11-5), atypical drug hypersensitivity reactions, and cutaneous reactions with a viral infection may lead to processes that are histologically similar to lymphomatoid papulosis. The clinical findings and identification of arthropod parts or viral inclusions are helpful for arriving at the appropriate diagnosis. The recently described EBV+ mucocutaneous ulcer, a lesion that may occur in a variety of extranodal sites, often in the setting of immunosuppression (most often related to advanced age), is characterized by a variable proportion of CD30+ large atypical cells in a reactive background, potentially mimicking lymphomatoid papulosis.[78] In contrast to lymphomatoid papulosis, however, the large cells express B-cell markers and harbor EBV.

Subcutaneous Panniculitis-Like T-Cell Lymphoma

Subcutaneous panniculitis-like T-cell lymphoma is a cytotoxic T-cell lymphoma of the alpha-beta type that preferentially involves subcutaneous fat.[79]

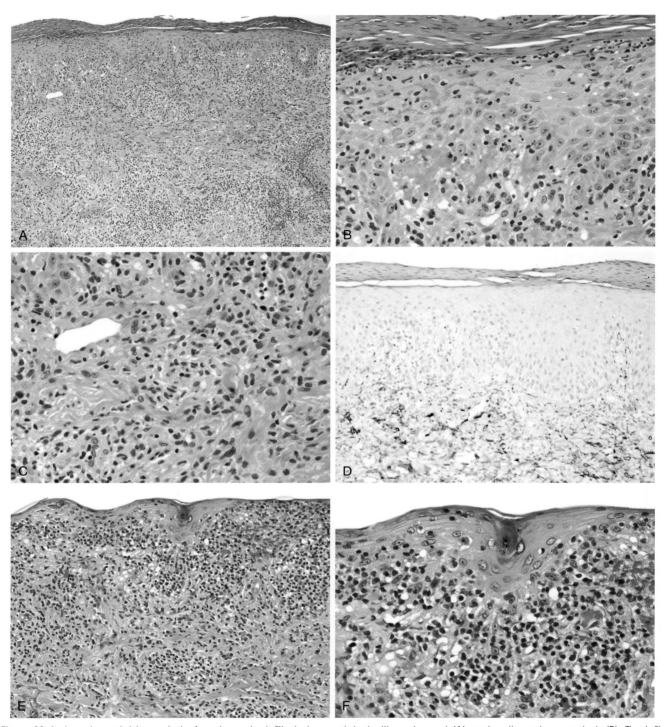

Figure 11-6 Lymphomatoid papulosis. A perivascular infiltrate is associated with scale crust **(A)** and erythrocyte exocytosis **(B)**. The infiltrate is composed of large cells admixed with scattered inflammatory cells **(C)**; the large cells stain positively for CD30 **(D)**. The differential diagnosis of lymphomatoid papulosis includes *pityriasis lichenoides et varioliformis acuta* (PLEVA), which may show a similar perivascular infiltrate and overlying epidermal changes **(E)**. Erythrocyte extravasation and dyskeratosis also are seen, and the infiltrate is composed of medium-sized, activated T cells without large anaplastic cells **(F)**.

Initially the name was used to describe any T-cell lymphoma predominantly involving the subcutaneous fat, with or without cytophagic histiocytic panniculitis.[80-82] However, researchers later recognized that alpha-beta T-cell–type lymphomas differed both morphologically and clinically from those with a gamma-delta phenotype; therefore gamma-delta tumors now are considered a distinct entity. Alpha-beta tumors are more clinically indolent than gamma-delta tumors and show less overlap with other clinical entities.[83-85] As a result, the WHO classification system restricts the designation of subcutaneous panniculitis-like T-cell lymphoma to lymphomas of alpha-beta T-cell lineage.

Clinical Features

Subcutaneous panniculitis-like T-cell lymphoma may occur in patients of all ages. The median age of onset is 35 years, and a slight female predominance is seen. The tumors present as nodules or plaques with areas of woody induration, usually on the legs and less commonly involving the trunk and arms. In cases with an associated hemophagocytic syndrome, patients also have fever, malaise, and weight loss; however, hemophagocytic syndrome is more commonly observed in cutaneous gamma-delta T-cell lymphoma.[84,86]

Although some authors suggest an association with lupus erythematosus, the relationship to autoimmune disease is not clear.[87,88] These tumors show histologic features that overlap with those of subcutaneous lupus (lupus profundus), and they may present with a clinical syndrome of fever, polyarthritis, and pericarditis that mimics an autoimmune disease.[86,89] No association with Epstein-Barr virus (EBV) or *Borrelia burgdorferi* infection has been shown[83,86,90]; EBV reported in subcutaneous panniculitis-like T-cell lymphoma likely represents extranodal natural killer (NK)/T-cell lymphoma, nasal type.[91,92]

Histologic Findings

Subcutaneous panniculitis-like T-cell lymphoma is characterized by a subcutaneous, lobular infiltrate of T cells with scant involvement of the overlying dermis. The neoplastic T cells are relatively monomorphic and have medium-sized to large, round to irregularly shaped, hyperchromatic nuclei and moderately abundant pale cytoplasm. The tumor cells form rims around the fat cells, often with associated karyorrhexis and histiocytes filled with karyorrhectic debris (Figure 11-7). Erythrophagocytosis is seen in rare cases, and occasionally histiocytic granulomas are present.[80,83,93,94] This cytotoxic T-cell lymphoma often displays vascular invasion associated with regions of necrosis.[83,85,90]

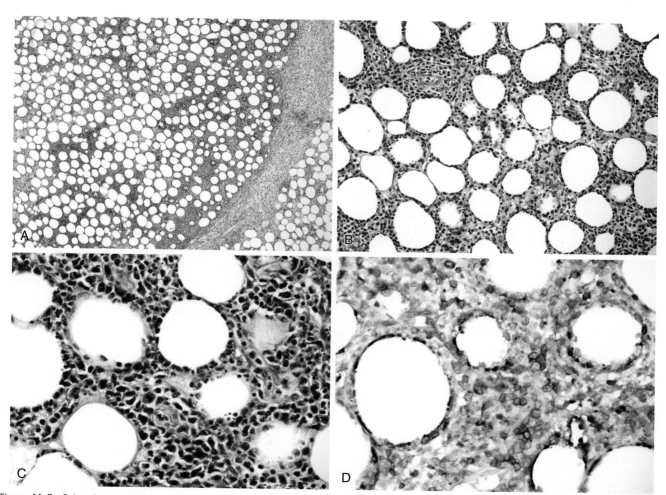

Figure 11-7 Subcutaneous panniculitis-like T-cell lymphoma. Note the lobular infiltrate with minimal involvement of the interlobular septae **(A)**. The tumor cells rim the fat spaces **(B)**. They have medium-sized hyperchromatic nuclei with moderate amounts of clear cytoplasm **(C)**, and they stain positively for CD3 **(D)**.

Continued

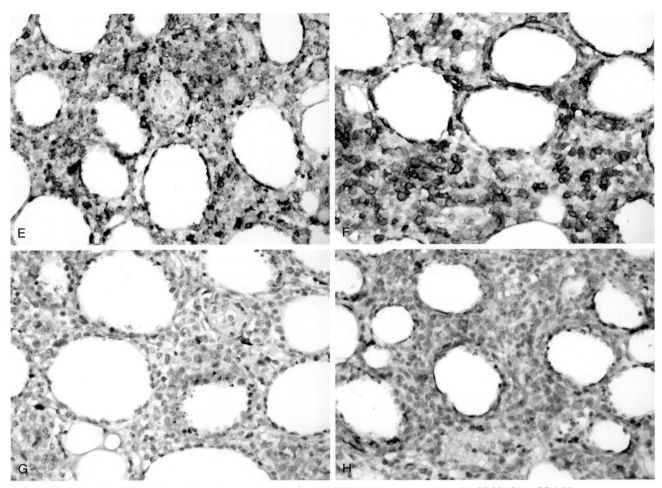

Figure 11-7, cont'd   They also stain positively for granzyme B **(E)** and CD8 **(F)**. They do not stain for CD20 **(G)** or CD4 **(H)**.

Subcutaneous panniculitis-like T-cell lymphoma is a tumor of cytotoxic CD3+, CD8+, TIA-1+, granzyme B+, perforin+, βF1+ T cells that do not express CD56 or CD30.[83,95] In rare cases co-expression of CD4 and CD8 is observed.[90] Clonal rearrangement of T-cell receptor genes is seen. Tumor cells are negative for EBV.

Staging, Treatment, and Outcome

The prognosis for subcutaneous panniculitis-like T-cell lymphoma is quite good; the 5-year disease-specific survival rate is 80%.[80,83,96] With time patients may experience local recurrences, but dissemination to lymph nodes and other organs is rare. In rare cases hemophagocytic syndrome may develop; it is the cause of death in most fatal cases.[80,86,97-99] Most previously reported cases of a rapidly fatal subcutaneous panniculitis-like T-cell lymphoma probably were actually cases of cutaneous gamma-delta T-cell lymphoma.[88,100] Multiagent chemotherapy historically has been the treatment for subcutaneous panniculitis-like T-cell lymphoma; however, less toxic therapies, including cyclosporine, steroids, and chlorambucil, may be effective.[96,101,102]

Differential Diagnosis

The differential diagnosis of subcutaneous panniculitis-like T-cell lymphoma is broad and includes other forms of lymphoma and connective tissue disease. Immunophenotyping often is helpful for distinguishing this disease from other forms of lymphoma. The absence of CD4, CD8, and βF1 and expression of CD56 support the diagnosis of gamma-delta T-cell lymphoma.[85] In addition, granzyme M is more often seen in tumors of the gamma-delta type.[93] Histologically, periadnexal and epidermal involvement is more characteristic of both gamma-delta T-cell lymphoma and lupus than of subcutaneous panniculitis-like T-cell lymphoma. Expression of CD56 and EBV supports a diagnosis of extranodal NK/T-cell lymphoma, nasal type. Prominent angiocentric, angiodestructive growth and effacement of the fat lobular architecture by the tumor are common in NK/T-cell lymphoma.

ALCL with prominent involvement of the subcutaneous tissue occasionally enters the differential diagnosis. Features that favor ALCL include diffuse infiltration of the dermis, ulceration, and diffuse, strong expression of CD30 by large atypical lymphoid cells of T lineage.

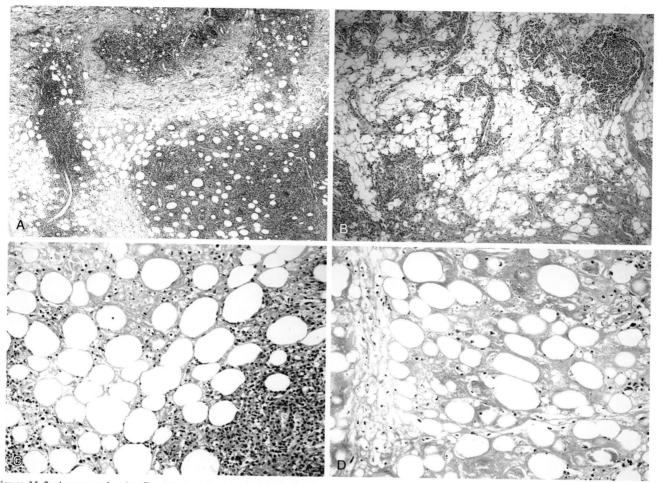

Figure 11-8 Lupus profundus. The lobular inflammatory infiltrate spares the interlobular fibrous septae **(A)**. Occasionally lymphoid follicles may be present **(B)**. The lymphocytes may have cytologic atypia but do not characteristically line the adipocyte spaces **(C)**. Eosinophilic acellular hyaline necrosis of the fat lobule may have a honeycomb-like appearance **(D)**.

As noted previously, subcutaneous panniculitis-like T-cell lymphoma and lupus profundus share many histologic features.[87,103,104] Both appear as a lobular panniculitis with a dense lobular proliferation of lymphoid cells that may include some large cells, and numerous histiocytes containing cellular debris. Two characteristic features of lupus profundus that are absent in subcutaneous panniculitis-like T-cell lymphoma are reactive lymphoid follicles and a honeycomb–like eosinophilic hyalinization of the fat lobule. Epidermal atrophy, follicular plugging, an interface dermatitis, increased dermal and subcutaneous connective tissue mucin deposits, infiltrates of plasma cells, and lymphocytic vasculitis also are findings more commonly observed in lupus profundus than in subcutaneous panniculitis-like T-cell lymphoma (Figure 11-8). Occasionally these distinguishing findings are absent. However, the characteristic rimming of adipocyte spaces by large atypical CD8+ cytotoxic T cells and the presence of erythrophagocytosis favor a diagnosis of lymphoma (Table 11-2). Because the degree of cytologic atypia can vary in subcutaneous panniculitis-like T-cell lymphoma, multiple biopsies may be necessary to arrive at a definitive diagnosis.[80,86,103]

The differential diagnosis of subcutaneous panniculitis-like T-cell lymphoma also includes a hypersensitivity reaction to an ingested antigen (e.g., a pharmaceutical agent) or an injected antigen (e.g., an arthropod bite). In an atypical drug reaction, the lymphocytic infiltrate more commonly displays Sézary cell–like atypia with small to medium-sized convoluted nuclei. In a bite reaction, the presence of polarizable arthropod parts, a dense infiltrate of eosinophils, and a careful clinical history may lead to the correct diagnosis. Both a drug reaction and a bite reaction may show epidermal changes, particularly dyskeratosis; epidermal changes are rare in subcutaneous panniculitis-like T-cell lymphoma.

Extranodal NK/T-Cell Lymphoma, Nasal Type

Extranodal NK/T-cell lymphoma, nasal type, is characterized by vascular damage and destruction, prominent necrosis, a cytotoxic phenotype, and association with EBV. It is designated NK/T-cell lymphoma because most cases are NK-cell neoplasms, but some cases show a cytotoxic T-cell phenotype.

TABLE 11-2

Histologic and Immunophenotypic Findings in Lupus Profundus and Subcutaneous Panniculitis-Like T-Cell Lymphoma

Findings	Lupus Profundus	Subcutaneous Lymphoma
Lobular panniculitis of atypical medium-sized lymphocytes	+	+
Fat necrosis	+	+
Debris-laden macrophages	+	+
Lymphoid aggregates with germinal centers	+	−
Eosinophilic hyaline change of fat (honeycomb-like appearance)	+	−
Hyaluronic acid deposition (connective tissue "mucin")	+	−
Epidermal pathologic condition (atrophy, vacuolar interface change, follicular plugs)	+	−
Erythrophagocytosis	−	+
Rimming of fat spaces by atypical T cells	−	+
CD8	+	+
CD56	−	−
CD30	−	−

+, Usually present; −, almost always absent.

Clinical Features

Extranodal NK/T-cell lymphoma, nasal type, most often occurs in the upper aerodigestive tract (see Lymphomas of the Nasal Cavity and Paranasal Sinuses in Chapter 3 for additional information). The skin is a common extranasal site of involvement. The lesions often take the form of a tumor nodule, which frequently is ulcerated. The tumors may present in the skin as solitary or multiple tumors; however, these patients usually are found to have widespread disease when staging is performed.[105]

Pathologic Features

When the tumors of extranodal NK/T-cell lymphoma, nasal type, occur in the skin, they display features similar to those seen in other sites of involvement. A diffuse infiltrate of lymphoid cells that are usually medium to large sized is seen, but the cytologic features may be quite variable, and atypia may be subtle. The tumor cells efface the dermis in an angiocentric and angiodestructive growth pattern, with fibrinoid necrosis of the vessel walls (Figure 11-9). Mitotic figures are easily identified. The overlying epidermis may be ulcerated or may display pseudoepitheliomatous hyperplasia, mimicking well-differentiated squamous cell carcinoma.

The tumor cells have a CD56+, granzyme B+, TIA+, perforin+, CD2+, cCD3+ immunophenotype, typically without staining for sCD3, CD4, CD5, CD8, βF1, CD43, CD25, or FAS.[105] Occasionally these tumors may express CD30 and may mimic ALCL. By definition, these tumors are EBV positive. Even in the absence of CD56, if cytotoxic molecules (granzyme B, TIA, perforin) and EBV are present, the tumor is classified as extranodal NK/T-cell lymphoma.

Staging, Treatment, and Outcome

Cutaneous involvement is associated with a poor prognosis and resistance to therapy.[106] Most patients who present with skin disease are found to have widespread disease. The mean survival is less than 1 year.[105]

Differential Diagnosis

The differential diagnosis includes other tumors that express NK-cell markers (Table 11-3). The histologic differential diagnosis of cutaneous extranodal NK/T-cell lymphoma, nasal type, also includes hydroa vacciniforme-like lymphoma, a recently described EBV+ lymphoma of T- or NK-cell lineage that is so named because of its shared features with hydroa vaccineforme, a disorder of unknown etiology that is related to photosensitivity. However, the clinical features of hydroa vacciniforme-like lymphoma are distinctive; it is a disease mainly of children from Asia and Central and South America who may be sensitive to arthropod bites.[106a,106b] The course of the disease is typically long, sometimes evolving over many years, although it does eventually result in death in some cases. The upper aerodigestive tract is rarely, if ever, involved in hydroa vacciniforme-like lymphoma.

Primary Cutaneous Peripheral T-Cell Lymphoma, Rare Subtypes

In the 2008 WHO Classification, the category of primary cutaneous peripheral T-cell lymphoma, rare subtypes, includes three entities: primary cutaneous gamma-delta T-cell lymphoma, primary cutaneous CD8+ aggressive epidermotropic cytotoxic T-cell lymphoma, and primary cutaneous CD4+ small/medium T-cell lymphoma; the second and third of these currently are designated provisional entities.[107]

Primary Cutaneous Gamma-Delta T-Cell Lymphoma

Primary cutaneous gamma-delta T-cell lymphoma is characterized by a clonal proliferation of mature activated gamma-delta T-cells with a cytotoxic phenotype. Now included in this category are cases previously classified as subcutaneous panniculitis-like T-cell lymphoma with a gamma-delta phenotype.[100,108,109] The relationship of this lymphoma to other T-cell lymphomas of gamma-delta T cells, such as hepatosplenic T-cell lymphoma, is uncertain (see Hepatosplenic T-Cell Lymphoma in Chapter 6 for additional information). However, as does hepatosplenic T-cell lymphoma of gamma-delta lineage, cutaneous gamma-delta T-cell lymphoma sometimes arises in the setting of immune dysregulation.

Clinical Features

Cutaneous gamma-delta T-cell lymphoma usually presents as ulcerated subcutaneous nodules on the extremities, particularly the thigh or buttocks. It usually occurs in adults and has no gender predilection.

Pathologic Features

Primary cutaneous gamma-delta T-cell lymphoma has heterogeneous histologic features; epidermotropic, dermal, or predominantly subcutaneous infiltrates may be seen. One or more patterns may be seen in the same biopsy specimen or in separate specimens from the same patient. The degree of epidermotropism varies from floridly pagetoid to minimal, as may be seen in gamma-delta lymphomas

with prominent subcutaneous involvement. The neoplastic cells have medium-sized to large nuclei with coarsely clumped chromatin; blastlike cells with prominent nucleoli are not characteristically observed. Often scattered cellular debris, tissue necrosis, and vascular invasion by the tumor cells are seen. In subcutaneous tumors, the neoplastic gamma-delta T cells rim the fat spaces in a pattern similar to that of subcutaneous panniculitis-like T-cell lymphoma (Figure 11-10).[96]

The tumor cells have a CD56+, CD3+, CD2+ immunophenotype and strongly express the cytotoxic proteins (granzyme B, TIA-1, and perforin). CD7 may be expressed but βF1, which detects expression of TCRαβ, is characteristically negative, and CD5, CD4, and CD8 usually are absent.[96] Among T-cell lymphomas, the absence of βF1 may serve as a surrogate for the gamma-delta phenotype.[110] Clonal rearrangement of the TCR gamma chain gene and the TCR delta chain gene is observed. Although the TCR beta chain gene may be rearranged or deleted, TCRαβ is not expressed at the protein level. These lymphomas are negative for EBV.

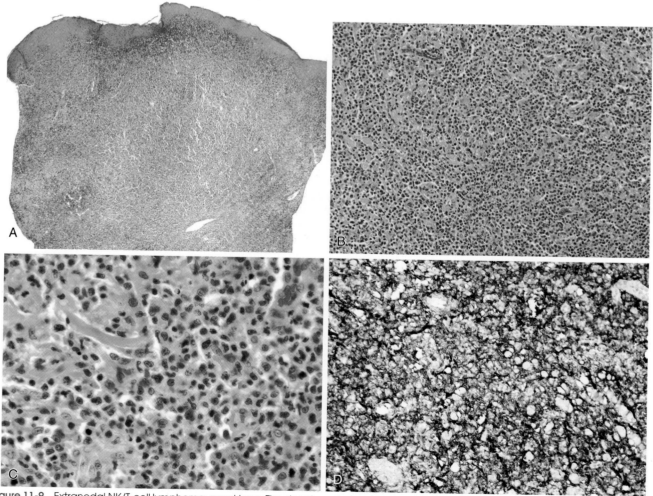

Figure 11-9 Extranodal NK/T-cell lymphoma, nasal type. The dermis and subcutaneous fat are diffusely infiltrated by neoplastic cells, often with ulceration of the overlying epidermis (A). The tumor cells display a broad cytologic spectrum and may be small, medium-sized, large, or anaplastic (B and C). They stain positively for CD56 (D).

Continued

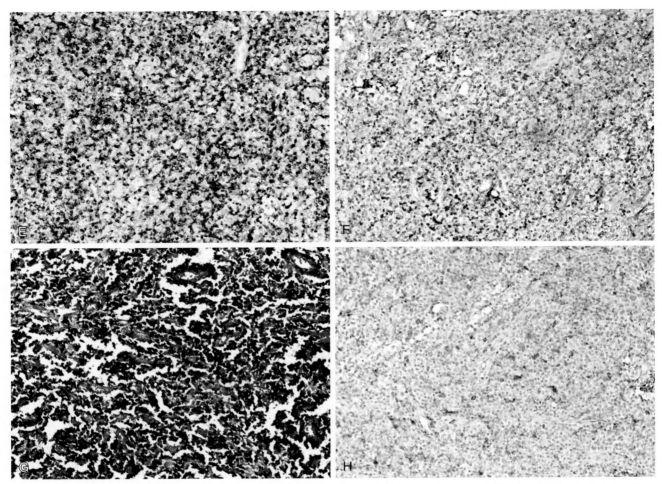

Figure 11-9   cont'd   They stain positively for granzyme B **(E)**, perforin **(F)**, and Epstein-Barr virus–encoded RNA (EBER) by in situ hybridization **(G)**. Scattered CD30+ cells may be present **(H)**.

TABLE 11-3

Differential Diagnosis of Cutaneous Neoplasms That Express T-Cell or NK-Cell Markers

Diagnosis	Clinical Appearance	CD3	CD4	CD8	CD56	TIA1, Granzyme B, or Perforin	EBV	Clonal TCR
Subcutaneous panniculitis-like T-cell lymphoma	Nodules on extremities and trunk	+	–	+	–	+	–	+
Primary cutaneous gamma-delta T-cell lymphoma	Nodules and plaques on extremities; occasionally ulcerated	+	–	–/+	+	+	–	+
Extranodal NK/T-cell lymphoma	Nodules on trunk and extremities	+	–	–	+	+	+	–
Primary cutaneous anaplastic large cell lymphoma	Nodules on trunk, face, extremities, and buttocks; frequently ulcerated	+	+	–	–	+	–	+
Mycosis fungoides	Patches, plaques, and nodules; predilection for sites protected from sunlight	+	+	–	–	–	–	+
Blastic plasmacytoid dendritic cell neoplasm	Nodules	–	+	–	+	–	–	–

Modified from Jaffe ES, Gaulard P, Ralfkiaer E et al: Subcutaneous panniculitis-like T-cell lymphoma. In Swerdlow SH, Campo E, Harris NL et al, editors: *WHO classification of tumours of haematopoietic and lymphoid tissues,* ed 4, Lyon, 2008, IARC.
EBV, Epstein-Barr virus; *TCR,* T-cell receptor genes; +, Typically positive; +/–, positive in many cases; –/+, usually negative; –, almost always negative.

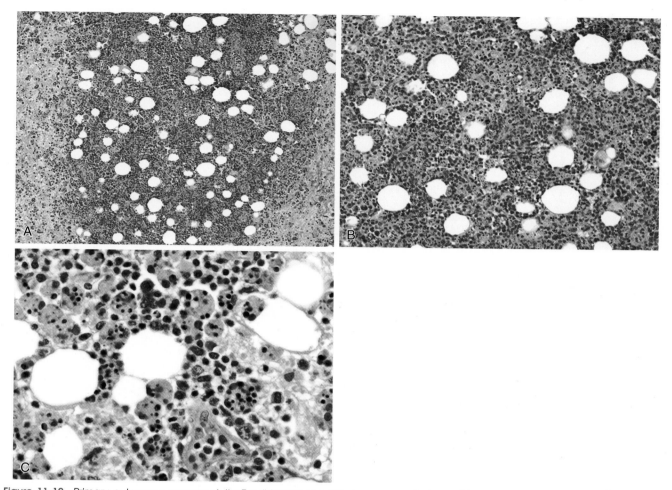

Figure 11-10 Primary cutaneous gamma-delta T-cell lymphoma. This tumor may display epidermotropic, dermal, and subcutaneous (**A**) patterns of growth. The subcutaneous form may show rimming of fat spaces (**B**) and numerous debris-laden macrophages with apoptosis and necrosis (**C**).

Staging, Treatment, and Outcome

Cutaneous gamma-delta T-cell lymphoma has a poor prognosis; the median survival time is approximately 1 year. Patients with involvement of the subcutaneous fat have a worse prognosis than those with tumors limited to the epidermis and dermis.[88,100] Patients with subcutaneous tumors may develop hemophagocytic syndrome; this is associated with a poor prognosis. Extracutaneous extranodal involvement is common, although the lymph nodes, spleen, and bone marrow usually are spared.[111] Nearly 50% of patients develop elevated liver enzymes and leukopenia; these findings are also associated with a poor prognosis.[112] Cutaneous gamma-delta T-cell lymphoma is generally resistant to radiotherapy and to multiagent chemotherapy.

Differential Diagnosis

In cases of cutaneous gamma-delta T-cell lymphoma involving the subcutaneous tissue, the neoplastic T cells rim the fat spaces, a finding also characteristic of subcutaneous panniculitis-like T-cell lymphoma of alpha-beta origin.[96] Immunohistochemical staining helps distinguish the alpha-beta and gamma-delta T-cell lymphomas, because gamma-delta T-cell lymphomas typically are CD56+, βF1−, and CD8−, whereas the alpha-beta subcutaneous panniculitis-like T-cell lymphomas typically are CD56−, βF1+, and CD8+.

Cutaneous gamma-delta T-cell lymphoma also should be distinguished from cutaneous lymphomas with a CD56+, CD8− immunophenotype, including extranodal NK/T-cell lymphoma, nasal type. Identification of EBV favors the latter diagnosis. Also in the differential diagnosis is CD4+, CD56+ blastic plasmacytoid dendritic cell tumor. Blastic plasmacytoid dendritic cell tumors (discussed later in the chapter) are composed of CD123+, CD4+, CD56+ tumor cells with ample cytoplasm and fine nuclear chromatin; they do not express T-cell–specific antigens, such as CD3.

Mycosis fungoides may resemble cutaneous gamma-delta T-cell lymphoma with epidermotropism; however, immunophenotyping can help determine the correct diagnosis. The CD56+, βF1− phenotype of cutaneous gamma-delta T-cell

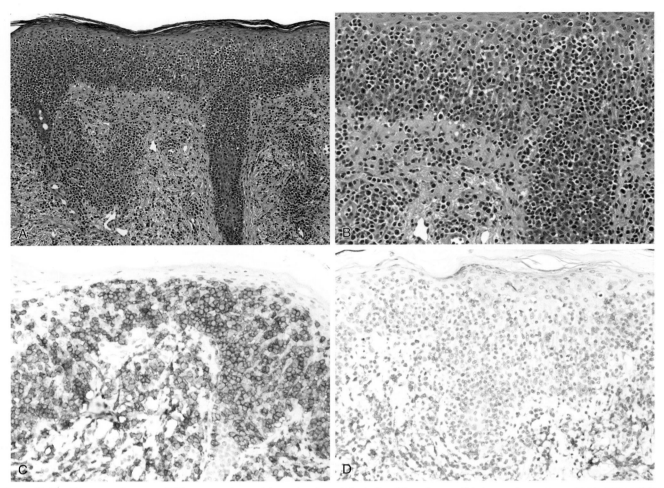

Figure 11-11 Primary cutaneous CD8+ aggressive epidermotropic cytotoxic T-cell lymphoma. This tumor shows a predominantly epidermotropic growth pattern with a pagetoid appearance **(A)**. The tumor cells form intraepidermal collections **(B)** and have a CD8+ **(C)** and CD4– **(D)** immunophenotype.

lymphoma is distinctive from the CD4+, CD56–, βF1+ immunophenotype of mycosis fungoides.

The differential diagnosis of cutaneous gamma-delta T-cell lymphoma also includes lupus panniculitis. Honeycomb-pattern eosinophilic hyalinization of the fat lobule, germinal center formation, and dermal and subcutaneous deposits of connective tissue mucin (hyaluronic acid) are findings often found in lupus panniculitis and not usually observed in subcutaneous lymphomas. However, these characteristic features may not be present in lupus, and the lobular panniculitis with necrosis and lymphoid atypia characteristic of lupus may closely resemble cutaneous gamma-delta T-cell lymphoma.[113]

Primary Cutaneous CD8+ Aggressive Epidermotropic Cytotoxic T-Cell Lymphoma (Provisional Entity)

Primary cutaneous CD8+ aggressive epidermotropic cytotoxic T-cell lymphoma is a rare cutaneous T-cell lymphoma characterized by the features embodied in its name; it is an aggressive lymphoma with a preferential intraepidermal proliferation of CD8+ T cells.[107]

Clinical Features

Primary cutaneous CD8+ aggressive epidermotropic cytotoxic T-cell lymphoma occurs in adults and is associated with an aggressive clinical course.[36,114] Tumors may be generalized or localized and appear as eruptive papules or nodules, often with ulceration. The lesions also may present as hyperkeratotic patches and plaques.[36,115,116]

Pathologic Features

CD8+ aggressive epidermotropic cytotoxic T-cell lymphoma is characterized by a dense epidermotropic infiltrate of CD8+ cells with a pagetoid pattern (Figure 11-11). The epidermotropic tumor cells may extend down adnexal structures. Neoplastic cells may be distributed in an angiocentric pattern, sometimes with angioinvasion. Epidermal changes include ulceration, dyskeratosis, spongiosis, and subepidermal edema, occasionally with blister formation, acanthosis, and hyperkeratosis.[36,117] The tumor cells have medium-sized to large, usually round nuclei.

CD8+ aggressive epidermotropic cytotoxic T-cell lymphoma is composed of CD8+, CD3+, granzyme

B+, TIA-1+, perforin+, βF1+ cells that sometimes express CD7 and CD45RA without CD4 expression and usually without CD45RO, CD2, or CD5. In rare cases these tumors may express CD15,[118] or CD30.[119] Clonal rearrangement of T-cell receptor genes is seen, and the tumors are negative for EBV. Nonneoplastic CD4+ T cells may be present.

Staging, Treatment, and Outcome

CD8+ aggressive epidermotropic cytotoxic T-cell lymphoma is associated with a poor prognosis; the median survival time is less than 3 years.[36] Although lymph node involvement is rare, the lymphoma may spread to the lungs, testes, oral mucosa, and central nervous system (CNS).[36,120]

Differential Diagnosis

The differential diagnosis of CD8+ aggressive epidermotropic cytotoxic T-cell lymphoma includes other forms of cutaneous lymphoma derived from CD8+ cytotoxic T cells.[85] The clinical presentation, clinical behavior, and extent of epidermotropism are helpful for distinguishing CD8+ aggressive epidermotropic cytotoxic T-cell lymphoma from mycosis fungoides and CD8+ variants of CD30+ lymphoproliferative disease, including the recently proposed lymphomatoid papulosis, type D (see earlier discussion).[69] Mycosis fungoides is associated with a prolonged clinical course with plaques and patches, unlike the rapidly progressive clinical course seen in CD8+ aggressive epidermotropic cytotoxic T-cell lymphoma. Unlike CD8+ aggressive epidermotropic cytotoxic T-cell lymphoma, which usually presents as multiple tumors, primary cutaneous ALCL usually presents as solitary nodules, frequently with ulceration. Lymphomatoid papulosis has an indolent course; therefore, clinicopathologic correlation is useful for preventing its misdiagnosis as an aggressive lymphoma.

The aggressive Ketron-Goodman variant of pagetoid reticulosis likely represents either CD8+ aggressive epidermotropic cytotoxic T-cell lymphoma or gamma-delta T-cell lymphoma. Clinical features of CD8+ aggressive epidermotropic cytotoxic T-cell lymphoma may resemble gamma-delta T-cell lymphoma insofar as gamma-delta T-cell lymphomas often present with disseminated plaques and ulcerated nodules on the extremities. Gamma-delta T-cell lymphoma usually is CD56+ and lacks CD4, CD8, and βF1; in contrast, CD8+ aggressive epidermotropic cytotoxic T-cell lymphoma typically has a CD8+, βF1+, CD56− immunophenotype.

CD8+ aggressive epidermotropic cytotoxic T-cell lymphoma also may occasionally involve the subcutaneous fat in a pattern similar to that of subcutaneous panniculitis-like T-cell lymphoma. These CD8+ tumors share a βF1+ phenotype with the expression of cytotoxic proteins. Nevertheless, extensive epidermotropism helps identify CD8+ aggressive epidermotropic cytotoxic T-cell lymphoma; epidermal involvement is rare in subcutaneous panniculitis-like T-cell lymphoma.

Primary Cutaneous CD4+ Small/Medium T-Cell Lymphoma (Provisional Entity)

Primary cutaneous CD4+ small/medium T-cell lymphoma, a provisional entity in the WHO classification system,[107] is an uncommon form of prognostically favorable cutaneous T-cell lymphoma. Distinguishing it from florid reactive processes can be challenging.

Clinical Features

Primary cutaneous CD4+ small/medium T-cell lymphoma most often presents as a solitary plaque or nodule on the face, neck, or upper trunk. Cutaneous CD4+ small/medium T-cell lymphomas rarely involve the lower extremities. Cases with cutaneous patches characteristic of mycosis fungoides are excluded.[121-125]

Pathologic Features

The disorder is characterized by a dense dermal infiltrate of small to medium-sized pleomorphic lymphocytes without significant epidermotropism; it occasionally extends into subcutaneous fat.[121-124] Scattered large neoplastic lymphoid cells comprising less than 30% of the tumor may be observed in rare cases. B cells, plasma cells, and histiocytes also are often present.[126] Some cases have been reported to show numerous eosinophils.[127]

CD4+ small/medium T-cell lymphoma is a neoplasm of CD3+, CD4+, CD8−, and CD30− T cells without expression of cytotoxic proteins. Occasionally loss of pan–T-cell markers is seen.[4,121] The atypical T cells co-express markers of T-follicular helper cells (T$_{FH}$), including PD1, CXCL13, and bcl6, a distinctive feature that may help set this disorder apart from other cutaneous lymphoid infiltrates.[128] Clonal rearrangement of T-cell receptor genes often is detected. These lymphomas are negative for EBV.

Staging, Treatment, and Outcome

CD4+ small/medium T-cell lymphomas are indolent; the 5-year survival rate exceeds 80%.[3,121-125] Solitary or localized tumors are associated with a better prognosis than is more widespread cutaneous disease.[127] Treatment includes surgical excision or local radiotherapy. In addition to the anatomic distribution and number of tumors, the extent of infiltration by CD8+ T cells and the proliferation rate correlate with disease progression. A low density of infiltrating CD8+ T cells and a high Ki67 proliferation index are associated with more rapid cutaneous dissemination.[127]

Differential Diagnosis

The differential diagnosis of CD4+ small/medium T-cell lymphomas includes cutaneous lymphoid hyperplasia. Both processes may have infiltrates that contain histiocytes and eosinophils, and the degree of atypia in the neoplastic cells of CD4+ small/medium T-cell lymphoma is often minimal, similar to that seen in activated T cells in drug reactions or other reactive processes. Immunophenotyping and molecular genetic analysis may not distinguish the two definitively, because pan–T-antigen loss is not consistently found in primary cutaneous CD4+ small/medium T-cell lymphoma and because clonal T-cell populations may be found by PCR in some instances in reactive processes.

The presence of a relatively monotonous diffuse dermal proliferation of slightly enlarged small to medium CD4+ T cells without a significant infiltrate of CD8+ cells or epidermotropism suggests the diagnosis of CD4+ small/medium T-cell lymphoma. How many of these cases may represent reactive infiltrates with a T-cell–detectable clone, rather than a bona fide T-cell neoplasm, remains unclear and somewhat controversial.

Clinical findings can help distinguish CD4+ small/medium T-cell lymphoma from mycosis fungoides; the presence of papules and nodules in the absence of patches favors the diagnosis of CD4+ small/medium T-cell lymphoma. Histologically mycosis fungoides is characterized by the presence of epidermotropism, whereas CD4+ small/medium T-cell lymphoma occurs in the dermis and subcutis with little epidermotropism.[126]

■ CUTANEOUS B-CELL LYMPHOMAS

Primary cutaneous B-cell lymphomas account for approximately 28% of all cutaneous lymphomas. Primary cutaneous follicle center lymphoma, cutaneous extranodal marginal zone B-cell lymphoma, and diffuse large B-cell lymphoma account for more than 90% of cutaneous B-cell lymphomas.[9] Although cutaneous B-cell lymphomas show morphologic and immunophenotypic overlap with their extracutaneous counterparts, there are important differences in the clinical presentation and outcome.[4]

Extranodal Marginal Zone Lymphoma of Mucosa-Associated Lymphoid Tissue (MALT Lymphoma)

Extranodal marginal zone lymphoma arises in a wide variety of extranodal sites, of which the skin is among the more common. Although cutaneous marginal zone lymphoma shares many clinical and pathologic features with marginal zone lymphomas arising in other sites, it has some distinctive features.

Clinical Features

The type of tumor commonly seen with cutaneous marginal zone lymphoma is an erythematous papule, plaque, or nodule, usually on the trunk or extremities. Occasionally multiple tumors may be seen, appearing as a confluent plaque or localized grouping of erythematous papules.[6,129-136,136a] Some investigators have suggested that *B. burgdorferi* infection may play a role in lymphomagenesis in a subset of patients with cutaneous marginal zone lymphoma,[137]

although most cases have no known underlying predisposing factor.

Pathologic Features

Cutaneous marginal zone lymphoma shares some histologic findings with extranodal marginal zone lymphoma at other sites. The lymphomas are characterized by the presence of a perivascular and periadnexal infiltrate, or larger aggregates or nodules or a diffuse proliferation of lymphoid cells, typically including reactive germinal centers surrounded by a proliferation of marginal zone cells, plasma cells, and admixed reactive T lymphocytes.[138-141] Epidermal involvement is rare; the infiltrate usually is separated from the epidermis by a zone of uninvolved papillary dermis (Figure 11-12). The infiltrate often extends from the dermis into the subcutaneous fat. The neoplastic cells range from small lymphocytes with scant cytoplasm to marginal zone or monocytoid B cells with more abundant cytoplasm. Plasma cells are often found ringing the periphery of aggregates of lymphoid cells; they may also be seen scattered among lymphoid cells or in a superficial perivascular distribution.

Cutaneous marginal zone lymphomas have a spectrum of histologic findings. In some cases, most of the neoplastic cells are marginal zone cells that form sheetlike aggregates around the germinal centers with few plasma cells; other cases are marked by zones of plasma cells in the interfollicular areas without many marginal zone cells.[142] The marginal zone B cells have small, round, oval or slightly irregular nuclei and ample pale cytoplasm. If neoplastic, the plasma cells may contain intranuclear pseudoinclusions of immunoglobulin, called *Dutcher bodies.* Increasing degrees of plasmacytic differentiation may be seen over time with serial biopsies.[143] Infiltration of the hair follicle epithelium by the neoplastic B cells is occasionally conspicuous, but lymphoepithelial lesions are overall uncommon.

Almost always, some evidence of pre-existing reactive lymphoid follicles is seen, either on routinely stained sections or on sections immunostained with antibodies to follicular dendritic cells. Two forms of germinal centers may be seen in cutaneous marginal zone lymphoma: reactive lymphoid follicles devoid of neoplastic cells, and reactive lymphoid follicles infiltrated or "colonized" by neoplastic B cells. The first type of follicle can often be identified. Follicular colonization is not present in all cases, but when conspicuous, it may impart a resemblance to cutaneous follicle center lymphoma.[135,144]

The density of the reactive T-cell infiltrate is quite variable; in many cases the T cells outnumber the neoplastic B cells.[142,145,146] CD123+ plasmacytoid dendritic cells may be identified in clusters in primary cutaneous marginal zone lymphomas[147]; they appear to be more commonly found in cutaneous marginal zone lymphomas than in other types of cutaneous B-cell lymphomas.

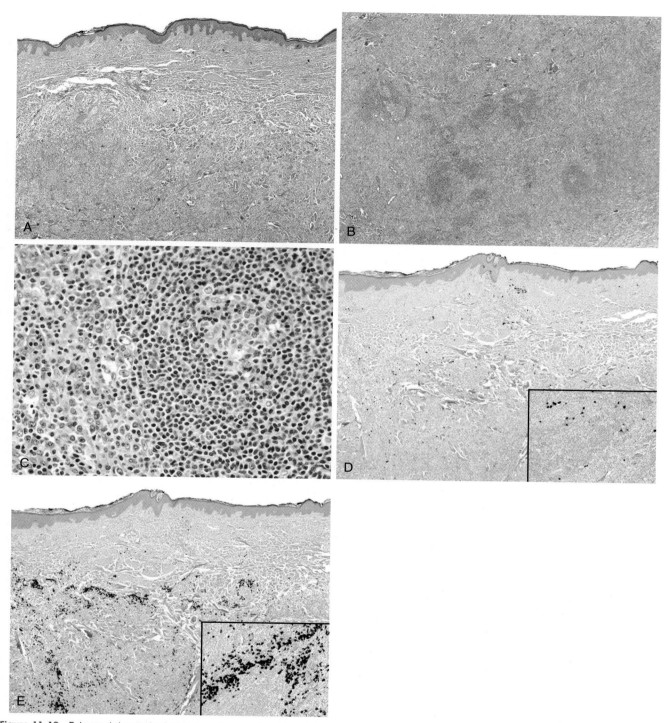

Figure 11-12 Extranodal marginal zone lymphoma of mucosa-associated lymphoid tissue (MALT lymphoma). **A,** The tumor presents as a dermally based proliferation separated from the epidermis by a grenz zone of uninvolved papillary dermis without epidermal changes. **B,** The neoplastic cells form sheets and aggregates surrounding benign reactive lymphoid follicles. Zones of plasma cells **(C)** or sheets of marginal zone B cells may be present. In situ hybridization demonstrates lambda light chain restriction in (kappa **(D)** and inset; lambda **(E)** and inset).

The neoplastic marginal zone cells express CD20 and bcl2 but usually not CD5, CD10, or bcl6.[144,148-150] Plasma cells usually are CD20– but express CD138, CD79a, and MUM1/IRF4. Many cases have plasmacytic differentiation, and cytoplasmic light chain restriction is identified by immunohistochemistry or in situ hybridization in more than 70% of cases.[138,139,151] Stains for bcl6, bcl2, and CD21 may highlight the lymphoid follicles. Most lymphoid follicles are revealed as round or oval collections of bcl6+, bcl2– reactive follicle center cells supported by a meshwork of CD21+ follicular dendritic cells (see Figure 11-12). In cases with colonized follicles, scattered bcl6− neoplastic B cells infiltrate and expand the follicles and disrupt the bcl6+, bcl2−, CD10+ reactive follicle center cells and CD21+ meshworks.[146] Neoplastic marginal zone cells usually express bcl2, but on colonization of a follicle, bcl2 expression may be lost; therefore lack of bcl2 alone does not exclude the presence of neoplastic cells infiltrating a reactive follicle.

Most cutaneous marginal zone lymphomas express class-switched immunoglobulin. IgG is expressed most frequently and IgA, IgE, and IgM less commonly. This is in contrast to marginal zone lymphomas arising in most other sites, in which expression of IgM is most common.[152] (Notable exceptions include thymic marginal zone lymphoma, which most often expresses IgA [see Lymphomas of the Thymus in Chapter 4] and immunoproliferative small intestinal disease, which characteristically expresses alpha heavy chain [see Immunoproliferative Small Intestinal Disease in Chapter 5]). In a few cases the lymphoma has been biclonal, with neoplastic populations expressing different heavy chains and/or different light chains. Some investigators suggest that cutaneous marginal zone lymphomas fit into one of two categories. The majority of cases express immunoglobulin with heavy chain class switch (usually IgG), contain numerous reactive T cells, often outnumbering B cells, typically lacking a diffuse confluent pattern of growth, and lacking evidence of extracutaneous involvement by lymphoma. A minority of cases express IgM; this group more often shows a diffuse pattern of growth with a predominance of B cells, more like marginal zone lymphomas arising in other sites. Indeed some patients with IgM+ cutaneous marginal zone lymphoma are reported to have extracutaneous lymphoma, raising the question of whether the skin may not be the primary site.[136a] In addition, some IgM+ cutaneous marginal zone lymphomas express CXCR3, a receptor for interferon gamma-induced chemokines, as is true of the majority of marginal zone lymphomas arising in other sites. CXCR3 expression has not been detected in the heavy chain class switched cutaneous marginal zone lymphomas.[136a,152]

Although most marginal zone lymphomas are associated with upregulation of Th1-type cytokines (e.g., IFNγ, CXCL10, and IL-12), cutaneous marginal zone lymphomas appear to be associated with a Th2-type cytokine milieu, with higher levels of IL-4 present.[152] CXCR3 expression, which appears absent in the B cells of heavy chain class switched cutaneous marginal zone lymphomas, is characteristic of activated T cells, particularly Th1 cells.[136a] These observations suggest a difference in the pathogenesis between primary cutaneous marginal zone lymphoma and marginal zone lymphomas arising in other sites.

AP12-MALT1 fusion [t(11;18)] is found in fewer than 20% of cases.[153-156] In one study, 25% of cases had a t(14;18) involving *IGH* and *MALT1*; the translocation appeared to be more common among cases with a monocytoid morphology, with a component of neoplastic B cells having abundant pale cytoplasm.[157] In most cases no chromosomal translocation is detected.[157]

Staging, Treatment, and Outcome

The clinical behavior of cutaneous marginal zone lymphoma is similar to that of extranodal marginal zone lymphoma arising in other sites.[6,130,140,141,158-160] The 5-year disease-specific survival rate is nearly 100%; nevertheless, up to 30% of patients experience extracutaneous relapse,[6,132,151,159,161] most commonly in other extranodal sites, including the breast, salivary glands, and orbit.[158,162] Although rare, transformation to large cell lymphoma has been reported.[132,151]

Treatment generally is localized and includes surgical excision, radiation therapy, and intralesional injection of steroids or interferon.[135,150,151] Systemic therapy, including rituximab and chemotherapy, may be used for patients with more widespread disease.[150]

Differential Diagnosis

The differential diagnosis of cutaneous marginal zone lymphoma includes primary cutaneous follicle center lymphoma, plasmacytoma, and reactive lymphoid infiltrates.

Primary cutaneous follicle center lymphoma may have a follicular and/or diffuse pattern of growth. Cutaneous marginal zone lymphoma usually takes the form of a diffuse or vaguely nodular proliferation; the latter pattern may be conspicuous if follicular colonization is present. Both types of lymphoma are characterized by the presence of lymphoid follicles (which are neoplastic in follicle center lymphoma, and intact, colonized, or overrun by neoplastic cells in marginal zone lymphoma) and by small to medium-sized neoplastic cells with irregular nuclei. Stains for CD21 highlight the follicular dendritic cell meshworks, indicating true follicular structures in both primary cutaneous follicle center lymphoma and cutaneous marginal zone lymphoma.

Histologic features that favor a diagnosis of cutaneous marginal zone lymphoma include zones of plasma cells and sheets of interfollicular marginal zone B cells. Germinal centers that appear to be irregularly shaped and spilling out into the interfollicular dermis with aggregates of centrocytes and large centroblasts in direct apposition to the reticular dermal collagen fibers without intervening small mature lymphocytes favor the diagnosis of follicle center lymphoma.

In some cases distinguishing neoplastic follicles of primary cutaneous follicle center lymphoma from reactive or colonized follicles of cutaneous marginal zone lymphoma may be difficult, because bcl6 and CD10 are expressed by both reactive and neoplastic follicles, and bcl2 usually is negative in primary cutaneous follicle center lymphoma.[144,163]

A combination of immunostaining for CD21, bcl6, CD10, and bcl2 may be useful for distinguishing primary cutaneous follicle center lymphoma from cutaneous marginal zone lymphoma based on the architecture of the follicles and the interfollicular areas (Table 11-4). In cases of cutaneous marginal zone lymphoma, the colonized follicles, when present, display aggregates of CD21+ follicular dendritic cells, similar to neoplastic follicles or reactive germinal centers; however, they also contain distinct clusters of bcl6−, bcl2+/− neoplastic B cells in addition to clusters of bcl6+, bcl2− germinal center cells (Figure 11-13). In contrast, the neoplastic follicles in primary cutaneous follicle center lymphoma contain a more uniform population of neoplastic bcl6+, CD10+, bcl2− cells. Finally, in contrast to primary cutaneous follicle center lymphoma, in which the bcl6+ cells form irregularly shaped follicles and aggregates in the interfollicular zones, bcl6+ and CD10+ cells are not observed in interfollicular and diffuse areas devoid of CD21+ cells in cutaneous marginal zone lymphoma.

In cases of cutaneous marginal zone lymphoma with a dominant population of neoplastic plasma cells, the differential diagnosis may include plasmacytoma. The presence of a component of B cells and of reactive lymphoid follicles favors marginal zone lymphoma over plasmacytoma. In general, expression of IgM favors marginal zone lymphoma over plasmacytoma; however, because most cutaneous marginal zone lymphomas are IgG positive, the class of immunoglobulin expressed is less helpful for making a distinction.

Reactive lymphoid infiltrates may also mimic cutaneous marginal zone lymphoma and may arise secondary to continued antigenic stimulation (e.g., arthropod bite, autoimmune disease, pharmaceutical agents, tattoos, or infectious organisms). When the etiology is unknown, these nonneoplastic infiltrates are preferably termed *cutaneous lymphoid hyperplasia;* however, many synonyms and related terms are used, including *pseudolymphoma, lymphocytoma cutis, lymphadenosis benigna cutis, pseudolymphoma of Spiegler-Fendt,* and *lymphadenoma granulosa.* The clinical presentation and histologic features overlap to such a degree that before the advent of immunohistochemical analysis, most cases of cutaneous marginal zone lymphoma probably were diagnosed as cutaneous lymphoid hyperplasia.[164,165] Reports of cutaneous lymphoid hyperplasia with monotypic plasma cells and immunocytoma now are considered to represent cutaneous marginal zone lymphoma.[27,129,166,167]

As mentioned, cutaneous marginal zone lymphoma and cutaneous lymphoid hyperplasia share many clinical features; both occur more commonly in women, and both often present as a solitary, slow-growing cutaneous nodule on the upper extremity or trunk. Histologically both manifest as a dermal lymphocytic infiltrate with a grenz zone, reactive follicles, and admixed inflammatory cells (Table 11-5). Nevertheless, the presence of epidermal changes (particularly epidermal atrophy or hyperplasia), exocytosis, spongiosis, or hyperkeratosis favors a diagnosis of cutaneous lymphoid hyperplasia, possibly because many cases of cutaneous lymphoid hyperplasia represent reactions to external antigens. On the other hand, sheets of marginal zone cells and zones of monotypic plasma cells in the interfollicular regions and around the superficial vascular plexus support a diagnosis of cutaneous marginal zone lymphoma.[139]

The observation that reactive lymphoid follicles are more commonly seen in cutaneous marginal lymphoma than in lymphoid hyperplasia led to a revision of the earlier concept that lymphoid follicles favored a nonneoplastic diagnosis.[168] The use of immunohistochemical stains for B cells and T cells reveals central zones of B cells and surrounding T cells similar to the pattern observed in many reactive

TABLE 11-4

Immunophenotype of Follicles in Cutaneous Follicle Center Lymphoma and Cutaneous Marginal Zone Lymphoma					
	Cutaneous Follicle Center Lymphoma		**Cutaneous Marginal Zone Lymphoma**		
	Neoplastic Follicles	**Interfollicular Areas**	**Reactive Follicles**	**Colonized Follicles**	**Interfollicular Areas**
CD21	+ Often irregular shapes	−	+ Usually round or oval	+ May appear splayed	−
Bcl6	+ Neoplastic cells	+/− Neoplastic cells	+ Nonneoplastic cells	−/+ Bcl6+ nonneoplastic cells with scattered Bcl6− neoplastic cells	−
CD10	+	−/+	+ (weak)	−	−
Bcl2	−/+ Neoplastic cells usually negative	−/+ Neoplastic cells;+ Nonneoplastic cells	− Nonneoplastic cells	+/− Bcl2− nonneoplastic cells with scattered Bcl2+/− neoplastic cells	+

+, Typically present; +/−, present in many cases; −/+, usually absent; −, almost always absent.

dermatoses. A panel of immunohistochemical stains often is helpful. In cases with inconspicuous follicles on hematoxylin and eosin staining, stains for bcl2 and CD21 identify focal nonstaining areas and aggregates of follicular dendritic cells, respectively, which correspond to lymphoid follicles.[144] In situ hybridization or immunohistochemistry reveals monotypic light chain expression by plasma cells in more than 70% of cases of marginal zone lymphoma but not in cutaneous lymphoid hyperplasia.[6] An infiltrate that is 75% or greater B cells and co-expression of CD43 and CD20 also support a diagnosis of B-cell lymphoma.[139,169]

In the past, the presence of a bottom-heavy infiltrate was thought to favor a diagnosis of lymphoma; however, this is not diagnostic. A dense superficial dermal or top-heavy infiltrate may be observed in marginal zone lymphoma, whereas hypersensitivity reactions to injected antigens and lymphomatoid drug reactions may both show deep dermal, bottom-heavy, lymphoid infiltrates. Although not completely specific, the presence of aggregates of eosinophils or of abundant neutrophils with nuclear dust tends to exclude a diagnosis of marginal zone lymphoma.[139]

Primary Cutaneous Follicle Center Lymphoma

Primary cutaneous follicle center lymphoma is the most common type of primary cutaneous B-cell lymphoma; it accounts for about 60% of cases.[4,143,170]

Clinical Features

Primary cutaneous follicle center lymphoma occurs slightly more often in men than in women, and the median age of onset is 65 years.[136] The disorder presents as solitary or multiple erythematous cutaneous papules, nodules, or plaques, sometimes as a central lesion with adjacent satellites. These tumors most commonly occur on the scalp or neck and less

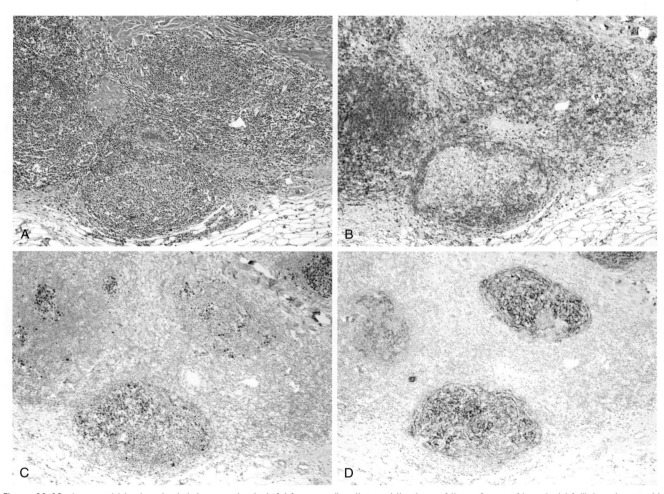

Figure 11-13 Immunohistochemical stains may be helpful for revealing the architecture of three forms of lymphoid follicles observed in cutaneous marginal zone lymphoma (cMZL) and cutaneous follicle center lymphoma (cFCL). Reactive follicles (**A**, *bottom of image*) are observed in cMZL and reveal an absence of bcl2 staining (**B**, *bottom of image*), with staining of the follicle center cells for bcl6 (**C**, *bottom*), supported by a tight collection of CD21+ follicular dendritic cells (**D**, *bottom*). Colonized follicles (**A**, *upper right*) may be observed in cMZL and display scattered neoplastic bcl2+ cells (**B**, *upper right*) splaying the bcl6+ follicle center cells (**C**, *upper right*), supported by CD21+ follicular dendritic cells (**D**, *upper right*).

Continued

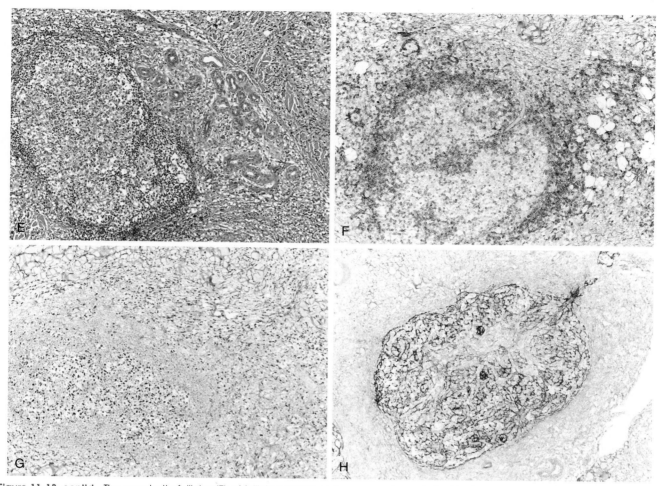

Figure 11-13, cont'd The neoplastic follicles **(E)** of follicle center lymphoma are characterized by irregularly shaped aggregates of bcl2– **(F)**, bcl6+ **(G)** tumor cells, in some cases supported by CD21+ meshworks of follicular dendritic cells **(H)**. Note that bcl6+ cells are also identified in diffuse areas **(G)**.

TABLE 11-5

Histologic and Immunophenotypic Findings in Cutaneous Lymphoid Hyperplasia, Primary Cutaneous Marginal Zone Lymphoma, and Primary Cutaneous Follicle Center Lymphoma			
Finding	**Cutaneous Lymphoid Hyperplasia**	**Primary Cutaneous Marginal Zone Lymphoma**	**Primary Cutaneous Follicle Center Lymphoma**
Epidermal pathologic condition (hyperkeratosis, parakeratosis, erythrocyte extravasation, ulceration, dyskeratosis, spongiosis)	+/–	–	–
Dermal eosinophils and neutrophils	+/–	–/+	–
Plasma cells in zones (perivascular and interfollicular)	–	+/–	–
Marginal zone cells in large aggregates (interfollicular)	–	+	–
Dutcher bodies (intranuclear immunoglobulin pseudoinclusions)	–	+/–	–
Light chain–restricted plasma cells	–	+/–	–
Light chain–restricted follicles	–	–	–
Follicle centers (reactive or neoplastic)	–/+	–	+
Grenz zone of uninvolved papillary dermis	+	+/–	+/–
		+	+

+, Usually present; +/–, present in many cases; –/+, usually absent; –, almost always absent.

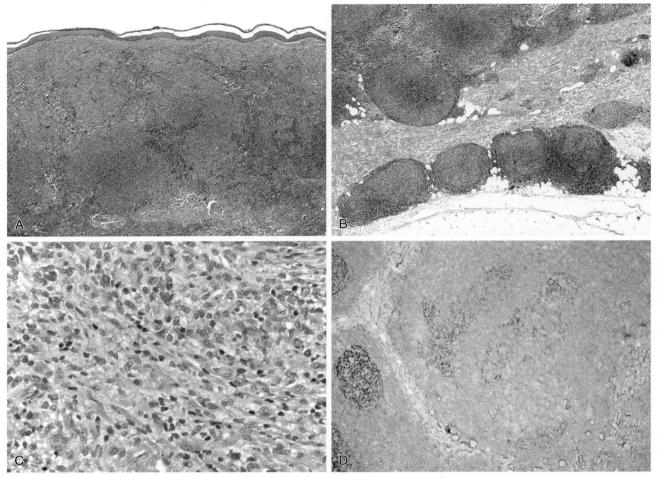

Figure 11-14 Primary cutaneous follicle center lymphoma. A dense dermal infiltrate may appear follicular, follicular and diffuse **(A)**, or diffuse on scanning magnification. The tumor cells are separated from the epidermis by a grenz zone of uninvolved papillary dermis and neoplastic cells abut reticular dermal collagen without intervening mantles **(A)** and often infiltrate throughout the dermis to involve the subcutaneous fat **(B)**. The neoplastic cells are irregular and often elongate **(C)**. The neoplastic follicles may be oval but also may form irregular shapes, with disruption of the CD21+ follicular dendritic cell meshworks **(D)**.

commonly on the trunk, but they may occur at any cutaneous site.[129,131,132,136,171-173]

Pathologic Features

Primary cutaneous follicle center lymphoma is characterized by a dermal proliferation of centrocytes and centroblasts in a follicular, follicular and diffuse, or diffuse pattern that often extends into the subcutaneous fat (Figure 11-14). The centrocytes have medium-sized or large, cleaved or irregular nuclei with dispersed chromatin, inconspicuous nucleoli, and scant cytoplasm. Large centrocytes generally are more plentiful in diffuse primary cutaneous follicle center lymphoma than in cases with a follicular component. The centrocytes may be elongated or spindle shaped.

The centroblasts, which typically are a minor population of the tumor, have large, round nuclei with peripherally located basophilic nucleoli and a rim of basophilic cytoplasm. Although centroblasts usually are present, by definition they do not form

confluent sheets in primary cutaneous follicle center lymphoma. The neoplastic cells usually appear as expanded, irregularly shaped, lymphoid follicles in the dermis. Occasionally the neoplastic cells spill out of the follicles and surround aggregates of benign small lymphocytes; these follicles are termed "inside-out follicles." The neoplastic cells also may form nodules that are in direct apposition to the reticular dermal collagen without a mantle zone of small lymphocytes; these follicles are called "naked follicles."

Numerous admixed small T cells and sclerosis often are present. Although other inflammatory cells, including eosinophils and granulocytes, and histiocytes may be present, plasma cells typically are absent or, if present, do not form aggregates or zones. Grading of primary cutaneous follicle center lymphoma is not recommended, because it has not been shown to have clinical relevance.

The neoplastic cells in primary cutaneous follicle center lymphoma are CD20+ and bcl6+ with variable expression of CD10. The tumor cells do not stain for CD5, CD43, or MUM1/IRF4.[144] In contrast to the bcl2+ nodal follicular lymphomas, primary cutaneous follicle center lymphomas usually do not express bcl2 protein, and when they do, it generally is dim.[174,175] CD21+, CD23+, CD35+ follicular dendritic cells usually are detected in irregularly shaped meshworks corresponding to the follicular areas.[176] Light chain restriction is difficult to demonstrate with immunohistochemical stains on paraffin sections or with in situ hybridization because neoplastic plasma cells are not a feature of primary cutaneous follicle center lymphoma. The proliferation fraction with Ki67 may be higher than expected for nodal follicular lymphoma, but this does not predict a more aggressive course.

Primary cutaneous follicle center lymphoma usually lacks the t(14;18) *(IGH/BCL2)* fusion observed in most nodal follicular lymphomas; however, evidence of the translocation sometimes is found with PCR or fluorescence in situ hybridization (FISH).[129,174,175,177] PCR techniques detect clonal rearrangement of immunoglobulin genes in approximately 50% of cases; the sensitivity of this assay may be diminished because of somatic hypermutation of immunoglobulin genes characteristic of follicle center cells.

Staging, Treatment, and Outcome

The 5-year disease-specific survival rate for patients with primary cutaneous follicle center lymphoma exceeds 97%.[4,143] Unlike most nodal follicular lymphomas, these tumors rarely spread to the lymph nodes, spleen, or bone marrow.[10,129,172] Excision, radiation therapy, and intralesional rituximab are standard therapies for localized lesions.[178] In patients with multifocal cutaneous disease, systemic rituximab has been suggested as the initial approach. Combination chemotherapy usually is not recommended because of the overall good prognosis associated with this tumor.[179]

Although factors other than site clearly play a role, primary cutaneous follicle center lymphoma that presents on the lower leg seems to follow a more aggressive clinical course than cases presenting on the head, neck, or trunk.[179,180] If the lymphoma expresses bright CD10 or bright bcl2 protein or if the t(14;18) translocation is present, staging for evidence of extracutaneous follicular lymphoma is especially important, because these findings are much more common in primary lymph nodal follicular lymphoma than in primary cutaneous follicle center lymphoma.

Differential Diagnosis

When primary cutaneous follicle center lymphoma has a prominently follicular or follicular and diffuse architecture, the differential diagnosis includes cutaneous marginal zone lymphoma, cutaneous lymphoid hyperplasia, and involvement of the skin by nodal follicular lymphoma. Both cutaneous marginal zone lymphoma and primary cutaneous follicle

center lymphoma may present on the scalp, trunk, or upper extremities.[*] Both types of lymphoma usually are localized at diagnosis and rarely disseminate to the lymph nodes or bone marrow.[6,130,181] Histologically, primary cutaneous follicle center lymphoma and cutaneous marginal zone lymphoma also have overlapping features. Both may display a follicular or nodular growth pattern and both contain lymphoid follicles.[131] Bcl2 is not a helpful marker in most cases, because both the neoplastic follicles in most primary cutaneous follicle center lymphomas and the reactive follicles in cutaneous marginal zone lymphoma are negative for bcl2.[129,174,182] The differential diagnosis of these tumors is discussed in detail in the section on primary cutaneous marginal zone lymphoma.

Lymph nodal follicular lymphoma occasionally involves the skin as a secondary site; in rare cases the cutaneous lymphoma is the first lesion biopsied. In contrast to primary cutaneous follicle center lymphoma, in which the neoplastic follicles often are bcl2– and variably express CD10, nodal follicular lymphomas often strongly express CD10 and bcl2. Although t(14;18) *(IGH/BCL2)* is not observed in most primary cutaneous follicle center lymphoma, it is identified in more than 75% of nodal follicular lymphomas.[183]

When primary cutaneous follicle center lymphoma has a diffuse pattern of growth, the differential diagnosis includes primary cutaneous large B-cell lymphoma, leg type. Tumors with a diffuse pattern composed entirely of centroblasts are excluded from the category of primary cutaneous follicle center lymphoma and usually are best classified as primary cutaneous large B-cell lymphoma, leg type. In addition, strong staining for bcl2 and MUM1/IRF4 with dim or no staining for bcl6 supports the diagnosis of large B-cell lymphoma, leg type, over cutaneous follicle center lymphoma, which usually is negative for both bcl2 and MUM1/IRF4 and expresses bcl6. Cytoplasmic expression of IgM or IgD or both is nearly always seen in diffuse large B-cell lymphoma, leg type, but is unusual in cutaneous follicle center lymphoma.[184]

Primary Cutaneous Diffuse Large B-Cell Lymphoma, Leg Type

Primary cutaneous diffuse large B-cell lymphoma, leg type, is a relatively aggressive lymphoma composed of large lymphoid cells that usually arises on the lower extremities. It accounts for a minority of primary cutaneous B-cell lymphomas.[185]

Clinical Features

Primary cutaneous diffuse large B-cell lymphoma, leg type, occurs more often in women than in men, and 80% of cases present in patients older than 70 years.[9] The disorder usually presents as solitary or multiple erythematous or violaceous nodules on one or both lower extremities below the knee, often with ulceration.[186] Although most common on the

---

*References 6, 10, 130, 131, 133, 159, 172, and 181.

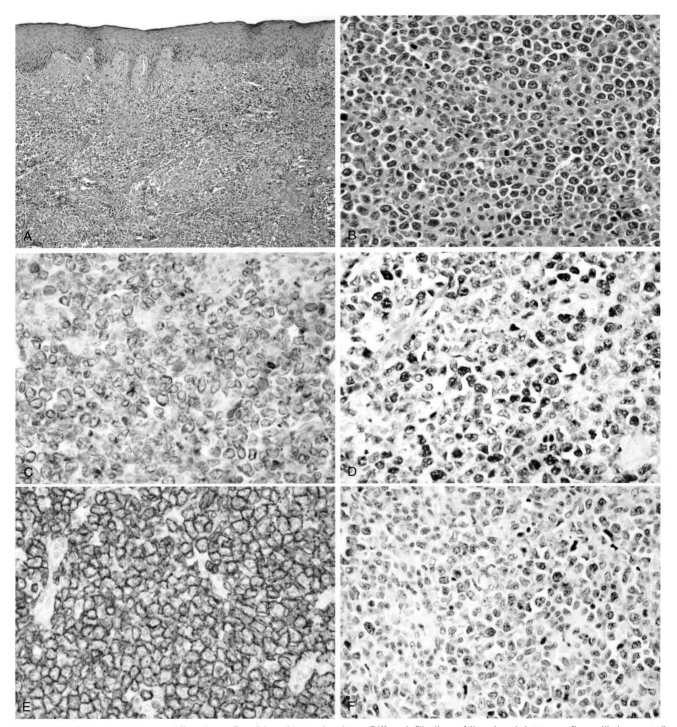

Figure 11-15   Primary cutaneous diffuse large B-cell lymphoma, leg type. Diffuse infiltration of the dermis is seen, often with tumor cells abutting the epidermis **(A)** and occasionally with ulceration. The neoplastic centroblasts and immunoblasts may have a striking round cell morphology **(B)**, and the immunophenotype is bcl2+ **(C)**, MUM1/IRF4+ **(D)**, CD20+ **(E)**, and bcl6−/+ **(F)**.

lower leg, primary cutaneous diffuse large B-cell lymphoma, leg type, can occur at any cutaneous site.

Pathologic Features

Primary cutaneous diffuse large B-cell lymphoma, leg type, is defined as a diffuse dermal infiltrate of round, monomorphic large B cells with prominent nucleoli and vesicular nuclei resembling immunoblasts and centroblasts (Figure 11-15). Few reactive cells are admixed.[180,187,188] Epidermotropism is absent, although the tumor cells may abut the dermal-epidermal junction. Although the overall growth pattern is diffuse, scanning magnification may reveal a vaguely nodular appearance.[186] When the criteria of the WHO-EORTC classification are

TABLE 11-6

Differential Diagnosis of Cutaneous Follicle Center Lymphoma and Diffuse Large B-Cell Lymphoma, Leg Type		
Parameter	Cutaneous Follicle Center Lymphoma	Cutaneous Diffuse Large B-Cell Lymphoma, Leg Type
Morphology	Predominance of centrocytes, often large, especially in diffuse lesions Centroblasts possible but not in sheets Follicular, follicular and diffuse, or diffuse pattern (a continuum) Admixed small lymphocytes Fibrosis	Predominance or confluent sheets of medium-sized to large B cells with round nuclei, prominent nucleoli, and coarse chromatin, resembling centroblasts and/or immunoblasts Diffuse growth pattern Minimal inflammatory background
Phenotype	bcl2−/+ bcl6 + CD10+/− MUM1/IRF4 −	Bcl2++ bcl6+/− CD10− MUM1/IRF4+
Clinical features	Middle-aged adults Lesions localized on head or trunk (90%) Multifocal lesions (rare)	Elderly, especially women Lesions localized on one or both legs, most often below the knee Lesions in site other than leg (rare; 10%)

+, Typically positive; ++, strongly positive; +/−, positive in many cases; −/+, usually negative; −, almost always negative.

used, most cases of primary cutaneous diffuse large B-cell lymphoma are classified as "leg type," regardless of whether they occur on the leg.

These lymphomas are characterized by a CD20+, bcl2+, MUM1/IRF4+ immunophenotype. Neoplastic cells also express CD19, CD22, CD79a, and FOXP1.[179,186,189] The intensity of tumor cell bcl2 staining often exceeds that of the nonneoplastic T cells and is a significant adverse prognostic factor.[187,190] Bcl6 is variably positive. The tumor cells do not stain for CD10 or CD138, and meshworks of CD21+ follicular dendritic cells generally are absent. The proliferation fraction as assessed by Ki67 exceeds 60%.

PCR techniques detect clonal rearrangement of immunoglobulin genes in most cases, and the t(14:18) translocation generally is absent.[174,190,191] Gene expression profiling studies have revealed similarities between primary cutaneous diffuse large B-cell lymphoma, leg type, and ABC-type of diffuse large B-cell lymphoma, in contrast to the germinal center B-cell profile observed in primary cutaneous follicle center lymphoma.[192] Primary cutaneous diffuse large B-cell lymphoma, leg type, also showed high levels of expression of genes associated with cellular proliferation, including PIM1, PIM2, and MYC.

Staging, Treatment, and Outcome

The 5-year survival rate for diffuse large B-cell lymphoma, leg type, approaches 50%.[179,193] Large studies of 100 or more patients reported that diffuse large B-cell lymphoma involving the lower extremity had a less favorable prognosis than diffuse large B-cell lymphoma arising at other cutaneous sites,[180,189,190] although a few studies did not support this conclusion.[186] The existence of multiple tumors at presentation is also a poor prognostic finding.[180,187]

Differential Diagnosis

The differential diagnosis of primary cutaneous diffuse large B-cell lymphoma, leg type, includes the entirely diffuse form of primary cutaneous follicle center lymphoma. The diffuse form of cutaneous follicle center lymphoma is a proliferation of large and small centrocytes and centroblasts. In contrast to diffuse large B-cell lymphoma, leg type, primary cutaneous follicle center lymphoma is composed of bcl6+, CD10+/−, bcl2−/dim, and MUM1/IRF4− tumor cells often associated with a CD21+ meshwork of follicular dendritic cells. Predominance of centroblasts or immunoblasts with strong expression of bcl2 and MUM1/IRF4 favors primary cutaneous diffuse large B-cell lymphoma, leg type (Table 11-6). Cytoplasmic IgM or IgD or both usually are observed in diffuse large B-cell lymphoma, leg type, but not in follicle center lymphoma.[184]

A diagnosis of primary cutaneous diffuse large B-cell lymphoma, other, is a diagnosis of exclusion and should be made rarely. These cases lack the features of either primary cutaneous follicle center lymphoma or primary cutaneous diffuse large B-cell lymphoma, leg type. They are composed of a monomorphic proliferation of centroblasts and immunoblasts but lack the characteristic immunophenotype of the leg type of lymphoma. These rare tumors behave more aggressively than diffuse forms of primary cutaneous follicle center lymphoma.[187] In rare cases, primary cutaneous diffuse large B-cell lymphoma displays a strikingly spindled cytomorphology; immunophenotyping confirms the diagnosis and excludes other spindle cell cutaneous neoplasms.[194-196]

T-cell/histiocyte-rich large B-cell lymphoma is a rare, morphologically distinct form of large B-cell lymphoma for which the differential diagnosis includes cutaneous lymphoid hyperplasia because of the relative scarcity of large neoplastic B cells in relation to a very dense T-cell and histiocytic infiltrate.[197-202]

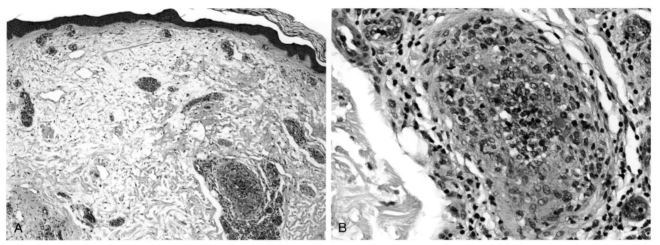

Figure 11-16   Intravascular large B-cell lymphoma. The intravascular tumor cells may be accompanied by a perivascular infiltrate of small reactive lymphocytes **(A)**. The tumor cells have large nuclei with scant cytoplasm and fill the vascular spaces **(B)**.

Immunoglobulin gene rearrangement and immuno-histochemistry for detection of CD20+ large atypical B cells that may show light chain–restriction are helpful in establishing a diagnosis.[203,204]

Intravascular Large B-Cell Lymphoma

Intravascular large B-cell lymphoma is a rare but distinct variant of diffuse large B-cell lymphoma characterized by the presence of large neoplastic B cells confined to vascular lumina (see Chapter 14).

Clinical Features

Intravascular large B-cell lymphoma presenting with cutaneous involvement appears to show a female preponderance. The skin and CNS are the most commonly involved sites. Cutaneous tumors appear as violaceous plaques on the trunk and lower extremities. CNS involvement is not infrequent and is associated with a poor outcome.

Pathologic Features

Intravascular large B-cell lymphoma of the skin is characterized by the presence of large lymphoid cells, often associated with fibrin thrombi, in the dermal vasculature (Figure 11-16).[205-207] The cells are cytologically atypical large cells that express B-cell antigens, including CD19, CD20, CD22, and CD79a.[205-207] Clonal rearrangement of immunoglobulin genes characteristically is present.

Staging, Treatment, and Outcome

Although intravascular large B-cell lymphoma may present in the skin, it is always considered to be systemic for therapeutic purposes,[208] even in the absence of documented extracutaneous disease. Nevertheless, one study found that female patients with disease limited to the skin who had normal platelet counts had a better prognosis.[209] This tumor usually is disseminated and involves the liver, kidneys, endocrine glands, lungs and, less frequently, lymph nodes. Treatment involves combination chemotherapy.

■ SECONDARY CUTANEOUS MANIFESTATIONS OF LYMPHOMA AND LEUKEMIA

Patients with leukemia/lymphoma may develop cutaneous lesions that represent lymphoma or leukemic infiltration of the skin (specific lesions) or non-neoplastic reactive infiltrates (nonspecific lesions). The incidence of leukemia cutis approaches 20% for patients with lymphoid leukemias; the disorder is seen even more frequently (up to 50% of cases in some series) in patients with myeloid leukemia and myeloproliferative disorders.[210] In rare cases a patient may present with leukemia in the skin that precedes diagnostic evidence of leukemia in the bone marrow and blood by a month or more. This form of primary extramedullary leukemia of the skin, which is quite rare, has been termed *aleukemic leukemia cutis*.[211-213] The clinical and histologic differential diagnosis of a specific cutaneous leukemic infiltrate includes a variety of reactive neutrophilic, lymphoid, and infectious processes that in rare cases may histologically mimic a leukemic infiltrate.

Lymphoblastic Leukemia/Lymphoma

Clinical Features

B-lymphoblastic and T-lymphoblastic neoplasms rarely present with cutaneous involvement.[214] The term *lymphoblastic lymphoma* is used when localized clinical disease is present without peripheral blood or bone marrow involvement; the term *lymphoblastic leukemia* indicates extensive bone marrow or peripheral blood involvement.

Among patients with widespread disease, cutaneous involvement is relatively common; it has been observed in 30% of patients with B-lymphoblastic leukemia/lymphoma, most of whom were children.[215,216] Cutaneous lesions of B-lymphoblastic lymphoma arise most commonly on the skin of the head, neck, upper back, chest, and abdomen. Tumors appear as a solitary erythematous or violaceous nodule or as multiple erythematous papules.

Pathologic Features

Lymphoblastic leukemia/lymphoma is characterized by a monomorphic dermal infiltrate of small to medium-sized lymphoid blasts that dissect through the reticular dermal collagen, forming a dermal-based nodule (Figure 11-17). The nuclei have dispersed nuclear chromatin and multiple nucleoli. Mitotic activity is brisk. The overlying epidermis may be attenuated, without infiltration by tumor cells. In early lesions, the tumor cells may be present in a perivascular distribution in the dermis.[217,218]

The tumor cells stain positively for terminal deoxynucleotidyl transferase (TdT) in both B- and T-lymphoblastic neoplasms. In B-lymphoblastic leukemia/lymphoma, CD79a, Pax5, CD19, and CD10 usually are expressed, whereas CD20 usually is negative. CD45 often is expressed but dimly. T-cell and myeloid-specific markers are not expressed, although the myeloid-associated antigens CD13 and CD33 may be detected,[217] if the specimen is evaluated by flow cytometry. In cases of T-lymphoblastic leukemia/lymphoma, the tumor cells usually stain for CD1a, CD2, CD3, CD5, CD7, and both CD4 and CD8. The presence of CD34 and CD99 also supports the precursor phenotype. T lymphoblasts may aberrantly express CD79a; the myeloid-associated markers CD13 and CD33 may also be expressed, as may CD56.

B-lymphoblastic neoplasms typically have clonally rearranged *IGH*. T-lymphoblastic leukemia/lymphoma is associated with clonal *TCR* rearrangement and occasionally with simultaneous clonal rearrangement of *IGH;* this apparent lineage promiscuity

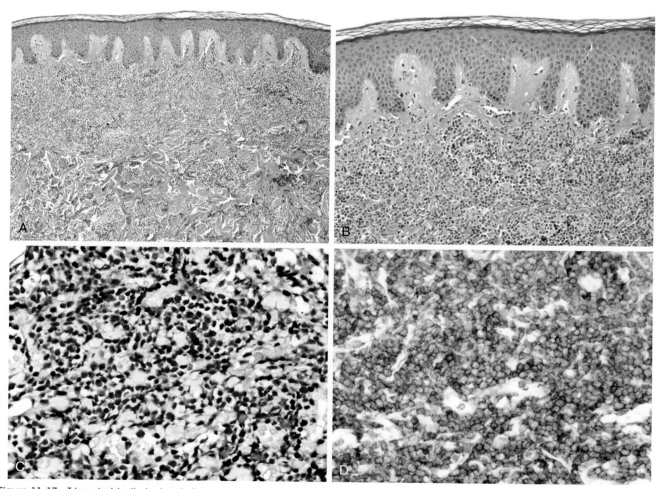

Figure 11-17   T-lymphoblastic leukemia/lymphoma. Tumor cells infiltrate the dermis in a perivascular and diffuse pattern (**A**). These cells, which have round blastic nuclei with a high nucleus to cytoplasm ratio, finely stippled chromatin, and inconspicuous nucleoli, spare the epidermis (**B**). TdT is expressed (**C**), as is CD43 (**D**).

Continued

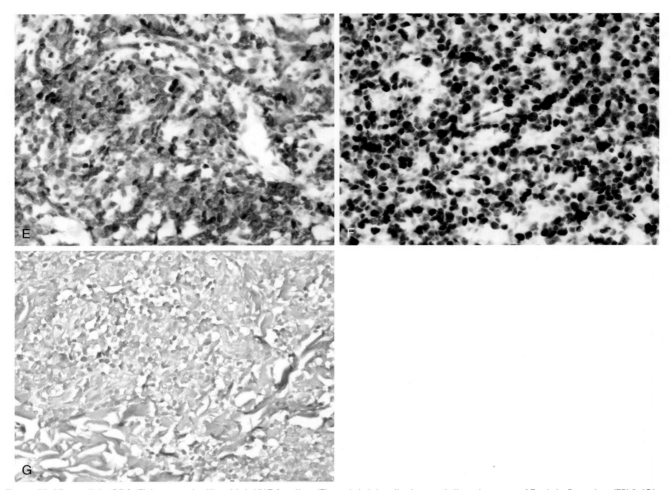

Figure 11-17, cont'd CD3 **(E)** is present with a high Ki67 fraction **(F)** and staining that reveals the absence of Epstein-Barr virus (EBV) **(G)**.

may be related to the primitive stage of differentiation of the neoplastic cells (see Lymphomas of the Thymus in Chapter 4 for additional information on T-lymphoblastic leukemia/lymphoma).

Staging, Treatment, and Outcome

In children, B-lymphoblastic leukemia/lymphoma is cured in more than 80% of cases.[219] Adults have a somewhat lower cure rate (60%), and their median survival time is 5 years. T-lymphoblastic leukemia/lymphoma is an aggressive disease. The prognosis largely depends on the extent of disease, the patient's age, and LDH levels. Multiagent chemotherapy with CNS prophylaxis has improved outcomes. The presence of minimal residual disease after therapy is a poor prognostic factor.

Differential Diagnosis

Histologically B lymphoblasts are indistinguishable from T lymphoblasts. Immunophenotyping allows differentiation of these tumors.

The differential diagnosis of lymphoblastic leukemia/lymphoma includes blastic plasmacytoid dendritic cell neoplasm, acute myelogenous leukemia/myeloid sarcoma, cutaneous involvement by blastoid mantle cell lymphoma, and poorly differentiated neuroendocrine carcinoma. The presence of TdT suggests a lymphoblastic process; however, TdT+ may also be seen in blastic plasmacytoid dendritic cell tumors. CD20 often is negative in B-lymphoblastic leukemia/lymphoma; therefore, other stains, such as CD79a and Pax5, may need to be used to demonstrate a B-cell lineage. The expression of CD68, myeloperoxidase, chloroacetate esterase, and lysozyme in the absence of B or T-cell specific markers supports the diagnosis of a myeloid neoplasm. Mantle cell lymphoma in the skin is characterized by the presence of CD20, CD5, CD43, bcl2, and bcl1/cyclin D1 and the absence of CD10, bcl6, and TdT. Although Pax5 may be expressed in neuroendocrine tumors, a diagnosis of neuroendocrine carcinoma (e.g., Merkel cell carcinoma) is confirmed by the presence of cytokeratin 20 in a punctate perinuclear pattern and the presence of other epithelial and neural markers.[220]

Adult T-Cell Leukemia/Lymphoma

HTLV-1–associated adult T-cell leukemia/lymphoma was the first human malignancy demonstrated to have a retroviral etiology. Originally described as a rapidly fatal disease in Japan,[221] adult T-cell leukemia/lymphoma has been identified in other geographic regions where HTLV-1 is endemic, including the Caribbean, central Africa, and the southeastern United States (see also Adult T-Cell Leukemia/Lymphoma in Chapter 13).[222,223,223a]

Clinical Features

Approximately half of patients with adult T-cell leukemia/lymphoma have cutaneous lesions. The four clinical groups of adult T-cell leukemia/lymphoma are acute, lymphomatous, chronic, and smoldering. Skin lesions are observed in all types; however, they are a principal finding in many cases of the smoldering type. In the smoldering form of adult T-cell leukemia/lymphoma, patients often present with cutaneous lesions without other disease manifestations, although some patients have pulmonary lesions. These patients do not have a peripheral blood lymphocytosis, lymphadenopathy, hypercalcemia, hepatosplenomegaly, or gastrointestinal or bone marrow involvement. Patients may have less than 5% abnormal lymphocytes in the peripheral blood, although in the absence of biopsy-proven cutaneous or lung involvement, more than 5% abnormal lymphocytes are required for a diagnosis of the smoldering form of adult T-cell leukemia/lymphoma. In cases of the chronic form, patients typically have more extensive disease. Cutaneous manifestations may be conspicuous, but there may also be lymphadenopathy, involvement of liver, spleen and lung, and more than 5% abnormal T lymphocytes in peripheral blood, without hypercalcemia, effusions or involvement of CNS, gastrointestinal tract, or bone marrow.[223a,223b,224] The lymphoma type is characterized by lymphadenopathy with or without extranodal involvement but with at most 1% abnormal T cells in peripheral blood, and the acute form is a rapidly progressive neoplasm with leukemic involvement.

The cutaneous lesions of the acute and lymphomatous forms have a variable appearance. They may present as a rash, a papular eruption, or as tumor nodules. The chronic form usually is associated with an exfoliative erythroderma, and the smoldering type may present as cutaneous erythema, a papular eruption or, in rare cases, as tumors. In contrast to mycosis fungoides, which is considered a primary cutaneous T-cell lymphoma even when it presents with nodal involvement at the time of diagnosis, adult T-cell leukemia/lymphoma is considered a leukemia with associated lymphoma, even in the smoldering form that presents with clinically evident disease limited to the skin and a sparse if not undetectable population of circulating tumor cells.

Pathologic Features

The skin lesions of adult T-cell leukemia/lymphoma are characterized histologically by a variably dense epidermotropic infiltrate of pleomorphic lymphocytes with hyperlobated nuclei. The atypical cells usually are accompanied by an infiltrate of small lymphocytes. Mitotic figures are common, and scattered large Reed-Sternberg–like cells with eosinophilic macronucleoli may be present. Overall the pattern is that of a lichenoid, or superficial, perivascular dermatosis. Notably, Pautrier collections are observed in more than 50% of cases. In the tumor stage, the neoplastic cells diffusely infiltrate through the dermis and extend into the subcutaneous fat, similar to the diffuse infiltration in the involved viscera.

The neoplastic T cells have a CD2+, CD3+, CD5+, CD25+ immunophenotype. CD4 usually is expressed, but occasionally a CD8+ immunophenotype is seen; in rare cases, both CD4 and CD8 are expressed.[225,226] Loss of CD7 is characteristic, and the large transformed cells may express CD30 but are negative for ALK. The tumor cells also express CCR4 and FOXP3, consistent with regulatory T cells.[227]

Staging, Treatment, and Outcome

Despite aggressive therapy, the mean survival time of patients with the acute form of adult T-cell leukemia/lymphoma is less than 6 months. The smoldering and chronic forms may behave in an indolent manner for a prolonged period, but they eventually may progress to the acute form. Clinical features associated with a poor prognosis include hypercalcemia, hyperbilirubinemia, and an elevated serum LDH level.

Differential Diagnosis

The differential diagnosis of smoldering adult T-cell leukemia/lymphoma includes mycosis fungoides. The cutaneous lesions of adult T-cell leukemia/lymphoma are similar to those observed in mycosis fungoides, appearing as erythematous papules, plaques, and/or nodules. However, the hepatosplenomegaly and frequent opportunistic infections characteristic of adult T-cell leukemia/lymphoma are rarely seen in mycosis fungoides. In addition, although adult T-cell leukemia/lymphoma does not occur in children, it occurs at a younger age than does mycosis fungoides; the peak incidence is seen in the fifth decade of life.

Chronic Lymphocytic Leukemia/Small Lymphocytic Lymphoma

Clinical Features

In rare cases chronic lymphocytic leukemia/small lymphocytic lymphoma may present with cutaneous involvement. More often the skin is secondarily involved in patients with an established diagnosis of chronic lymphocytic leukemia. Cutaneous infiltrates of chronic lymphocytic leukemia may be found in association with scars, with other cutaneous neoplasms, or as a specific papular eruption on the trunk, head, or neck.[228]

Pathologic Features

The cutaneous infiltrate of chronic lymphocytic leukemia/small lymphocytic lymphoma characteristically is composed of a monomorphic population of small, round, mature lymphocytes. The infiltrate usually displays a superficial and mid-dermal perivascular pattern and rarely forms an expansile nodule in the dermis. Epidermal changes are absent, and the neoplastic B cells do not infiltrate the epidermis or adnexal epithelium. Lymphoid follicles are not present, nor is a significant infiltrate of histiocytes, eosinophils, or neutrophils observed.

In cutaneous involvement by chronic lymphocytic leukemia/small lymphocytic lymphoma, the neoplastic B cells display a CD5+, CD23+, CD43+, CD19+, CD79a+ immunophenotype. CD20 expression often is dim. The tumor cells do not stain for CD10 or cyclin D1.

Nonleukemic cases are termed *small lymphocytic lymphoma*. A cutaneous infiltrate of neoplastic small, round CD5+, CD23+ B cells is diagnosed as "small lymphocytic lymphoma" in patients without known leukemia and as "cutaneous involvement by chronic lymphocytic leukemia" in patients with peripheral blood or marrow involvement (see also Chronic Lymphocytic Leukemia, Chapter 13).

Differential Diagnosis

The differential diagnosis of chronic lymphocytic leukemia/small lymphocytic lymphoma in the skin includes the T-cell lymphomas composed of small cells, other low-grade B-cell lymphomas, and reactive lymphoid infiltrates. In cutaneous chronic lymphocytic leukemia/small lymphocytic lymphoma, the monomorphic cytology of the small, round lymphocytes is distinct from the convoluted nuclei of mycosis fungoides. Mycosis fungoides also is characterized by epidermotropism, a rare finding in cutaneous involvement by chronic lymphocytic leukemia/small lymphocytic lymphoma. The absence of lymphoid follicles helps exclude cutaneous marginal zone lymphoma and primary cutaneous follicle center lymphoma.

Immunohistochemical studies can readily identify the distinctive immunophenotype of chronic lymphocytic leukemia/small lymphocytic lymphoma and distinguish it from other B-cell lymphomas, T-cell lymphomas, and reactive infiltrates. An important finding is the presence of both CD5 and CD43 (often used as pan–T-cell markers in the skin) on the neoplastic B cells of chronic lymphocytic leukemia/small lymphocytic lymphoma. Also, CD20 staining may be weak or absent. Staining for other B-cell antigens, including Pax5 and CD19, is positive in chronic lymphocytic leukemia/small lymphocytic lymphoma; these antigens are not present in the T-cell lymphomas. Strong staining for CD23 without cyclin D1 supports the diagnosis of chronic lymphocytic leukemia/small lymphocytic lymphoma and excludes the diagnosis of mantle cell lymphoma. In some cases of chronic lymphocytic leukemia, CD23 expression is not readily detected on paraffin sections; in this context, cyclin D1 staining is important for differentiating chronic lymphocytic leukemia from mantle cell lymphoma.

Mantle Cell Lymphoma

Mantle cell lymphoma is a B-cell neoplasm that rarely presents with cutaneous involvement; it is not considered a form of primary cutaneous lymphoma as patients typically have widespread extracutaneous disease on staging.[228a] The hallmark of mantle cell lymphoma is nuclear expression of cyclin D1 as a result of an underlying chromosomal translocation involving *IGH* and *CCND1* [t(11;14)] (see Mantle Cell Lymphoma of the Gastrointestinal Tract, Chapter 5, and Mantle Cell Lymphoma, Chapter 13, for additional information on mantle cell lymphoma).

Clinical Features

When involvement by mantle cell lymphoma occurs in the skin, it presents as cutaneous lesions, usually without ulceration and without obvious preferential anatomic distribution. The disease shows a male predominance, and the median age is in the seventh decade of life.

Pathologic Features

The cutaneous infiltrates of mantle cell lymphoma form a middermal and subcutaneous dense diffuse nodule, and sometimes a less confluent perivascular and periadnexal infiltrate, composed of small to medium-sized (rarely large) monomorphic lymphoid cells with slightly to moderately irregular, dark nuclei and scant cytoplasm that typically lacks distinct nucleoli. Interspersed plasma cells may be seen, but they are not part of the neoplastic clone and are not immunoglobulin light chain restricted. The tumor cells typically express CD20, IgM/IgD, CD5, FMC7, bcl2, cyclin D1, and CD43. CD10 and BCL6 are absent. CD23 may be weakly positive. Rare cases may lack CD5, but cyclin D1 expression is retained.

Differential Diagnosis

The differential diagnosis of mantle cell lymphoma involving the skin includes marginal zone lymphoma, lymphoblastic leukemia/lymphoma, and chronic lymphocytic leukemia/small lymphocytic lymphoma. Immunophenotypic identification of cyclin D1 is helpful for identifying the tumor cells of mantle cell lymphoma.

Lymphomatoid Granulomatosis

After the lung, the skin is one of the sites more commonly involved by lymphomatoid granulomatosis; it is typically found in conjunction with involvement of lung and sometimes other sites as well, rather than as an isolated finding. Cutaneous involvement by lymphomatoid granulomatosis is characterized by dermal and/or subcutaneous involvement by lesions that usually take the form of papules or nodules. Microscopic examination reveals an atypical lymphohistiocytic infiltrate typically with angiocentric, angiodestructive growth and necrosis, with a predominance of CD4+ T cells similar to lymphomatoid granulomatosis in other sites. A variable number of EBV+ large B cells are present, although they tend to be fewer than found in pulmonary lesions.[228b] (See also Pulmonary Lymphomas in Chapter 4 for additional information on Lymphomatoid Granulomatosis.)

Plasmablastic Lymphoma

Clinical Features

Plasmablastic lymphoma often arises in the oral cavity and is discussed in more detail in Lymphomas of the Oral Cavity in Chapter 3. It is mentioned here because the skin is one of the favored extranodal sites of involvement. These tumors usually arise in immunosuppressed patients.[229-232]

Pathologic Features

Plasmablastic lymphoma is a proliferation of large cells that resemble immunoblasts and have an immunophenotype of plasma cells. They are EBV positive in most cases. The neoplastic cells stain positively for CD138, CD38, and MUM1/IRF4. CD79a is positive in most cases, and monotypic expression of light chains is detected in more than 50% of cases. EMA and CD30 frequently are identified. EBV is readily detected using in situ hybridization for Epstein Barr virus–encoded RNA (EBER); LMP1 is rarely expressed. The tumors cells do not stain for (or stain weakly for) CD20, Pax5, CD45, and CD56.

Staging, Treatment, and Outcome

Because patients usually are in an advanced stage of the disease when the cutaneous lesions are identified, overall survival is extremely poor. Most patients die within 1 year of diagnosis. In rare cases a patient may have a more protracted course.[233]

Differential Diagnosis

The differential diagnosis of plasmablastic lymphoma is broad; it is discussed in detail in Lymphomas of the Oral Cavity in Chapter 3.

Blastic Plasmacytoid Dendritic Cell Neoplasm

Blastic plasmacytoid dendritic cell neoplasms are derived from the precursors of plasmacytoid dendritic cells. This disorder is not considered a lymphoma, but it may enter the differential diagnosis of lymphoid neoplasms and was previously thought to be a lymphoma. It is discussed here because patients initially may present with cutaneous involvement, but most have or subsequently develop widespread disease. This rare tumor has a distinctive morphology and immunophenotype and has variably been termed "CD4+ CD56+ hematodermic neoplasm" and "blastic NK-cell lymphoma." The disorder has a poor prognosis, and it is important to distinguish it from other tumors and reactive infiltrates in the skin.[234]

Clinical Features

The lesions of blastic plasmacytoid dendritic cell neoplasm present on the skin as solitary or multiple papules, plaques, or nodules or occasionally as bruised-appearing lesions. The disorder most commonly occurs in elderly men, but it may be seen in children and women. Involvement of the bone marrow typically is found at diagnosis or shortly thereafter.

Pathologic Features

Blastic plasmacytoid dendritic cell neoplasm is characterized by a diffuse dermal infiltrate of relatively monomorphous, medium-sized cells with finely dispersed nuclear chromatin and small nucleoli (Figure 11-18). The cytoplasm is scant and somewhat amphophilic. The epidermis is spared. No significant necrosis or vasculitis is seen, and mitotic activity is not brisk.

The tumor cells express CD4, CD56, and CD43 and the plasmacytoid dendritic cell–associated antigen CD123. CD68 and CD7 often are expressed. TdT is present in approximately one third of cases. CD33 may be expressed. CD34, CD117, TIA1, perforin, CD19, CD20, CD79a, CD3, CD5, lysozyme, myeloperoxidase, and EBV are not expressed; expression of any of these markers is strong evidence against a diagnosis of blastic plasmacytoid dendritic cell neoplasm.

Staging, Treatment, and Outcome

Regional lymphadenopathy is present in 20% of patients when they present with skin lesions. Progression leads to the involvement of the peripheral blood and bone marrow, with a leukemic phase. Patients may develop a myelomonocytic leukemia or acute myeloid leukemia. The median survival time is about 1 year.

Differential Diagnosis

Blastic plasmacytoid dendritic cell neoplasm may resemble other types of infiltrates of primitive hematologic cells found in cutaneous involvement by lymphoblastic lymphoma/leukemia, acute myeloid leukemia, myeloid sarcoma, and monocytic sarcoma. The histologic appearance of these tumors also may occasionally resemble histiocytic infiltrates in the skin. Immunohistochemical findings in blastic plasmacytoid dendritic cell neoplasm are distinctive; the tumor cells express CD4, CD123, CD56, and CD43. It should be noted that this immunophenotype, although distinctive, is not completely specific. Neoplastic monoblasts, in particular, can have a similar immunophenotype, including expression of CD123. Expression of lysozyme by neoplastic cells supports a diagnosis of monocytic sarcoma or acute monocytic leukemia and excludes blastic plasmacytoid dendritic cell tumor. Clusters of nonneoplastic plasmacytoid dendritic cells (CD123+) may be found in cutaneous B-cell lymphomas (most commonly in marginal zone lymphomas) and in cases of cutaneous pseudolymphomas.[147] Therefore, the presence of plasmacytoid dendritic cells alone is not specific for blastic plasmacytoid dendritic cell neoplasm; this cell type may be found in association with a variety of neoplastic and reactive conditions in the skin and in other sites.

Hodgkin's Lymphoma

Classical Hodgkin's lymphoma may involve the skin, which in rare cases may be the presenting site of the lymphoma.[235,236] Cutaneous involvement may occur through direct extension from underlying lymph nodal involvement or with widespread disease. The histologic features are similar to those of Hodgkin's lymphoma at other sites. The neoplastic cells in classical Hodgkin's lymphoma express CD30 and usually CD15. They typically are Pax5 dim+. CD20, if expressed at all, typically is weak and of variable intensity. CD45 usually is negative. Neoplastic cells in approximately half of all cases harbor EBV.

Differential Diagnosis

The differential diagnosis includes the CD30+ lymphoproliferative disorders and transformed cases of mycosis fungoides. These disorders show staining for CD4 and/or CD30 without expression of CD15, Pax5 or EBV, which differentiates them from cutaneous involvement by classical Hodgkin's lymphoma.[235]

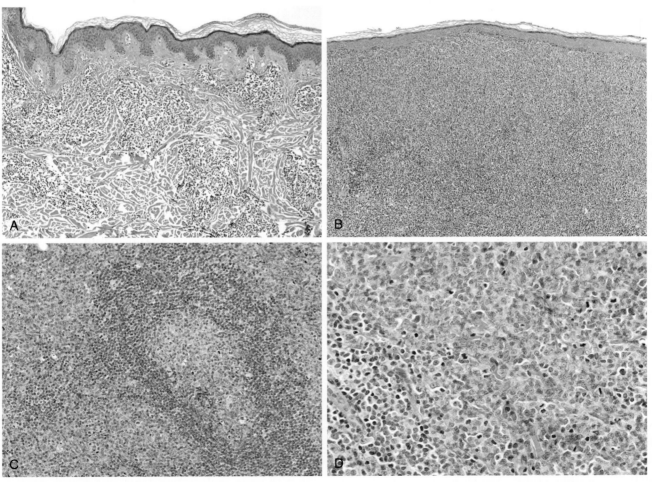

Figure 11-18 Blastic plasmacytoid dendritic cell neoplasm. These tumors present as a perivascular (A) or diffuse (B) infiltrate in the dermis with sparing of the epidermis. In rare cases, reactive lymphoid follicle centers are present with sheets of interfollicular monomorphic neoplastic cells (C). The tumor cells are medium-sized blasts with irregular nuclei, fine chromatin, and small nucleoli (D).

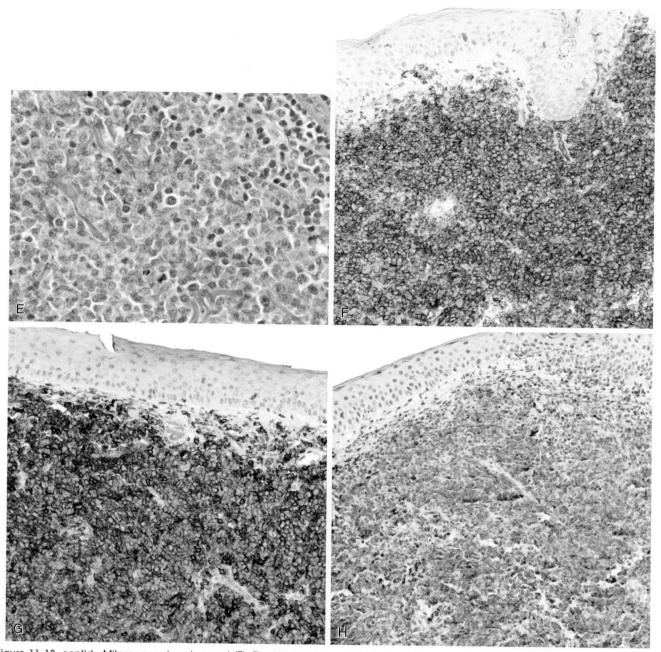

Figure 11-18, cont'd   Mitoses may be observed **(E)**. The blastic plasmacytoid dendritic cells usually have a CD123+ **(F)**, CD4+ **(G)**, and CD56+ **(H)**.

Continued

EBV+ mucocutaneous ulcer, noted above in the differential diagnosis of lymphomatoid papulosis, has a cellular composition that may mimic classical Hodgkin's lymphoma and an immunophenotype that overlaps with that of classical Hodgkin's lymphoma, although large atypical cells in EBV+ mucocutaneous ulcer are less often CD15+, and more often positive for CD20, CD79a, Oct2, and Bob1 than Reed-Sternberg cells and variants. EBV+ mucocutaneous ulcer typically forms a well circumscribed ulcerated lesion, which could help in the differential diagnosis of Hodgkin's lymphoma. Only about half of classical Hodgkin's lymphomas have tumor cells that contain EBV, although by definition EBV is present in EBV+ mucocutaneous ulcer. The distinction is important, as the natural history of the two diseases is very different, with a subset of cases of EBV+ mucocutaneous ulcer showing spontaneous healing.[78]

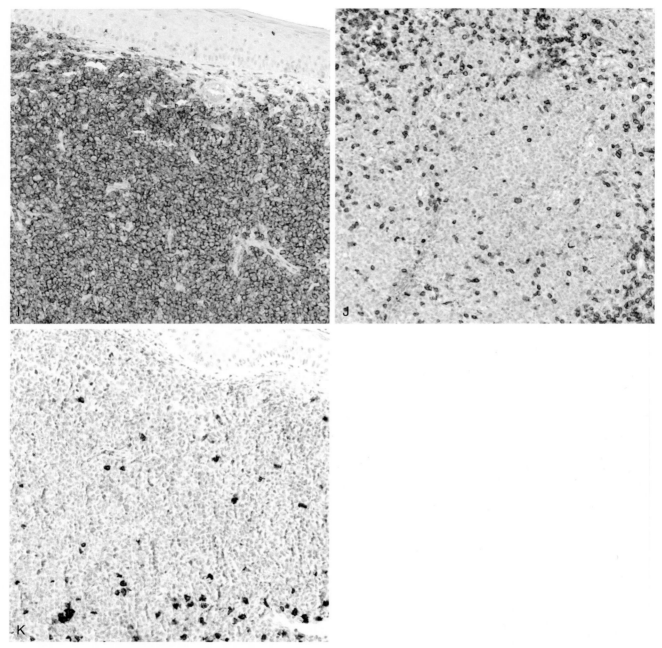

Figure 11-18, cont'd There is also CD43+ **(I)** immunophenotype without staining for CD3 **(J)** or CD79a **(K)**.

REFERENCES

1. Harris NL, Jaffe ES, Stein H et al: A revised European-American classification of lymphoid neoplasms: a proposal from the International Lymphoma Study Group, *Blood* 84:1361-1392, 1994.
2. Swerdlow SH, Campo E, Harris NL et al, editors: *WHO classification of tumours of haematopoietic and lymphoid tissues,* ed 4, Lyon, 2008, IARC.
3. Willemze R, Jaffe ES, Burg G et al: WHO-EORTC classification for cutaneous lymphomas, *Blood* 105:3768-3785, 2005.
4. Willemze R, Kerl H, Sterry W et al: EORTC classification for primary cutaneous lymphomas: a proposal from the Cutaneous Lymphoma Study Group of the European Organization for Research and Treatment of Cancer, *Blood* 90:354-371, 1997.
5. LeBoit PE, Burg G, Weedon D, Sarasin A, editors: *Pathology and genetics of skin tumours,* Lyon, 2006, IARC.
6. Bailey EM, Ferry JA, Harris NL et al: Marginal zone lymphoma (low-grade B-cell lymphoma of mucosa-associated lymphoid tissue type) of skin and subcutaneous tissue, *Am J Surg Pathol* 8:1011-1023, 1996.
7. Vergier B, Beylot-Barry M, Pulford K et al: Statistical evaluation of diagnostic and prognostic features of CD30+ cutaneous lymphoproliferative disorders: a clinicopathologic study of 65 cases, *Am J Surg Pathol* 22:1192-1202, 1998.
8. Kadin ME: Anaplastic large cell lymphoma and its morphological variants, *Cancer Surv* 30:77-86, 1997.
9. Bradford PT, Devesa SS, Anderson WF, Toro JR: Cutaneous lymphoma incidence patterns in the United States: a population-based study of 3884 cases, *Blood* 113:5064-5073, 2009.

10. Santucci M, Pimpinelli N, Arganini L: Primary cutaneous B-cell lymphoma: a unique type of low-grade lymphoma—clinicopathologic and immunologic study of 83 cases, *Cancer* 67:2311-2326, 1991.

11. Veelken H, Wood GS, Sklar J: Molecular staging of cutaneous T-cell lymphoma: evidence for systemic involvement in early disease, *J Invest Dermatol* 104:889-894, 1995.

12. Wood GS: Using molecular biologic analysis of T-cell receptor gene rearrangements to stage cutaneous T-cell lymphoma, *Arch Dermatol* 134:221-223, 1998.

13. Wood GS, Haeffner A, Dummer R, Crooks CF: Molecular biology techniques for the diagnosis of cutaneous T-cell lymphoma, *Dermatol Clin* 12:231-241, 1994.

14. Ralfkiaer E, Cerroni L, Sander C et al: Mycosis fungoides. In Swerdlow S, Campo E, Harris N et al, editors: *WHO classification of tumours of haematopoietic and lymphoid tissues,* ed 4, Lyon, 2008, IARC.

15. Cerroni L, Rieger E, Hodl S, Kerl H: Clinicopathologic and immunologic features associated with transformation of mycosis fungoides to large-cell lymphoma, *Am J Surg Pathol* 16:543-552, 1992.

16. Kadin ME: Lymphomatoid papulosis and associated lymphomas: how are they related? *Arch Dermatol* 129:351-353, 1993.

17. Menagé Hdu P, Sattar NK, Haskard DO et al: A study of the kinetics and pattern of E-selectin, VCAM-1 and ICAM-1 expression in chronic actinic dermatitis, *Br J Dermatol* 134:262-268, 1996.

18. Davis T, Morton C, Miller-Cassman R et al: Hodgkin's disease, lymphomatoid papulosis, and cutaneous T-cell lymphoma derived from a common T-cell clone, *N Engl J Med* 326:1115, 1992.

19. Shapiro PE, Pinto FJ: The histologic spectrum of mycosis fungoides/Sézary syndrome (cutaneous T-cell lymphoma), *Am J Surg Pathol* 18:645-667, 1994.

20. Fung M: "Epidermotropism" vs "exocytosis" of lymphocytes 101: definition of terms, *J Cutan Pathol* 37:525-529, 2010.

21. Smoller BR, Bishop K, Glusac E et al: Reassessment of histologic parameters in the diagnosis of mycosis fungoides, *Am J Surg Pathol* 19:1423-430, 1995.

22. Ralfkiaer E: Immunohistologic markers for the diagnosis of cutaneous lymphomas, *Semin Diagn Pathol* 8:62-72, 1991.

23. Wood GS: Benign and malignant cutaneous lymphoproliferative disorders including mycosis fungoides. In Knowles DM, editor: *Neoplastic hematopathology,* Baltimore, 1992, Williams & Wilkins.

24. Burg G, Kempf W, Cozzio A et al: WHO/EORTC classification of cutaneous lymphomas 2005: histological and molecular aspects, *J Cutan Pathol* 32:647-674, 2005.

25. Hastrup N, Ralfkiaer E, Pallesen G: Aberrant phenotypes in peripheral T cell lymphomas, *J Clin Pathol* 42:398-402, 1989.

26. Edinger JT, Clark BZ, Pucevich BE et al: CD30 expression and proliferative fraction in nontransformed mycosis fungoides, *Am J Surg Pathol* 33:1860-1868, 2009.

27. Wood G, Ngan B-Y, Tung R et al: Clonal rearrangements of immunoglobulin genes and progression to B-cell lymphoma in cutaneous lymphoid hyperplasia, *Am J Pathol* 135:13-19, 1989.

28. Kern DE, Kidd PG, Moe R et al: Analysis of T-cell receptor gene rearrangement in lymph nodes of patients with mycosis fungoides: prognostic implications, *Arch Dermatol* 134:158-164, 1998.

29. Fraser-Andrews EA, Mitchell T, Ferreira S et al: Molecular staging of lymph nodes from 60 patients with mycosis fungoides and Sézary syndrome: correlation with histopathology and outcome suggests prognostic relevance in mycosis fungoides, *Br J Dermatol* 155:756-762, 2006.

30. van Doorn R, Van Haselen CW, van Voorst Vader PC et al: Mycosis fungoides: disease evolution and prognosis of 309 Dutch patients, *Arch Dermatol* 136:504-510, 2000.

31. Magro CM, Crowson AN: Drug-induced immune dysregulation as a cause of atypical cutaneous lymphoid infiltrates: a hypothesis, *Hum Pathol* 27:125-132, 1996.

32. Wood GS, Weiss LM, Hu CH et al: T-cell antigen deficiencies and clonal rearrangements of T-cell receptor genes in pagetoid reticulosis (Woringer-Kolopp disease), *N Engl J Med* 318:164-167, 1988.

33. Woringer PK: Lesion erythemato-squameuse polycyclique de l'avant-bras evoluant dupis 6 ans chez un garconnet de 13 ans: histolgiquement infiltrat intra-epidermique d'apparence tumorale, *Anals Derm Syph* 10:945-958, 1939.

34. Haghighi B, Smoller BR, LeBoit PE et al: Pagetoid reticulosis (Woringer-Kolopp disease): an immunophenotypic, molecular, and clinicopathologic study, *Mod Pathol* 13:502-510, 2000.

35. Braun-Falco O, Schmoeckel C, Burg G, Ryckmanns F: Pagetoid reticulosis: a further case report with a review of the literature, *Acta Derm Venereol Suppl (Stockh)* 59:11-21, 1979.

36. Berti E, Tomasini D, Vermeer MH et al: Primary cutaneous CD8-positive epidermotropic cytotoxic T cell lymphomas: a distinct clinicopathological entity with an aggressive clinical behavior, *Am J Pathol* 155:483-492, 1999.

37. LeBoit PE: Granulomatous slack skin, *Dermatol Clin* 12:375-389, 1994.

38. van Haselen CW, Toonstra J, van der Putte SJ et al: Granulomatous slack skin: report of three patients with an updated review of the literature, *Dermatology* 196:382-391, 1998.

39. Tannous Z, Baldassano MF, Li VW et al: Syringolymphoid hyperplasia and follicular mucinosis in a patient with cutaneous T-cell lymphoma, *J Am Acad Dermatol* 41:303-308, 1999.

40. Tomaszewski MM, Lupton GP, Krishnan J et al: Syringolymphoid hyperplasia with alopecia, *J Cutan Pathol* 21:520-526, 1994.

41. Lehman JS, Cook-Norris RH, Weed BR et al: Folliculotropic mycosis fungoides: single-center study and systematic review, *Arch Dermatol* 146:607-613, 2010.

42. Cerroni L: Pilotropic mycosis fungoides: a clinicopathologic variant of mycosis fungoides yet to be completely understood, *Arch Dermatol* 146:662-664, 2010.

43. Rappaport H, Thomas LB: Mycosis fungoides: the pathology of extracutaneous involvement, *Cancer* 34:1198-1229, 1974.

44. Lutzner M, Edelson R, Schein P et al: Cutaneous T-cell lymphomas: the Sézary syndrome, mycosis fungoides, and related disorders, *Ann Intern Med* 83:534-552, 1975.

45. Fletcher V, Zackheim HS, Beckstead JH: Circulating Sézary cells: a new preparatory method for their identification and enumeration, *Arch Pathol Lab Med* 108:954-958, 1984.

46. Ralfkiaer E, Willemze R, Whittaker S: Sézary syndrome. In Swerdlow S, Campo E, Harris N et al, editors: *WHO classification of tumours of haematopoietic and lymphoid tissues,* ed 4, Lyon, 2008, IARC.

47. Trotter MJ, Whittaker SJ, Orchard GE, Smith NP: Cutaneous histopathology of Sézary syndrome: a study of 41 cases with a proven circulating T-cell clone, *J Cutan Pathol* 24:286-291, 1997.

48. Fierro MT, Comessatti A, Quaglino P et al: Expression pattern of chemokine receptors and chemokine release in inflammatory erythroderma and Sézary syndrome, *Dermatology* 213:284-292, 2006.

49. Sokolowska-Wojdylo M, Wenzel J, Gaffal E et al: Absence of CD26 expression on skin-homing CLA+ CD4+ T lymphocytes in peripheral blood is a highly sensitive marker for early diagnosis and therapeutic monitoring of patients with Sézary syndrome, *Clin Exp Dermatol* 30:702-706, 2005.

50. Campbell JJ, Clark RA, Watanabe R, Kupper TS: Sézary syndrome and mycosis fungoides arise from distinct T cell subsets: a biologic rationale for their distinct clinical behaviors, *Blood* 116:767-771, 2010.

51. Arulogun SO, Prince HM, Ng J et al: Long-term outcomes of patients with advanced-stage cutaneous T-cell lymphoma and large cell transformation, *Blood* 112:3082-3087, 2008.

52. Ralfkiaer E, Willemze R, Paulli M, Kadin M: Primary cutaneous CD30-positive T-cell lymphoproliferative disorders. In Swerdlow S, Campo E, Harris N et al, editors: *WHO classification of tumours of haematopoietic and lymphoid tissues,* ed 4, Lyon, 2008, IARC.

53. Krishnan J, Tomaszewski M, Kao G: Primary cutaneous CD30-positive anaplastic large-cell lymphoma: report of 27 cases, *J Cutan Pathol* 20:193-202, 1992.

54. De Bruin PC, Beljaards RC, Van Heerde P et al: Differences in clinical behavior and immunophenotype between primary cutaneous and primary nodal anaplastic large cell lymphoma of T-cell or null cell phenotype, *Histopathology* 23:127-135, 1993.

55. Sandlund JT, Pui C-H, Santana VM et al: Clinical features and treatment outcome for children with CD30+ large cell non-Hodgkin's lymphoma, *J Clin Oncol* 12:895-898, 1994.

56. Willemze R, Beljaards RC: Spectrum of primary cutaneous CD30 (Ki-1)-positive lymphoproliferative disorders: a proposal for classification and guidelines for management and treatment, *J Am Acad Dermatol* 28:973-980, 1993.

57. Beljaards RC, Kaudewitz P, Berti E et al: Primary cutaneous CD30-positive large cell lymphoma: definition of a new type of cutaneous lymphoma with a favorable prognosis—a European Multicenter Study of 47 patients, *Cancer* 71:2097-2104, 1993.

58. Paulli M, Berti E, Rosso R et al: CD30/Ki-1—positive lymphoproliferative disorders of the skin: clinicopathologic correlation and statistical analysis of 86 cases—a multicentric study from the European Organization for Research and Treatment of Cancer Cutaneous Lymphoma Project Group, *J Clin Oncol* 13:1343-1354, 1995.

59. MacGrogan G, Vergier B, Dubus P et al: CD30 positive cutaneous large cell lymphomas: a comparative study of clinicopathologic and molecular features of 16 cases, *Am J Clin Pathol* 105:440-450, 1996.

60. Beylot-Barry M, Lamant L, Vergier B et al: Detection of t(2;5) (p23;q35) translocation by reverse transcriptase polymerase chain reaction and in situ hybridization in CD30-positive primary cutaneous lymphoma and lymphomatoid papulosis, *Am J Pathol* 149:483-492, 1996.

61. DeCoteau JF, Butmarc JR, Kinney MC, Kadin ME: The t(2;5) chromosomal translocation is not a common feature of primary cutaneous CD30+ lymphoproliferative disorders: comparison with anaplastic large-cell lymphoma of nodal origin, *Blood* 87:3437-3441, 1996.

62. Ott G, Katzenberger T, Siebert R et al: Chromosomal abnormalities in nodal and extranodal CD30+ anaplastic large cell lymphomas: infrequent detection of the t(2;5) in extranodal lymphomas, *Genes Chromosomes Cancer* 22:114-121, 1998.

63. Pulford K, Lamant L, Morris SW et al: Detection of anaplastic lymphoma kinase (ALK) and nucleolar protein nucleophosmin (NPM)-ALK proteins in normal and neoplastic cells with the monoclonal antibody ALK1, *Blood* 89:1394-1404, 1997.

64. Bernier M, Bagot M, Broyer M et al: Distinctive clinicopathologic features associated with regressive primary CD30 positive cutaneous lymphomas: analysis of 6 cases, *J Cutan Pathol* 24:157-163, 1997.

65. Guitart J, Querfeld C: Cutaneous CD30 lymphoproliferative disorders and similar conditions: a clinical and pathologic prospective on a complex issue, *Semin Diagn Pathol* 26:131-140, 2009.

66. Werner B, Massone C, Kerl H, Cerroni L: Large CD30-positive cells in benign, atypical lymphoid infiltrates of the skin, *J Cutan Pathol* 35:1100-1107, 2008.

67. Cepeda LT, Pieretti M, Chapman SF, Horenstein MG: CD30-positive atypical lymphoid cells in common non-neoplastic cutaneous infiltrates rich in neutrophils and eosinophils, *Am J Surg Pathol* 27:912-918, 2003.

68. Macaulay WL: Lymphomatoid papulosis: a continuing self-healing eruption, clinically benign—histologically malignant, *Arch Dermatol* 97:23-30, 1968.

69. Saggini A, Gulia A, Argenyi Z et al: A variant of lymphomatoid papulosis simulating primary cutaneous aggressive epidermotropic CD8+ cytotoxic T-cell lymphoma: description of 9 cases, *Am J Surg Pathol* 34:1168-1175, 2010.

70. Demierre M-F, Goldberg LJ, Kadin ME, Koh HK: Is it lymphoma or lymphomatoid papulosis? *J Am Acad Dermatol* 36:765-772, 1997.

71. Basarab T, Fraser-Andrews EA, Orchard G et al: Lymphomatoid papulosis in association with mycosis fungoides: a study of 15 cases, *Br J Dermatol* 139:630-638, 1998.

72. LeBoit PE: Lymphomatoid papulosis and cutaneous CD30+ lymphoma, *Am J Dermatopathol* 18:221-235, 1996.

73. McCarty MJ, Vukelja SJ, Sausville EA et al: Lymphomatoid papulosis associated with Ki-1—positive anaplastic large cell lymphoma: a report of two cases and a review of the literature, *Cancer* 74:3051-3058, 1994.

74. Zackheim HS, LeBoit PE, Gordon BI, Glassberg AB: Lymphomatoid papulosis followed by Hodgkin's lymphoma, *Arch Dermatol* 129:86-91, 1993.

75. Beylot-Barry M, Groppi A, Vergier B et al: Characterization of t(2;5) reciprocal transcripts and genomic breakpoints in CD30+ cutaneous lymphoproliferations, *Blood* 91:4668-4676, 1998.

76. el-Azhary RA, Gibson LE, Kurtin PJ et al: Lymphomatoid papulosis: a clinical and histopathologic review of 53 cases with leukocyte immunophenotyping, DNA flow cytometry, and T-cell receptor gene rearrangement studies, *J Am Acad Dermatol* 30:210-218, 1994.

77. Li G, Salhany KE, Rook AH, Lessin SR: The pathogenesis of large cell transformation in cutaneous T-cell lymphoma is not associated with t(2;5)(p23;q35) chromosomal translocation, *J Cutan Pathol* 24:403-408, 1997.

78. Dojcinov SD, Venkataraman G, Raffeld M et al: EBV positive mucocutaneous ulcer: a study of 26 cases associated with various sources of immunosuppression, *Am J Surg Pathol* 34:405-417, 2010.

79. Jaffe E, Gaulard P, Ralfkiaer E et al: Subcutaneous panniculitis-like T-cell lymphoma. In Swerdlow S, Campo E, Harris N et al, editors: *WHO classification of tumours of haematopoietic and lymphoid tissues,* ed 4, Lyon, 2008, IARC.

80. Gonzalez CL, Medeiros LJ, Braziel RM, Jaffe ES: T-cell lymphoma involving subcutaneous tissue: a clinicopathologic entity commonly associated with hemophagocytic syndrome, *Am J Surg Pathol* 15:17-27, 1991.

81. Alegre VA, Winkelmann RK: Histiocytic cytophagic panniculitis [see comment], *J Am Acad Dermatol* 20:177-185, 1989.

82. Winkelmann RK, Bowie EJ: Hemorrhagic diathesis associated with benign histiocytic, cytophagic panniculitis and systemic histiocytosis, *Arch Intern Med* 140:1460-1463, 1980.

83. Salhany KE, Macon WR, Choi JK et al: Subcutaneous panniculitis-like T-cell lymphoma: clinicopathologic, immunophenotypic, and genotypic analysis of alpha/beta and gamma/delta subtypes, *Am J Surg Pathol* 22:881-893, 1998.

84. Weenig RH, Ng CS, Perniciaro C: Subcutaneous panniculitis-like T-cell lymphoma: an elusive case presenting as lipomembranous panniculitis and a review of 72 cases in the literature, *Am J Dermatopathol* 23:206-215, 2001.

85. Santucci M, Pimpinelli N, Massi D et al: Cytotoxic/natural killer cell cutaneous lymphomas: report of EORTC Cutaneous Lymphoma Task Force Workshop, *Cancer* 97:610-627, 2003.

86. Marzano AV, Berti E, Paulli M, Caputo R: Cytophagic histiocytic panniculitis and subcutaneous panniculitis-like T-cell lymphoma: report of 7 cases [see comment], *Arch Dermatol* 136:889-896, 2000.

87. Magro CM, Crowson AN, Kovatich AJ, Burns F: Lupus profundus, indeterminate lymphocytic lobular panniculitis and subcutaneous T-cell lymphoma: a spectrum of subcuticular T-cell lymphoid dyscrasia, *J Cutan Pathol* 28:235-247, 2001.

88. Willemze R, Jansen PM, Cerroni L et al: Subcutaneous panniculitis-like T-cell lymphoma: definition, classification, and prognostic factors: an EORTC Cutaneous Lymphoma Group study of 83 cases, *Blood* 111:838-845, 2008.

89. von den Driesch P, Staib G, Simon M Jr, Sterry W: Subcutaneous T-cell lymphoma, *J Am Acad Dermatol* 36:285-289, 1997.

90. Kumar S, Krenacs L, Medeiros J et al: Subcutaneous panniculitic T-cell lymphoma is a tumor of cytotoxic T lymphocytes, *Hum Pathol* 29:397-403, 1998.

91. Cho KH, Oh JK, Kim CW et al: Peripheral T-cell lymphoma involving subcutaneous tissue, *Br J Dermatol* 132:290-295, 1995.

92. Iwatsuki K, Harada H, Ohtsuka M et al: Latent Epstein-Barr virus infection is frequently detected in subcutaneous lymphoma associated with hemophagocytosis but not in non-fatal cytophagic histiocytic panniculitis [comment], *Arch Dermatol* 133:787-788, 1997.

93. Krenacs L, Smyth MJ, Bagdi E et al: The serine protease granzyme M is preferentially expressed in NK-cell, gamma delta T-cell, and intestinal T-cell lymphomas: evidence of origin from lymphocytes involved in innate immunity, *Blood* 101:3590-3593, 2003.

94. Scarabello A, Leinweber B, Ardigo M et al: Cutaneous lymphomas with prominent granulomatous reaction: a potential pitfall in the histopathologic diagnosis of cutaneous T- and B-cell lymphomas, *Am J Surg Pathol* 26:1259-1268, 2002.

95. Kumar S, Krenacs L, Raffeld M, Jaffe ES: Subcutaneous panniculitis-like T-cell lymphoma is a tumor of cytotoxic T lymphocytes, *Lab Invest* 76:129a, 1997.

96. Massone C, Chott A, Metze D et al: Subcutaneous, blastic natural killer (NK), NK/T-cell, and other cytotoxic lymphomas of the skin: a morphologic, immunophenotypic, and molecular study of 50 patients, *Am J Surg Pathol* 28:719-735, 2004.

97. Romero LS, Goltz RW, Nagi C et al: Subcutaneous T-cell lymphoma with associated hemophagocytic syndrome and terminal leukemic transformation, *J Am Acad Dermatol* 34:904-910, 1996.

98. Aronson IK, West DP, Variakojis D et al: Panniculitis associated with cutaneous T-cell lymphoma and cytophagocytic histiocytosis, *Br J Dermatol* 112:87-96, 1985.

99. Wang CY, Su WP, Kurtin PJ: Subcutaneous panniculitic T-cell lymphoma, *Int J Dermatol* 35:1-8, 1996.

100. Toro JR, Liewehr DJ, Pabby N et al: Gamma-delta T-cell phenotype is associated with significantly decreased survival in cutaneous T-cell lymphoma, *Blood* 101:3407-3412, 2003.

101. Hoque SR, Child FJ, Whittaker SJ et al: Subcutaneous panniculitis-like T-cell lymphoma: a clinicopathological, immunophenotypic and molecular analysis of six patients, *Br J Dermatol* 148:516-525, 2003.

102. Tsukamoto Y, Katsunobu Y, Omura Y et al: Subcutaneous panniculitis-like T-cell lymphoma: successful initial treatment with prednisolone and cyclosporin A, *Intern Med* 45:21-24, 2006.

103. Gonzalez EG, Selvi E, Lorenzini S et al: Subcutaneous panniculitis-like T-cell lymphoma misdiagnosed as lupus erythematosus panniculitis, *Clin Rheumatol* 26:244-246, 2007.

104. Magro CM, Crowson AN, Byrd JC et al: Atypical lymphocytic lobular panniculitis [see comment], *J Cutan Pathol* 31:300-306, 2004.

105. Yu JB, Zuo Z, Tang Y et al: Extranodal nasal-type natural killer/T-cell lymphoma of the skin: a clinicopathologic study of 16 cases in China, *Hum Pathol* 40:807-816, 2009.

106. Chan JK, Sin VC, Wong KF et al: Nonnasal lymphoma expressing the natural killer cell marker CD56: a clinicopathologic study of 49 cases of an uncommon aggressive neoplasm, *Blood* 89:4501-4513, 1997.

106a. Quintanilla-Martinez L, Kimura H, Jaffe E: EBV-positive T-cell lymphoproliferative disorders of childhood. In Swerdlow S, Campo E, Harris N et al, editors: *WHO classification of tumours of haematopoietic and lymphoid tissues*, ed 4, Lyon, 2008, IARC.

106b. Rodriguez-Pinilla SM, Barionuevo C, Garcia J et al: EBV-associated cutaneous NK/T-cell lymphoma: review of a series of 14 cases from Peru in children and young adults, *Am J Surg Pathol* 34:1773–1782, 2010.

107. Gaulard P, Berti E, Willemze R, Jaffe E: Primary cutaneous T-cell lymphomas: rare subtypes. In Swerdlow S, Campo E, Harris N et al, editors: *WHO classification of tumours of haematopoietic and lymphoid tissues*, ed 4, Lyon, 2008, IARC.

108. Berti E, Cerri A, Cavicchini S et al: Primary cutaneous gamma/delta T-cell lymphoma presenting as disseminated pagetoid reticulosis, *J Invest Dermatol* 96:718-723, 1991.

109. de Wolf-Peeters C, Achten R: Gamma/delta T-cell lymphomas: a homogeneous entity? *Histopathology* 36:294-305, 2000.

110. Jones D, Vega F, Sarris AH, Medeiros LJ: CD4– CD8– "double-negative" cutaneous T-cell lymphomas share common histologic features and an aggressive clinical course, *Am J Surg Pathol* 26:225-231, 2002.

111. Arnulf B, Copie-Bergman C, Delfau-Larue MH et al: Non-hepatosplenic gamma/delta T-cell lymphoma: a subset of cytotoxic lymphomas with mucosal or skin localization, *Blood* 91:1723-1731, 1998.

112. Ghobrial IM, Weenig RH, Pittlekow MR et al: Clinical outcome of patients with subcutaneous panniculitis-like T-cell lymphoma, *Leuk Lymphoma* 46:703-708, 2005.

113. Aguilera P, Mascaro JM Jr, Martinez A et al: Cutaneous gamma/delta T-cell lymphoma: a histopathologic mimicker of lupus erythematosus profundus (lupus panniculitis), *J Am Acad Dermatol* 56:643-647, 2007.

114. Agnarsson BA, Vonderheid EC, Kadin ME: Cutaneous T cell lymphoma with suppressor/cytotoxic (CD8) phenotype: identification of rapidly progressive and chronic subtypes, *J Am Acad Dermatol* 22:569-577, 1990.

115. Csomor J, Bognar A, Benedek S et al: Rare provisional entity: primary cutaneous aggressive epidermotropic CD8+ cytotoxic T-cell lymphoma in a young woman, *J Clin Pathol* 61:770-772, 2008.

116. Fika Z, Karkos PD, Badran K, Williams RE: Primary cutaneous aggressive epidermotropic CD8 positive cytotoxic T-cell lymphoma of the ear, *J Laryngol Otol* 121:503-505, 2007.

117. Liu V, Cutler CS, Young AZ: Case records of the Massachusetts General Hospital: case 38-2007—a 44-year-old woman with generalized, painful, ulcerated skin lesions, *N Engl J Med* 357:2496-2505, 2007.

118. Yoshizawa N, Yagi H, Horibe T et al: Primary cutaneous aggressive epidermotropic CD8+ T-cell lymphoma with a CD15(+)CD30(-) phenotype, *Eur J Dermatol* 17:441-442, 2007.

119. Gelfand JM, Wasik MA, Vittorio C et al: Progressive epidermotropic CD8+/CD4– primary cutaneous CD30+ lymphoproliferative disorder in a patient with sarcoidosis, *J Am Acad Dermatol* 51:304-308, 2004.

120. Marzano AV, Ghislanzoni M, Gianelli U et al: Fatal CD8+ epidermotropic cytotoxic primary cutaneous T-cell lymphoma with multiorgan involvement, *Dermatology* 211:281-285, 2005.

121. Bekkenk MW, Vermeer MH, Jansen PM et al: Peripheral T-cell lymphomas unspecified presenting in the skin: analysis of prognostic factors in a group of 82 patients, *Blood* 102:2213-2219, 2003.

122. Beljaards RC, Meijer CJ, Van der Putt SC et al: Primary cutaneous T-cell lymphoma: clinicopathological features and prognostic parameters of 35 cases other than mycosis fungoides and CD30-positive large cell lymphoma, *J Pathol* 172:53-60, 1994.

123. Friedmann D, Wechsler J, Delfau MH et al: Primary cutaneous pleomorphic small T-cell lymphoma: a review of 11 cases—the French Study Group on Cutaneous Lymphomas, *Arch Dermatol* 131:1077-1080, 1995.

124. Sterry W, Siebel A, Mielke V: HTLV-1–negative pleomorphic T-cell lymphoma of the skin: the clinicopathological correlations and natural history of 15 patients, *Br J Dermatol* 126:456-462, 1992.

125. von den Driesch P, Coors EA: Localized cutaneous small to medium-sized pleomorphic T-cell lymphoma: a report of 3 cases stable for years, *J Am Acad Dermatol* 46:531-535, 2002.

126. Grogg KL, Jung S, Erickson LA et al: Primary cutaneous CD4-positive small/medium-sized pleomorphic T-cell lymphoma: a clonal T-cell lymphoproliferative disorder with indolent behavior, *Mod Pathol* 21:708-715, 2008.

127. Garcia-Herrera A, Colomo L, Camos M et al: Primary cutaneous small/medium CD4+ T-cell lymphomas: a heterogeneous group of tumors with different clinicopathologic features and outcomes, *J Clin Oncol* 26:3364-3371, 2008.

128. Rodriguez Pinilla SM, Roncador G, Rodriguez-Peralto JL et al: Primary cutaneous CD4+ small/medium-sized pleomorphic T-cell lymphoma expresses follicular T-cell markers, *Am J Surg Pathol* 33:81-90, 2009.

129. Cerroni L, Arzberger E, Putz B et al: Primary cutaneous follicle center cell lymphoma with follicular growth pattern, *Blood* 95:3922-3928, 2000.

130. Cerroni L, Signoretti S, Hofler G et al: Primary cutaneous marginal zone B-cell lymphoma: a recently described entity of low-grade malignant cutaneous B-cell lymphoma, *Am J Surg Pathol* 21:1307-1315, 1997.

131. Garcia CF, Weiss LM, Warnke RA, Wood G: Cutaneous follicular lymphoma, *Am J Surg Pathol* 10:454, 1986.

132. Gronbaek K, Moller PH, Nedergaard T et al: Primary cutaneous B-cell lymphoma: a clinical, histological, phenotypic and genotypic study of 21 cases, *Br J Dermatol* 142:913-923, 2000.

133. Tomaszewski MM, Abbondanzo SL, Lupton GP: Extranodal marginal zone B-cell lymphoma of the skin: a morphologic and immunophenotypic study of 11 cases, *Am J Dermatopathol* 22:205-211, 2000.

134. Yang B: Clinicopathologic reassessment of primary cutaneous B-cell lymphomas with immunophenotypic and molecular genetic characterization [comment], Am J Surg Pathol 24:694-702, 2000.

135. Kiyohara T, Kumakiri M, Kobayashi H et al: Cutaneous marginal zone B-cell lymphoma: a case accompanied by massive plasmacytoid cells, *J Am Acad Dermatol* 48:S82-S85, 2003.

136. Storz MN: Gene expression profiles of cutaneous B cell lymphoma [comment], *J Invest Dermatol* 120:865-870, 2003.

136a. Edinger JT, Kant JA, Swerdlow SH: Cutaneous marginal zone lymphomas have distinctive features and include 2 subsets, *Am J Surg Pathol* 34:1830-1841, 2010.

137. Goodlad JR, Davidson MM, Hollowood K et al: *Borrelia burgdorferi*–associated cutaneous marginal zone lymphoma: a clinicopathological study of two cases illustrating the temporal progression of *B. burgdorferi*–associated B-cell proliferation in the skin, *Histopathology* 37:501-508, 2000.

138. Bailey EM, Ferry JA, Harris NL et al: Marginal zone lymphoma (low-grade B-cell lymphoma of mucosa-associated lymphoid tissue type) of skin and subcutaneous tissue: a study of 15 patients [see comment], *Am J Surg Pathol* 20:1011-1023, 1996.

139. Baldassano MF, Bailey EM, Ferry JA et al: Cutaneous lymphoid hyperplasia and cutaneous marginal zone lymphoma: comparison of morphologic and immunophenotypic features, *Am J Surg Pathol* 23:88-96, 1999.

140. Harris NL: Extranodal lymphoid infiltrates and mucosa-associated lymphoid tissue (MALT): a unifying concept, *Am J Surg Pathol* 15:879-884, 1991.

141. Isaacson P, Wright DH: Malignant lymphoma of mucosa-associated lymphoid tissue: a distinctive type of B-cell lymphoma, *Cancer* 52:1410-1416, 1983.

142. Geyer JT, Ferry JA, Longtine JA et al: Characteristics of cutaneous marginal zone lymphomas with marked plasmacytic differentiation and a T cell-rich background, *Am J Clin Pathol* 133:59-69, 2010.

143. Sander CA, Kind P, Kaudewitz P et al: The revised European-American classification of lymphoid neoplasms (REAL): a new perspective for the classification of cutaneous lymphomas, *J Cutan Pathol* 24:329-341, 1997.

144. de Leval L, Harris NL, Longtine J, Duncan LM: Cutaneous B-cell lymphomas of follicular and marginal zone types: use of bcl-6, CD10 and CD21 in differential diagnosis and classification, *Am J Surg Pathol* 25:732-741, 2001.

145. LeBoit PE, McNutt NS, Reed JA et al: Primary cutaneous immunocytoma: a B-cell lymphoma that can easily be mistaken for cutaneous lymphoid hyperplasia, *Am J Surg Pathol* 18:969-978, 1994.

146. Sander C, Kaudewitz P, Schirren C et al: Immunocytoma and marginal zone B-cell lymphoma (MALT lymphoma) presenting in skin: different entities or a spectrum of disease? *J Cutan Pathol* 23:59a, 1996.

147. Kutzner H, Kerl H, Pfaltz MC, Kempf W: CD123-positive plasmacytoid dendritic cells in primary cutaneous marginal zone B-cell lymphoma: diagnostic and pathogenetic implications, *Am J Surg Pathol* 33:1307-1313, 2009.

148. Salama S: Primary cutaneous B-cell lymphoma and lymphoproliferative disorders of skin: current status of pathology and classification, *Am J Clin Pathol* 114(Suppl):S104-S128, 2000.

149. Li C, Inagaki H, Kuo TT et al: Primary cutaneous marginal zone B-cell lymphoma: a molecular and clinicopathologic study of 24 Asian cases, *Am J Surg Pathol* 27:1061-1069, 2003.

150. Streubel B, Lamprecht A, Dierlamm J et al: t(14;18)(q32;q21) involving IGH and MALT1 is a frequent chromosomal aberration in MALT lymphoma, *Blood* 101:2335-2339, 2003.

151. Servitje O, Gallardo F, Estrach T et al: Primary cutaneous marginal zone B-cell lymphoma: a clinical, histopathological, immunophenotypic and molecular genetic study of 22 cases, *Br J Dermatol* 147:1147-1158, 2002.

152. van Maldegem F, van Dijk R, Wormhoudt TA et al: The majority of cutaneous marginal zone B-cell lymphomas expresses class-switched immunoglobulins and develops in a T-helper type 2 inflammatory environment, *Blood* 112:3355-3361, 2008.

153. Takino H, Li C, Hu S et al: Primary cutaneous marginal zone B-cell lymphoma: a molecular and clinicopathological study of cases from Asia, Germany, and the United States, *Mod Pathol* 21:1517-1526, 2008.

154. Palmedo G, Hantschke M, Rutten A et al: Primary cutaneous marginal zone B-cell lymphoma may exhibit both the t(14;18)(q32;q21) IGH/BCL2 and the t(14;18)(q32;q21) IGH/MALT1 translocation: an indicator for clonal transformation towards higher-grade B-cell lymphoma? *Am J Dermatopathol* 29:231-236, 2007.

155. Cho-Vega JH, Vega F, Rassidakis G, Medeiros LJ: Primary cutaneous marginal zone B-cell lymphoma, *Am J Clin Pathol* 125(Suppl):S38-S49, 2006.

156. Wongchaowart NT, Kim B, Hsi ED et al: t(14;18)(q32;q21) involving IGH and MALT1 is uncommon in cutaneous MALT lymphomas and primary cutaneous diffuse large B-cell lymphomas, *J Cutan Pathol* 33:286-292, 2006.

157. Schreuder MI, Hoefnagel JJ, Jansen PM et al: FISH analysis of MALT lymphoma–specific translocations and aneuploidy in primary cutaneous marginal zone lymphoma, *J Pathol* 205:302-310, 2005.

158. Mattia AR, Ferry JA, Harris NL: Breast lymphoma: a B-cell spectrum including the low grade B-cell lymphoma of mucosa associated lymphoid tissue, *Am J Surg Pathol* 17:574-587, 1993.

159. de la Fouchardiere A, Balme B, Chouvet B et al: Primary cutaneous marginal zone B-cell lymphoma: a report of 9 cases, *J Am Acad Dermatol* 41:181-188, 1999.

160. Pelstring RJ, Essel JH, Kurtin PJ et al: Diversity of organ site involvement among malignant lymphomas of mucosa-associated tissues, *Am J Clin Pathol* 96:738-745, 1991.

161. Bailey EM, Harris NL, Ferry JA, Duncan LM: Cutaneous B-cell lymphoma at the Massachusetts General Hospital, 1972-1994, *Lab Invest* 74:39A, 1996.

162. White WL, Ferry JA, Harris NL, Grove AS Jr: Ocular adnexal lymphoma: a clinicopathologic study with identification of lymphomas of mucosa-associated lymphoid tissue type, *Ophthalmology* 102:1994-2006, 1995.

163. Leinweber B, Colli C, Chott A et al: Differential diagnosis of cutaneous infiltrates of B lymphocytes with follicular growth pattern, *Am J Dermatopathol* 26:4-13, 2004.

164. Sangueza OP, Yadav S, White C, Braziel R: Evolution of B-cell lymphoma from pseudolymphoma: a multidisciplinary approach using histology, immunohistochemistry, and Southern blot analysis, *Am J Dermatopathol* 14:408-415, 1992.

165. Rijlaarsdam J, Meijer C, Willemze R: Differentiation between lymphadenosis benigna cutis and primary cutaneous follicular center cell lymphomas: a comparative clinicopathologic study of 57 patients, *Cancer* 65:2301-2306, 1990.

166. Duncan LM, LeBoit PE: Are primary cutaneous immunocytoma and marginal zone lymphoma the same disease? [comment], *Am J Surg Pathol* 21:1368-1372, 1997.

167. Schmid U, Eckert F, Griesser H et al: Cutaneous follicular lymphoid hyperplasia with monotypic plasma cells: a clinicopathologic study of 18 patients, *Am J Surg Pathol* 19:12-20, 1995.

168. Caro W, Helwig E: Cutaneous lymphoid hyperplasia, *Cancer* 24:487-502, 1969.

169. Ritter J, Adesokan P, Fitzgibbon J, Wick M: Paraffin section immunohistochemistry as an adjunct to morphologic analysis in the diagnosis of cutaneous lymphoid infiltrates, *J Cutan Pathol* 21:481-493, 1994.

170. Willemze R, Swerdlow SH, Harris N, Vergier B: Primary cutaneous follicle centre lymphoma. In Swerdlow S, Campo E, Harris N et al, editors: *WHO classification of tumours of haematopoietic and lymphoid tissues,* ed 4, Lyon, 2008, IARC.

171. Nagatani T, Miyazawa M, Matsuzaki T et al: Cutaneous B-cell lymphoma: a clinical, pathological and immunohistochemical study, *Clin Exp Dermatol* 18:530-536, 1993.

172. Willemze R, Meijer CJLM, Sentis HJ et al: Primary cutaneous large cell lymphomas of follicular center cell origin, *J Am Acad Dermatol* 16:518, 1987.

173. Willemze R, Kruyswijk MR, De Bruin CD et al: Angiotropic (intravascular) large cell lymphoma of the skin previously classified as malignant angioendotheliomatosis, *Br J Dermatol* 116:393-399, 1987.

174. Cerroni L, Volkenandt M, Rieger E et al: Bcl-2 protein expression and correlation with the interchromosomal 14;18 translocation in cutaneous lymphomas and pseudolymphomas, *J Invest Dermatol* 102:231-235, 1994.

175. Triscott JA, Ritter JH, Swanson PE, Wick MR: Immunoreactivity for bcl-2 protein in cutaneous lymphomas and pseudolymphomas, *J Cutan Pathol* 22:2, 1995.

176. Liu YJ, Grouard G, de Bouteiller O, Banchereau J: Follicular dendritic cells and germinal centers, *Int Rev Cytol* 166:139-179, 1996.

177. Yang B, Tubbs RR, Finn W et al: Clinicopathologic reassessment of primary cutaneous B-cell lymphomas with immunophenotypic and molecular genetic characterization, *Am J Surg Pathol* 24:694-702, 2000.

178. Senff NJ, Noordijk EM, Kim YH et al: European Organization for Research and Treatment of Cancer and International Society for Cutaneous Lymphoma consensus recommendations for the management of cutaneous B-cell lymphomas, *Blood* 112:1600-1609, 2008.

179. Senff NJ, Hoefnagel JJ, Jansen PM et al: Reclassification of 300 primary cutaneous B-cell lymphomas according to the new WHO-EORTC classification for cutaneous lymphomas: comparison with previous classifications and identification of prognostic markers, *J Clin Oncol* 25:1581-1587, 2007.

180. Grange F, Bekkenk MW, Wechsler J et al: Prognostic factors in primary cutaneous large B-cell lymphomas: a European multicenter study, *J Clin Oncol* 19:3602-3610, 2001.

181. Pandolfino TL, Siegel RS, Kuzel TM et al: Primary cutaneous B-cell lymphoma: review and current concepts, *J Clin Oncol* 18:2152-2168, 2000.

182. Isaacson PG, Wotherspoon AC, Diss T, Pan LX: Follicular colonization in B-cell lymphoma of mucosa-associated lymphoid tissue, *Am J Surg Pathol* 15:819-828, 1991.

183. Kim BK, Surti U, Pandya A et al: Clinicopathologic, immunophenotypic, and molecular cytogenetic fluorescence in situ hybridization analysis of primary and secondary cutaneous follicular lymphomas, *Am J Surg Pathol* 29:69-82, 2005.

184. Koens L, Vermeer MH, Willemze R, Jansen PM: IgM expression on paraffin sections distinguishes primary cutaneous large B-cell lymphoma, leg type, from primary cutaneous follicle center lymphoma, *Am J Surg Pathol* 34:1043-1048, 2010.

185. Meijer C, Vergier B, Duncan L, Willemze R: Primary cutaneous DLBCL, leg type. In Swerdlow S, Campo E, Harris N et al, editors: *WHO classification of tumours of haematopoietic and lymphoid tissues,* ed 4, Lyon, 2008, IARC.

186. Paulli M, Viglio A, Vivenza D et al: Primary cutaneous large B-cell lymphoma of the leg: histogenetic analysis of a controversial clinicopathologic entity, *Hum Pathol* 33:937-943, 2002.

187. Grange F, Petrella T, Beylot-Barry M et al: Bcl-2 protein expression is the strongest independent prognostic factor of survival in primary cutaneous large B-cell lymphoma, *Blood* 103:3662-3668, 2004.

188. Lair G, Parant E, Tessier MH et al: Primary cutaneous B-cell lymphomas of the lower limbs: a study of integrin expression in 11 cases, *Acta Derm Venereol* 80:367-369, 2000.

189. Vermeer MH, Geelen FA, van Haselen C et al: Primary cutaneous large B-cell lymphomas of the legs: a distinct type of cutaneous B-cell lymphoma with an intermediate prognosis—Dutch Cutaneous Lymphoma Working Group, *Arch Dermatol* 132:1304-1308, 1996.

190. Geelen FA, Vermeer MH, Meijer CJ et al: bcl-2 protein expression in primary cutaneous large B-cell lymphoma is site related, *J Clin Oncol* 16:2080-2085, 1998.

191. Delia D, Borrello MG, Berti E et al: Clonal immunoglobulin rearrangements and normal T-cell receptor, bcl-2 and c-myc in primary cutaneous B-cell lymphomas, *Cancer Res* 49:4901-4905, 1989.

192. Hoefnagel JJ, Dijkman R, Basso K et al: Distinct types of primary cutaneous large B-cell lymphoma identified by gene expression profiling, *Blood* 105:3671-3678, 2005.

193. Goodlad JR, Krajewski AS, Batstone PJ et al: Primary cutaneous diffuse large B-cell lymphoma: prognostic significance of clinicopathological subtypes, *Am J Surg Pathol* 27:1538-1545, 2003.

194. Ferrara G, Bevilacqua M, Argenziano G: Cutaneous spindle B-cell lymphoma: a reappraisal, *Am J Dermatopathol* 24:526-527, 2002.

195. Cerroni L, El-Shabrawi-Caelen L, Fink-Puches R et al: Cutaneous spindle-cell B-cell lymphoma: a morphologic variant of cutaneous large B-cell lymphoma, *Am J Dermatopathol* 22:299-304, 2000.

196. Goodlad JR: Spindle-cell B-cell lymphoma presenting in the skin, *Br J Dermatol* 145:313-317, 2001.

197. Dommann SN, Dommann-Scherrer CC, Zimmerman D et al: Primary cutaneous T-cell–rich B-cell lymphoma: a case report with a 13-year follow-up, *Am J Dermatopathol* 17:618-624, 1995.

198. Krishnan J: T-cell–rich large B-cell lymphoma: a study of 30 cases, supporting its histologic heterogeneity and lack of clinical distinctiveness, *Am J Surg Pathol* 18:455-465, 1994.

199. Sander CA, Kaudewitz P, Kutzner H et al: T-cell–rich B-cell lymphoma presenting in skin: a clinicopathologic analysis of six cases, *J Cutan Pathol* 23:101-108, 1996.

200. Take H, Kubota K, Fukuda T et al: An indolent type of Epstein-Barr virus–associated T-cell–rich B-cell lymphoma of the skin: report of a case, *Am J Hematol* 52:221-223, 1996.

201. Li S, Griffin CA, Mann RB, Borowitz MJ: Primary cutaneous T-cell–rich B-cell lymphoma: clinically distinct from its nodal counterpart? *Mod Pathol* 14:10-13, 2001.

202. Ramsay AD, Smith WJ, Isaacson PG: T-cell–rich B-cell lymphoma, *Am J Surg Pathol* 12:433-443, 1988.

203. Osborne BM: The value of immunophenotyping on paraffin sections in the identification of T-cell rich B-cell large-cell lymphomas: lineage confirmed by JH rearrangement, *Am J Surg Pathol* 14:933-938, 1990.

204. Dunphy CH, Nahass GT: Primary cutaneous T-cell–rich B-cell lymphomas with flow cytometric immunophenotypic findings: report of 3 cases and review of the literature, *Arch Pathol Lab Med* 123:1236-1240, 1999.

205. Chang A, Zic JA, Boyd AS: Intravascular large cell lymphoma: a patient with asymptomatic purpuric patches and a chronic clinical course, *J Am Acad Dermatol* 39:318-321, 1998.

206. DiGiuseppe JA, Nelson WG, Seifter EJ et al: Intravascular lymphomatosis: a clinicopathologic study of 10 cases and assessment of response to chemotherapy, *J Clin Oncol* 12:2573-2579, 1994.

207. Ferry JA, Harris NL, Picker LJ et al: Intravascular lymphomatosis (malignant angioendotheliomatosis): a B-cell neoplasm expressing surface homing receptors, *Mod Pathol* 1:444-452, 1988.

208. Rubin MA, Cossman J, Freter CE, Azumi N: Intravascular large cell lymphoma coexisting within hemangiomas of the skin, *Am J Surg Pathol* 21:860-864, 1997.

209. Ferreri AJ, Campo E, Seymour JF et al: Intravascular lymphoma: clinical presentation, natural history, management and prognostic factors in a series of 38 cases, with special emphasis on the "cutaneous variant," *Br J Haematol* 127:173-183, 2004.

210. Su WP: Clinical, histopathologic, and immunohistochemical correlations in leukemia cutis, *Semin Dermatol* 13:223-230, 1994.

211. Chang H, Shih LY, Kuo TT: Primary aleukemic myeloid leukemia cutis treated successfully with combination chemotherapy: report of a case and review of the literature, *Ann Hematol* 82:435-439, 2003.

212. Byrd JC, Edenfield WJ, Shields DJ, Dawson NA: Extramedullary myeloid cell tumors in acute nonlymphocytic leukemia: a clinical review, *J Clin Oncol* 13:1800-1816, 1995.

213. Husak R, Blume-Peytaki U, Orfanos CE: Aleukemic leukemia cutis in an adolescent boy, *N Engl J Med* 340:893-894, 1999.

214. Gallagher G, Chhanabhai M, Song KW, Barnett MJ: Unusual presentation of precursor T-cell lymphoblastic lymphoma: involvement limited to breasts and skin, *Leuk Lymphoma* 48:428-430, 2007.

215. Maitra A, McKenna RW, Weinberg AG et al: Precursor B-cell lymphoblastic lymphoma: a study of nine cases lacking blood and bone marrow involvement and review of the literature, *Am J Clin Pathol* 115:868-875, 2001.

216. Schmitt IM, Manente L, Di Matteo A et al: Lymphoblastic lymphoma of the pre-B phenotype with cutaneous presentation, *Dermatology* 195:289-292, 1997.

217. Mori N, Oka K, Yoda Y et al: Predominant expression of lambda light chain in adult cases with non-T-cell acute lymphocytic and chronic myelogenous leukemia in lymphoid blast crisis, *Cancer* 68:776-780, 1991.

218. Jaing TH, Hsueh C, Chiu CH et al: Cutaneous lymphocytic vasculitis as the presenting feature of acute lymphoblastic leukemia, *J Pediatr Hematol Oncol* 24:555-557, 2002.

219. Muljono A, Graf NS, Arbuckle S: Primary cutaneous lymphoblastic lymphoma in children: a series of eight cases with review of the literature, *Pathology* 41:223-228, 2009.

220. Torlakovic E, Slipicevic A, Robinson C et al: Pax-5 expression in nonhematopoietic tissues, *Am J Clin Pathol* 126:798-804, 2006.

221. Uchiyama T, Yadoi J, Sagawa K et al: Adult T-cell leukemia: clinical and hematologic features of 16 cases, *Blood* 50:481-492, 1977.

222. Swerdlow S, Habeshaw J, Rohatiner A et al: Caribbean T-cell lymphoma/leukemia, *Cancer* 54:687, 1984.

223. Jaffe E, Blattner W, Blayney D et al: The pathologic spectrum of adult T-cell leukemia/lymphoma in the United States, *Am J Surg Pathol* 8:263, 1984.

223a. Ohshima K, Jaffe E, Kikuchi M: Adult T-cell leukemia/lymphoma In Swerdlow S, Campo E, Harris N, et al, editors: *WHO classification of tumours of haematopoietic and lymphoid tissues,* ed 4. Lyon, 2008, IARC.

223b. Shimoyama M: Diagnostic criteria and classification of clinical subtypes of adult T-cell leukaemia- lymphoma: a report from the Lymphoma Study Group (1984-1987), *Br J Haematol* 79:428-437, 1991.

224. Takatsuki K, Yamaguchi K, Kawano F et al: Clinical aspects of adult T-cell leukemia/lymphoma (ATL). In Miwa M, editor: *Retroviruses in human lymphoma/leukemia,* Tokyo, 1985, VNU Science Press.

225. Uchiyama T, Hori T, Tsudo M et al: Interleukin-2 receptor (Tac antigen) expressed on adult T-cell leukemia cells, *J Clin Invest* 76:446-453, 1985.

226. Watanabe S, Mukai K, Shimoyama M: Adult T cell leukemia/lymphoma. In Knowles D, editor: *Neoplastic hematopathology,* Baltimore, 1992, Williams & Wilkins.

227. Karube K, Ohshima K, Tsuchiya T et al: Expression of FoxP3, a key molecule in CD4CD25 regulatory T cells, in adult T-cell leukaemia/lymphoma cells, *Br J Haematol* 126:81-84, 2004.

228. Albregts T, Orengo I, Salasche S et al: Squamous cell carcinoma in a patient with chronic lymphocytic leukemia: an intraoperative diagnostic challenge for the Mohs surgeon, *Dermatol Surg* 24:269-272, 1998.

228a. Sen F, Medeiros L, Lu D et al: Mantle cell lymphoma involving skin: cutaneous lesions may be the first manifestation of disease and tumors often have blastoid cytologic features, *Am J Surg Pathol* 26:1312-1318, 2002.

228b. Beaty MW, Toro J, Sorbara L et al: Cutaneous lymphomatoid granulomatosis: correlation of clinical and biologic features, *Am J Surg Pathol* 25:1111-1120, 2001.

229. Hernandez C, Cetner AS, Wiley EL: Cutaneous presentation of plasmablastic post-transplant lymphoproliferative disorder in a 14-month-old, *Pediatr Dermatol* 26:713-716, 2009.

230. Arbiser JL, Mann KP, Losken EM et al: Presence of p16 hypermethylation and Epstein-Barr virus infection in transplant-associated hematolymphoid neoplasm of the skin, *J Am Acad Dermatol* 55:794-798, 2006.

231. Liu W, Lacouture ME, Jiang J et al: KSHV/HHV8–associated primary cutaneous plasmablastic lymphoma in a patient with Castleman's disease and Kaposi's sarcoma, *J Cutan Pathol* 33(Suppl 2):46-51, 2006.

232. Hausermann P, Khanna N, Buess M et al: Cutaneous plasmablastic lymphoma in an HIV-positive male: an unrecognized cutaneous manifestation, *Dermatology* 208:287-290, 2004.

233. Gilaberte M, Gallardo F, Bellosillo B et al: Recurrent and self-healing cutaneous monoclonal plasmablastic infiltrates in a patient with AIDS and Kaposi sarcoma, *Br J Dermatol* 153:828-832, 2005.

234. Facchetti F, Jones D, Petrella T: Blastic plasmacytoid dendritic cell neoplasm. In Swerdlow S, Campo E, Harris N et al, editors: *WHO classification of tumours of haematopoietic and lymphoid tissues,* ed 4, Lyon, 2008, IARC.

235. Khalifeh I, Hughey LC, Huang CC et al: Solitary plaque on the scalp as a primary manifestation of Hodgkin lymphoma: a case report and review of the literature, *J Cutan Pathol* 36(Suppl 1):80-85, 2009.

236. Hsia CC, Howson-Jan K, Rizkalla KS: Hodgkin lymphoma with cutaneous involvement, *Dermatol Online J* 15:5, 2009.

CHAPTER 12

Lymphomas of Bone

Judith A. Ferry

PRIMARY LYMPHOMA OF BONE

SECONDARY OSSEOUS INVOLVEMENT
BY LYMPHOMA

■ PRIMARY LYMPHOMAS OF BONE

Introduction

Primary lymphoma of bone was first described in 1928 by Oberling.[1] In 1939 its existence was confirmed, and the first series of this type of neoplasm was published by Parker and Jackson.[2] Primary lymphoma of bone usually is defined as lymphoma that arises in bone with or without extension into adjacent soft tissue but without lymphoma elsewhere on staging, although some series have included cases that also have regional lymph node involvement.[3-6] Fewer than 1% of all lymphomas arise in bone.[3,7] Primary lymphoma of bone accounts for 3% of primary osseous neoplasms[8,9] and for approximately 5%[10] of extranodal non-Hodgkin's lymphomas. Among children, primary lymphoma of bone accounts for a higher proportion of all non-Hodgkin's lymphomas, or about 3% to 6%.[11]

Clinical Features

Primary lymphoma of bone shows a male preponderance. In most Western series, the male to female ratio, on average, is approximately 2:1[3-9,12-21]; it is overall higher in several Asian series, ranging from 2:1 to 12:1.[22-24] Primary lymphoma of bone can affect patients of any age, from toddlers to individuals in the tenth decade of life; however, these patients mainly are adults, and the median age in most series is in the 40s or 50s.[*] Nearly all these lymphomas arise sporadically, but a few patients have been HIV positive,[19,22] and rare patients have had previous long-standing osteomyelitis[15,26] or Paget's disease.[15]

Patients almost always present with pain localized to the involved bone.[†] A minority of patients also have swelling or a palpable mass, fracture, or loss of neurologic function.[7,8,20] Pathologic fracture is most common in the long, weight-bearing bones of the lower extremities. Patients with vertebral involvement may develop spinal cord or nerve root compression if the involved bone fractures or if epidural extension occurs.[3] On average, only about 10% of patients have constitutional symptoms.[‡]

The bones of the axial skeleton and the appendicular skeleton are affected with roughly equal frequency, although the proportion varies substantially from one series to another. The bones of the lower half of the body are more often involved than those of the upper half.[22] The femur is the bone most often involved, followed by the spine, the bones of the pelvis, the tibia, the humerus, the skull and bones of the jaw, and the ribs. The scapula, other long bones (ulna, radius, fibula), and the clavicle occasionally are affected.[§] Involvement of the small bones of the hands and feet is exceptional.[16,30] In most cases the disease is monostotic; in approximately one fourth of cases in adults, it is polyostotic.[*] Polyostotic disease appears to be more common among children.[11,27,28] Constitutional symptoms appear to be much more common in the setting of polyostotic disease.[15]

Radiographic examination typically shows a poorly demarcated lytic lesion, but occasionally a mixed lytic and sclerotic appearance and in rare cases an entirely sclerotic lesion. Up to about half of cases show radiographic evidence of soft tissue extension, which may be associated with a periosteal reaction (Figure 12-1). In a minority of cases, a pathologic fracture is seen.[†] Open biopsy, needle biopsy, or curettage may be performed to obtain diagnostic tissue.

Pathologic Features and Clinicopathologic Correlates

Diffuse Large B-Cell Lymphoma

Diffuse large B-cell lymphoma is by far the most common type of primary lymphoma of bone in adults (Table 12-1). Most diffuse large B-cell lymphomas are composed of large atypical cells with irregular or multilobated nuclei; a minority are composed of centroblasts with round to oval nuclei, immunoblasts, or bizarre anaplastic cells (Figures 12-2 through 12-4).[‡] Large lymphoid cells may become elongate and resemble spindle cells.[9,15] In some cases, neoplastic cells may resemble signet ring cells or may grow in an Indian-file pattern or an alveolar or nested pattern, resembling adenocarcinoma.[15] Crush artifact may be prominent, and foci diagnostic of lymphoma may be identified only focally (see Figure 12-3). An admixture of small lymphocytes and histiocytes and foci with reactive woven bone often are present, particularly at the periphery of the lesion. If there is an associated pathologic fracture, fracture callus may be seen (see Figure 12-2). Lymphoma of bone often is associated with sclerosis.[9,15] In rare cases, diffuse large B-cell lymphoma of the plasmablastic type (see Lymphomas of the Oral Cavity in Chapter 3) presents with bony involvement.[31,32]

The immunophenotype of primary diffuse large B-cell lymphomas of bone is similar to that of diffuse large B-cell lymphoma arising in other sites (Table 12-2). These lymphomas are virtually always CD20+. They express IgG more often than IgM,[9] in contrast to most B-cell lymphomas, which usually express IgM; this is consistent with origin from a B cell that has already undergone heavy chain class switch. In most series, CD10 is expressed in about 40% to 50% of cases (see Figure 12-4, C).[20,33,34] Bcl6 expression varies widely among series, from 30%[13] to 80%[21] or 85%[33] in some, whereas others report an intermediate proportion to be bcl6+.[20,34] In most series, bcl2 and MUM1/IRF4 are each expressed in most cases.[13,20,33,34]

[*]References 3, 5, 7, 9, 12-16, 21, and 25.
[†]References 3, 4, 7, 9, 11, 20, and 21.
[‡]References 4, 7, 8, 11, 14, 19, and 22.
[§]References 4-9, 11-13, 16, 17, 19-21, 23, 24, and 27-29.

[*]References 3, 4, 6, 13-15, 21-23, and 29.
[†]References 3, 8, 9, 12, 14, 22, and 24.
[‡]References 5, 9, 12, 13, 16, 17, 21, 25, and 29.

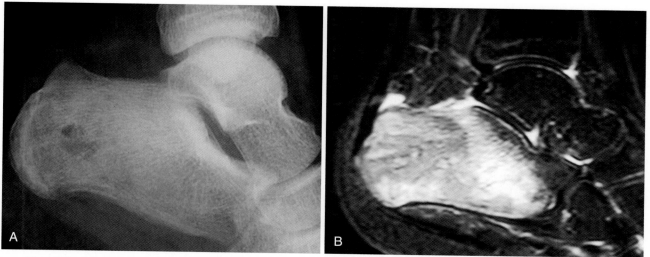

Figure 12-1 Diffuse large B-cell lymphoma of the calcaneus. **A,** Plain x-ray film shows a poorly defined, mixed lytic and sclerotic lesion involving the posterior half of the calcaneus. A periosteal reaction is present along the inferior aspect of the bone. **B,** T2-weighted MRI scan shows diffuse high signal throughout most of the medullary cavity of the bone.

TABLE 12-1

Principal Features of Primary Lymphoma of Bone	
Parameter	**Features**
Patients affected	Broad age range, but most are adults (median age, about 50 yr); males affected more often than females; almost always arises sporadically, with no associated predisposing illness
Clinical manifestations	Common: Pain in the involved bone almost always present Less common: palpable mass, pathologic fracture, constitutional symptoms
Anatomic distribution of tumor	*Most frequently involved:* Femur *Commonly involved:* Vertebral column, pelvis, tibia, humerus, bones in the head *Infrequently involved:* Scapula, radius, ulna, fibula, clavicle *Rarely involved:* Small bones of the hands and feet Monostotic disease more common than polyostotic disease
Pathologic features	*Adults:* Diffuse large B-cell lymphoma predominates; other types of lymphoma are rare *Children:* Diffuse large B-cell lymphoma is slightly more common than B-lymphoblastic lymphoma, which is more common than Burkitt's lymphoma and anaplastic large cell lymphoma
Response to therapy and outcome	With optimal therapy, almost all patients achieve complete remission, and the prognosis is very good.

The proportion of lymphomas with a germinal center B-cell immunophenotype, as opposed to a non-germinal center type (according to the criteria of Hans and colleagues[35]), also varies from one series to another. In one series, lymphomas of the non-germinal center type were slightly more frequent than those of the germinal center type[20]; in other series, there were roughly twice as many cases of the germinal center type as there were of the non-germinal center type.[21,33,34] Therefore, although the immunophenotype of diffuse large B-cell lymphoma of bone varies somewhat from one series to another, all agree that both the germinal center B-cell type and the non-germinal center B-cell type of diffuse large B-cell lymphoma may be encountered in this site.

The genetic features of primary lymphoma of bone have not been studied extensively. However, as in other B-cell lymphomas, rearrangement of the immunoglobulin heavy chain gene *(IGH)* usually can be demonstrated.[13] When the lymphomas are evaluated using polymerase chain reaction (PCR), chromosomal translocation involving *IGH* and *BCL2* [t(14;18)] is uncommon.[13,33] When t(14;18) has been sought using fluorescence in situ hybridization (FISH), however, approximately 25% of cases have been positive.[20,34] Translocations involving *BCL6* are uncommon[20,34] and appear to be less common than mutations within the *BCL6* gene. In one study, 31% of diffuse large B-cell lymphomas primary in bone harbored mutations of the 5' noncoding region of the *BCL6* gene[29]; such mutations may lead to deregulation of *BCL6* and thus contribute to the development of lymphoma. The *BCL6* mutations were more common among stage I cases compared with cases with spread to lymph nodes (stage II) or cases with polyostotic disease (stage IV).

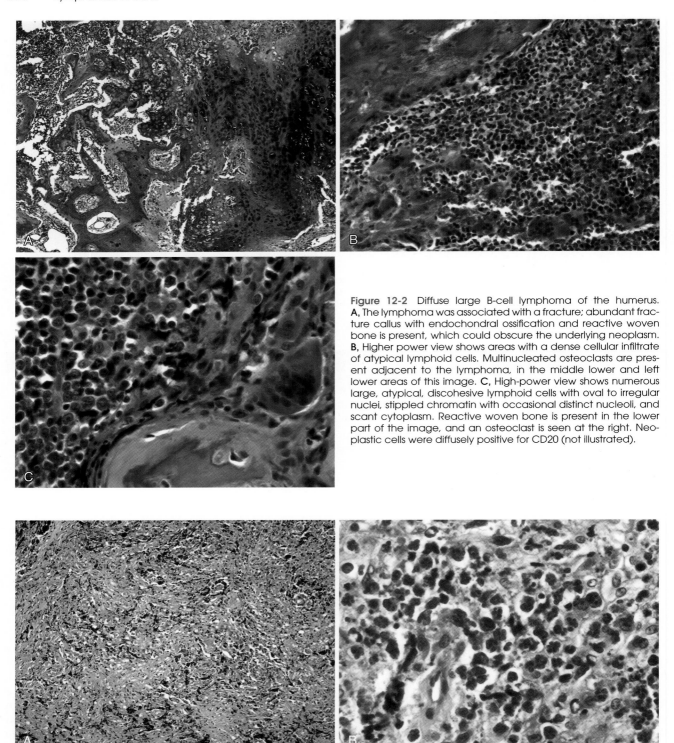

Figure 12-2 Diffuse large B-cell lymphoma of the humerus. **A,** The lymphoma was associated with a fracture; abundant fracture callus with endochondral ossification and reactive woven bone is present, which could obscure the underlying neoplasm. **B,** Higher power view shows areas with a dense cellular infiltrate of atypical lymphoid cells. Multinucleated osteoclasts are present adjacent to the lymphoma, in the middle lower and left lower areas of this image. **C,** High-power view shows numerous large, atypical, discohesive lymphoid cells with oval to irregular nuclei, stippled chromatin with occasional distinct nucleoli, and scant cytoplasm. Reactive woven bone is present in the lower part of the image, and an osteoclast is seen at the right. Neoplastic cells were diffusely positive for CD20 (not illustrated).

Figure 12-3 Diffuse large B-cell lymphoma of the skull. **A,** The lymphoma is poorly preserved, with prominent crush artifact. **B,** In a few small foci, intact large atypical lymphoid cells with prominently multilobated nuclei are present. Tumor cells were diffusely CD20+ (not illustrated).

Cases with mutations of *BCL6* showed a trend toward a better outcome. When FISH was used, approximately 9% of cases harbored rearrangements of *MYC*,[20,34] including one case with concurrent *BCL2* and *MYC* rearrangement.[34] Epstein-Barr virus is not often found in primary diffuse large B-cell lymphoma of bone, although the rare plasmablastic lymphomas usually harbor Epstein-Barr virus, as is true of plasmablastic lymphoma in other sites.[31,32] The rare cases of diffuse large B-cell lymphoma arising in association with chronic osteomyelitis that have been tested also contain Epstein-Barr virus[26,36];

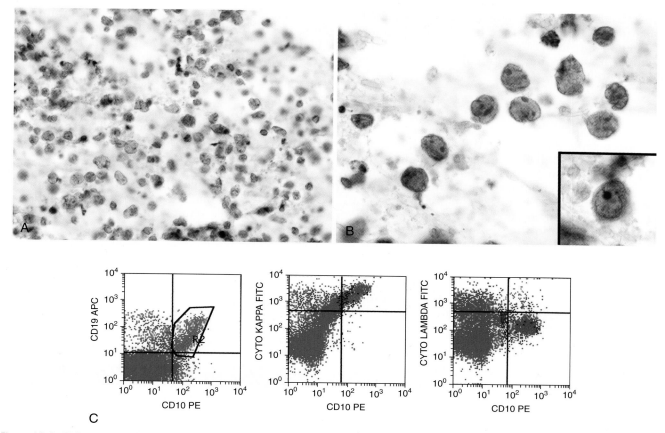

Figure 12-4 Diffuse large B-cell lymphoma involving the first cervical vertebra. Because of the location, the lesion was difficult to biopsy, but a fine needle aspiration biopsy was performed. **A,** The aspiration yielded multiple atypical discohesive cells. **B,** High-power view shows medium-sized to large atypical cells with oval, irregular, or lobated nuclei; smooth chromatin; distinct nucleoli; and scant cytoplasm. Occasional cells have prominent nucleoli *(inset)* (*A* and *B,* Papanicolaou stain). **C,** Flow cytometry disclosed a small population of abnormal B cells (CD19+, CD20+, and CD10+ with a suggestion of monotypic expression of surface kappa light chain); the small size of the population is likely due to loss of the delicate large lymphoid cells during processing. The population highlighted in blue represents CD19+, CD10+ cells. Permeabilization to assess cytoplasmic light chain expression discloses that the target population is monotypic cytoplasmic kappa light chain positive. Immunohistochemical stains also were performed on tiny cores obtained by fine needle aspiration; these showed atypical cells that were CD20+, CD10+, Pax-5+, and TdT− (not illustrated).

these are considered to belong to the group of diffuse large B-cell lymphomas associated with chronic inflammation.[36]

The information given on staging and outcome is based on reports of cases classified as diffuse large B-cell lymphoma and on cases diagnosed using earlier classification systems but presumed to be diffuse large B-cell lymphoma. Most patients have localized disease, but staging occasionally reveals more widespread disease, most often involving regional lymph nodes or other bones[5,14,33] or occasionally the bone marrow.[12] Primary diffuse large B-cell lymphoma of bone has a better prognosis than most other malignancies arising in bone.[6] Local recurrences are uncommon if radiation greater than 50 Gy is delivered to the primary site[37]; however, patients receiving local treatment alone (surgery, radiation) are at risk for distant relapse.[6,7,38] For adult patients, a combination of chemotherapy and radiation usually is recommended to increase the chance of cure.[5,7,38] Nearly all patients achieve complete remission.[5,7,21] In patients with localized

disease who are optimally treated, the prognosis is very good.[*]

A variety of clinical and pathologic features have been found to affect the prognosis. The prognosis is worse with higher stage, polyostotic disease, extension into soft tissue, a lymphoma that is primary in the pelvis or spine, and older age. Lymphoma that arises in a long bone has a better prognosis.[5,7,11,12,21] Among diffuse large B-cell lymphomas, a better outcome has been associated with age under 60 years,[20,21] lymphomas composed of large irregular cells or multilobated cells,[12,16,17,25] a germinal center–like phenotype,[33] and complete response to initial therapy.[20] A worse outcome is associated with noncleaved, immunoblastic, or pleomorphic cells.[12,16]

If patients develop relapses, the most common sites are other bones and lymph nodes.[†] Less often, lymphoma relapses in the lungs, bone marrow, and central nervous system.[9,17] A tendency to spread to

---

[*]References 5, 9, 11, 21, 22, and 29.
[†]References 5, 9, 12-14, 17, 21, 22, and 28.

other bones before extraosseous spread occurs has been noted.[12] The tendency of primary lymphoma of bone to spread to other bones suggests that it has homing properties that distinguish it from primary nodal lymphoma.[4]

Anaplastic Large Cell Lymphoma of Bone

Anaplastic large cell lymphoma primary in bone, including both ALK+ and ALK− cases, has been described. Although it is a rare tumor, it is probably the most common type of T-cell lymphoma to arise in bone. Based on the limited number of cases reported, both ALK+ and ALK− anaplastic large cell lymphomas appear to be characterized by a higher male to female ratio than is found in cases of diffuse large B-cell lymphoma (approximately 90% of patients are male), and by a stronger predilection to affect the axial skeleton.[17,23,24,29,39]

ALK+ anaplastic large cell lymphoma mainly affects children and young adults, although occasionally middle-aged or older adults are affected.[17,24,39] The histologic and immunophenotypic features are similar to those in other sites (Table 12-2 and Figure 12-5). Patients have usually been treated with combination chemotherapy with or without radiation. In contrast to ALK+ anaplastic large cell lymphoma in most other sites, the prognosis is not favorable. Persistent disease and spread to other sites after treatment, including the lungs, central nervous system, and lymph nodes, is common. Most reported patients died of lymphoma.[17,24,39]

ALK− anaplastic large cell lymphoma affects adults over a wide age range. As in ALK+ anaplastic large cell lymphoma, the prognosis is poor, and most patients succumb to the lymphoma.[17,23,24]

Miscellaneous B-Cell and T-Cell Lymphomas of Bone

Other types of B-cell lymphoma, including Burkitt's lymphoma,[12,18] B-lymphoblastic lymphoma (Figure 12-6),[40] and low-grade B-cell lymphomas[4,5,12,23]

TABLE 12-2

Lymphomas of Bone and Their Differential Diagnosis

Diagnosis	Typical Morphology	Usual Immunophenotype
Diffuse large B-cell lymphoma	Diffuse infiltrate of irregular or multilobated cells, centroblasts, or immunoblasts	CD45+, CD20+, CD10+/−, bcl6+/−, bcl2+/−, MUM1/IRF4+/−, sIg+ (often IgG)
B-lymphoblastic lymphoma	Diffuse infiltrate of medium-sized, oval or irregular cells with fine chromatin and scant cytoplasm	CD45+/−, CD19+, Pax5+, CD20−, CD10+, TdT+, sIg−
Burkitt's lymphoma	Diffuse infiltrate of uniform, medium-sized cells with round nuclei, clumped chromatin, several nucleoli per cell, and a moderate amount of cytoplasm with numerous mitoses and tingible body macrophages	CD45+, CD20+, CD10+, bcl6+, bcl2−, Ki67 100%, sIgM+
Anaplastic large cell lymphoma	Diffuse infiltrate of large cells with oval or indented nuclei, relatively abundant cytoplasm, and hallmark cells	CD30+, Alk1+ or −, T antigen +/−, EMA+/−
Osteomyelitis	Acute and/or chronic inflammation with bony necrosis, often with reactive woven bone	Lymphocytes are a mixture of B and T cells; plasma cells are polytypic.
Metastatic carcinoma	Cords, aggregates, or sheets of atypical, variably cohesive cells, often associated with reactive fibrosis	Cytokeratin+, CD45−, CD20−, CD3−
Osteogenic sarcoma	Large, pleomorphic cells that produce osteoid	Vimentin+, smooth muscle actin+/−
Langerhans cell histiocytosis	Large cells with pale nuclei that may be oval or have longitudinal or complex nuclear folds and a moderate amount of pale cytoplasm	S-100+, CD1a+, CD20−, CD3−, cytokeratin−
Plasmacytoma	Pure population of mature or immature plasma cells growing in sheets	CD45−/+, CD20−, CD138+, sIg−, cIg+
Ewing's sarcoma/ peripheral neuroectodermal tumor (PNET)	Diffuse infiltrate of small, uniform cells with pale, glycogen-rich cytoplasm and distinct cell borders	Vimentin+, CD99+, FLI-1+, NSE−/+, synaptophysin−/+, chromogranin−/+, cytokeratin−/+
Metastatic neuroblastoma	Diffuse or nested infiltrate of small round or oval nuclei with dark nuclei and variable amount of interstitial fibrillar material, often with Homer-Wright rosettes	Vimentin−, neurofilament+, NSE+, synaptophysin+, CD99−, FLI-1−
Rhabdomyosarcoma (usually metastatic)	Small cells with round or oval nuclei and scant cytoplasm, with a few cells with eosinophilic cytoplasm with cross-striations	Desmin+, myogenin+, Myo-D1+
Myeloid sarcoma	Diffuse infiltrate of round or irregular cells, usually slightly smaller and with finer chromatin than large lymphoid cells, and with scant to moderate amount of cytoplasm	CD45+/−, lysozyme+, myeloperoxidase+/−, CD68+/−, CD34+/−, CD117+/−

+, Positive in the vast majority of cases; +/−, positive in most cases; −/+, positive in a minority of cases; −, negative in the vast majority of cases.

occur but are very infrequent. The small numbers of T-cell lymphomas (other than anaplastic large cell lymphoma) that have been reported have mostly been peripheral T-cell lymphomas, not otherwise specified, or peripheral T-cell lymphomas that have not been subclassified.[3,5,17-19,23,29] Rare cases of adult T-cell lymphoma (positive for human T-cell leukemia virus type 1 [HTLV-1]) that apparently arose in bone have been described.[41,42] Peripheral T-cell lymphoma of bone appears to be more prevalent in series from the Far East.[23]

Classical Hodgkin's Lymphoma of Bone

Rare cases of classical Hodgkin's lymphoma presenting in bone have been reported,[8,43,44] and although workup reveals lymph node involvement in most cases,[44] some are convincing cases of primary osseous Hodgkin's lymphoma.[43] Unifocal and multifocal Hodgkin's lymphoma primary in bone has been described.[43]

Primary Lymphoma of Bone in Children

Among children, the frequency of different types of lymphoma deviates from that encountered in adults. Diffuse large B-cell lymphoma is still the most common type, but it accounts for only about half of pediatric primary lymphoma of bone. Lymphoblastic lymphoma (B-lineage when immunophenotyping has been performed) is next most common, making up close to 40% of cases (see Figure 12-5). The remainder are Burkitt's lymphoma and anaplastic large cell lymphoma, ALK+ (see Figure 12-6; also see Tables 12-1 and 12-2).[11,27,28,39,45]

Currently, chemotherapy alone is the preferred treatment for children, because it allows for a good outcome and may prevent complications, such as secondary sarcomas in the radiated bone.[28,45] Aside from ALK+ anaplastic large cell lymphoma, which, as noted previously, does not appear to have a good prognosis, lymphomas arising in bone in children have a very good to excellent prognosis with therapy

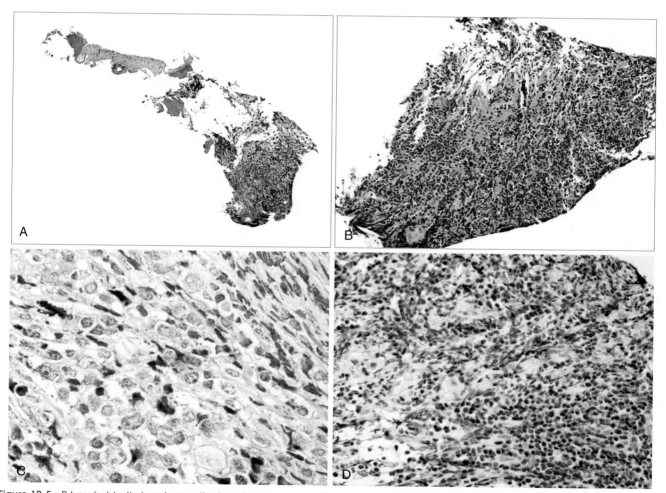

Figure 12-5 B-lymphoblastic lymphoma; the lymphoma was an infiltrative lesion that involved nearly the entire sacrum. **A,** The specimen consists of tiny fragments of bone and soft tissue. **B,** Despite the small size of the specimen, some areas have well preserved; monotonous tumor cells. **C,** The atypical cells are small to medium sized and have finely dispersed chromatin and scant cytoplasm. (Giemsa stain, oil immersion.) Some atypical cells are Pax5+ **(D).**

Continued

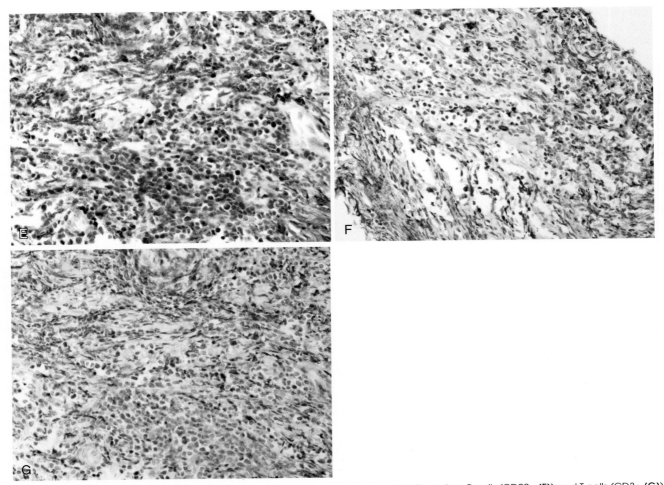

Figure 12-5, cont'd   Other atypical cells are TdT+ **(E)**, with few scattered non-neoplastic mature B cells (CD20+ **(F)**) and T cells (CD3+ **(G)**). They also were positive for CD10, CD34, and CD79a and negative for myeloid markers and cytokeratin. (Immunoperoxidase technique on paraffin sections.)

selected according to the pathologic type of the lymphoma.[11,28,45] Patients with lymphoblastic lymphoma may relapse in the form of acute lymphoblastic leukemia.[11,28]

Differential Diagnosis

The clinical and radiographic features of primary lymphoma of bone are not specific; therefore, the clinical differential diagnosis is broad (see Table 12-2). The differential diagnosis can include osteomyelitis, Langerhans' cell histiocytosis (eosinophilic granuloma, histiocytosis X), Ewing's sarcoma, and other malignant round cell neoplasms. With multiple lesions, particularly among older patients, the possibility of multiple myeloma or metastasis to bone can be considered.[17,24,27,39]

Rendering the correct diagnosis may be difficult for the pathologist because of associated fibrosis, crush artifact, overdecalcification, small sample size, and admixture of many reactive cells.[9,11] In many series, cases of lymphoma initially were misdiagnosed as other types of neoplasms or as reactive inflammatory processes.[8,11,12,15,37] Bone lymphoma can be misdiagnosed as a reactive process, such as chronic osteomyelitis,[8,11,15] or as a simple fracture[8] if there is a large component of reactive cells and if neoplastic cells are present in small numbers or are not well preserved.

Primary lymphoma of bone can mimic a variety of other neoplasms, but in general, careful attention to cytologic details and judicious use of immunostains generally can establish a diagnosis. Because in some cases, particularly (as noted previously) in association with sclerosis, neoplastic cells are elongate and resemble spindle cells or grow in nests or cords, sarcoma and metastatic carcinoma can enter the differential diagnosis.[9,15] Because bone lymphoma (and other neoplasms involving bone) can be associated with reactive woven bone formation, it may be misinterpreted as osteogenic sarcoma.[11,12]

A plasmacytoma composed of immature plasma cells can be difficult to distinguish from a diffuse large B-cell lymphoma arising in bone, particularly if that lymphoma is composed of immunoblasts. However, plasmacytomas are diffusely CD138+, typically lack expression of B-cell–associated antigens CD20

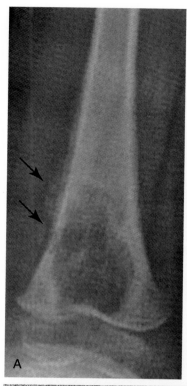

Figure 12-6   Anaplastic large cell lymphoma, ALK+, in a 2-year-old boy. **A,** Plain x-ray film reveals an oval lytic lesion in the distal femoral metaphysis. The tumor has eroded the lateral cortex and has elicited a circumferential layer of periosteal new bone, which is most prominent laterally *(arrows)*. **B,** Low-power view shows a dense, diffuse infiltrate disrupting bone. **C,** Higher power view shows a cellular tumor with interspersed maturing myeloid elements. The atypical cells have oval to indented nuclei and moderately abundant pink to amphophilic cytoplasm. **D,** With a Giemsa stain, neoplastic cells have deep blue-purple cytoplasm, often with a distinct paranuclear hof. **E,** Occasional neoplastic cells have kidney-shaped, indented nuclei with eosinophilic paranuclear regions, consistent with the hallmark cells *(arrows)* characteristic of anaplastic large cell lymphoma. (Oil immersion.)

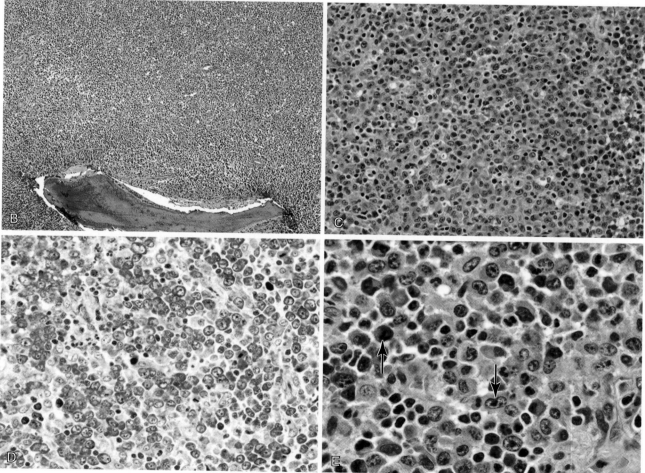

Continued

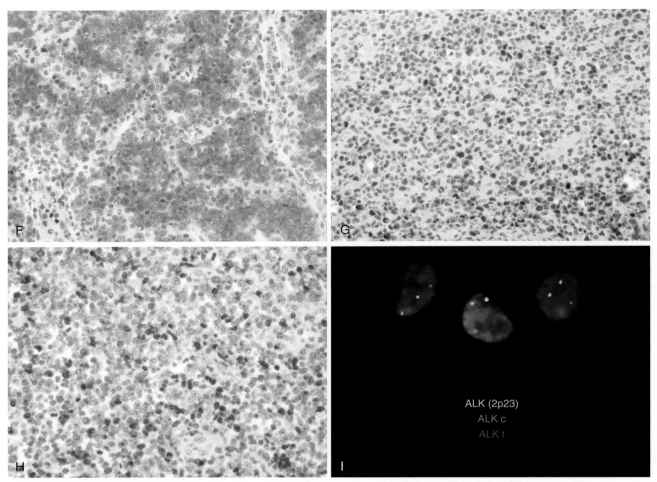

Figure 12-6, cont'd Neoplastic cells are CD30+ **(F)** and Alk1+ **(G)**; they also were CD45+ and EMA+, with limited expression of T-cell antigens. Lysozyme highlights nonneoplastic myeloid elements **(H)** (immunoperoxidase technique on paraffin sections). I, Fluorescence in situ hybridization (FISH) using a break-apart probe for *ALK* shows three cells, each with *ALK* rearrangement (one green and one red signal) and one intact *ALK* (yellow signal) **(A,** from Ferry JA: Diagnosis of lymphoma in extranodal sites other than skin. In Jaffe ES, Harris NL, Vardiman JW, editors: *Hematopathology,* St. Louis, 2010, Saunders, 991-1020. I, courtesy Dr. Paola dal Cin, Cytogenetics Laboratory, Brigham and Women's Hospital, Boston, Massachusetts).

and Pax5, and often express strong monotypic cytoplasmic immunoglobulin light chain on paraffin sections (Figure 12-7); diffuse large B-cell lymphomas, on the other hand, usually are positive for pan–B-cell markers, negative for CD138, and negative or occasionally weakly positive for cytoplasmic light chain. Individuals with plasmacytomas may have diffuse bone marrow involvement by plasma cell myeloma and a serum paraprotein, in contrast to patients with diffuse large B-cell lymphoma of bone.

Lymphoma also may raise consideration of a small round cell tumor, but Ewing's sarcoma has cytoplasmic glycogen and a more cohesive growth pattern and less pleomorphic nuclei than does lymphoma.[12] Neuroblastoma may present with bony metastases, but its tumor cells are pear or carrot shaped with denser chromatin than lymphoma; they may form rosettes. Myeloid sarcomas composed of primitive cells with scant cytoplasm can mimic lymphoblastic lymphoma. Myeloid sarcomas with a component of immature monocytes with irregular nuclei can resemble diffuse large B-cell lymphomas with large cleaved or multilobated cells.[12,15]

We have seen a pediatric case of ALK+ anaplastic large cell lymphoma of bone in which the characteristic indented nuclei and eosinophilic cytoplasm of the tumor cells led to a resemblance to immature myeloid cells and thus to an initial misdiagnosis of myeloid sarcoma (see Figure 12-6). Neuron-specific enolase expression by anaplastic large cell lymphoma has been described; this could result in confusion with non-lymphoid small round cell tumors (see Table 12-2).[39]

For the rare patients with Hodgkin's lymphoma that presents with involvement of bone, the differential diagnosis includes acute or chronic osteomyelitis, depending on the composition of the reactive population, particularly if large neoplastic cells are present in small numbers.[43]

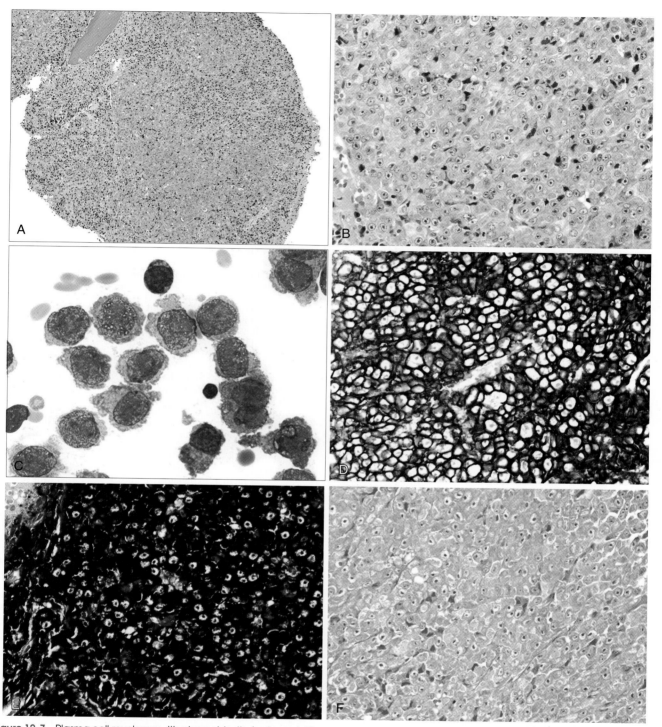

Figure 12-7   Plasma cell myeloma with plasmablastic features. **A,** The marrow is diffusely involved by tumor. **B,** Neoplastic cells are a monotonous population of large cells with oval nuclei, vesicular chromatin, prominent central nucleoli, and a moderate amount of amphophilic cytoplasm, consistent with plasmablasts. **C,** The aspirate in this case shows enlarged, immature plasma cells with prominent nucleoli. (Wright stain.) **D,** Neoplastic cells are diffusely positive for CD138 (immunoperoxidase technique on a paraffin section). In situ hybridization for kappa **(E)** and lambda **(F)** immunoglobulin light chain shows strong monotypic staining for kappa light chain.

■ SECONDARY OSSEOUS INVOLVEMENT BY LYMPHOMA

Secondary involvement of bone by lymphoma is much more common than primary lymphoma of bone. Skeletal involvement occurs in 10% of disseminated non-Hodgkin's lymphomas.[3] Lymphoma with secondary osseous involvement is more likely to involve the axial skeleton than the appendicular skeleton, compared with primary lymphoma of bone.[30] A wide variety of lymphoma types can affect the bones secondarily. The prognosis is poor.[3]

REFERENCES

1. Oberling C: Les reticuloendotheliosarcomes de la moelle osseuse, *Bull Assoc Fr Etud Cancer* 17:259-296, 1928.
2. Parker F, Jackson M: Primary reticulum cell sarcoma of bone, *Surg Gynecol Obstet* 68:45-53, 1939.
3. Brousse C, Baumelou E, Morel P: Primary lymphoma of bone: a prospective study of 28 cases, *Joint Bone Spine* 67:446-451, 2000.
4. Christie DR, Barton MB, Bryant G et al: Osteolymphoma (primary bone lymphoma): an Australian review of 70 cases—Australasian Radiation Oncology Lymphoma Group (AROLG), *ANZ J Med* 29:214-219, 1999.
5. Barbieri E, Cammelli S, Mauro F et al: Primary non-Hodgkin's lymphoma of the bone: treatment and analysis of prognostic factors for stage I and stage II, *Int J Radiat Oncol Biol Phys* 59:760-764, 2004.
6. Lucraft H: Primary lymphoma of bone: a review of 13 cases emphasizing orthopaedic problems, *Clin Oncol (R Coll Radiol)* 3:265-269, 1991.
7. Fairbanks R, Bonner J, Inwards C et al: Treatment of stage IE primary lymphoma of bone, *Int J Radiat Oncol Biol Phys* 28:363-372, 1993.
8. Limb D, Dreghorn C, Murphy J, Mannion R: Primary lymphoma of bone, *Int Orthop* 18:180-183, 1994.
9. Pettit C, Zukerberg L, Gray M et al: Primary lymphoma of bone: a B cell tumor with a high frequency of multilobated cells, *Am J Surg Pathol* 14:329-334, 1990.
10. Freeman C, Berg J, Cutler S: Occurrence and prognosis of extranodal lymphomas, *Cancer* 29:252-260, 1972.
11. Furman W, Fitch S, Hustu O, Callihan T: Primary lymphoma of bone in children, *J Clin Oncol* 7:1275-1280, 1989.
12. Clayton F, Butler J, Ayala A et al: Non-Hodgkin's lymphoma in bone, *Cancer* 60:2494-2501, 1987.
13. Huebner-Chan D, Fernandes B, Yang G: An immunophenotypic and molecular study of primary large B-cell lymphoma of bone, *Mod Pathol* 14:1000-1007, 2001.
14. Mendenhall N, Jones J, Kramer B et al: The management of primary lymphoma of bone, *Radiother Oncol* 9:137-145, 1987.
15. Ostrowski M, Unni K, Banks P et al: Malignant lymphoma of bone, *Cancer* 58:2646-2655, 1986.
16. Dosoretz D, Raymond A, Murphy G et al: Primary lymphoma of bone: the relationship of morphologic diversity to clinical behavior, *Cancer* 50:1009-1014, 1982.
17. Jones D, Kraus M, Dorfman D: Lymphoma presenting as a solitary bone lesion, *Am J Clin Pathol* 111:171-178, 1999.
18. Pileri S, Montanari M, Falini B et al: Malignant lymphoma involving the mandible: clinical morphologic, and immunohistochemical study of 17 cases, *Am J Surg Pathol* 14:652-659, 1990.
19. Pires de Camargo O, dos Santos Machado T, Croci A et al: Primary bone lymphoma in 24 patients treated between 1955 and 1999, *Clin Orthop Relat Res* 397:271-280, 2002.
20. Bhagavathi S, Micale MA, Les K et al: Primary bone diffuse large B-cell lymphoma: clinicopathologic study of 21 cases and review of literature, *Am J Surg Pathol* 33:1463-1469, 2009.
21. Heyning FH, Hogendoorn PC, Kramer MH et al: Primary lymphoma of bone: extranodal lymphoma with favourable survival independent of germinal centre, post-germinal centre or indeterminate phenotype, *J Clin Pathol* 62:820-824, 2009.
22. Deshmukh C, Bakshi A, Parikh P et al: Primary non-Hodgkin's lymphoma of the bone, *Med Oncol* 21:263-267, 2004.
23. Hsieh PP, Tseng HH, Chang ST et al: Primary non-Hodgkin's lymphoma of bone: a rare disorder with high frequency of T-cell phenotype in southern Taiwan, *Leuk Lymphoma* 47:65-70, 2006.
24. Nagasaka T, Nakamura S, Medeiros L et al: Anaplastic large cell lymphomas presented as bone lesions: a clinicopathologic study of six cases and review of the literature, *Mod Pathol* 13:1143-1149, 2000.
25. Lewis VO, Primus G, Anastasi J et al: Oncologic outcomes of primary lymphoma of bone in adults, *Clin Orthop Relat Res* 15:90-97, 2003.
26. Copie-Bergman C, Niedobitek G, Mangham D et al: Epstein-Barr virus in B-cell lymphoma associated with chronic suppurative inflammation, *J Pathol* 183:287-292, 1997.
27. Glotzbecker M, Kersun L, Choi J et al: Primary non-Hodgkin's lymphoma of bone in children, *J Bone Joint Surg* 88A:583-594, 2006.
28. Lones M, Perkins S, Sposto R et al: Non-Hodgkin's lymphoma arising in bone in children and adolescents is associated with an excellent outcome: a children's cancer group report, *J Clin Oncol* 20:2293-2301, 2002.
29. Gianelli U, Ponzoni M, Moro A et al: Mutations of the 5' noncoding region of the BCL-6 gene in primary bone lymphomas, *Ann Hematol* 82:691-695, 2003.
30. Dunn N, Grahame-Smith H, Doherty M: Disappearing foot disease: an unusual presentation of primary lymphoma of bone, *J R Soc Med* 82:302-303, 1989.
31. Dong HY, Scadden DT, de Leval L et al: Plasmablastic lymphoma in HIV-positive patients: an aggressive Epstein-Barr virus–associated extramedullary plasmacytic neoplasm, *Am J Surg Pathol* 29:1633-1641, 2005.
32. Schichman S, McClure R, Schaefer R, Mehta P: HIV and plasmablastic lymphoma manifesting in sinus, testicles and bones: a further expansion of the disease spectrum, *Am J Hematol* 77:291-295, 2004.
33. de Leval L, Braaten KM, Ancukiewicz M et al: Diffuse large B-cell lymphoma of bone: an analysis of differentiation-associated antigens with clinical correlation, *Am J Surg Pathol* 27:1269-1277, 2003.
34. Lima FP, Bousquet M, Gomez-Brouchet A et al: Primary diffuse large B-cell lymphoma of bone displays preferential rearrangements of the c-MYC or BCL2 gene, *Am J Clin Pathol* 129:723-726, 2008.
35. Hans CP, Weisenburger DD, Greiner TC et al: Confirmation of the molecular classification of diffuse large B-cell lymphoma by immunohistochemistry using a tissue microarray, *Blood* 103:275-282, 2004.
36. Chan J, Aozasa K, Gaulard P: DLBCL associated with chronic inflammation. In Swerdlow S, Campo E, Harris N et al, editors: *WHO classification: tumours of haematopoietic and lymphoid tissues*, ed 4, Lyon, 2008, IARC.
37. Dosoretz D, Murphy G, Raymond A et al: Radiation therapy for primary lymphoma of bone, *Cancer* 51:44-46, 1983.
38. Zinzani PL, Carrillo G, Ascani S et al: Primary bone lymphoma: experience with 52 patients, *Haematologica* 88:280-285, 2003.
39. Bakshi N, Ross C, Finn W et al: ALK-positive anaplastic large cell lymphoma with primary bone involvement in children, *Am J Clin Pathol* 125:57-63, 2006.
40. Lin P, Jones D, Dorfman DM, Medeiros LJ: Precursor B-cell lymphoblastic lymphoma: a predominantly extranodal tumor with low propensity for leukemic involvement, *Am J Surg Pathol* 24:1480-1490, 2000.
41. Hara T, Wakatsuki S, Ozaki S et al: Primary adult T-cell leukemia/lymphoma of bone, *Int J Hematol* 79:157-160, 2004.

42. Takemoto S, Matsuoka M, Sakata K et al: Primary adult T-cell leukemia of bone: two patients with primary bone lesion showing monoclonal integration of HTLV-I proviral DNA, *Leukemia* 10:333-337, 1996.
43. Gebert C, Hardes J, Ahrens H et al: Primary multifocal osseous Hodgkin disease: a case report and review of the literature, *J Cancer Res Clin Oncol* 131:163-168, 2005.
44. Ozdemirli M, Mankin H, Aisenberg A, Harris N: Hodgkin's disease presenting as a solitary bone tumor, *Cancer* 77:79-88, 1996.
45. Loeffler J, Tarbell N, Kozakewich H et al: Primary lymphoma of bone in children: analysis of treatment results with Adriamycin, prednisone, oncovin (APO), and local radiation therapy, *J Clin Oncol* 4:496-501, 1986.

CHAPTER 13

Lymphomas of the Bone Marrow

Robert P. Hasserjian

■ INTRODUCTION

The bone marrow is sampled to evaluate for lymphoma in three main clinical scenarios:

1. To establish a diagnosis and specific classification for a lymphoid leukemia (typically manifesting as peripheral blood lymphocytosis)
2. To establish a primary diagnosis and (if possible) specific classification for lymphoma suspected clinically because of lymphadenopathy, splenomegaly, an extramedullary mass, and/or a paraprotein
3. To stage a lymphoma for which the diagnosis and classification already have been established on a biopsy specimen of extramedullary tissue

The pathologist interpreting the bone marrow should know which of these situations applies, because the specific clinical scenario can influence the approach to diagnosis and the type of information that should be communicated in the pathology report.

In the first scenario, it is particularly critical to review the peripheral smear; in many lymphoid leukemias, the diagnostic features are more obvious in the peripheral blood than in the bone marrow. Flow cytometry is important for distinguishing among the various lymphoid leukemias, and cytogenetic analysis can provide clinically relevant diagnostic and prognostic information.

In the second scenario, the pathologist must exercise particular caution, because a lymphoma's appearance in the bone marrow may differ from that seen in the primary extramedullary site. Moreover, considerable overlap may exist in the morphologic and immunophenotypic features of different lymphomas involving the marrow, and precise classification can be difficult. In addition, sampling artifact caused by bone marrow fibrosis or inadequate material can result in a false-negative result. For these reasons, in this clinical scenario, the primary involved extramedullary tissue may need to be biopsied to definitively classify some lymphomas, even if the marrow is involved.

In the third scenario, because a diagnosis of lymphoma has already been established, the pathologist's main role is to determine whether the marrow is involved and to comment on any differences between the appearance of the marrow lymphoma that that of the extramedullary lymphoma. Often, reviewing the original diagnostic biopsy specimen can be helpful for comparing the morphologic features with the bone marrow lymphoma.

Many of the lymphomas described in the following sections have prominent manifestations in extranodal sites other than the bone marrow; these lymphomas are also discussed in the chapter corresponding to that extranodal site. This chapter focuses on the features and differential diagnosis of lymphomas in the bone marrow.

■ PATTERNS OF NEOPLASTIC AND REACTIVE BONE MARROW INFILTRATES

Lymphomas may involve the bone marrow biopsy specimen in various patterns, which can be helpful in narrowing the differential diagnosis; however, some reactive lymphoid infiltrates can have patterns that overlap with those of lymphomas. The factors that contribute to the varied patterns of lymphoma growth in the bone marrow are largely unknown, but they may relate to aspects of the bone marrow microenvironment. For example, the cells of follicular lymphoma typically grow in a paratrabecular pattern and are in close association with CD4+ small T cells, as well as stromal reticular cells that express high levels of low-affinity nerve growth factor receptor (LNGFR) and often co-express CD35. Marrow infiltrates of lymphoplasmacytic and mantle cell lymphoma also contain LNGFR+ stromal cells, but they do not show as bright LNGFR expression as those in follicular lymphoma and do not co-express CD35.[1] In contrast, the aggregates of chronic lymphocytic leukemia and marginal zone lymphomas do not show such close association with stromal cells and appear to merely displace the marrow stromal elements. Although these microenvironmental components likely play a role in intramedullary tumor cell homing and growth patterns, the factors that drive specific tumor cell growth in the bone marrow are unknown, nor is it clear whether these stromal cells derive from marrow elements or are "imported" from peripheral blood progenitors.[2]

Five primary histologic patterns of bone marrow involvement by lymphoma have been described.

- *Nodular nonparatrabecular pattern.* In this pattern (Figure 13-1, *A*), the lymphocytes form confluent collections that displace the fat cells to form spherical aggregates. Nonparatrabecular aggregates may occur adjacent to bone trabeculae and may even be closely opposed to the bone surface; however, unlike true paratrabecular aggregates, they have a spherical rather than a linear configuration and do not extend along the trabecular surface. Nodular aggregates can occur in nearly all lymphoma subtypes.

  It is important to distinguish lymphomas that exhibit the nodular nonparatrabecular pattern from reactive, nonneoplastic lymphoid aggregates. Reactive lymphoid aggregates are more common in elderly patients and also can be seen in bone marrow from patients with autoimmune diseases, infections (including the human immunodeficiency virus [HIV]), aplastic anemia, and various myeloid neoplasms.[3,4] Features that favor neoplastic aggregates include a large number of aggregates, large size, and poor circumscription with infiltration of lymphocytes into the adjacent interstitium.[4,5] The presence of aggregates within subcortical fatty marrow (nonhematopoietic marrow immediately underlying the superficial iliac cortex) also favors a neoplastic etiology.[4] Reactive lymphoid aggregates have a mixture of T cells and

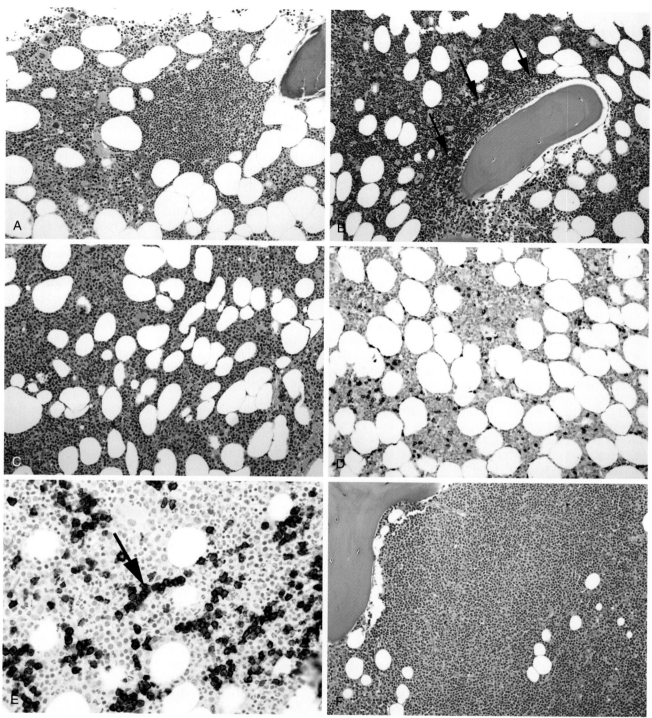

Figure 13-1 Patterns of lymphoid infiltrates in the bone marrow. **A,** Nonparatrabecular nodule with a round shape that pushes away adjacent adipocytes. **B,** Paratrabecular infiltrate *(arrows),* representing an elongated array of neoplastic lymphocytes that is closely applied to the bone's trabecular surface. **C,** Interstitial pattern of lymphoma, in which the neoplastic small lymphocytes percolate among the hematopoietic elements but do not form discrete nodules and do not disturb the randomly distributed adipocytes. **D,** Normal interstitial pattern of bone marrow T cells (CD3 immunostain) that are randomly dispersed among the hematopoietic elements. **E,** Intrasinusoidal pattern of bone marrow lymphoma highlighted by CD20 immunostain. Linear arrays of neoplastic B cells *(arrow)* correspond to lymphoma cells in bone marrow sinusoids. **F,** Diffuse lymphomatous infiltrate, in which the neoplastic lymphocytes form sheets that obliterate both adipocytes and areas of hematopoiesis.

B cells, but lymphomatous nodules also may contain a mixed cell population. Therefore the use of immunohistochemistry for T- and B-cell markers alone often is insufficient to differentiate reactive from neoplastic aggregates. Occasional reactive marrow lymphoid aggregates, particularly when located adjacent to small blood vessels, may contain germinal centers. These resemble the germinal centers in lymph nodes, with intact mantle zones and germinal center cells that express CD10 and bcl6 and lack bcl2, as well as investment by CD21+ follicular dendritic cells; in addition, frequent intrafollicular T cells may be observed, including some that express CD57.[6,7] In contrast, most lymphomatous aggregates, except for those of marginal zone lymphomas, lack germinal centers. Increased reticulin fibrosis is associated with most neoplastic lymphoid aggregates,[8] but it also is present in reactive lymphoid aggregates and generally is unhelpful for distinguishing reactive from neoplastic aggregates.

- *Paratrabecular pattern.* In this pattern, the lymphocytes form confluent, linear collections that extend along the surface of the bone trabecula; these collections typically taper off at the edges of the aggregates (see Figure 13-1, *B*). The lymphocytes are directly in contact with the bone surface, without intervening hematopoietic elements, fat cells, or blood vessels. Paratrabecular aggregates invariably are longer than they are wide. They must be distinguished from nonparatrabecular aggregates that may contact the bone trabecula focally (discussed previously); the latter are more rounded and do not display the "avidity" for the bone surface that characterizes paratrabecular aggregates. Varying degrees of fibrosis, sometimes with collagen deposition or admixed fibroblasts and relative paucicellularity, may occur, particularly after therapy.[9]

  Paratrabecular aggregates are almost always indicative of lymphoma, because this pattern is extremely rare in reactive bone marrow; it has been reported to occur in systemic lupus erythematosus, sarcoidosis, and some systemic infections.[10] Paratrabecular aggregates can occur in many lymphoma subtypes but are most prominent in follicular lymphoma and are exceedingly rare in chronic lymphocytic leukemia.

- *Interstitial pattern.* The lymphocytes in this pattern (see Figure 13-1, *C*) occur as single cells or small cell clusters scattered randomly among the hematopoietic elements and do not form visible aggregates that displace hematopoietic elements and fat cells. This pattern is can be difficult to appreciate on routine histology, and immunohistochemical stains may be required to identify and quantify the lymphoma cells. Normal resident lymphocytes in the bone marrow occupy the marrow in an interstitial pattern and comprise 10% to 20% of the marrow cells; lymphocytes are more numerous in children and can comprise up to 40% of all bone marrow cells in healthy infants.[11]

Distinguishing between normal interstitial lymphocytes and interstitial-pattern lymphoma can be difficult. Most lymphomas that involve the marrow have a predominantly B-cell lineage. In contrast, normal marrow lymphocytes are predominantly T cells (typically with a 2:1 to 3:1 ratio of T cells to B cells) and lack the cytologic atypia that characterizes many lymphomas (see Figure 13-1, *D*).[12,13] The number of normal bone marrow B-cell precursors (hematogones) can be increased in reactive states (e.g., post chemotherapy), and they may mimic an interstitial-pattern B-cell lymphoma. The immunophenotypic heterogeneity of hematogones, which show variable CD20 and TdT expression by flow cytometry, is a helpful clue to their benign nature.

- *Intrasinusoidal pattern.* The lymphocytes in this pattern (see Figure 13-1, *E*) are located within small bone marrow sinusoids. As in some cases of the interstitial pattern, intrasinusoidal involvement is very difficult or impossible to identify on routine histology and usually requires immunohistochemistry. The involved sinusoids, which are seldom dilated, can be revealed by applying immunohistochemistry for vascular endothelial markers such as CD34 or Factor VIII. In addition, the presence of a linear array of several lymphocytes is considered to represent intrasinusoidal involvement, even if a vascular structure cannot be clearly identified. Such linear arrays of lymphoma cells are best visualized using immunohistochemistry for lineage-specific antigens (CD3 for T-cell lymphomas and CD20 for B-cell lymphomas). Intrasinusoidal involvement can be seen as a minor component in almost all B-cell lymphomas that involve the bone marrow, but it is most often seen in splenic marginal zone lymphoma.[14] It also may be seen as a major pattern in some T-cell leukemias and is usually the exclusive pattern in intravascular large B-cell lymphoma.

- *Diffuse pattern.* The lymphocytes in this pattern (see Figure 13-1, *F*) form confluent sheets of cells that displace the fat and hematopoietic cells and completely occupy at least one intertrabecular marrow space. Intervening hematopoietic cells may be present, but they make up the minority of the cells; adipocytes are rare or absent in the involved areas. The diffuse pattern of involvement is associated with more aggressive lymphomas or advanced disease.

  It is important to recognize that diffuse lymphohistiocytic infiltrates may occur in florid reactive processes, most often as a result of systemic autoimmune diseases or HIV infection. The presence of a polymorphous cell mixture (versus the usually monomorphous appearance of lymphomas that involve the marrow in a diffuse pattern) can be a helpful clue to a reactive diffuse infiltrate; this often includes lymphocytes with varied nuclear sizes and shapes and admixed polyclonal plasma cells, histiocytes, mast cells, and eosinophils. Reactive lymphohistiocytic infiltrates often show increased reticulin fiber deposition.[6]

Although none of these patterns of involvement is specific for any type of lymphoma, they can provide important clues that ultimately lead to a precise diagnosis. For example, identifying a lymphoma with a prominent intrasinusoidal pattern may stimulate clinical correlation (investigation for splenomegaly) and peripheral blood flow cytometry that lead to a diagnosis of splenic marginal zone lymphoma.

■ LYMPHOMAS PRESENTING IN THE BONE MARROW AND BLOOD

Precursor Lymphoid Neoplasms

Precursor lymphoid neoplasms encompass malignant proliferations of B or T lymphocytes that may present as leukemia, with predominant involvement of peripheral blood, or as lymphoma, with predominant involvement of lymph nodes or extranodal tissues. The distinction of leukemia versus lymphoma does not appear to have biologic relevance and is somewhat arbitrarily based on the clinical presentation. Patients with extramedullary disease at presentation (lymphadenopathy or an extranodal mass lesion) but in whom lymphoblasts make up fewer than 25% of the bone marrow cells and are absent or infrequent in the blood are classified as having lymphoma; all other patients are classified as having leukemia, regardless of whether extramedullary disease is present.

It is important to note that, unlike the clear blast cutoff of 20% that defines acute myeloid leukemia, no blast cutoff has been designated to define a primary diagnosis of lymphoblastic leukemia in the absence of extramedullary tissue involvement. However, in most patients, bone marrow blasts exceed 20%, and the classification system established by the World Health Organization (WHO) in 2008 recommends that a diagnosis of B- or T-acute lymphoblastic leukemia in the absence of documented extramedullary disease should require at least 20% bone marrow blasts.[15] The pathologic classification of lymphoblastic neoplasms includes B-lymphoblastic leukemia/lymphoma (B-ALL/LBL) and T-lymphoblastic leukemia/lymphoma (T-ALL/LBL).

B-Lymphoblastic Leukemia/Lymphoma

Most cases of B-ALL/LBL present as acute leukemia. The peak incidence occurs between 2 and 5 years of age, and a slight male predominance is seen.[16] Patients usually present with symptoms related to bone marrow replacement, such as fever, fatigue, bone pain, and bleeding, and variable numbers of circulating lymphoblasts are present. Some patients are aleukemic, and a small subset show hyperleukocytosis (a white blood cell [WBC] count above 100 × 10⁹/L); however, symptoms related to leukostasis are rare. Cases of B-ALL/LBL that present as lymphoma represent only about 10% of B-lymphoblastic neoplasms and predominantly occur in children.

The main sites of involvement are the skin, lymph nodes, and bone; unlike in T-ALL/LBL, mediastinal involvement is rare in B-lymphoblastic lymphoma.[17,18] By definition, lymphoblasts comprise fewer than 25% of the bone marrow aspirate smear cells, and about half of patients have no detectable marrow involvement.[18]

The leukemic blasts in the blood and bone marrow aspirate smears usually are small to intermediate in size and have characteristically scant cytoplasm (Figure 13-2, A). Often the cytoplasm is so reduced that it appears as a small tag applied to the nucleus (so-called "hand mirror cell"). The nucleus may be round or irregular and has delicate, dispersed chromatin and indistinct nucleoli. Some cases are characterized by larger blasts and more prominent nucleoli. However, abundant basophilic cytoplasm or prominent nucleoli should raise the differential of a high-grade lymphoma, such as Burkitt's lymphoma, or a myeloid leukemia.

The bone marrow biopsy specimen usually is diffusely infiltrated, although cases of B-lymphoblastic lymphoma involving the marrow may show an interstitial infiltration pattern. Lymphoblastic lymphoma is one of the few lymphoid neoplasms in which the cells may be more easily detected in the bone marrow aspirate than in the biopsy specimen, particularly if the marrow is minimally involved.[19] In the biopsy specimen, the neoplastic cells are medium sized and have very scant cytoplasm and fine chromatin; mitotic figures usually are frequent, and interspersed phagocytic histiocytes may impart a starry sky appearance (see Figure 13-2, B). Currently, no morphologic variants of B-ALL/LBL have been recognized. A subset of leukemic cases may show prominent peripheral and bone marrow eosinophilia and relatively low-level blast infiltration. This presentation usually is associated with a t(5;14)(q31;q32) translocation that juxtaposes the IL3 and IGH genes, resulting in a paraneoplastic eosinophilia.

Although the morphology of the bone marrow and peripheral blood may strongly suggest a precursor lymphoid neoplasm, immunophenotyping is required to distinguish B-ALL/LBL from acute myeloid leukemia (AML) as well as mature lymphoid neoplasms and to determine whether a B- or T-cell phenotype is present. B-ALL/LBL expresses CD19, CD79a, and PAX5 and is variably positive for CD20 and CD34. CD45 usually is dim in intensity compared to normal lymphocytes and may be negative. TdT is almost invariably positive, surface immunoglobulin is negative, and most cases express CD10. Rare cases may express monotypic surface immunoglobulin, but these cases should have morphologic and other immunophenotypic features of B-ALL/LBL, and mature B-cell lymphomas (e.g., Burkitt's lymphoma, diffuse large B-cell lymphoma) must be excluded.[20] The myeloid antigens CD13 and/or CD33 may be expressed; in the absence of the lineage-specific myeloid marker myeloperoxidase (MPO) or monocytic markers (lysozyme, nonspecific

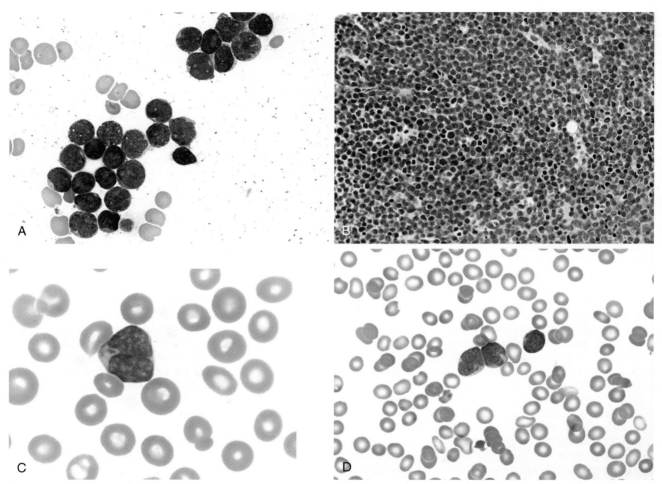

Figure 13-2 Precursor lymphoid neoplasms. **A,** Lymphoid blasts of B-acute lymphoblastic leukemia in a bone marrow aspirate. Although often small, lymphoid blasts are distinguishable from small mature lymphocytes by their finely dispersed chromatin. Nuclear membrane convolutions, present in this case, also can be a helpful feature. **B,** Diffuse sheets of lymphoid blasts from a case of B-acute lymphoblastic leukemia in a bone marrow biopsy specimen. **C,** Blasts in B-acute lymphoblastic leukemia may occasionally contain azurophilic cytoplasmic crystals; these should not be confused with Auer rods. **D,** The circulating lymphoblasts of T-acute lymphoblastic leukemia often are relatively small and have highly irregular nuclei and very scant cytoplasm.

esterase [NSE], CD14, CD64, and/or CD11c), they do not qualify a case as a mixed-lineage leukemia.

Cytogenetic analysis is critical for risk stratification of B-ALL/LBL, and several cytogenetic subgroups define distinct entities in the WHO classification system.[21] Gene rearrangement studies are rarely needed to establish the diagnosis, but almost all cases show clonal *IGH* rearrangement despite failure to express immunoglobulin protein on the cell surface.

The prognosis of B-ALL/LBL is excellent in children, in whom long-term remission rates of up to 80% are seen. In adults, however, the long-term survival rate is only 40% to 50%. The outcome depends significantly on the specific cytogenetic subgroup; favorable prognostic factors include age between 1 and 10 years and a WBC count below 50×10^9/L.[22] Rapid response to initial therapy (a low or undetectable level of minimal residual disease at various time points after the initial induction chemotherapy) is an important and independent predictor of relapse in childhood B-ALL/LBL; however, it requires specialized flow cytometric

evaluation tailored to detect very low levels of malignant lymphoblasts.[23]

Because of the broad morphologic spectrum of B-ALL/LBL, there is a broad differential diagnosis. Diagnostic difficulties can arise even with the use of immunophenotyping. AML and mixed-lineage leukemias should be excluded by demonstration of lack of MPO expression and lack of monocytic markers such as CD11c, CD64, and CD14. The presence of Auer rods normally would exclude B-ALL/LBL and establish a finding of a malignant myeloid proliferation. However, B-ALL/LBL sometimes shows cytoplasmic granules or even crystalline structures that superficially resemble Auer rods (Figure 13-2, *C*); careful examination reveals that these structures are rhomboidal and azurophilic rather than needlelike and eosinophilic. An MPO cytochemical stain can be helpful in such cases, because Auer rods are MPO+, whereas lymphoblasts should show no or only very faint MPO staining. It is important to note that CD19, PAX5, and TdT may be expressed in some cases of AML, and (as mentioned previously) CD13 and

CD33 can be expressed in B-ALL/LBL.[24,25] Therefore, a broad panel of immunophenotypic markers often must be used to distinguish among B-ALL/LBL, mixed-lineage leukemias, and AML. Gene rearrangement studies should not be used to establish lymphoid versus myeloid lineage or T- versus B-lineage, because "promiscuous" rearrangements of TCR may occur in a high proportion of B-ALL/LBL cases[26]; IGH and TCR rearrangements also may occur in AML.

Burkitt's lymphoma often has a blastic appearance and in fact was classified as a subtype of B-ALL in the French-American-British classification (so-called "L3 type"). Although Burkitt's lymphoma, like B-ALL/LBL, expresses CD20 and CD10, Burkitt's lymphoma is CD34− and TdT−, and most cases express surface immunoglobulin. Rare cases of leukemias resembling B-ALL/LBL but with a t(8;14) translocation involving the MYC gene have been reported, as have blastic leukemias that bear concurrent translocations of MYC, BCL2, and/or BCL6 genes; these cases also may show mixed immunophenotypic features of B-ALL/LBL and a mature B-cell lymphoma, including surface immunoglobulin light chain expression.[27-29] The classification of these cases is controversial. Blastoid mantle cell lymphoma may be morphologically indistinguishable from B-ALL/LBL, but it is easily identified by its distinctive immunophenotype (cyclin D1+, CD5+, TdT−). Other small round blue cell tumors of childhood, such as Ewing's sarcoma, may enter into the morphologic differential diagnosis. Caution should be used in relying only on CD45 to exclude lymphoid neoplasms in the workup of such tumors, because B-ALL/LBL may be CD45 weak or negative.[30]

Finally, it is important to recognize that benign B lymphoblasts (hematogones) have a morphology and immunophenotype similar to those of B-ALL/LBL cells. Hematogones normally comprise fewer than 5% of all marrow cells, but their numbers may increase in response to marrow stress (e.g., chemotherapy recovery), particularly in pediatric patients.[31] This may present diagnostic difficulties, mainly in the post-treatment setting in patients with a history of B-ALL/LBL. Hematogones are essentially indistinguishable from mature lymphocytes or small lymphoblasts in the bone marrow trephine and appear as small to medium-sized cells, often with a long cleft in the nucleus, with cytologic features intermediate between small lymphocytes and blasts. Flow cytometry is critical for distinguishing benign hematogone populations from malignant B lymphoblasts. Hematogones usually show a heterogeneous pattern of CD34, TdT, CD10, and CD20 expression, as they comprise various stages of maturation, although this pattern may be distorted after chemotherapy or the use of anti-CD20 antibody therapy.[32] Neoplastic lymphoblasts also usually show immunophenotypic aberrancies, such as inappropriate antigen combinations and/or expression of CD13 or CD33, that can be helpful in distinguishing them from hematogones.[33]

T-Lymphoblastic Leukemia/Lymphoma

In contrast to the more common B-ALL/LBL, T-ALL/LBL usually presents with a large anterior mediastinal mass representing thymic involvement, often with leukocytosis with numerous circulating blasts, peripheral lymphadenopathy, and hepatosplenomegaly.[34] On average, patients are older than in B-ALL/LBL; the median age is 20 to 30 years. The lymphoblasts of T-ALL/LBL are morphologically similar to those of B-ALL/LBL; these two neoplasms are distinguished by their immunophenotype and distinct genetic features. The prognosis of T-ALL/LBL in children appears to be somewhat inferior to that of B-ALL/LBL.[35] The prognostic factors are similar to those in B-ALL/LBL except for the WBC count, which does not appear to be an important prognostic factor in T-ALL/LBL.

Although both T- and B-lymphoblastic leukemias/lymphomas show a range of cell sizes, T-ALL/LBL is more likely to show small blasts with relatively condensed chromatin that may be difficult to distinguish from mature lymphocytes (Figure 13-2, D). The blasts of T-ALL/LBL express CD7, TdT, and cytoplasmic CD3; they variably express other T-cell markers such as surface CD3, CD4, CD8, and CD2. Assessment of cytoplasmic CD3 is critical, because CD3 is the only true T-lineage–specific marker, and many cases may lack surface CD3 expression.[36] Many cases express CD1a and CD99 and co-express CD4 and CD8, a phenotype resembling cortical thymocytes. CD34 is positive in about half of cases.[37, 38] As in B-ALL/LBL, a large panel of immunophenotyping markers should be applied, because subsets of T-ALL/LBL may express B-cell markers (e.g., CD79a) and/or myeloid markers (e.g., CD13, CD33, or CD117). Only the expression of MPO, monocytic markers, or sufficient markers specific for B-lineage (CD19 in addition to CD79a and/or cytoplasmic CD22) qualifies such a case as a mixed-lineage leukemia.[36]

Unlike B-ALL/LBL and AML, T-ALL/LBL has no distinct cytogenetic subgroups. However, many cases show recurrent translocations, including those involving TCR loci at 14q11.2, 7q35, and 7p14-15 with numerous partner oncogenes.[39] About half of the cases show activating point mutations of the NOTCH1 gene that appear to contribute to leukemogenesis through C-MYC activation and/or upregulation.[40] The TCR genes are clonally rearranged, even though TCRαβ or TCRγδ proteins are undetectable in most cases. Rare cases show a precursor natural killer (NK) phenotype. These "precursor NK-cell" ALL/LBL cases lack TCR rearrangement and express the CD94 lectin-like NK antigen receptor but lack the expression of CD56 that characterizes mature NK cells. Similar to T-ALL/LBL, they are TdT+, express cytoplasmic CD3, and occur in adolescents and young adults.[41]

The main differential diagnosis of T-ALL/LBL in the bone marrow is peripheral T-cell lymphomas that may share some immunophenotypic features, such as expression of CD10 and/or co-expression of CD4 and CD8. Recognition of the blastic morphology of T-ALL/LBL in well-prepared smears and assessment for TdT expression are helpful in this differential diagnosis. Blastoid plasmacytoid dendritic cell neoplasm expresses CD4, may be TdT+, and has a blastic morphology resembling that of T-ALL/LBL; however, it is negative for cytoplasmic CD3 and expresses CD123. Cases with eosinophilia should be evaluated by cytogenetics or fluorescence in situ hybridization (FISH) for a translocation involving the *FGFR1* gene located at 8p11. Such cases are classified separately as myeloid and lymphoid neoplasms with *FGFR1* abnormalities, even if they present with a picture resembling T-ALL/LBL.

Chronic Lymphocytic Leukemia

Chronic lymphocytic leukemia (CLL) is a relatively common B-cell leukemia of adults. The median age at diagnosis is 60 to 70 years, and a male predominance is seen. Patients often are asymptomatic and are diagnosed when lymphocytosis is found on routine blood testing. Symptomatic patients usually present with fatigue, symptoms related to splenomegaly, and/or lymphadenopathy.[42] Autoimmune thrombocytopenia, hemolytic anemia, or both (Evans syndrome) may be present at diagnosis or may develop later in the course of the disease. By definition, absolute lymphocytosis is present; by flow cytometry, the absolute level of clonal CLL cells must be at least 5×10^9/L in the peripheral blood. The range of lymphocyte counts at diagnosis varies and the count may exceed 100×10^9/L in some patients. A diagnosis of CLL may be made with a peripheral blood B-cell count below 5×10^9/L, provided the patient has cytopenias or other symptoms that can be attribute to the neoplastic B-cell population[43]; in such cases, a bone marrow examination should be performed, and other B-cell lymphomas should be excluded. A diagnosis of small lymphocytic lymphoma (SLL) may be made in patients who have lymphadenopathy as a result of a neoplastic infiltrate of CLL cells but fewer than 5×10^9/L CLL cells in the blood.

The diagnosis of CLL usually can be established on the basis of a clonal B-cell population in the peripheral blood (absolute count above 5×10^9/L) with characteristic morphology and flow cytometry immunophenotype; therefore a bone marrow sample is not required for a primary diagnosis of CLL. However, bone marrow biopsy is recommended before therapy is started to establish the baseline level of disease and to evaluate the success of subsequent therapeutic interventions. Marrow examination also may be performed in patients with CLL who develop thrombocytopenia, which may occur secondary to either extensive bone marrow infiltration or a paraneoplastic immune thrombocytopenic purpura.[44]

On peripheral blood smears, CLL cells resemble small lymphocytes. They have regularly condensed chromatin, absent or small nucleoli, and scant, pale cytoplasm (Figure 13-3, *A* and *B*). The regular "checkerboard" pattern of chromatin condensation in CLL cells is subtly different from the more irregularly condensed chromatin of normal circulating lymphocytes, but this may be difficult to appreciate on many smear preparations. Smudge cells (ruptured cell nuclei devoid of cytoplasm) frequently are seen in peripheral blood smears in patients with CLL and may comprise most of the white cells in the smear. Preparing the smear by hand rather than by an automated method, or adding albumin to the blood, abrogates the tendency of the CLL cells to smudge, allowing a more accurate peripheral blood white cell differential count. Smudge cells are by no means specific to CLL and frequently can be seen with other circulating lymphoma cells, blasts, or even reactive atypical lymphocytes.

Prolymphocytes represent the proliferating cell component in CLL and usually are present at low levels in the peripheral blood of patients with CLL. Prolymphocytes are at least twice the diameter of small lymphocytes and have a round nucleus; somewhat dispersed nuclear chromatin (less condensed than that of small lymphocytes but less finely dispersed than that of blasts); and a prominent central nucleolus; the cytoplasm is moderately abundant and usually basophilic. Although prolymphocytes are rare in the blood in most CLL cases, they should be enumerated, because increased numbers of prolymphocytes are associated with more aggressive disease. If prolymphocytes comprise more than 55% of the circulating lymphocytes at presentation, a diagnosis of prolymphocytic leukemia is made.

Some cases of CLL show cells intermediate in size between small lymphocytes and prolymphocytes, with variably prominent nucleoli; however, a strict definition of prolymphocytes should be used, and such cells should not be counted among the prolymphocytes. Although the CLL lymphocytes usually have round nuclear contours, a subset of cases contains cells with irregular or even clefted nuclei and/or distinct nucleoli. These cases, which have been called "atypical CLL" by some authors, may have a more aggressive course.[45] Other cases may have unusually abundant, pale cytoplasm. Despite the wide cytomorphologic spectrum manifested by CLL, atypical morphologic features do not appear to have an independent impact on the prognosis when genetic prognostic markers are taken into account. The WHO classification system does not recognize morphologic subtypes of CLL; the previous category of CLL/PL (CLL with 10% to 55% prolymphocytes) has been eliminated.[43]

In the bone marrow biopsy sample, CLL may manifest any infiltration pattern (nodular nonparatrabecular, interstitial, diffuse or, occasionally, intrasinusoidal) except the paratrabecular pattern.[46] The nodular and interstitial patterns are the most common. The nodules in CLL consist of monotonous small lymphocytes with occasional admixed larger, nucleolated cells. Unlike in many types of lymphomatous infiltrates, reticulin staining usually is not significantly increased in the lymphoid nodules in CLL.[4] A diffuse pattern of involvement is seen in about 20% of patients biopsied and has been associated with an adverse prognosis,[46,47] but this does not appear to be independent of other risk factors, such as genetic features.[48] The CLL cells appear as small, round lymphocytes that percolate among the hematopoietic elements singly or as small clusters in an interstitial pattern and/or form nonparatrabecular aggregates (see Figure 13-3, *C* and *D*). Proliferation centers are collections of enlarged CLL cells (medium-sized prolymphocytes and large paraimmunoblasts with vesicular nuclei) that appear pale on low-power examination among the small, dark blue CLL lymphocytes. Proliferation centers commonly are seen in extramedullary tissues involved by CLL; in the bone marrow, they may be seen in the diffuse pattern of involvement and to a lesser degree within nodular aggregates (see Figure 13-3, *E*).[49]

Immunophenotypic analysis of blood and/or bone marrow is a cornerstone of CLL diagnosis. CLL has a characteristic immunophenotype, typically showing expression of CD19; dim expression of CD20, CD22, and monotypic surface immunoglobulin light chain; and co-expression of CD5 (usually at a somewhat dimmer level than that of benign T cells) and CD23. Rare CLL cases (0.5% to 3%) may co-express the T-cell marker CD8.[50] FMC7, which recognizes an epitope of CD20 and is associated with bright expression of this protein, usually is dim or negative, as is CD79b.[51,52] CD20 and surface immunoglobulin expression may be so low that they are undetectable by flow cytometry; investigation of permeabilized cells by flow cytometry usually discloses monotypic expression of cytoplasmic immunoglobulin in such cases. The hairy cell markers CD103 and CD25 are negative, although CD11c may be expressed in a subset of cases.

Because CLL is a common disease, the existence of some immunophenotypic variability is not surprising. Atypical immunophenotypes that can occur in otherwise typical CLL cases include lack of CD5, lack of CD23, and strong CD20 and/or surface immunoglobulin expression. Scoring systems have been developed to reconcile such deviations from the classical CLL phenotype.[52] In ambiguous

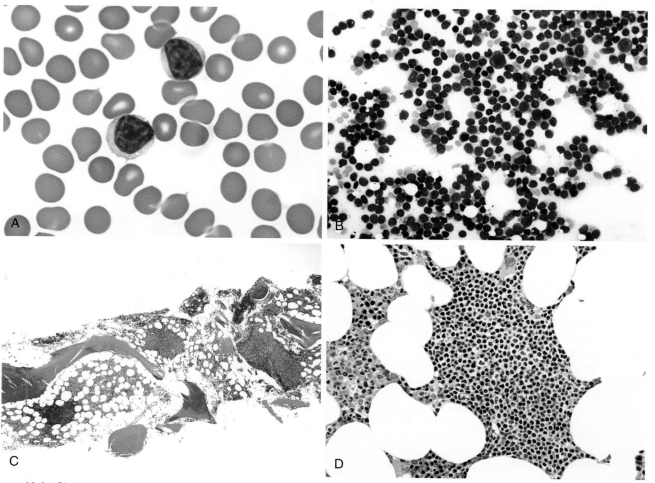

Figure 13-3   Chronic lymphocytic leukemia (CLL) and B-cell prolymphocytic leukemia (B-PLL). **A,** Peripheral blood appearance of CLL small lymphocytes, with condensed chromatin that forms large clumps within a round or ovoid nucleus; small nucleoli may be present. **B,** CLL extensively involving the bone marrow aspirate. **C,** Bone marrow biopsy specimen from a patient with CLL shows the typical nodular, nonparatrabecular pattern. **D,** The nodules are composed of monotonous, small, round to slightly irregular lymphocytes with condensed chromatin.

Continued

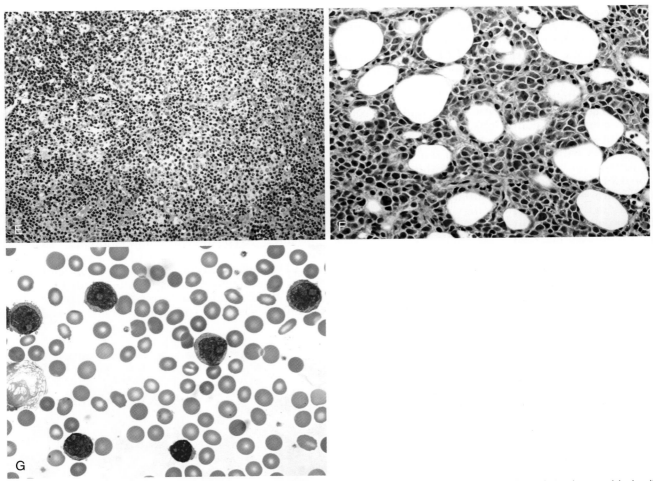

Figure 13-3, cont'd E, Proliferation centers, which appear pale because of the presence of prolymphocytes and paraimmunoblasts with vesicular nuclei, may be observed in diffuse areas of involvement. **F,** In this case of Richter's transformation involving the bone marrow, the marrow is infiltrated by large, pleomorphic lymphoid cells with prominent nucleoli. **G,** B-PLL in the peripheral blood. The lymphoid cells are larger than small lymphocytes and have prominent nucleoli.

cases, assessment for characteristic CLL aberrations by FISH (see below) may prove useful. Immunohistochemistry usually is not required if full flow cytometric immunophenotyping has been performed. However, performing cyclin D1 immunostaining is prudent if mantle cell lymphoma has not been excluded by cytogenetics or FISH for a t(11;14) translocation. Some cases of mantle cell lymphoma may express CD23 or demonstrate other immunophenotypic features resembling CLL.[53]

The traditional Rai and Binet clinical staging systems have been used for decades to stratify the risk for patients with CLL.[42,54] These clinical staging systems, which are based on the presence or absence of lymphadenopathy (and the number of sites affected), organomegaly, and cytopenias, correlate with patient survival. More recently, cytogenetic and molecular genetic features have been increasingly used as prognostic factors at diagnosis. Routine cytogenetic analysis of CLL often is uninformative because of the poor growth of CLL cells in culture. An interphase FISH study on the neoplastic lymphocytes from the blood, bone marrow, or involved extramedullary tissues can identify several recurring abnormalities associated with CLL that have important prognostic implications; 80% of CLL cases exhibit at least one such abnormality.[55] The most common abnormality is del(13q), which is associated with a favorable prognosis provided it is the only detected abnormality. The less frequent abnormalities del(11q), del(17p), and del(6q) are associated with an inferior prognosis, and trisomy 12 is associated with an intermediate prognosis.[55] In particular, del(17p) that results in loss of the *TP53* gene predicts a relatively aggressive clinical course. Adverse cytogenetic markers not present at diagnosis may develop in patients as the disease progresses.[56]

An important molecular genetic prognostic marker is the mutational status of the *IGH* gene variable region. About half of CLL cases show high levels of somatic hypermutation (less than 98% homology with the germline variable region, implying origin from a lymphocyte that is germinal center or post-germinal center). These cases have a significantly better prognosis than cases that lack somatic hypermutation (implying origin from a naïve, pre-germinal center lymphocyte).[57] Use of the *IGH* variable V_H3-21 family also is a marker for a poorer prognosis, irrespective of the mutational status.[58] Assessment of mutational status, a specialized test that requires sequencing, is not available in most laboratories. Immunophenotypic surrogates that correlate with unmutated CLL (and a poor prognosis) include expression of ZAP-70 on more than 20% of the tumor cells[59,60] and CD38 expression on more than 30% of the tumor cells.[61] Although these markers do not correlate perfectly with the mutational status, they do provide significant prognostic information.

CLL is an indolent disease, and patients often die of unrelated causes. The median survival time is 15 years or longer, and patients with favorable prognostic features have a median survival time of more than 20 years. Adverse events include the development of a predominant population of prolymphocytes in the blood and Richter's transformation. Richter's transformation represents progression of CLL to a diffuse large B-cell lymphoma, usually accompanied by abruptly worsening clinical symptoms and lymphadenopathy; it is associated with an aggressive clinical course and a poor prognosis.[62] A diagnosis of Richter's transformation can be made from the bone marrow biopsy sample if the marrow has been replaced by sheets of large B cells (see Figure 13-3, F). Rare cases of CLL may transform to a picture resembling classical Hodgkin's lymphoma, with Reed-Sternberg cells that often are positive for the Epstein-Barr virus (EBV). Interestingly, in Richter's or Hodgkin transformations of CLL, the transformed neoplasm frequently is clonally unrelated to the background CLL.[63]

The differential diagnosis of CLL includes other small B-cell lymphomas and some nonmalignant conditions. Among the lymphomas, mantle cell lymphoma can bear a close morphologic resemblance to CLL and can present as a leukemia; the proliferation centers that are a clue to CLL diagnosis in lymph nodes often are lacking in CLL involving the bone marrow. Immunophenotypic analysis is critical for showing bright (as opposed to dim) expression of CD20 and surface immunoglobulin in mantle cell lymphoma and, typically, lack of CD23. The gold standard of mantle cell lymphoma diagnosis is demonstration of cyclin D1 expression by immunohistochemistry and/or a t(11;14) by cytogenetics, FISH, or polymerase chain reaction (PCR) on a bone marrow or blood sample. Of note, some cyclin D1 expression may be detected within the proliferation centers of CLL, but it is not strong and uniform, as is the cyclin D1 expression in mantle cell lymphoma.[64] Marginal zone lymphomas rarely demonstrate CD5 expression, mimicking CLL,[65] whereas some CLL cases have abundant cytoplasm, mimicking the villous lymphocytes of splenic marginal zone lymphoma; splenomegaly also is relatively common in CLL. The lymphocyte count in CLL usually is higher than in splenic marginal zone lymphoma, and on well-prepared smears, the characteristic regularly condensed chromatin of CLL is a helpful clue. In difficult cases, FISH analysis can be very helpful, because splenic marginal zone lymphomas do not show the common cytogenetic abnormalities of CLL and may show other abnormalities, such as del(7q). Cases of CLL with abundant cytoplasm on smear preparations may raise the differential of hairy cell leukemia. However, CLL cases in bone marrow sections do not show the abundant, pale cytoplasm that characterize almost all hairy cell leukemia cases and also lack expression of CD103 and CD25. Table 13-1 presents the pathologic features that aid in the differential diagnosis of CLL with other B-cell leukemias.

The main nonmalignant disorder that may be confused with CLL is monoclonal B-lymphocytosis (MBL). This is a clonal or oligoclonal proliferation of B cells that usually have an immunophenotype similar to that of CLL but are present in insufficient numbers (fewer than 5×10^9/L in the blood, without extramedullary tissue involvement) to warrant a diagnosis of CLL. MBL is relatively common and is analogous to monoclonal gammopathy of undetermined significance (MGUS). The incidence of MBL increases with age and 3.5% of adults over age 40 have a detectable B-cell clone in the blood.[66] These circulating B-cell clones often are discovered incidentally when peripheral blood is subjected to flow cytometry for other reasons.

MBL likely is related to CLL and may represent a precursor of the disease. Its incidence is higher in first-degree relatives of patients with CLL,[67] and a small but significant percentage of patients with MBL (about 1% per year) progress to CLL.[68] The bone marrow findings for patients with MBL have not been well studied. It is uncertain whether patients with fewer than 5×10^9/L CLL cells in the blood but with bone marrow infiltrates resembling CLL should be classified as CLL or as MBL. The International Workshop on Chronic Lymphocytic Leukemia (IWCLL) recommends that the marrow should contain at least 30% lymphoid cells to qualify for CLL, but this is an arbitrary figure.[69]

If confirmatory peripheral blood or bone marrow flow cytometry is not available, the nonparatrabecular aggregates in CLL may overlap with reactive lymphoid aggregates. Small T cells may be admixed with the neoplastic aggregates of CLL, but close inspection of the CD5 stain relative to the stains for B-cell and other T-cell markers, such as CD3, can be helpful for disclosing the malignant B-cell population in CLL; the latter usually shows dimmer staining for CD5 than the admixed normal T cells.[70,71]

B-Cell Prolymphocytic Leukemia

As defined by the WHO classification system, B-cell prolymphocytic leukemia (B-PLL) is a de novo leukemia in which prolymphocytes comprise at least 55% of the peripheral blood lymphoid cells. Defined as such, B-PLL is a rare disease. The clinicopathologic features of B-PLL are not well characterized, because most publications have included cases of CLL with increased prolymphocytes that are now encompassed within CLL, as well as cases with

TABLE 13-1

Differential Diagnosis of B-Cell Leukemias

Feature	HCL	SMZL	HCL-v	CLL	B-PLL	B-ALL
White blood count	Usually low	Low, normal, or high	High	High	Very high	Low, normal, or high
Cell morphology in smears						
Nuclei	Medium sized, oval or indented	Small to medium sized, round	Medium sized, round or oval	Small, round	Large, round	Medium sized, round or irregular
Chromatin	Finely stippled	Condensed	Variable	Condensed	Moderately dispersed	Finely dispersed
Nucleoli	Absent	Small or absent	Present	Small or absent	Prominent	Usually small
Cytoplasm	Abundant, pale blue	Moderate amount, pale blue	Abundant	Scant, pale	Abundant, pale blue	Very scant
Cell surface	Circumferential projections	Polar projections	Present, variable	Smooth	Smooth	Smooth
Marrow infiltration pattern	Diffuse and interstitial	Nodular, interstitial, intrasinusoidal	Diffuse and interstitial	Nodular, interstitial, diffuse	Nodular, interstitial, diffuse	Diffuse and interstitial
Immuno-phenotype	CD20br+, FMC7+	CD20br+, FMC7+	CD20br+, FMC7+	CD20dim+, FMC7−	CD20br+, FMC7−	CD20− or +
	CD5−, CD10−, CD23−, sIg+	CD5−, CD10−, CD23−/+, sIg+	CD5−, CD10−, CD23−, sIg+	CD5+, CD10−, CD23+, sIg dim+ or −	CD5−/+, CD10−, CD23−, sIg+	CD5−, CD10+, CD23−, sIg−
	CD103+, CD25+, CD11c+	CD103−, CD25−/+, CD11c+/−	CD103+/−, CD25−, CD11c−	CD103−, CD25−, CD11c−/+	CD103−, CD25−, CD11c−/+	CD103−, CD25−, CD11c−
	CD123+, annexin A1+, cyclin D1+/−	CD123−, annexin A1−, cyclin D1−	CD123−, annexin A1−, cyclin D1−	CD123−/+, annexin A1−, cyclin D1−	CD123−, annexin A1−, cyclin D1−	CD123−/+
	TdT−	TdT−	TdT−	TdT−	TdT−	TdT+, CD34+/−

B-ALL, B-lymphoblastic leukemia/lymphoma; *B-PLL,* B-cell prolymphocytic leukemia; *br,* bright; *CLL,* chronic lymphocytic leukemia; *HCL,* hairy cell leukemia; *HCL-v,* hairy cell leukemia variant; *sIg,* surface immunoglobulin (kappa or lambda); *SMZL,* splenic marginal zone lymphoma.

t(11;14) translocation that are now considered to represent mantle cell lymphoma.[72] B-PLL affects older adults. The median age is 60 to 70 years, and a slight male preponderance is seen. Patients usually present with systemic symptoms and splenomegaly, but, in contrast to most cases of leukemic mantle cell lymphoma, without significant lymphadenopathy. A marked leukocytosis with a rapid lymphocyte doubling time is characteristic.[73]

In the blood, the vast majority of the lymphoid cells are prolymphocytes, resembling those seen in much smaller numbers in CLL. Although the prolymphocyte nucleus usually is round, some cases may show prominent nuclear irregularities or lobulations. A uniform feature of B-PLL is a prominent "punched out" nucleolus (see Figure 13-3, *G*).[73] The bone marrow is involved in all cases and shows an interstitial, nodular, or diffuse pattern of involvement.

Immunophenotypically, B-PLL shows expression of CD19 and strongly expresses CD20, CD22, CD79a, and CD79b. Unlike in CLL, FMC7 is strongly expressed. B-PLL also differs from CLL in its relatively infrequent expression of CD5 and CD23, seen in only a minority of cases.[73,74] Cytogenetic and FISH analysis shows some genetic relationship with CLL; del(17p) is present in half the cases, *TP53* mutations are frequent, and del(13q) also is common.[74,75] However, usage of the *IGH* variable region family in B-PLL appears distinct from that seen in CLL cases with increased prolymphocytes, which supports the separation of B-PLL from CLL advocated in the WHO classification system.[74]

B-PLL has a poor prognosis; the median survival time is 2 to 4 years. No clinical or pathologic prognostic markers have been identified. These patients do not respond well to standard CLL therapies, and the appropriate therapy is uncertain at this time.[73]

The main differential diagnosis with B-PLL is CLL with increased prolymphocytes. Figure 13-4 shows the spectrum of small lymphocytes and prolymphocytes seen in B-PLL and CLL. The prolymphocytes in CLL show CD5 expression more often than is seen in B-PLL, although CD23 may be lost when CLL cases develop an increase in prolymphocytes. Eliciting a previous history of CLL is critical for excluding a diagnosis of de novo B-PLL in such cases.

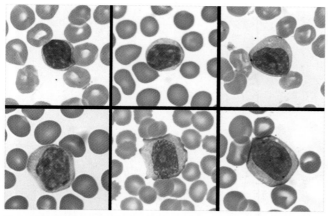

Figure 13-4 The spectrum of cells in CLL and B-PLL, ranging from small lymphocytes *(top left panel)* to prolymphocytes *(lower three panels)*. The top middle and top right panels demonstrate cells that are slightly enlarged but do not qualify as prolymphocytes.

Assessment for t(11;14) by FISH in a blood sample and/or for cyclin D1 expression in tissue sections is important for excluding a leukemic presentation of mantle cell lymphoma. Like B-PLL, hairy cell leukemia variant, considered a subcategory of unclassifiable splenic B-cell lymphoma/leukemia in the WHO classification system, shows prominent splenomegaly and leukocytosis at presentation. The neoplastic cells in the peripheral blood usually are somewhat enlarged compared to small lymphocytes, but they are smaller than B-PLL cells and have less prominent nucleoli. Hairy cell leukemia variant may lack many characteristic markers of hairy cell leukemia, such as CD25 and annexin A1, but unlike B-PLL, it usually is CD103+.[76] Distinguishing between B-PLL and hairy cell leukemia variant may be difficult or impossible in some cases; an intrasinusoidal infiltrate in the bone marrow may be a helpful clue that suggests the hairy cell leukemia variant.[77] Features that aid the differential diagnosis of B-PLL with other B-cell leukemias are listed in Table 13-1.

Lymphoplasmacytic Lymphoma

Lymphoplasmacytic lymphoma is an uncommon B-cell neoplasm. It arises from a post-germinal center B cell, shows plasmacytic differentiation, and in most cases secretes an IgM paraprotein (fewer than 10% of cases secrete IgG or IgA).[78] The IgM paraprotein may result in hyperviscosity and/or cryoglobulinemia. The clinical syndrome of lymphoplasmacytic lymphoma involving the bone marrow accompanied by an IgM paraprotein is called *Waldenström's macroglobulinemia*. Although many lymphoplasmacytic lymphoma cases are not associated with hyperviscosity at diagnosis, it may develop later in the course of disease. Lymphoplasmacytic lymphoma affects older adults, and a male predominance is seen. Most patients present with symptoms related to bone marrow infiltration, such as anemia or infections, or hyperviscosity.[79] Patients who present with

hyperviscosity have a particularly high serum IgM level: the median level in these patients is 3.8 to 5.1 g/dL, whereas the reported median IgM level in lymphoplasmacytic lymphoma overall is 1.5 to 2.2 g/dL.[78-81] Some cases may be associated with hepatitis C infection, commonly with concomitant type II cryoglobulinemia.[82]

The bone marrow is involved in almost all cases at presentation, and bone marrow sampling is the main modality by which the diagnosis is made[80,81]; 5% to 30% of patients may have concurrent lymphadenopathy and/or splenomegaly.[79,83] The reported infiltration patterns in the bone marrow biopsy sample vary: the interstitial and nodular nonparatrabecular patterns are consistently the most commonly seen, and paratrabecular nodular infiltrates have been reported to occur in 4% to 31% of cases.[78,81,84] Diffuse infiltration patterns are reported to occur in 4% to 58% of cases.[80,81] The pattern or degree of bone marrow involvement does not appear to correlate with the prognosis,[80] and surprisingly, the level of IgM paraprotein at diagnosis correlates with neither the prognosis nor the extent of bone marrow infiltration.[81,85]

The neoplastic infiltrates include small lymphocytes, plasma cells, and plasmacytoid lymphocytes that represent "hybrids" between lymphocytes and plasma cells. In most cases, lymphocytes outnumber the plasma cell component in the bone marrow, although plasma cells predominate in a minority of cases. Plasmacytoid lymphocytes are seen in a spectrum of forms, frequently including cells with condensed, "clock face" chromatin that resembles that of plasma cells but is accompanied by the scant, pale cytoplasm of a lymphocyte. Also seen are cells with the more dispersed nuclear chromatin of lymphocytes combined with variably abundant basophilic plasmacytoid cytoplasm (Figure 13-5, *A*). Plasmacytoid lymphocytes cells may be identified in the peripheral blood but usually are present in relatively low numbers.[86] Intranuclear eosinophilic immunoglobulin pseudoinclusions (Dutcher bodies) are identified in about half of the cases,[78] whereas cytoplasmic immunoglobulin inclusions (Russell bodies) are seen in fewer than 10%.[80] The plasma cells may be intimately admixed with the lymphocyte component or, when nodules are present, may be located at the periphery of the lymphoid nodules (see Figure 13-5, *B* and *C*).[78] Following therapy, mature plasma cells may represent the main neoplastic cell population in some cases, and clonal B cells may be lacking.[87] Large cells usually are infrequent; however, some cases may have more frequent large cells, imparting a polymorphous appearance. Transformation to diffuse large B-cell lymphoma, reported to occur in 5% to 13% of patients, often is heralded by the onset of extramedullary disease and profound cytopenias and is associated with poor survival.[88,89] Mast cells frequently are admixed with the lymphoma cells and have been postulated to play a role in tumor growth through CD154/CD40 signaling.[90] However,

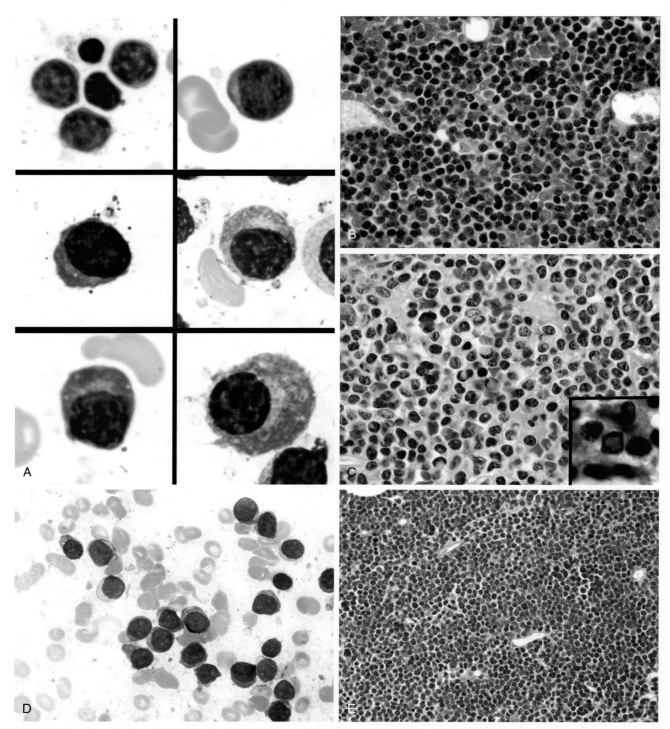

Figure 13-5   Lymphoplasmacytic lymphoma (LPL). **A,** The spectrum of cells in bone marrow aspirates from cases of LPL, ranging from small lymphocytes *(upper panels)* to plasma cells *(lower right panel),* with many intermediate lymphoplasmacytoid cells; the relative distribution of the cells across this spectrum varies widely from case to case. **B,** The bone marrow biopsy specimen shows small lymphocytes, often with clumped "clock face" chromatin resembling that of plasma cells, as well as variable numbers of admixed mature plasma cells. **C,** Dutcher bodies, dense eosinophilic intranuclear immunoglobulin pseudoinclusions, often are seen in the lymphocytes, plasma cells, and/or lymphoplasmacytoid cells of LPL; these pseudoinclusions can be highlighted with periodic acid Schiff (PAS) staining *(inset).* **D,** Plasma cell myeloma may show small cell morphology, mimicking LPL; however, the cells have a more uniform cytologic appearance in the bone marrow aspirate smear and lack the cell spectrum seen in LPL. **E,** Small cell myeloma can appear very lymphocyte-like in the bone marrow biopsy specimen.

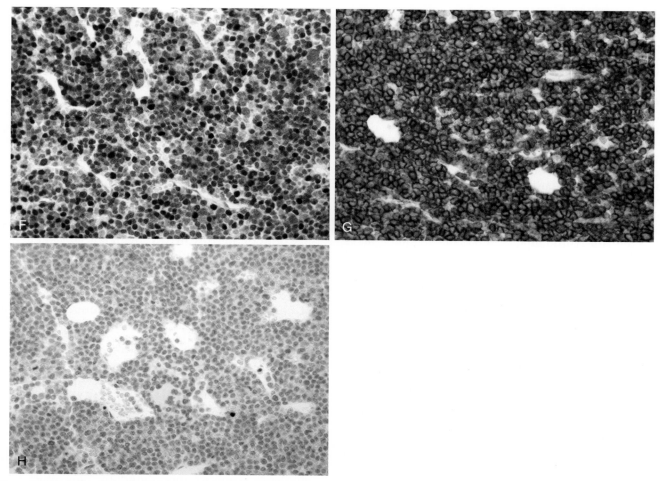

Figure 13-5, cont'd   F, Cyclin D1 immunostaining frequently is positive in small cell myeloma; this finding excludes a diagnosis of LPL and can be helpful in the differential diagnosis. Unlike the lymphocytes in LPL, small cell myeloma cells are strongly, uniformly CD138+ **(G)** and PAX5– **(H).**

mast cells also can be frequent in other bone marrow lymphomas and are not specific to lymphoplasmacytic lymphoma.

A clonal B-cell component is always detectable at diagnosis by flow cytometry (although this B-cell component may be lacking in patients after therapy with anti-CD20 immunotherapy) and is characteristically CD20+, CD5–, CD10–, and CD23–. Up to 20% of cases may express CD5, and up to 61% can express CD23.[91,92] Unlike in CLL, CD5 and/or CD23 usually are only weakly expressed in lymphoplasmacytic lymphoma.[78] CD10 expression is exceedingly rare.[53] The B-lymphocytes express monotypic surface IgM, and the plasma cells and lymphoplasmacytic cells express cytoplasmic IgM. Rare cases express IgG or other heavy chain types.[86]

Lymphoplasmacytic lymphoma is overall an indolent disease; the median survival time is 5 to 10 years. Transformation to diffuse large B-cell lymphoma occurs infrequently.[89] No defining associated cytogenetic or molecular abnormality has been identified. About 50% of cases bear a 6q deletion, a finding that has been associated with an adverse prognosis.[93]

It is important to recognize that not all lymphomas presenting with an IgM paraprotein represent lymphoplasmacytic lymphoma: CLL/SLL, marginal zone lymphomas, follicular lymphoma, diffuse large B-cell lymphoma, and even angioimmunoblastic T-cell lymphoma also may present with an IgM paraproprotein. Although rare patients with other types of lymphoma may have high IgM levels and hyperviscosity, the serum IgM level in these other lymphomas usually is much lower (median, 0.4 to 0.9 g/dL) than in lymphoplasmacytic lymphoma (median, 2.2 g/dL).[79,94,95] Although a high IgM paraprotein level (over 3 g/dL) nearly always indicates lymphoplasmacytic lymphoma, only 36% of patients had such a high IgM level at diagnosis in one recent series, and a diagnosis of lymphoplasmacytic lymphoma can be made with lower IgM levels if the typical pathologic features are present.[79] Conversely, MGUS may be an IgM type. Usually, the paraprotein level in IgM MGUS is relatively low. In the absence of a neoplastic lymphoid infiltrate of clonal small lymphocytes and lymphoplasmacytoid cells, a diagnosis of lymphoplasmacytic lymphoma should not be made in the setting of an IgM paraprotein, even if a bone marrow monotypic plasma cell component is present. Unlike plasma cell myeloma, there is no standardized cut-off in the level of lymphoplasmacytic infiltrate that would establish a diagnosis of lymphoma in the setting of an IgM paraprotein; some investigators have suggested a level of 10% or more of the bone marrow cellularity as qualifying for a diagnosis of lymphoplasmacytic lymphoma, whereas lower levels of infiltration would represent IgM MGUS.[96]

The main pathologic differential diagnosis of lymphoplasmacytic lymphoma is with plasma cell myeloma and with other lymphomas that may show plasmacytic differentiation. Some cases of plasma cell myeloma express CD20 and have a small cell appearance that mimics lymphoplasmacytic lymphoma (see Figure 13-5, D and E). However, unlike lymphoplasmacytic lymphoma, plasma cell myeloma lacks a surface immunoglobulin-positive clonal B-cell component. The plasma cell component of lymphoplasmacytic lymphoma almost always expresses IgM heavy chain and is CD19+/CD45+, whereas plasma cells in myeloma are CD19−/CD45−; also, IgM plasma cell myeloma is exceedingly rare.[97] CD20+ plasma cell myelomas often express cyclin D1 and bear a t(11;14) translocation, findings that exclude a diagnosis of lymphoplasmacytic lymphoma[98] (see Figure 13-5, F). Myelomas, including CD20+ cases, also should co-express CD138 but lack PAX5 expression (see Figure 13-5, G and H).

Distinction from other lymphomas with plasmacytic differentiation may be problematic, particularly when an IgM paraprotein is present. Although CD5 may be expressed in lymphoplasmacytic lymphoma, it usually lacks the uniform moderate to bright expression level characteristic of chronic lymphocytic leukemia and mantle cell lymphoma and has brighter CD20 and surface immunoglobulin expression than chronic lymphocytic leukemia.[78] Extranodal, nodal, and splenic marginal zone lymphomas often show plasmacytic differentiation; intrasinusoidal involvement can be a clue to diagnosis of the latter.[99] Although considerable morphologic and immunophenotypic overlap is seen between these marginal zone lymphomas and lymphoplasmacytic lymphoma, correlation with clinical and radiographic features (e.g., the presence or absence of splenomegaly, lymphadenopathy, or an extranodal mass) and the paraprotein level allow classification in most cases. Finally, angioimmunoblastic T-cell lymphoma may show a marked reactive bone marrow plasmacytic infiltrate, as well as an IgM paraprotein.[100]

Hairy Cell Leukemia

Hairy cell leukemia is a mature B-cell neoplasm that primarily involves the blood, bone marrow, and splenic red pulp. Hairy cell leukemia is relatively rare and represents only 2% of all leukemias.[101] The median age at diagnosis is 50 years, and a marked male predominance is seen. Patients present most often with symptoms related to cytopenias, such as

infection or fatigue. Notably, monocytopenia is seen in almost all cases and is considered one of the most sensitive markers of disease. More than three fourths of patients have palpable splenomegaly at diagnosis, but peripheral lymphadenopathy is uncommon.[102-104] In up to one fourth of patients, hairy cell leukemia is diagnosed incidentally as a result of routine hematologic screening in asymptomatic patients.[102] Most patients are leukopenic or pancytopenic at presentation. Leukocytosis is present in only 10% of cases, and when marked, it raises the possibility of hairy cell leukemia variant (discussed later) or another lymphoma.[103] Although a diagnosis usually can be made based on the peripheral blood morphology and immunophenotype, examination of bone marrow is recommended in all newly diagnosed cases to assess the extent of marrow involvement and to establish a baseline for assessment of the response to treatment. Obtaining a good bone marrow core biopsy sample is essential, because the bone marrow aspirate often is poorly cellular or unobtainable.[105] If an aspirate cannot be obtained, the diagnostic immunophenotype usually can be demonstrated in the peripheral blood, because almost all patients have circulating neoplastic cells, even when they are difficult to identify on the smears.[106]

The morphology is ideally represented on well-prepared peripheral blood smears. Hairy cells are one and one half to two times the size of small lymphocytes and are characterized by oval or bean-shaped nuclei, dispersed chromatin with features intermediate between a mature lymphocyte and a blast, and absent or inconspicuous small nucleoli. Hairy cell cytoplasm is moderately abundant, pale blue, and flocculent and often has a ruffled or ragged surface showing wispy, hairlike projections (Figure 13-6, A).[107,108] The hairy projections are best seen in thin areas of the smears, and when well demonstrated, they are present all around the cell membrane. The cellular trauma induced in preparing the bone marrow aspirate renders the characteristic hairy cell cytomorphology more difficult to appreciate in the aspirate smears or touch preparations than in peripheral smears.[109] Therefore, the peripheral blood smear should be examined in conjunction with the bone marrow specimen in the primary diagnosis of hairy cell leukemia.

The bone marrow infiltrate is mainly interstitial and/or diffuse and does not form the well-defined aggregates that characterize most other small B-cell lymphomas (see Figure 13-6, B). In most cases, at diagnosis the bone marrow is hypercellular and has diffuse sheets of hairy cells.[107] However, in early stages of the disease, the bone marrow may be normocellular or even hypocellular and have a subtle interstitial infiltrate that is not readily apparent on routine stains.[110] On a higher power view, the hairy cells appear monotonous and have oval or bean-shaped nuclei set in an abundant, clear to pale pink cytoplasm that holds the nuclei equidistant, imparting the characteristic "fried egg" appearance (see Figure 13-6, C and D).[109,111] Hairy projections usually are not evident on routine stains, although they may be visualized with DBA 44 immunohistochemistry.[112] In up to 70% of the cases, immunohistochemical stains for CD20 or DBA 44 may also reveal an intrasinusoidal component of the infiltrate.[113,114] In some cases with extensive involvement, the neoplastic cell infiltrate may appear spindled (see Figure 13-6, *E*).[111] The extent of marrow cellularity and intertrabecular space occupied by hairy cells should be given in the pathology report, both in the primary diagnosis of hairy cell leukemia (to provide a baseline) and in samples obtained after therapy (to determine effectiveness of therapy). The amount of residual hematopoiesis varies, but a reduction in normal hematopoietic cells, particularly of the myeloid lineage, often is seen.[115,116] Hematopoietic elements may manifest morphologic dysplasia, mimicking a myelodysplastic syndrome,[116,117] and in some cases the marrow may appear markedly hypoplastic, mimicking aplastic anemia.[110] Not infrequently, a modest increase in the number of plasma cells and mast cells is seen.[118] Significant reticulin fibrosis is found in almost all cases, which explains the poor aspirate

smears or inaspirable marrow characteristic of the disease (see Figure 13-6, *F*).[119]

Neoplastic cells express CD45, CD20, and surface immunoglobulin, all at bright intensity, as well as the B-cell markers CD19, FMC-7, CD22, and CD79a. CD5, CD10, and CD23 usually are negative. Although CD5 is positive in fewer than 5% of cases, CD10 can be positive in 10% to 26% of cases, and CD23 has been reported to be positive in up to 17% of cases.[120-124] Bright expression of CD11c, CD25, and CD103 is characteristic,[122] and these markers should be added to the flow cytometry panels in all cases of possible hairy cell leukemia. CD123 is expressed in 95% of cases of hairy cell leukemia, but it is not expressed in hairy cell leukemia variant, splenic marginal zone lymphoma, or other small B-cell lymphomas[125]; therefore, CD123 may be helpful in differentiating other diseases with "hairy" or "villous" morphology from hairy cell leukemia. If the hairy cells are not recognized on the peripheral smear, the characteristic high forward and side light scatter qualities of hairy cells on flow cytometry may be helpful clues.

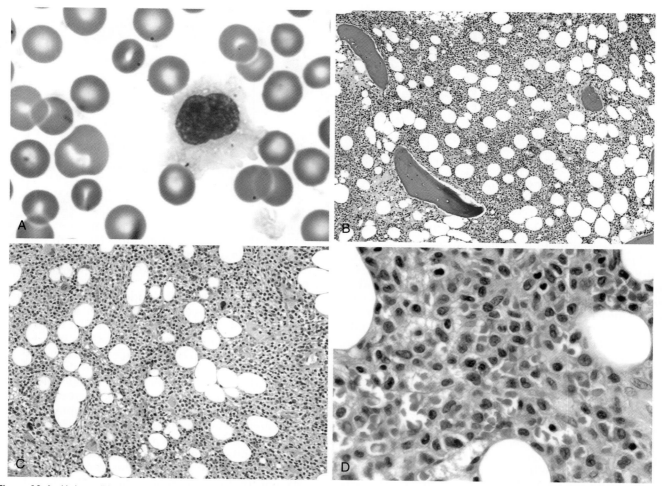

Figure 13-6   Hairy cell leukemia. **A,** Hairy cell on a peripheral smear, with an indented nucleus, dispersed chromatin, and abundant, flocculent cytoplasm with a ragged surface border. **B,** The infiltrate of hairy cell leukemia is characteristically interstitial and does not form nodules. **C,** The cells have a "fried egg" appearance because of the abundant, clear or pale cytoplasm. **D,** High-power view shows the characteristic oval, indented, and often bean-shaped nuclei.

Continued

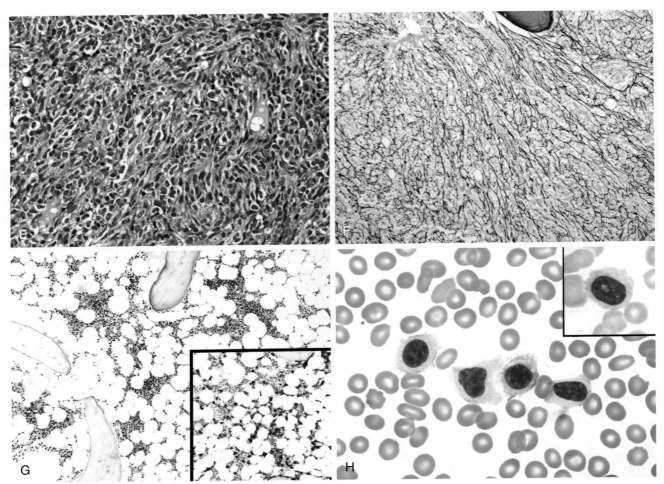

Figure 13-6, cont'd **E,** In some cases with extensive, diffuse involvement, the hairy cells may have a spindled appearance. **F,** Reticulin fibers usually are increased to a moderate or marked level and may result in an inaspirable marrow. **G,** In some patients, involvement may be subtle, particularly when the marrow is hypocellular; in such cases, CD20 immunohistochemical staining can help disclose the neoplastic cells *(inset)*. **H,** Hairy cell variant cells typically are far more numerous than conventional hairy cell leukemia cells in the peripheral blood; the nucleoli often are prominent *(inset)*.

The diagnosis of hairy cell leukemia should rest on the integration of bone marrow biopsy specimen and peripheral blood morphologic findings with the clinical features and immunophenotype. Most cases of hairy cell leukemia (and only rare cases of other B-cell lymphomas) express at least three of the four characteristic hairy cell leukemia markers (CD11c, CD103, CD25, and CD123 [or the less commonly used marker HC2]).[76,125-127] Cases with an atypical immunophenotype, such as CD10 or CD5 expression or lack of CD103 or CD25 expression, may still be diagnosed as hairy cell leukemia if the clinical features, marrow infiltration pattern, and cytomorphology are otherwise typical.[121] The use of tartrate-resistant acid phosphatase (TRAP) cytochemical staining has declined recently with the widespread use of flow cytometry to evaluate lymphoproliferative disorders and with the development of a reliable antibody to detect TRAP. However, the TRAP antibody may stain other B-cell neoplasms and therefore is less specific than cytochemistry.[128] If the characteristic HCL immunophenotype can be demonstrated

in peripheral blood or bone marrow aspirate samples, paraffin section immunohistochemistry on the biopsy sample usually is unnecessary, except to help quantify involvement in morphologically subtle or treated cases.

Hairy cells can be readily identified in tissue sections by routine B-cell markers such as CD20 and CD79a, and these markers often reveal far more hairy cells than are evident on routine stains (see Figure 13-6, *G*). CD25 and CD123 co-expression can be demonstrated by immunohistochemistry, although these antigens also are expressed in other marrow cells. DBA 44 stains hairy cells in bone marrow trephine sections, but it may not stain all the neoplastic cells, and it is expressed in other neoplasms.[129] Cyclin D1 is overexpressed in most cases of hairy cell leukemia and can be detected by immunohistochemistry in paraffin sections; however, the staining usually is weak and/or focal compared to the strong, diffuse staining in mantle cell lymphoma,[130] and no translocation involving the *CCND1* locus is seen.[131,132] Antibodies to CD11c (5D11)[133] and the annexin A1 protein[134] have been shown to be highly sensitive and specific markers for hairy cell leukemia in the bone marrow biopsy specimen.

About 10% of patients who present with peripheral blood lymphocytes reminiscent of hairy cell leukemia display morphologic, immunophenotypic, and clinical features that deviate significantly from typical hairy cell leukemia. The WHO classification system includes these cases in a provisional subgroup of unclassifiable splenic B-cell lymphomas/leukemias and has designated them *hairy cell leukemia variant* (HCL-v). In contrast to patients with classical hairy cell leukemia, patients with HCL-v are older (median age is 70 years) and have massive splenomegaly and usually marked leukocytosis (the median WBC count is 116×10^9/L) with numerous circulating neoplastic cells.[135,136] The leukemic cells resemble hairy cells but have prominent central nucleoli, which are not typically seen in classical hairy cell leukemia (see Figure 13-6, *H*).[135] Monocytopenia is not seen, and there is relatively little marrow fibrosis.[135] The pattern of bone marrow infiltration is similar to that in typical hairy cell leukemia. Immunophenotypically, HCL-v is CD103+, but it is usually CD25,TRAP, CD123, and annexin A1 negative.[136] The clinical course is somewhat more aggressive than in classical hairy cell leukemia, and about 50% of these patients are resistant to the purine analog therapy used to treat classical hairy cell leukemia.[135,136]

The clinical course of hairy cell leukemia has changed dramatically over the past several decades with advances in therapy: long-term survival, with current therapies, is excellent (96% at 13 years).[137] Accurate diagnosis and differentiation from other types of B-cell lymphoma are critical for ensuring that patients receive disease-appropriate therapy. Hairy cell leukemia usually can be diagnosed accurately with the proper workup, as long as it is considered in the differential diagnosis. However, if the neoplastic infiltrate is subtle, the cytopenic presentation, relative erythroid hyperplasia, and reactive dysplastic changes in bone marrow hematopoietic elements may lead to an erroneous diagnosis of myelodysplasia or, in hypoplastic cases, aplastic anemia.[110] Immunostaining of the bone marrow biopsy specimen with a B-cell marker (e.g., CD20) is recommended in cases in which myelodysplasia or aplastic anemia is considered but hairy cell leukemia remains a possibility. Splenic marginal zone lymphoma is the most common differential diagnostic consideration. Although both splenic marginal zone lymphoma and hairy cell leukemia may show an intrasinusoidal pattern of marrow infiltration, the former usually also shows lymphoid nodules, which are absent in hairy cell leukemia. Circulating splenic marginal zone lymphoma cells have less prominent and blunter hairy projections, which are "polarized" to one section of the cell surface, unlike the encircling hairy projections present in hairy cells.[138] Although splenic marginal zone lymphoma is also negative for CD5 and CD10, it does not typically manifest the

CD103+, CD25+, CD11c+ phenotype characteristic of hairy cell leukemia; it also is CD123− and negative for annexin A1 and cyclin D1. Morphologic and clinical features that help in the differential diagnosis of hairy cell leukemia with other B-cell leukemias and lymphomas are listed in Table 13-1. Splenic diffuse red pulp small B-cell lymphoma, a provisional neoplasm recognized in the WHO classification system, has a splenic infiltration pattern similar to that of hairy cell leukemia, but also bone marrow intrasinusoidal involvement similar to that seen in splenic marginal zone lymphoma. The immunophenotype appears to be more similar to splenic marginal zone lymphoma, although some cases can express CD123 or CD103,[139] and DBA 44 frequently is positive.[140] Some overlap also exists between this entity and HCL-v.[113,140] This entity is discussed further in Chapter 6, Lymphomas of the Spleen.

Large Granular Lymphocytic Leukemia

Large granular lymphocytic leukemia is an indolent peripheral T-cell leukemia that involves bone marrow and peripheral blood, often with associated splenomegaly. The median age at presentation is 55 to 60 years, and men and women are equally affected. Patients may be asymptomatic or may present with symptoms related to associated cytopenias, particularly infections resulting from neutropenia. Patients often manifest symptoms for several years before the diagnosis is made, which attests to the chronic, indolent nature of this disease.[141,142] At diagnosis about one half of patients have splenomegaly, but lymphadenopathy is rare.[143] Large granular lymphocytic leukemia is associated with autoimmune diseases, particularly rheumatoid arthritis, but also various autoimmune diseases that affect the endocrine organs, such as ulcerative colitis, immune thrombocytopenic purpura (ITP), and pure red cell aplasia.[144] Most patients have an absolute lymphocytosis, although some may lack lymphocytosis but have a relative increase in large granular lymphocytes. The median survival time after diagnosis is about 10 years.

Large granular lymphocytic leukemia cells are indistinguishable from normal large granular lymphocytes cytologically. They are medium-sized lymphoid cells with round nuclei that lack conspicuous nucleoli, and they have abundant, pale to clear cytoplasm that contains discrete azurophilic granules (Figure 13-7, *A*).[145] Large granular lymphocytes are increased; the absolute count usually exceeds 2×10^9/L (the absolute count in normal individuals is 0.1×10^9 to 0.3×10^9/L), and that level is sustained for at least 6 months.[144] Because of a frequently associated neutropenia, the large granular lymphocytes often comprise most of the peripheral blood leukocytes; in contrast, in normal individuals they account for only about 2% to 3% of all blood leukocytes.

Flow cytometry in both blood and bone marrow characteristically demonstrates a CD3+, CD8+, CD57+, CD16+, CD94+, TCRαβ immunophenotype.

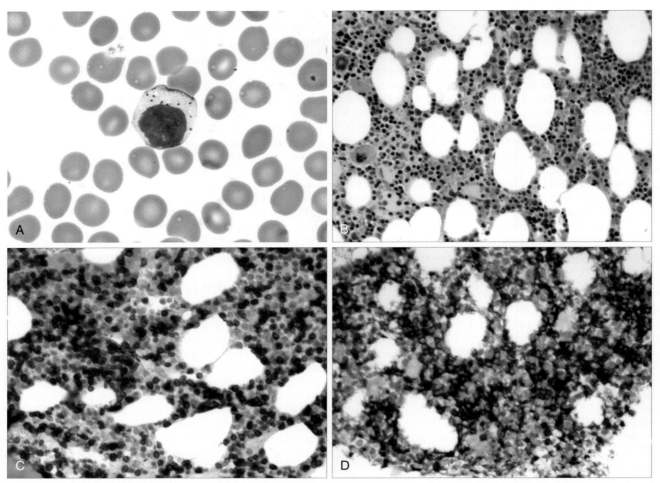

Figure 13-7 Large granular lymphocytic (LGL) leukemia. **A,** LGL leukemia cells are slightly larger than small lymphocytes and have abundant cytoplasm containing distinct granules. **B,** The interstitial lymphoid infiltrate in the bone marrow often is subtle but is revealed by immunostains for T-cell markers such as CD3 **(C)** and CD8 **(D)**.

CD5 and/or CD7 are frequently absent or dimly expressed. CD56 is detected in about one third of cases. Rare phenotypic variants include CD4+, CD8– cases and variants that express TCRγδ, which can be either CD8+, CD4– or double negative (CD4–, CD8–).[145,146] CD4+ large granular lymphocytic leukemia does not appear to be associated with autoimmune diseases; affected patients have less prominent neutropenia and splenomegaly and more commonly have lymphadenopathy than do patients with CD8+ large granular lymphocytic leukemia.[147] About 5% of all cases are TCRγδ+. These patients have clinicopathologic features and an indolent clinical course similar to those of TCRαβ large granular lymphocytic leukemia, but they are more frequently anemic than the latter patients and can have associated hemolytic anemia or pure red cell aplasia.[148,149] The clonality of the T cells may be demonstrated by either PCR detection of a *TCR* gene rearrangement or by restricted expression of the TCR variable region (TCR-Vbeta) as detected by flow cytometry.[150,151] Most cases also show restricted expression of killer cell immunoglobulin-like receptors (KIR), detectable by flow cytometry; this finding correlates with the clonality

and is similar to the restricted KIR expression found in NK-cell leukemias (discussed later).[152] However, PCR testing for *TCR* rearrangement is the most commonly used method to prove clonality in large granular lymphocytic leukemia, because immunophenotypic analyses of TCR-Vbeta and KIR expression profiles are not available in most laboratories.

The diagnosis usually can be made by examination of a peripheral smear combined with peripheral blood flow cytometry (demonstration of the characteristic CD3+, CD8+, CD57+, CD16+ immunophenotype) and PCR (demonstration of a clonal *TCR* rearrangement), thus obviating the need for a diagnostic bone marrow sample. However, because of the cytopenic presentation and often minimal lymphocytosis, bone marrow biopsy may be performed to address a clinical suspicion of myelodysplastic syndrome or aplastic anemia. The marrow in large granular lymphocytic leukemia is usually normocellular. An interstitial lymphoid infiltrate is seen in all cases and an intrasinusoidal infiltration in about half of the cases.[14,153] As with many lymphomas with a predominantly interstitial pattern, the bone marrow infiltrate in large granular lymphocytic leukemia usually is subtle, often requiring immunostains to reveal its presence (see Figure 13-7, *B* to *D*).[154] Nonparatrabecular nodules are also present in about half of the cases, but these represent reactive rather than neoplastic lymphoid aggregates. The nonparatrabecular nodules have a central CD20+, polyclonal B-cell core surrounded by nonneoplastic CD4+ T cells that are distinct from the interstitial and intrasinusoidal CD8+ neoplastic cells; germinal centers often are present.[145,153] Other frequently associated findings include moderately increased reticulin fibrosis and relative eosinophilia in the hematopoietic elements.[153]

Although large granular lymphocytes invariably are present in the bone marrow aspirate, the cytoplasm usually is not well-displayed, and they can be indistinguishable from normal marrow T cells; this emphasizes the importance of peripheral smear review.[145] The surrounding bone marrow often shows erythroid hyperplasia, sometimes with increased early erythroid forms.[145] A subset of cases may show dysplastic changes in one or more hematopoietic lineages, resembling a myelodysplastic syndrome. These changes are frequently associated with anemia, but it is unclear whether they represent true concomitant myelodysplasia or a reactive paraneoplastic phenomenon related to the lymphoma.[155]

Immunostaining of the bone marrow biopsy specimen reveals CD3+, CD8+ lymphocytes that occur in small interstitial clusters and also as linear arrays within vascular sinuses. They comprise an average of 35% of the bone marrow cellularity, often much higher than the estimate of involvement based on routine histology.[145,153] The neoplastic cells express the cytotoxic proteins TIA-1, perforin, and granzyme B. They can express CD57 and show aberrantly weak CD5 expression, but they usually are CD56−.

The main differential diagnosis is with reactive, nonneoplastic proliferations of large granular lymphocytes. Because the latter may be transient, at least a 6-month interval of elevated levels of large granular lymphocytes is required to establish a diagnosis of large granular lymphocytic leukemia (unless prominent leukocytosis is present, which would exclude a reactive etiology). Nonneoplastic increases in large granular lymphocytes may occur after splenectomy, solid organ transplantation, or bone marrow transplantation and also may be seen in association with viral infections.[144] Elderly patients may show persistent clonal CD8+ lymphocytosis without symptoms or cytopenias; these cases are not considered equivalent to large granular lymphocytic leukemia.[156] A lack of neutropenia and/or splenomegaly can be a helpful clue to the nonneoplastic nature of such large granular lymphocytoses. However, Felty's syndrome is characterized by neutropenia and splenomegaly and often shows an increase in large granular lymphocytes. Complicating matters, rheumatoid arthritis and Felty's syndrome can occur together with large granular lymphocytic leukemia.[145] In contrast to most cases of large granular lymphocytic leukemia, normal and reactive CD3+, CD8+ T cells lack CD16

expression and show variable rather than uniformly strong CD57 expression.[145] Loss or dim expression of CD5 and/or CD7 also may be helpful clues to a neoplastic T-cell population. Bone marrow examination can be helpful for disclosing the interstitial and intrasinusoidal cytotoxic CD8+ T-cell infiltrates that characterize large granular lymphocytic leukemia, although the spectrum of bone marrow findings that may occur in reactive large granular lymphocyte proliferations is not well-defined. Ultimately, given the significant morphologic and some immunophenotypic overlap with normal large granular lymphocytes, assessment for T-cell clonality by PCR in a bone marrow or peripheral blood specimen, considered in the context of the typical clinical features (cytopenias with or without splenomegaly), is critical for establishing a definitive diagnosis. T-cell prolymphocytic leukemia also presents with a T-cell lymphocytosis, but its immunophenotype and morphology are distinct from those of large granular lymphocytic leukemia (discussed below).

T-Cell Prolymphocytic Leukemia

T-cell prolymphocytic leukemia (T-PLL) is a rare, highly aggressive leukemic peripheral T-cell lymphoma of adults that involves the blood and bone marrow, usually with associated diffuse lymphadenopathy and hepatosplenomegaly. The median age is 60 to 70 years, and men and women are affected equally. Patients present with leukocytosis that is rapidly progressive: the median lymphocyte doubling time is only 9 months. The leukocytosis of T-PLL historically has been characterized as marked (in most cases exceeding 100×10^9/L). However, a more recent study that used the 2001 WHO classification system reported a median presenting lymphocyte count of 40×10^9/L.[157,158] About one third of patients are diagnosed on the basis of a routine complete blood count (CBC) and do not have disease-related symptoms. However, most patients present with a relatively abrupt onset of systemic symptoms, such as weight loss, fatigue, fever, and/or lymphadenopathy. Skin lesions, such as edema, maculopapular lesions, and erythroderma, are seen in 20% to 30% of patients, and serous effusions also are relatively common.[157,158] Most patients have splenomegaly, but unlike in B-PLL, diffuse lymphadenopathy is common.[73]

The morphology of T-PLL cells in peripheral blood and bone marrow aspirate smears is reminiscent of the prolymphocytes of CLL or B-PLL, but the cells are medium sized rather than large, the cytoplasm is more scant, and the nucleolus is visible but not usually prominent (Figure 13-8, *A* and *B*). The cytoplasm is pale and basophilic and usually lacks granules. Surface cytoplasmic protrusions or blebs may be seen, although this finding is not specific to T-PLL. Some cases may show predominantly small cells with an inconspicuous nucleolus, and a subset of cases may show cerebriform nuclear contours.[159,160] These small cell variants previously were included in the older diagnostic category of "T-cell chronic

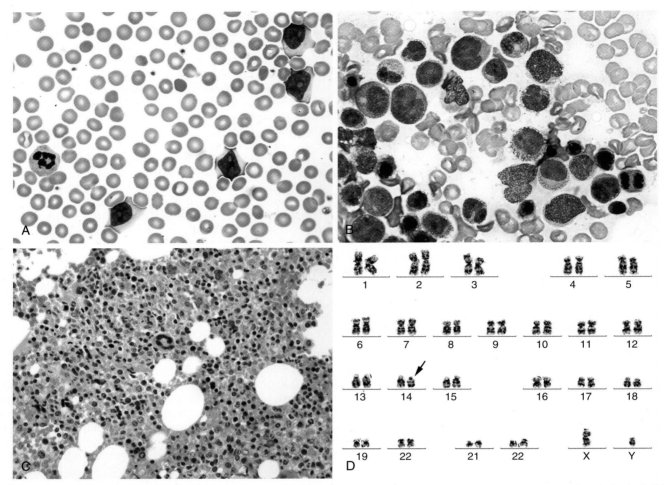

Figure 13-8   T-cell and NK-cell leukemias. **A,** T-cell prolymphocytic leukemia (T-PLL) cells in the peripheral blood appear similar to B-PLL cells but are generally smaller and may have less prominent nucleoli. **B,** In the aspirate smear, T-PLL cells often have a more pleomorphic appearance, with irregular nuclei and cytoplasm containing vacuoles and surface "tags." **C,** The bone marrow biopsy specimen in T-PLL shows a heavy interstitial infiltrate of large, irregular lymphocytes. **D,** Karyotype from bone marrow involved by T-PLL, showing the inv(14) abnormality *(arrow)* present in most cases.

lymphocytic leukemia," which no longer exists in the current 2008 WHO classification system.[161]

The bone marrow is involved in all cases of T-PLL, although the distinctive features usually allow a diagnosis to be made based on peripheral blood examination. The infiltration pattern in the bone marrow typically is heavily interstitial, but a minority of cases can show nodular or diffuse patterns of involvement (see Figure 13-8, *C*).[157] Bone marrow reticulin fiber staining usually is increased.[73]

T-PLL cells are mature T cells that express CD2 and CD3. They also express TCRαβ but not TCRγδ, and they are negative for the precursor T-cell markers TdT and CD1a and for cytotoxic markers, such as TIA-1 and granzyme.[162] Unlike in many peripheral T-cell lymphomas, loss of CD5 or CD7 is very infrequent in T-PLL.[142] Most cases are CD4+/CD8−, and smaller subsets may show a CD4−/CD8+ or CD4+/CD8+ phenotype.[158] The latter "double positive" T-cell phenotype characterizes about one third of T-PLL cases; provided a precursor T-cell neoplasm is excluded, the presence of a CD4+/CD8+ phenotype in a peripheral T-cell leukemia strongly suggests a

diagnosis of T-PLL. TCL1 expression, not present on normal mature T cells, can be demonstrated by immunohistochemistry in 70% to 80% of cases.[142,157]

About 90% of T-PLL cases show rearrangements of chromosome 14q11 and 14q32 loci, most frequently manifesting as inv(14)(q11;q32.1) and less commonly as t(14;14)(q11;q32.1) (see Figure 13-8, *D*). These rearrangements juxtapose the T-cell leukemia 1 (*TCL1*) gene with the T-cell receptor (*TCR*) locus, resulting in overexpression of the TCL1 protein.[163,164] Some cases bear a t(X;14)(q28;q11) translocation the involves the *MTCP1* gene, a *TCL1* homolog.[165,166] Abnormalities of chromosomes 6, 8, 11, and 17, including deletion of the ataxia telangiectasia mutated (*ATM*) gene at 11q23 and the *TP53* gene at 17p13.1, also can be seen.

T-PLL has a poor prognosis; the median survival time is only 27 months. In a subset of cases, the disease can show a relatively indolent behavior.[157,167] Factors associated with an adverse outcome include a WBC count over 40×10^9/L at presentation, a lymphocyte doubling time of less than 6 months, and age over 62 years.[157]

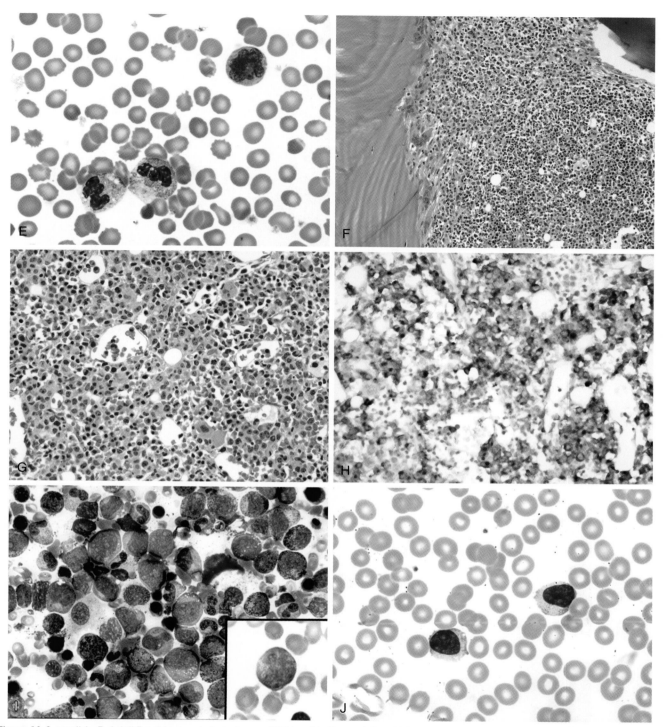

Figure 13-8, cont'd   E, Adult T-cell leukemia/lymphoma (ATLL) cell in the peripheral blood with a highly lobulated nucleus. **F,** ATLL involving the bone marrow, with prominent osteoclastic activity on bone trabecula. The medium to large tumor cells infiltrate the marrow in an interstitial pattern **(G),** and express CD25 **(H)** as well as T-cell markers and CD4 (*not shown*). **I,** Aggressive NK-cell leukemia cells in the bone marrow aspirate and blood (*inset*). The cells are pleomorphic and have abundant basophilic cytoplasm containing occasional fine granules. **J,** Chronic NK lymphoproliferative disorder involving the peripheral blood, with medium-sized lymphoid cells that resemble large granular lymphocytes. (**D** courtesy Aurelia Meloni-Ehrig, Quest Diagnostics, Chantilly, Va.)

The differential diagnosis of T-PLL includes other peripheral T-cell lymphomas that can present with a leukemic picture; features that aid in this differential are listed in Table 13-2. Large granular lymphocytic leukemia usually has a much lower level of lymphocytosis and has neoplastic cells that lack distinct nucleoli and have more abundant, pale cytoplasm that contains granules. The large granular lymphocytes usually are CD8+ rather than CD4+ and, unlike in T-PLL, usually show dim or absent CD5

TABLE 13-2

Differential Diagnosis of T-Cell Leukemias

Feature	T-PLL	T-ALL	ATLL	ANKL	CNKL	LGL
White blood count	Very high	Variable	High in leukemic form	Variable	Low to mildly elevated	Low to mildly elevated
Cell morphology on smears						
Nuclei	Medium sized, round to cerebriform	Small to medium sized, irregular	Medium sized, convoluted and lobated	Medium sized to large, variable shape	Small to medium sized, round	Small to medium sized, round
Chromatin	Moderately dispersed	Finely dispersed	Condensed	Variable, often finely dispersed blastic	Condensed	Condensed
Nucleoli	Small	Absent or small	Absent	Absent or prominent	Absent	Absent
Cytoplasm	Abundant, pale basophilic	Scant	Scant, basophilic	Abundant, basophilic with granules	Abundant, pale to clear with granules	Abundant, pale to clear with granules
Cell surface	Smooth or with blebs	Smooth	Smooth	Smooth	Smooth	Smooth
Marrow infiltration pattern	Interstitial, diffuse, nodular	Diffuse and interstitial	Interstitial and diffuse	Interstitial	Interstitial and intrasinusoidal	Interstitial and intrasinusoidal
Immunophenotype	CD2+, CD3+ CD5+, CD7+ CD4+, sometimes CD4+/CD8+ or CD8+ TCRαβ+ CD56−, CD57−, CD16− TdT−, CD1a−, CD34− TIA-1−, GranB−, CD25− TCL1+/−	CD2+/−, CD3−/+ CD5+, CD7+ Usually CD4+/CD8+ TCRαβ−/+ CD56−/+ TdT+, CD1a+, CD34+/−, CD10+/−, CD99+, CD45dim+ TIA-1−/+, GranB−/+ CytoCD3+	CD2+, CD3+ CD5+, CD7−/+ CD4+, rarely CD4+/CD8+ TCRαβ+ CD57−, CD56−, CD16− TdT−, CD1a−, CD34− TIA-1−, GranB−, CD25+ CD30+/− CytoCD3+	CD2+, CD3− CD5−, CD7+/− CD4−, CD8−/+ TCRαβ−/γδ− CD57−, CD56+, CD16+, CD94+ TdT−, CD1a−, CD34− TIA-1+, GranB+, CD25− CytoCD3+ EBV+	CD2+/−, CD3− CD5−/+, CD7+/− CD4−, CD8−/+ TCRαβ−/γδ− CD57+/−, CD56−/+, CD16+, CD94+ TdT−, CD1a−, CD34− TIA-1+, GranB+ CytoCD3+	CD2+, CD3+ CD5+/−, CD7+/− CD8+ TCRαβ+, rarely TCRγδ+ CD57+/−, CD56−/+, CD16+, CD94+ TdT−, CD1a−, CD34− TIA-1+, GranB+, CD25−
Other helpful findings	Translocations involving TCL1 gene	Various translocations involving TCR locus, mutations in NOTCH1 gene	HTLV-1+ serology	EBV+	Restricted or absent KIR expression	Clonal TCR arrangement, restricted KIR expression

ANKL, Aggressive NK-cell leukemia; *ATLL*, adult T-cell leukemia/lymphoma; *CNKL*, chronic NK-cell lymphoproliferative disorders; *CytoCD3*, CD3 ε epitope; *EBV*, Epstein-Barr virus; *GranB*, granzyme B; *HTLV-1*, human T-cell leukemia virus type 1; *KIR*, killer cell immunoglobulin-like receptor; *LGL*, large granular lymphocyte leukemia; *T-ALL*, T-lymphoblastic leukemia/lymphoma; *TCR*, T-cell receptor; *T-PLL*, T-cell prolymphocytic leukemia.

expression and lack TCL1 expression. Sézary syndrome, a cutaneous T-cell lymphoma with a leukemic component, can resemble T-PLL by manifesting marked leukocytosis in some cases and has a similar CD4+ phenotype[160]; moreover, a subset of T-PLL cases may show erythroderma and neoplastic cutaneous T-cell infiltrates with cerebriform nuclear contours. However, unlike T-PLL, the neoplastic cells of Sézary syndrome are uniformly TCL1–. Also, eosinophilia is common in Sézary syndrome but uncommon in T-PLL.[142] The characteristic lobulated nuclei of adult T-cell leukemia/lymphoma, positive serology for human T-cell leukemia virus type 1 (HTLV-1), and frequently associated hypercalcemia help distinguish this neoplasm from T-PLL.[73] In contrast to T-PLL, hepatosplenic T-cell lymphoma shows a prominently intrasinusoidal pattern in the marrow and has neoplastic cells that usually express TCRγδ. When present, circulating leukemic cells are seen at a much lower level than in T-PLL (median, 1.5 × 10^9/L).[142] Finally, peripheral T-cell lymphoma not otherwise specified (NOS) may manifest a leukemic picture, but this almost always occurs as a feature of disease progression and is accompanied by massive, diffuse lymphadenopathy.

Adult T-Cell Leukemia/Lymphoma

Adult T-cell leukemia/lymphoma (ATLL) is a mature peripheral T-cell leukemia of adults associated with infection by the human retrovirus HTLV-1. The median age at presentation with lymphoma is about 60 years, and men and women are affected equally.[168] ATLL is most prevalent in Japan, the Caribbean, and parts of South America and Africa, areas that are endemic for infection with HTLV-1; by definition, all patients with ATLL have positive serology for HTLV-1.

The clinical presentation of ATLL is highly varied.[169] About 75% of patients present with leukemia, usually manifesting with a rapid onset of systemic symptoms, diffuse lymphadenopathy, hepatosplenomegaly, and leukocytosis with numerous circulating neoplastic cells ("acute" form of disease). A smaller proportion of leukemic cases may present with chronic lymphocytosis of months to years in duration and lacking significant lymphadenopathy or organomegaly; this group of patients usually also shows cutaneous manifestations of the disease (see Chapter 11). About 25% of patients present with lymphoma, showing lymphadenopathy and organomegaly and lacking significant lymphocytosis. Occasional cases present with only an erythematous skin rash, with or without pulmonary infiltration, and fewer than 5% circulating ATLL cells ("smoldering" form of disease).[169] Hypercalcemia, sometimes associated with lytic bone lesions, is common in ATLL and is present at diagnosis or develops during the course of the disease in most patients with the acute leukemic form of disease.[170] Hemophagocytic syndrome also may occur.[171]

In leukemic forms of ATLL, the circulating neoplastic lymphoid cells are pleomorphic. Most are medium sized and have a characteristically convoluted, highly lobated nucleus, described as "flower cells" (see Figure 13-8, E). In contrast to lymphoblasts, the chromatin is condensed and nucleoli are inconspicuous, although a small subpopulation of cells with more dispersed chromatin, resembling blasts, may be present.[169] The cytoplasm usually is basophilic. Cases with chronic or smoldering presentations may have lymphocytes that show less prominent atypia.

The bone marrow aspirate usually shows abnormal cells similar to those seen in the peripheral smear; however, involvement may be subtle or difficult to detect in the bone marrow biopsy specimen.[170] The infiltration pattern is interstitial or diffuse. Concordant with the frequent hypercalcemia, prominent osteoclastic activity on the bone trabeculae may be seen [172] (see Figure 13-8, F and G).

ATLL cells have a mature T-cell phenotype, with expression of the T-cell markers CD2, CD3, and CD5; loss of CD7 is frequent. Most cases are CD4+/CD8–, but rare cases are CD4–/CD8+. Interestingly, a rare "double positive" CD4+/CD8+ phenotypic variant of ATLL, similar to a subset of T-PLL, appears to be associated with more aggressive clinical behavior.[173] Strong expression of CD25 is a characteristic but nonspecific finding, because CD25 may be expressed in other T-cell leukemias (see Figure 13-8, H). In bone marrow sections, the cells may express CD30 but are CD15– and ALK1–.[174] The tumor cells also express FOXP3, which suggests a relationship with regulatory T cells; however, ATLL cells express FOXP3 at lower levels than normal CD4+, CD25+ regulatory T cells.[175] No specific cytogenetic or molecular genetic abnormality is associated with ATLL. The tumor cells contain clonally integrated HTLV-1, indicating the important role of this virus in ATLL leukemogenesis.[168,176]

A diagnosis of leukemic ATLL can be established by examination of the peripheral smear to demonstrate the characteristic "flower cells," in the context of the immunophenotype and positive serology for HTLV-1. A bone marrow biopsy is not necessary in most cases, and bone marrow examination plays no role in staging the leukemic forms of the disease. Diagnosis of smoldering ATLL can be more challenging, because the cells are often infrequent in the peripheral blood, and many healthy patients from endemic regions have positive HTLV-1 serology.

The acute leukemic form of ATLL has a poor prognosis; the median survival time is less than 1 year. The chronic leukemic and smoldering forms of ATLL have a more indolent course but may progress to a more aggressive acute phase of disease.[170,177] A high Ki67 proliferation index in the peripheral blood (greater than 18% Ki67+ T cells) is associated with more aggressive behavior in the chronic leukemic form of ATLL.[178]

Aggressive NK-Cell Leukemia

Aggressive NK-cell leukemia is a rare, highly aggressive EBV+ leukemia that predominantly affects Asians. The median age is 40 to 50 years, and men and women are affected equally.[179] Patients usually present with fever, hepatosplenomegaly, and cytopenias, with or without lymphadenopathy; almost all have B-symptoms and a high or high-intermediate International Prognostic Index (IPI) score.[179,180] An associated hemophagocytic syndrome may be seen.[181,182] The "leukemic" designation is somewhat of a misnomer, because fewer than half of the patients manifest leukocytosis at presentation. The WBC count is highly variable, ranging from 1.5 × 10^9/L to 232 × 10^9/L in one relatively large series.[179] Although aggressive NK-cell leukemia usually is a de novo disease, some cases have been reported that appear to represent transformations from an indolent chronic NK-cell lymphoproliferative disorder (discussed later).[182] The prognosis for aggressive NK-cell leukemia is extremely poor; the median survival time is only 1 to 2 months.[179]

On peripheral blood and bone marrow smear preparations, the neoplastic cells of aggressive NK-cell leukemia have a highly variable appearance that ranges from innocuous-appearing large granular lymphocytes to large lymphoid cells with folded nuclei, vesicular chromatin, and prominent nucleoli. Irrespective of the nuclear morphology, pale cytoplasm with fine cytoplasmic granulation is a characteristic feature. Cells in the aspirate smears are described as having a "comet-like" trailing, deeply basophilic, granulated cytoplasm (see Figure 13-8, I).[183,184] The tumor cells may be abundant or rare in the peripheral blood, ranging from 0 to 92% of all peripheral leukocytes; patients who are cytopenic as a result of hemophagocytic syndrome may have very low numbers of circulating neoplastic cells. The bone marrow shows variable infiltration that comprises a median of 30% of all aspirate cells and can be subtle in some cases.[184] The bone marrow biopsy specimen may be hypercellular or hypocellular with an interstitial infiltrate of neoplastic cells. Associated changes in the nonneoplastic marrow elements include hemophagocytosis and dyserythropoiesis, as well as serous fat atrophy and variable reticulin fibrosis.[184]

The neoplastic cells are CD2+, CD56+ NK cells that lack expression of surface CD3 or TCR. However, CD3 can be detected by paraffin section immunohistochemistry for cytoplasmic CD3.[185] The tumor cells are CD56+ and CD94+ and express cytotoxic proteins such as granzyme B and TIA-1. About 75% of cases express CD16, and most cases express CD7, whereas CD57, CD4, CD5, and CD25 are negative; CD8 is expressed in 29% of cases.[179] Unlike in T-cell lymphomas, immunohistochemistry for the TCRβ chain using the βF1 antibody is negative.[185] No specific cytogenetic finding is seen, and because NK cells do not undergo antigen-receptor gene rearrangements, no TCR gene rearrangement is present. Almost all cases are positive for Epstein-Barr virus–encoded

RNA (EBER) and have been shown to harbor EBV in a clonal episomal form, proving the clonal nature of this disease and its close relationship to EBV.[186]

The main differential diagnosis is with extranodal NK/T-cell lymphoma, nasal type, an EBV+ neoplasm with a similar immunophenotype and morphology that may involve the bone marrow in some cases. Patients with aggressive NK-cell leukemia have more prominent hepatosplenomegaly and lack the skin lesions occasionally found with extranodal NK/T-cell lymphoma.[187] Expression of CD16 also is helpful, because this marker is negative in extranodal NK/T-cell lymphoma.[183] Comparative genomic hybridization has shown genetic changes in aggressive NK-cell leukemia that are different from those of extranodal NK/T-cell lymphoma; this supports the categorization of these two neoplasms as distinct disease entities despite their morphologic and immunophenotypic overlap and shared association with EBV.[188]

The morphology of blastic plasmacytoid dendritic cell neoplasm can overlap with that of aggressive NK-cell leukemia. Although both disorders are CD56+, blastic plasmacytoid dendritic cell neoplasm is negative for EBV and expresses CD4. About 20% of myeloid leukemias express CD56, and some cases can express CD7 as well.[189] Therefore it is important to demonstrate absence of myeloid antigen and CD34 expression in cases of aggressive NK-cell leukemia with a blastic morphology. A subset of T-ALL/LBL cases may express CD56 and/or CD16, as well as cytotoxic markers,[190] and "true NK-cell" cases of CD56– T-ALL/LBL can express the NK-cell marker CD94 and/or KIR.[41] In contrast to aggressive NK-cell leukemia, these cases are TdT+ and should be EBV–. Large granular lymphocytic leukemia can show some morphologic overlap with cases of aggressive NK-cell leukemia showing small cell morphology; however, its phenotype is distinct, and it lacks EBV expression. Features that help differentiate aggressive NK-cell leukemia from other T-cell leukemias are listed in Table 13-2.

Chronic Lymphoproliferative Disorders of NK Cells

Rare indolent proliferations of NK cells that do not show the aggressive clinical behavior of aggressive NK-cell leukemia may occur in adults. Some of these cases previously were considered to represent variants of large granular lymphocytic leukemia. These disorders, also called "chronic NK-cell lymphocytosis," predominantly affect older adults. The median age is 60 years, and a marked male predominance is seen.[191,192] Patients often are asymptomatic or may present with neutropenia, anemia, and/or fever; associated autoimmune phenomena also can occur, such as pure red cell aplasia, vasculitis, or rheumatoid arthritis.[193] The diagnosis is established by demonstrating an unexplained and sustained increase (lasting at least 6 months) in peripheral blood NK cells.

No consensus has been reached regarding the minimum number of NK cells in the peripheral blood required for the diagnosis. Most patients have an absolute NK-cell count higher than 2×10^9/L (the median is about 5×10^9/L; in normal individuals, the median absolute NK-cell count is 0.2×10^9/L). Some authors have advocated using a minimum count of 0.6×10^9/L.[145,192,194]

The morphology of cells in the peripheral blood resembles that of normal large granular lymphocytes. The cells have moderately abundant, pale cytoplasm that contains azurophilic granules (see Figure 13-8, *J*). The phenotype of the neoplastic cells is surface CD3– and CD56+ and CD16+, with variable expression of CD2, CD57, and CD7. Some cases may show aberrant expression of CD5, which is not present on normal NK cells. Other helpful phenotypic deviations from NK cells include abnormally dim expression of CD56 or abnormally bright expression of CD16 and/or CD94.[97,195] No *TCR* gene rearrangement is seen, but KIR antigen expression is restricted in most cases, indicating a clonal proliferation.[192] Some cases may lack KIR expression entirely, an aberrant finding, because all normal NK cells should express this antigen.[195] EBV has been demonstrated in most cases from one series from Japan[187] but does not appear to be present in Western cases.[196]

Involvement of the bone marrow usually is subtle, with interstitial and intrasinusoidal infiltration by small cells that often only can be demonstrated by immunohistochemistry.[197] The bone marrow morphology is similar to that of large granular lymphocytic leukemia, and the neoplastic cells express cytotoxic markers TIA-1 and granzyme B.[195] Bone marrow granulomas may be observed.[198] No specific cytogenetic abnormalities are seen, and most cases have a normal bone marrow karyotype.

Chronic NK lymphoproliferative disorders have an indolent course, although rare cases may transform to aggressive NK-cell leukemia.[194] Similar to patients with large granular lymphocytic leukemia, these patients may develop complications secondary to leukemia-related cytopenias, such as infections. Although chronic NK lymphoproliferative disorders are morphologically identical to large granular lymphocytic leukemia and have similar clinical features at presentation, their NK phenotype is distinct (particularly the lack of surface CD3 expression, because CD56 may be expressed in large granular lymphocytic leukemia). The lack of systemic symptoms and indolent disease course distinguish this disease from aggressive NK-cell leukemia.

Reactive, transient NK proliferations may occur in response to infections, neoplasms (including lymphoma, myelodysplastic syndromes, and solid tumors), or autoimmune diseases. Therefore for a diagnosis of chronic NK lymphoproliferative disorder, the NK lymphocytosis must be sustained and the possibility of a secondary etiology must be eliminated. Uniformly bright CD16 and CD94 expression associated with aberrantly low CD56 and CD57 expression may be helpful clues to a neoplastic NK population; normal NK cells usually show a spectrum of CD16 and CD94 intensity and exhibit intact CD56 and CD57 expression.[185] Compared to normal NK cells, the neoplastic proliferations also may show aberrantly low or absent CD2 or CD7 expression and/or aberrant acquisition of CD5 expression. Because *TCR* is in the germline configuration in all NK proliferations, gene rearrangement studies cannot be used to establish clonality. Clonality can be proven by X-inactivation studies, by demonstrating restricted expression of isoforms of the KIR family of NK-cell receptors, and/or by EBV clonality studies in EBV+ cases; however, these studies are not available in most practices.[187,191,195]

■ LYMPHOMAS SECONDARILY INVOLVING THE BONE MARROW

Mantle Cell Lymphoma

Mantle cell lymphoma is a systemic disease that usually presents with diffuse lymphadenopathy. It involves the bone marrow in nearly all cases at diagnosis and circulating lymphoma cells can be detected in the peripheral smear and by flow cytometry immunophenotyping in most patients.[199] However, only about one quarter of patients have peripheral lymphocytosis (a level exceeding 5×10^9/L).

In bone marrow biopsy sections, most cases show a nodular pattern of involvement that includes paratrabecular infiltrates in almost half of the cases. Interstitial and diffuse patterns also are common, although an exclusively diffuse pattern is rare.[84,199,200] Extensive bone marrow involvement (greater than 50% of biopsy cellularity) is an adverse prognostic feature.[199,201,202] In biopsy sections, the neoplastic cells are small to medium sized with irregular nuclei. The blastoid variant has somewhat larger cells with more dispersed chromatin (Figure 13-9, *A*). The appearance in aspirate and peripheral smears is heterogeneous. Although the neoplastic cells often vary in size in smear preparations and may or may not have prominent nucleoli, the chromatin tends to be more dispersed than that of the cells of CLL, and the nuclei usually have irregular or cleaved nuclear borders (see Figure 13-9, *B*). A common feature that can be a helpful clue to the diagnosis is the presence of a small subset of binucleated or trinucleated cells.[198] In some cases of the blastoid variant, the cells have finely dispersed chromatin and inconspicuous nucleoli resembling lymphoblasts; in other cases, prominent nucleoli resembling myeloblasts or prolymphocytes may be seen (see Figure 13-9, *C*).[203,204]

Five percent to 10% of cases manifest a frankly leukemic presentation with marked leukocytosis.[199] Such "mantle cell leukemia" patients usually present with symptoms related to splenomegaly and/or cytopenias; unlike in CLL, incidental discovery of leukemic mantle cell lymphoma on a routine blood count evaluation is rare.[205] The median lymphocyte count in leukemic cases is 58×10^9/L, and one third

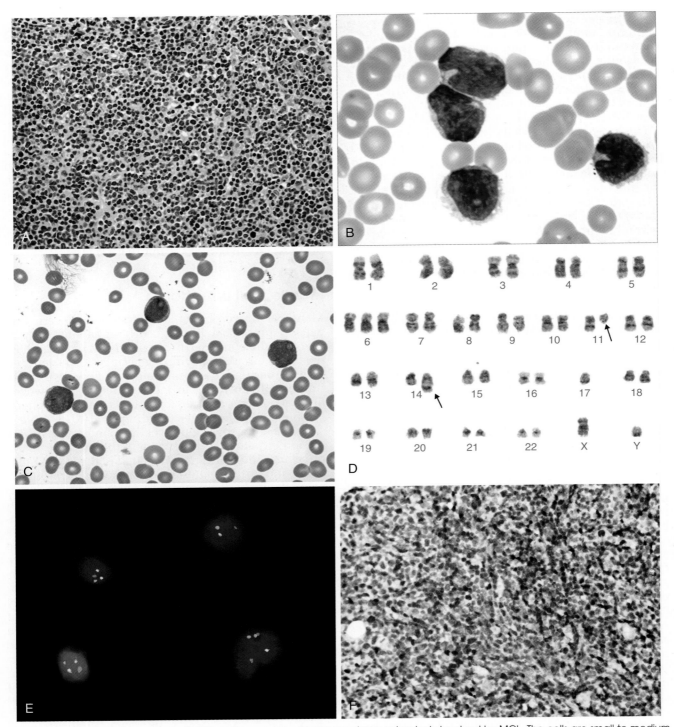

Figure 13-9 Mantle cell lymphoma (MCL). **A,** Bone marrow biopsy specimen extensively involved by MCL. The cells are small to medium sized and have irregular nuclei with monotonously dispersed nuclear chromatin. **B,** MCL involving the blood often manifests as small lymphocytes with irregular or notched nuclei. **C,** The blastoid variant of MCL in the blood frequently shows prominent nucleoli, mimicking prolymphocytic leukemia; however, the cytoplasm usually is less abundant than that of prolymphocytes. **D,** Karyotype of involved bone marrow shows a t(11;14) translocation *(arrows)*. **E,** Fluorescence in situ hybridization (FISH) demonstrates rearrangement of the *CCND1* gene, indicated by a yellow fused signal, as a result of juxtaposition of probes targeting the CCND1 *(red)* and IGH *(green)* loci. **F,** Cyclin D1 immunohistochemistry is strongly, diffusely positive.

of patients present with a lymphocyte count greater than 100 × 10⁹/L.[205] Like nodal-based mantle cell lymphoma involving the marrow, leukemic mantle cell lymphoma often shows a mixed pattern in the bone marrow; however, diffuse and heavy interstitial infiltration is more common, and nodules are less common.[205] Rare leukemic cases may show a prominent intrasinusoidal growth pattern.[206] In one study, the survival of patients with the leukemic presentation of mantle cell lymphoma appeared to be similar to that for nonleukemic patients and was not affected by the level of lymphocytosis or the presence of blastoid morphology.[205] However, another smaller study found very poor overall survival in leukemic cases presenting with marked leukocytosis.[203] Leukemic cases showing smaller cells that resemble those of CLL and lack significant lymphadenopathy often are associated with hypermutation of the *IGH* variable region and a more indolent clinical behavior.[207]

By flow cytometry, a CD20bright+, CD10−, CD5+, CD23− phenotype is characteristic; a small subset of cases may be CD5− or CD23+.[205] Identification of a t(11;14) involving the *CCND1* locus by cytogenetics or FISH analysis and/or demonstration of cyclin D1 expression by immunohistochemistry is critical for differentiating mantle cell lymphoma from CLL and other small B-cell lymphomas (see Figure 13-9, *D* to *F*). Demonstrating surface immunoglobulin expression and lack of TdT is helpful for distinguishing the blastoid variant of mantle cell lymphoma from B-ALL/LBL. Cyclin D1 immunostaining has simplified the differential diagnosis of mantle cell lymphoma with other small B-cell lymphomas. Other features that help distinguish mantle cell lymphoma from other small B-cell lymphomas involving the bone marrow are listed in Table 13-3. Of note, hairy cell leukemia and plasma cell myeloma frequently express cyclin D1, but the characteristic morphologic and other immunophenotypic features of these neoplasms allow their distinction from mantle cell lymphoma. When presenting as a leukemia, mantle cell lymphoma often shows prominent nucleoli and dispersed chromatin and may mimic an acute myeloid or lymphoid leukemia morphologically.[203,208] In such cases, the cells in the bone marrow trephine section often lack the prominent nucleoli present in the blood smears. Immunophenoptyping can readily distinguish mantle cell lymphoma from acute leukemias. The prominent nucleoli, marked leukocytosis, and splenomegaly that often characterize mantle cell lymphoma with a leukemic presentation have led to previous classification of some cases with B-PLL.[209,210] However, mature B-cell leukemias with t(11;14) now are considered to represent mantle cell lymphomas, irrespective of any morphologic resemblance to B-PLL.

Follicular Lymphoma

Bone marrow examination is performed to stage patients with follicular lymphoma in whom the diagnosis already has been established in an extramedullary tissue; it involves the bone marrow in 40% to 70% of patients. The staging bone marrow examination usually is performed to document disease that appears clinically to be stage I or II if bone marrow involvement would result in upstaging of the disease and possibly an alteration in therapy.[211] Whether a staging bone marrow examination should be performed in an apparently localized cutaneous follicular lymphoma is controversial. One recent study found bone marrow involvement as the only extracutaneous manifestation in 6% of cases of

follicular lymphoma presenting in the skin, and these patients had an inferior survival compared to patients lacking bone marrow involvement; these data suggest that bone marrow staging may identify a small subset of patients with cutaneous follicular lymphoma who have clinically relevant, unexpected systemic disease.[212] Bilateral bone marrow samples appear to be no more likely to detect bone marrow involvement than do unilateral samples.[213]

Rare cases of follicular lymphoma may present as leukemia with a high WBC count, clinically mimicking CLL. These patients almost always have concurrent splenomegaly and generalized lymphadenopathy.[214] A clue to the diagnosis of leukemia follicular lymphoma and distinction from CLL is its cytomorphology: the circulating cells in leukemic follicular lymphoma are small and have characteristic deep nuclear clefts or grooves ("buttock cells"), as well as markedly irregular nuclear contours (Figure 13-10, *A* and *B*).[214,215]

In most cases, at least some paratrabecular aggregates are observed in the bone marrow,[84,213] although nonparatrabecular nodules also are frequently seen. Exclusively nonparatrabecular involvement has been reported to occur in up to 14% of cases,[213] whereas interstitial and diffuse patterns of involvement are rare.[84] A high level of bone marrow lymphomatous involvement (10% or more of the marrow space) and a diffuse infiltration pattern are associated with poorer survival.[216] On close inspection, the lymphoid aggregates in follicular lymphoma contain cells with nuclear irregularity and angulation; however, these characteristic nuclear irregularities may be less marked in the bone marrow than in extramedullary follicular lymphoma. The neoplastic cells are arranged in parallel linear arrays immediately adjacent to the bone trabeculae and extending along the trabecular surface, which suggests a strong avidity for the bony surface (see Figure 13-10, *C* to *E*). The paratrabecular lymphomatous aggregates after therapy may be hypocellular, with relatively few lymphoma cells embedded in an area of fibrosis along the bone trabecula.[9]

Neoplastic follicles resembling those present in involved lymph nodes are uncommon in grade 1 and grade 2 follicular lymphoma involving the bone marrow, but they are seen more frequently in grade 3 follicular lymphoma.[84] Unlike germinal centers, which may occur in the bone marrow in reactive conditions and in other lymphomas (e.g., marginal zone lymphomas), the neoplastic follicles in grade 3 follicular lymphoma characteristically lack mantle zones and usually are bcl2+.[84,114] However, some grade 3 cases may be bcl2−, and cases have been reported that show a prominent nonparatrabecular pattern with intact mantle zones.[217]

The follicular lymphoma grade in the staging marrow may be is different from that of the primary extramedullary site; occasional cases of grade 3 follicular lymphoma and even diffuse large B-cell lymphoma are diagnosed in the staging bone marrow of grade 1 or grade 2 follicular lymphoma.[84] The

TABLE 13-3

Differential Diagnosis of Small B-Cell Lymphomas Involving the Bone Marrow

Feature	CLL/SLL	LPL	MCL	N/ENMZL	FL
Percentage of patients with marrow involvement	>90%	>90%	>80%	10% to 40%	40% to 70%
Marrow infiltration pattern	Nodular (nonparatrabecular), interstitial, or diffuse	Any pattern	Diffuse, nodular (often paratrabecular)	Nodular (sometimes paratrabecular), interstitial, intrasinusoidal	Paratrabecular and nonparatrabecular nodules
Cell morphology	Small, round to irregular nuclei; condensed chromatin	Spectrum of small round lymphocytes to mature plasma cells	Small to medium sized, irregular nuclei; moderately dispersed chromatin	Small, round to oval nuclei; condensed chromatin, often plasmacytoid	Small, angulated nuclei; condensed chromatin; variable large cells
Immunophenotype	CD20dim+ CD5+, CD10−, CD23+ Cyclin D1− bcl6−	CD20+ CD5−/+, CD10−, CD23−/+ Cyclin D1− bcl6− IgM+ clonal plasma cells	CD20+ CD5+, CD10−, CD23−/− Cyclin D1+ bcl6−	CD20+ CD5−, CD10−, CD23−/+ Cyclin D1− bcl6−	CD20+ CD5−, CD10+/−, CD23−/+ Cyclin D1− bcl6+
Paraprotein	Usually low or absent	High; almost always IgM	Usually absent	Usually low or absent	Usually absent
Other helpful findings	del(13q), del(11q), del(17q), del(6q), +12	Lymphoplasmacytoid cells on aspirate smears; del(6q)	t(11;14)(q13;q32)	Reactive germinal centers within nodules	t(14;18)

CLL/SLL, Chronic lymphocytic leukemia/small lymphocytic lymphoma; *FL*, follicular lymphoma; *LPL*, lymphoplasmacytic lymphoma; *MCL*, mantle cell lymphoma; *N/ENMZL*, nodal and extranodal marginal zone lymphomas.

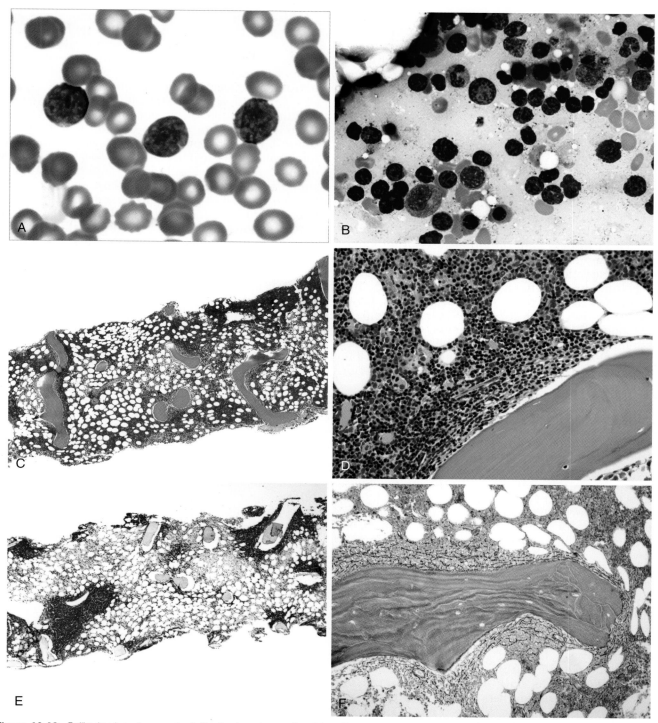

Figure 13-10 Follicular lymphoma. **A,** Follicular lymphoma involving the peripheral blood; small lymphocytes display nuclear clefts, grooves, and convolutions. **B,** Cleaved small lymphocytes may be observed in the bone marrow aspirate in heavily involved cases. **C,** Typical paratrabecular pattern of bone marrow lymphomatous infiltration. **D,** Paratrabecular aggregates comprise elongated arrays of irregular lymphocytes that are closely applied to the bone's trabecular surface and are relatively few cell layers thick. **E,** The neoplastic paratrabecular cells stain for CD20, highlighting their tropism for the trabecular bone surface. **F,** Reticulin fibers are increased in association with the aggregates, which may result in false-negative results by flow cytometry.

specific bone marrow grade (based on the centroblast count) should be reported, regardless of the grade of the extramedullary lymphoma.

Flow cytometry of bone marrow aspirate detects a clonal B-cell population in most cases with bone marrow biopsy involvement,[213] but false-negative results can be seen in up to half of the cases, most likely as a result of reticulin fibrosis associated with the paratrabecular lymphomatous aggregates (see Figure 13-10, *F*).[1,218,219] Conversely, flow cytometry may detect clonal B-cell populations in 1% to 8% of histologically negative staging marrows.[213,219,220] In the absence of histologic confirmation of involvement in the bone marrow biopsy specimen, such cases conventionally are considered negative for staging purposes.[221] Even in the absence of a confirmatory lymph node biopsy specimen, the combination of the characteristic immunophenotype (CD20bright+, CD10+, CD5−, cyclin D1−) with a predominantly or exclusively paratrabecular marrow involvement pattern would favor a diagnosis of follicular lymphoma; one recent study found that 90% of bone marrow lymphoma cases with an exclusively paratrabecular pattern proved to be follicular lymphoma.[84] Demonstrating co-expression of bcl2 and bcl6 and/or CD10 by immunohistochemistry in the bone marrow lymphocytes can help confirm a diagnosis of follicular lymphoma.[222] A t(14;18) involving the *BCL2* gene is characteristic of follicular lymphoma and may be helpful in its differential diagnosis with other lymphomas that involve the bone marrow. However, detection of an *IGH-BCL2* rearrangement in the blood or bone marrow of patients with follicular lymphoma is not considered diagnostic of involvement in the absence of morphologically identifiable lymphoma and does not appear to predict an inferior outcome.[223]

Splenic Marginal Zone Lymphoma

Splenic marginal zone lymphoma involves the bone marrow in most cases: the reported incidence of involvement is as high as 100%.[114] Patients usually present with splenomegaly and lymphocytosis, often with other cytopenias as a result of hypersplenism. Up to 25% may have lymphadenopathy, but this usually is localized to the abdomen, and peripheral lymphadenopathy at presentation is rare.[224]

Bone marrow involvement usually is seen as non-paratrabecular nodules, sometimes surrounding reactive germinal centers, and as intrasinusoidal infiltration (Figure 13-11, *A* to *C*); paratrabecular and interstitial infiltrates also are common.[99,114] Intrasinusoidal lymphoma involvement is characterized by small chains or clusters of neoplastic lymphoid cells within blood vessels, usually clearly identifiable only through immunohistochemistry for B-cell markers such as CD20 or PAX5 (see Figure 13-1, *E;* also Figure 13-11, *D* and *E*). Although commonly observed in splenic marginal zone lymphoma, intrasinusoidal involvement is not present in all cases and can be seen in other types of lymphoma.[114,225] An exclusively intrasinusoidal pattern, which may be overlooked on routine histology, is present in about 10% of cases of splenic marginal zone lymphoma.[10] Monotypic plasma cells are found in some cases.[99] Immunohistochemistry for follicular dendritic cell markers such as CD21 and CD23 may disclose colonized germinal center remnants within the lymphomatous nodules.[99,114]

Most patients have absolute lymphocytosis and rare patients may present with lymphocytosis before the development of splenomegaly.[226] Even in patients lacking lymphocytosis at presentation, neoplastic cells usually can be identified on the peripheral smear and/or detected by flow cytometry. Circulating neoplastic cells are medium sized and have oval nuclei, inconspicuous nucleoli, and a moderate amount of pale, basophilic cytoplasm; some appear plasmacytoid.[138] Cytoplasmic villous projections usually are located at one aspect of the cell surface ("polarized") and are relatively short compared to the longer villi present all around the cell surface in hairy cell leukemia.[227,228] In the bone marrow aspirate, the neoplastic cells appear heterogeneous and show a range of cell sizes and nuclear shapes. Monocytoid cells with moderately abundant, clear cytoplasm; small plasmacytoid cells; and occasional large cells that resemble centroblasts may be observed.[229] As with hairy cell leukemia, the villous projections of splenic marginal zone lymphoma usually are not as well-displayed in the bone marrow aspirate as in the peripheral blood smear.[226]

The immunophenotype of splenic marginal zone lymphoma is CD19+, CD20bright+, CD10−, and usually CD5−, CD103− and CD25−. CD11c and CD23 can be positive or negative DBA 44 can be positive by immunohistochemistry, although DBA 44 staining is more uniform and intense in splenic diffuse red pulp small B-cell lymphoma.[140] Expression of CD5 at variable levels can be seen in 10% to 15% of cases, and this finding alone does not exclude the diagnosis, provided CLL and mantle cell lymphoma can be ruled out. CD5 expression in splenic marginal zone lymphoma may be more frequent in the bone marrow than in the spleen, possibly because of influences within the bone marrow microenvironment.[230]

The combination of a nodular marrow infiltrate (often with intrasinusoidal infiltration, disclosed by CD20 staining), the typical immunophenotype, and characteristic morphology of the circulating neoplastic cells often allows a diagnosis of splenic marginal zone lymphoma in a patient with splenomegaly without the need for splenectomy.[226] The main differential diagnosis in such a context usually is lymphoplasmacytic lymphoma. Although about one third of patients with splenic marginal zone lymphoma have a serum paraprotein, the level usually is relatively low (less than 2 g/dL), and the paraprotein may be IgM or some other heavy chain type.[231] In contrast, the paraprotein in lymphoplasmacytic lymphoma is almost always IgM, and the level usually is higher than 2 g/dL. Also, lymphoplasmacytic lymphoma involvement of the bone marrow typically is more extensive, and intrasinusoidal involvement is uncommon.[226] Cases with heavy bone marrow involvement and a prominent intrasinusoidal pattern may raise the differential of splenic diffuse red pulp small B-cell lymphoma, an entity that

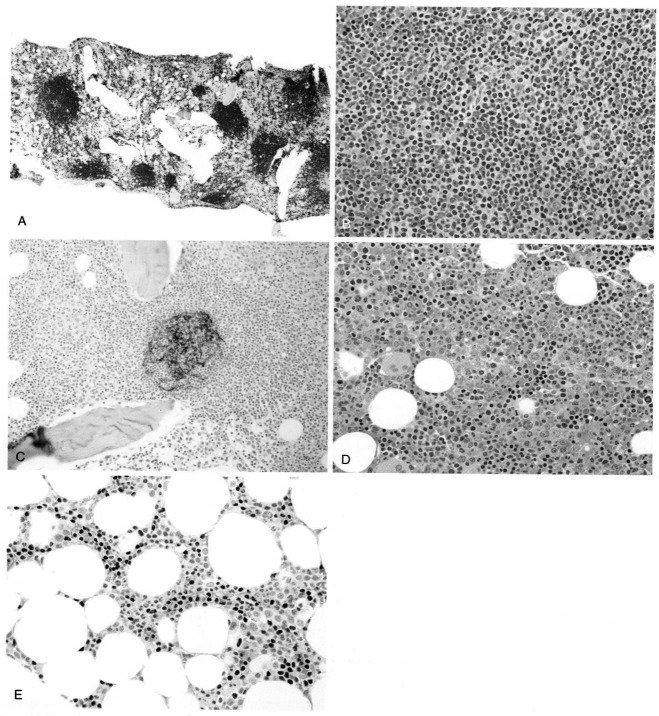

Figure 13-11 Splenic marginal zone lymphoma. **A,** CD20 staining of this bone marrow biopsy specimen highlights nonparatrabecular nodules, as well as numerous linear arrays and single, scattered lymphoma cells. **B,** The nodules are composed of small cells with oval or irregular nuclei and moderately abundant, pale cytoplasm. **C,** Some nodules may have germinal centers or infiltrated follicular structures highlighted by CD21 immunostain. **D,** Intrasinusoidal involvement usually is subtle on hematoxylin and eosin stain but is highlighted by immunohistochemical staining for B-cell markers such as PAX5 **(E)**; an example of CD20 staining illustrating intrasinusoidal involvement by SMZL is also shown in Figure 13-1, *E.*

can be difficult or impossible to distinguish from splenic marginal zone lymphoma on bone marrow histology alone.[140] In ambiguous cases, splenectomy may be required for definitive diagnosis (see Chapter 6). After splenectomy, the extent of bone marrow involvement by splenic marginal zone lymphoma may either increase or decrease. Nodular and interstitial involvement tends to predominate over intrasinusoidal infiltrates later in the course of the disease.[99,232]

Nodal and Extranodal Marginal Zone Lymphomas

Extranodal marginal zone lymphomas of mucosa-associated lymphoid tissue (MALT lymphomas) involve the bone marrow in 10% to 35% of cases; MALT lymphomas of the lung and ocular adnexa involve the bone marrow more frequently than those of the stomach or skin.[233,234] Because bone marrow involvement is not necessarily associated with an adverse clinical outcome, bone marrow sampling is not always performed to stage marginal zone lymphomas at diagnosis.[114,212,233] However, one study did find that bone marrow involvement was associated with an adverse outcome in nongastric marginal zone lymphomas in a multivariate analysis.[235] The National Comprehensive Cancer Network (NCCN) recommends that bone marrow staging be performed in patients with marginal zone lymphoma who have multifocal disease, which may indicate a higher likelihood of bone marrow involvement.[236]

Any bone marrow involvement usually is minimal (the median is 5% of the marrow space), and nodular (including paratrabecular), interstitial, and intrasinusoidal patterns can be seen.[114] About half of patients diagnosed with nodal marginal zone lymphoma have bone marrow involvement and, similar to splenic marginal zone lymphoma and extranodal marginal zone lymphomas, the pattern of bone marrow involvement usually is mixed. The tumor cells in most cases of marginal zone lymphoma are negative for CD5, CD23, CD10, and cyclin D1.[114,229] A small subset of extranodal marginal zone lymphomas express CD5, and these cases may have a higher propensity for bone marrow involvement.[237]

Diffuse Large B-Cell Lymphomas

A staging bone marrow examination is performed in nearly all cases of diffuse large B-cell lymphoma, because the tumor stage is an important component of the prognostically relevant IPI. The primary modality for diagnosing marrow involvement is histology of the bone marrow biopsy specimen; the bone marrow is involved in 11% to 27% of cases.[238-241] Some investigators have suggested that the bone marrow examination can be eliminated in stage I and stage II disease. In one series, the incidence of bone marrow involvement in patients at such a limited clinical stage was low (3.6%) and could be predicted in almost all cases by clinical parameters, such as leukopenia, anemia, and bulky disease.[242] Documenting bone marrow involvement by lymphoma not only categorizes the disease as stage IV, it also may result in an increase in the IPI because of documentation of an additional involved extranodal site.[243] In rare cases, a primary diagnosis of diffuse large B-cell lymphoma may be made from a bone marrow sample in a patient not known to have lymphoma; these patients often are elderly or immunosuppressed and present with fever and cytopenias.[244] Primary bone marrow diffuse large B-cell lymphoma may be more common in Asian patients. Although many such cases likely represent intravascular large B-cell lymphoma (discussed later in this chapter), one recent Asian series reported cases of primary bone marrow diffuse large B-cell lymphoma that showed a nodular and interstitial growth pattern rather than an intrasinusoidal one. These nonintrasinusoidal primary bone marrow lymphomas shared many features with intravascular large B-cell lymphomas, such as severe systemic symptoms at presentation, hemophagocytosis, CD5 expression in a subset of cases, and a short survival time (median, 15 months).[245] Figure 13-12, A, shows an example of a primary bone marrow diffuse large B-cell lymphoma in an HIV-positive patient.

Diffuse large B-cell lymphoma may involve the bone marrow in any pattern. Diffuse and interstitial patterns are most common, but nodular nonparatrabecular and occasionally paratrabecular involvement also may be seen.[84] Flow cytometry and molecular genetic studies to assess clonality can increase the sensitivity of detection, and some studies have shown that patients with negative bone marrow histology but clonal B cells detected by PCR have inferior survival to those lacking a demonstrable B-cell clone.[246] However, histologic diagnosis remains the gold standard for establishing bone marrow involvement.

Immunohistochemistry can be helpful for revealing involvement in rare cases in which the lymphoma cells are scattered among hematopoietic elements. This type of subtle interstitial infiltration pattern may be missed on routine histology and has been shown to have a significant impact on the outcome in histologically occult cases.[239] However, it is controversial whether immunohistochemistry should be performed on all cases of staging bone marrows for diffuse large B-cell lymphoma, and one recent study found no utility in CD20 staining to reveal involvement that was not detected on routine histology.[247] Nevertheless, it is reasonable to use immunohistochemistry for CD20 and/or other B-cell markers in cases that have large cells of uncertain linage (e.g., those with an apparent left-shift of myeloid and/or erythroid elements).

The bone marrow, even when uninvolved by lymphoma, may show reactive dysplastic maturation and left-shift, particularly in the erythroid series, and these may be difficult to distinguish morphologically from large cell lymphoma cells on the biopsy and aspirate specimens (see Figure 13-12, B to D).[244,248] In addition, rare cases of diffuse large B-cell lymphoma diffusely involving the splenic red pulp have been reported to involve the bone marrow in a subtle interstitial and intrasinusoidal pattern that may be obscured by erythroid hyperplasia and left-shift, which require B-cell marker immunohistochemistry for detection.[249] Flow cytometry has a general lack of sensitivity for detecting diffuse large B-cell lymphoma[250]; therefore, a negative flow cytometry result does not obviate the benefit of performing immunohistochemistry. Due to the more patchy involvement

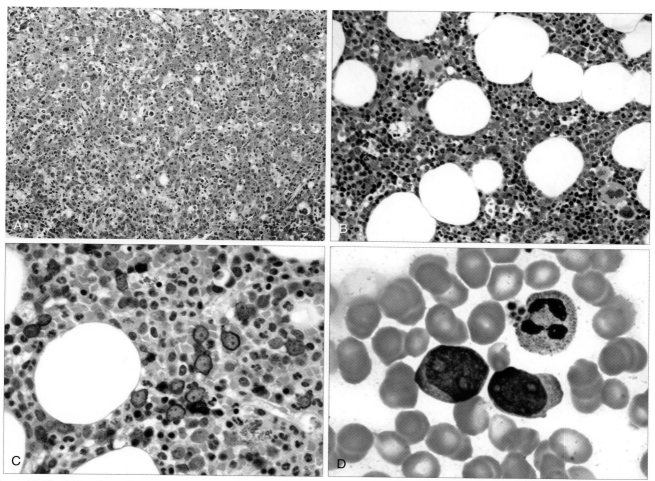

Figure 13-12 Diffuse large B-cell lymphoma (DLBCL). **A,** Extensive primary marrow involvement by DLBCL in an HIV-positive patient who presented with pancytopenia. **B,** Subtle involvement by DLBCL, appearing as large cells that can mimic early erythroid elements. **C,** CD20 immunohistochemical stain discloses the large neoplastic B cells. **D,** Large cells in the aspirate smear may resemble early erythroid elements or blasts, potentially leading to an erroneous diagnosis of a myeloid neoplasm or reactive erythroid hyperplasia.

Continued

seen in diffuse large B-cell lymphoma compared to the low-grade B-cell lymphomas, a larger trephine biopsy sample may be optimal to enhance sensitivity. One study suggested a core longer than 2 cm and examination of multiple histologic levels for optimal staging.[251] Some investigators have suggested that bilateral bone marrow sampling can increase the detection rate for diffuse large B-cell lymphoma by up to 20%, but this practice is not widespread.[252,253]

Of great importance in staging is distinguishing between "concordant" bone marrow involvement, in which the marrow lymphoma is composed predominantly of large cells, and "discordant" involvement, in which the bone marrow contains small neoplastic lymphoid cells with the appearance of a low-grade lymphoma, discordant from the primary diffuse large B-cell lymphoma diagnosed in extramedullary tissue (see Figure 13-12, *E*). Discordant involvement is relatively common, occurring in about half of cases of diffuse large B-cell lymphoma with involved bone marrow.[241,254] Concordant (i.e., large cell) involvement, a diffuse infiltration pattern, and involvement of more than 15% of the marrow space all are

associated with an adverse outcome.[240,241,255] Concordant marrow involvement also is associated with an increased risk of central nervous system relapse and is used by some as an indication for administration of prophylactic intrathecal chemotherapy.[254] Discordant involvement appears to be associated with an increased risk of late relapse but not with poorer overall survival compared to cases lacking any bone marrow involvement.[241,254] In most cases of discordant involvement, the marrow lymphoma can be shown to be clonally related to the extramedullary diffuse large B-cell lymphoma; in about 75% of such clonally-related cases, the marrow lymphoma has the appearance of follicular lymphoma, with paratrabecular aggregates and often an *IGH-BCL2* rearrangement, suggesting that the diffuse large B-cell lymphoma arose as transformation from an occult systemic follicular lymphoma.[250] An alternate hypothesis is that the discordant small cell appearance may reflect changes induced by the bone marrow microenvironment on the large cell lymphoma. In one third of discordant cases, the low-grade bone marrow lymphoma is clonally distinct from the primary diffuse

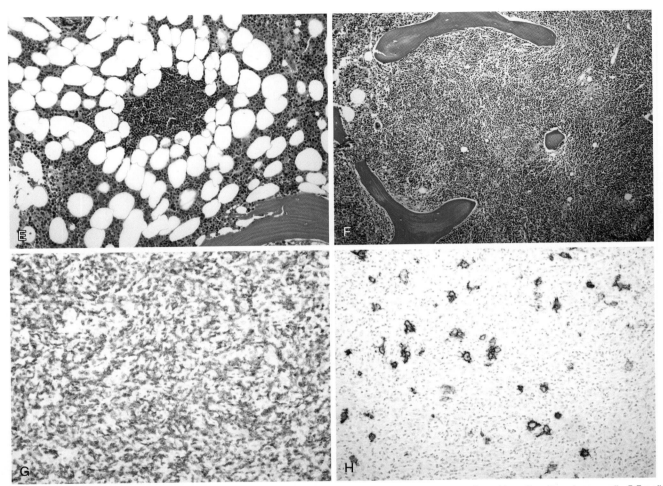

Figure 13-12, cont'd **E,** Discordant marrow involvement by DLBCL, with aggregates of small lymphocytes rather than large cells. **F,** T-cell/histiocyte-rich large B-cell lymphoma, with a diffuse infiltrate of predominantly small lymphocytes and scattered large, nucleolated cells. By immunohistochemistry, the small cells are CD3+ T cells **(G),** whereas the large neoplastic cells are CD20+ B cells **(H).**

large B-cell lymphoma, and in such cases the relationship of the marrow to the extramedullary lymphoma is uncertain.[250] The current convention is to report any type of lymphomatous involvement in the staging marrow and to specify whether the involvement is concordant or discordant.

The 2008 WHO classification system recognizes several distinct variants of diffuse large B-cell lymphoma. Among these, EBV+ diffuse large B-cell lymphoma and T-cell/histiocyte-rich large B-cell lymphoma can show distinct histologic features in involved bone marrow. EBV+ diffuse large B-cell lymphoma affects immunosuppressed patients and elderly nonimmunosuppressed patients. Bone marrow involvement appears to be more common in EBV+ diffuse large B-cell lymphoma than in conventional (EBV-) diffuse large B-cell lymphoma, occurring in almost 40% of cases.[256] EBV+ diffuse large B-cell lymphoma often shows a prominently nodular pattern in the bone marrow, whereas a nodular pattern is relatively uncommon in concordantly involved conventional diffuse large B-cell lymphoma.[257] These bone marrow nodules have a polymorphous appearance, with admixed histiocytes,

plasma cells, and variable numbers of large neoplastic cells that occasionally are located at the periphery of the nodules. The large cells often express CD30, occasionally include Reed-Sternberg-like cells, and are EBV+, as in the primary tumors.[257] In contrast to EBV+ diffuse large B-cell lymphomas of the elderly and immunosuppressed, lymphomatoid granulomatosis, another EBV+ diffuse large B-cell lymphoma, only rarely involves the bone marrow.[258]

T-cell/histiocyte-rich large B-cell lymphoma also may show a higher incidence of marrow involvement (up to 62% in one series) as compared with conventional diffuse large B-cell lymphoma.[259] Paratrabecular nodular and diffuse patterns are common (see Figure 13-12, *F*). In most cases, the histology resembles that of T-cell/histiocyte-rich large B-cell lymphoma in extramedullary sites, with scattered large neoplastic B cells in a predominant background of small T lymphocytes and/or histiocytes (see Figure 13-12, *G* and *H*). However, at relapse in the marrow or in some synchronous staging marrow samples, the tumor may manifest as sheets of large B cells, resembling conventional diffuse large B-cell lymphoma.[260,261]

Intravascular Large B-Cell Lymphoma

Intravascular large B-cell lymphoma (IVLBL) is a rare, highly aggressive lymphoma of adults in which the tumor cells almost exclusively exist within small vascular lumina of various organs, including the bone marrow vascular sinusoids. Three main clinical subtypes have been recognized, based on the pattern of presentation: the *classical*, or *Western form*, in which patients present most often with fever of unknown origin, skin rash, and/or neurologic symptoms; an *isolated cutaneous form*, in which the tumor is limited to skin blood vessels and has a more indolent behavior; and an *Asian variant*, characterized by hepatosplenomegaly, cytopenias, and an often rapid clinical decline because of an associated hemophagocytic syndrome.[262] Despite their intravascular growth pattern, tumor cells are rare in peripheral blood smears (particularly in the classical form), although the neoplastic cells may extravasate into tissues adjacent to involved small vessels. The clinicopathologic features of intravascular large B-cell lymphoma are discussed in more detail in Chapter 14.

The bone marrow is involved in about 75% of cases of the Asian variant of IVLBL, and the diagnosis often is made from a bone marrow biopsy specimen. Only about one third of cases of the classical form of IVLBL have marrow involvement.[263,264] About 38% of the cases are CD5+, and these are more likely to show bone marrow involvement, as well as tumor cells in the peripheral blood.[264] IVLBL often is unsuspected clinically; bone marrow examination may be performed to investigate fever of unknown origin in Western cases and cytopenias and hepatosplenomegaly in Asian variant cases.

In the bone marrow biopsy specimen, the tumor cells are large and have variably abundant cytoplasm; vesicular, often irregular nuclei; and prominent nucleoli. These cells fill dilated bone marrow sinuses but usually are absent from extravascular marrow tissue. Because of their characteristic intrasinusoidal location, neoplastic cells may be sparse or absent in the bone marrow aspirate.[265] They express CD45 as well as pan–B-cell antigens such as CD79a and CD20 but are negative for EBV.[264] In the Asian variant, an associated hemophagocytic syndrome is present in 61% of the cases, and histiocytes containing engulfed erythrocytes and nucleated hematopoietic cells are identified in the extravascular marrow space.[264,265] Histologically negative bone marrow samples from patients with extramedullary IVLBL may show a clonal *IGH* gene rearrangement, suggesting the presence of occult disease.[266] Moreover, subtle intrasinusoidal infiltrates may be revealed by an immunostain for CD20, and some authors suggest that bone marrow involvement may be underrecognized in the classical form of IVLBL.[263,267]

The differential diagnosis of IVLBL in the bone marrow includes other lymphomas that may have an intrasinusoidal growth pattern, such as splenic marginal zone lymphoma, large granular lymphocytic leukemia, and other peripheral T-cell lymphomas. The large cell size; vesicular, highly atypical nuclei; and frequent dilatation of the vascular sinusoids that characterize IVLBL help distinguish it from splenic marginal zone lymphoma.[14] The expression of B-cell markers distinguishes this entity from T-cell lymphomas with an intrasinusoidal growth pattern. Finally, a rare disorder of polyclonal B-cell lymphocytosis may exhibit intravascular collections of B cells. This benign disorder typically affects young female smokers who have splenomegaly, increased polyclonal IgM levels, and a mild lymphocytosis of often binucleated B cells that are polyclonal.[268] The bone marrow from these patients shows an intravascular and mild interstitial accumulation of small B cells that are CD5, CD23, CD43, and CD10 negative but express BCL2. In all cases, the B cells are polyclonal by flow cytometric analysis, and PCR study shows no monoclonal *TCR* or *IGH* gene rearrangements.[269] Interestingly, in most cases an *IGH-BCL2* rearrangement can be demonstrated in the B cells, without other features of follicular lymphoma.[269,270] The characteristic clinical features of polyclonal B-cell lymphocytosis (young females, smokers, lack of systemic symptoms) and small cell size help distinguish this benign disorder from intravascular large B-cell lymphoma.

Burkitt's Lymphoma

Burkitt's lymphoma is a highly aggressive B-cell lymphoma that presents in children, young adults, and occasionally older adults, usually with lymphadenopathy and/or an extranodal mass. The bone marrow is involved in 40% to 60% of patients overall, whereas involvement is present in only about 25% of children with Burkitt's lymphoma.[271,272] Unlike in many other lymphomas, the bone marrow aspirate is at least as useful as the biopsy specimen for detecting involvement, because the cells usually are well-represented in the aspirate smears.[19]

When involved, the bone marrow usually is extensively infiltrated (more than 70% of the marrow space) and shows a diffuse pattern, frequently with areas of geographic necrosis.[84] Bone marrow involvement constitutes Ann Arbor stage IV disease and, similar to diffuse large B-cell lymphoma, is associated with involvement of the central nervous system in both adult and pediatric patients.[271] Involvement of the bone marrow also is an independent poor prognostic marker in children with Burkitt's lymphoma.[272]

Burkitt's lymphoma cells appear in both the biopsy and aspirate as medium-sized cells with dispersed nuclear chromatin, round to slightly irregular nuclei, and multiple small nucleoli (Figure 13-13, *A*). The cytoplasm in air-dried Wright-Giemsa-stained bone marrow aspirate or peripheral blood smears is deeply basophilic and characteristically contains numerous small vacuoles (Figure 13-13, *B*). In biopsy sections, scattered phagocytic histiocytes impart a "starry sky" appearance similar to that seen in Burkitt's lymphoma

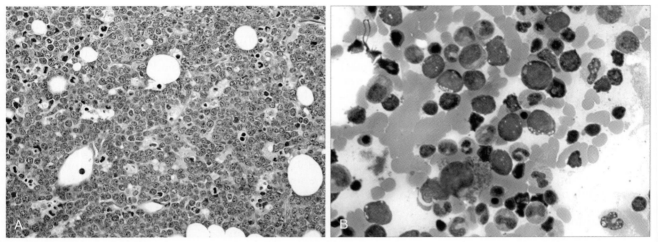

Figure 13-13 Burkitt's lymphoma. **A,** The pattern of marrow involvement usually is diffuse and has a "starry sky" appearance. **B,** The cells characteristically have vacuolated, basophilic cytoplasm on aspirate smears.

involving extramedullary tissues. Neoplastic cells express pan-B-cell markers CD19, CD20, and PAX5 and are bcl6+, brightly CD10+, and bcl2−, with expression of monotypic surface immunoglobulin. The Ki67 proliferation index is nearly 100%. Rearrangement of the *MYC* gene, usually resulting from a t(8;14) translocation involving the *IGH* locus, is a hallmark of Burkitt's lymphoma and is present in almost all cases.

Given the characteristic histologic appearance and immunophenotype, diagnosis of lymphomatous involvement in staging marrow from patients known to have Burkitt's lymphoma is relatively straightforward. However, Burkitt's lymphoma can present as a leukemia in about 15% of cases,[271] and in such cases it may mimic a myeloid or lymphoid leukemia. AML may have a basophilic and vacuolated cytoplasm; flow cytometry and/or immunohistochemical demonstration of myeloid rather than B-cell marker expression are helpful in this distinction.

Differentiating Burkitt's lymphoma from B-ALL can be more problematic, because considerable morphologic overlap may be seen (B-ALL can also have a "starry sky" appearance and a high proliferation index) and, like Burkitt's lymphoma, B-ALL expresses CD19 and can express CD10 and CD20. However, unlike Burkitt's lymphoma, B-ALL is negative for surface immunoglobulin, is TdT+, and often expresses CD34. A subset of childhood B-ALL cases with t(1;19) translocation involving *E2A-PBX1* rearrangement can be CD34−, but these cases are TdT+.[273] The differential diagnosis of Burkitt's lymphoma is discussed further in Burkitt's Lymphoma of the Gastrointestinal Tract in Chapter 5.)

T-Cell Lymphomas

Diagnosis of peripheral T-cell lymphomas in the bone marrow poses a special problem, because these lymphomas are rare, and the bone marrow infiltration pattern often is subtle. In addition, many T-cell lymphomas cause reactive changes in the nonneoplastic marrow elements that may camouflage the

neoplastic infiltrate and lead to diagnosis of another neoplasm or reactive condition.[146] Immunohistochemistry using pan-T-cell markers can be helpful for detecting the often subtle bone marrow infiltrates; among the various T-cell markers, CD2 appears to be the most ubiquitously preserved in T-cell lymphomas.[37] Moreover, patterns of aberrant antigen expression and/or loss can help distinguish lymphomatous infiltrates from reactive bone marrow T-cell populations. Features that aid in the differential diagnosis of T-cell lymphomas that commonly involve the bone marrow are listed in Table 13-4.

Angioimmunoblastic T-Cell Lymphoma

The bone marrow is involved in 54% to 80% of cases of angioimmunoblastic T-cell lymphoma.[100,146,274,275] Patients with anemia at presentation are more likely to have bone marrow involvement.[274] The infiltration pattern is most commonly nodular and often is paratrabecular, but interstitial infiltration also can be present.[100,274] Unlike most other lymphomas with a nodular pattern, the nodules in angioimmunoblastic T-cell lymphoma are often poorly circumscribed and include numerous admixed nonneoplastic epithelioid histiocytes and eosinophils (Figure 13-14, *A*).[100] The neoplastic lymphocytes show the cytologic spectrum seen in involved lymph nodes, including cells with clear cytoplasm (Figure 13-14, *B*).

By immunohistochemistry, the neoplastic lymphocytes stain with pan-T-cell markers such as CD2, CD3, and CD5. Co-expression of CD10 and BCL6 is variable and is seen less often in bone marrow than in the involved lymph nodes. Most cases show co-expression of the follicular chemokine CXCL13 in at least a subset of the neoplastic cells.[100,274] A proliferation of CD21+ follicular dendritic cells, which characterizes nodal angioimmunoblastic T-cell lymphoma, usually is not seen in involved bone marrow.[276]

Because patients often present with systemic symptoms such as fevers and cytopenias, a bone

TABLE 13-4

Differential Diagnosis of T-Cell Lymphomas Involving the Bone Marrow

Feature	AITL	ALCL	PTCL-U	HSTCL
Percentage of patients with marrow involvement	54% to 80%	15%	30% to 40%	>90%
Marrow infiltration pattern	Nodular (often paratrabecular), minor interstitial	Interstitial, sometimes diffuse or nodular	Variably mixed patterns	Intrasinusoidal and interstitial
Cell morphology	Small to medium sized, moderate amount of clear cytoplasm	Small to large; hallmark cells	Variable	Small to large, irregular nuclei, dispersed chromatin, scant cytoplasm
Immunophenotype in marrow	CD2+, CD3+	CD2+/−, CD3+/−	CD2+, CD3+	CD2+, CD3+
	CD5+, CD7+/−	CD5+/−, CD7−/+	CD5+/−, CD7+/−	CD5−/+, CD7+/−
	CD4+, rarely CD8+	Usually CD4+, rarely CD8+	CD4+ or CD8+; may also be CD4−/CD8− or CD4+/CD8+	CD4−/CD8−
	TIA-1−, GranB−, CD25−	TIA-1+, GranB+, CD25+	TIA−/+, GranB−/+, CD25−/+	TIA-1+, GranB−, CD25−
	TCRαβ+	TCRαβ+	TCR αβ+	TCR γδ+
	CXCL13+, CD10−/+, BCL6−/+	CD30+, EMA+, ALK+/−		CD56+
Other helpful findings	Frequent admixed plasma cells, sometimes EBV+ large B cells	Translocations involving ALK gene		iso(7q)

AITL, Angioimmunoblastic T-cell lymphoma; *ALCL:* anaplastic large cell lymphoma; *EBV,* Epstein-Barr virus; *GranB,* granzyme B; *HSTCL,* hepatosplenic T-cell lymphoma; *PTCL-U,* peripheral T-cell lymphoma, unspecified.

marrow biopsy may precede a diagnostic lymph node biopsy. This can create a diagnostic pitfall, because the bone marrow characteristically shows prominent reactive features even when uninvolved by lymphoma. There is usually a marked increase in polytypic plasma cells that can comprise nearly half of the marrow cells.[100] Other findings include hypercellularity, relative erythroid hyperplasia, and reticulin fibrosis; pure red cell aplasia and hemophagocytosis also have been reported.[100,274] Because these features can distract from the neoplastic T-cell infiltrate, misdiagnosis has been reported to occur in approximately half of cases in which a bone marrow biopsy precedes the diagnostic lymph node biopsy. Reported misdiagnoses include myeloproliferative neoplasms, plasma cell neoplasms, hemolytic anemia, and ITP.[100,274,277] The presence of scattered large CD20+ B cells in a subset of angioimmunoblastic T-cell lymphoma can mimic a T-cell/histiocyte-rich large B-cell lymphoma. Expression of EBER in these CD20+ B cells is a hallmark of angioimmunoblastic T-cell lymphoma in the lymph nodes but is seen less frequently in involved bone marrow.[100] Close attention to the morphologic atypia of the aggregated T cells and their characteristic immunophenotype (sometimes CD10+ or BCL6+, usually CXCL13+) can be helpful in raising the possibility of angioimmunoblastic T-cell lymphoma and leading to a confirmatory lymph node biopsy. The neoplastic

cells frequently co-express CD56 by flow cytometry, which can be a helpful clue to the diagnosis.[37] Paratrabecular location of the neoplastic lymphoid nodules, present in many cases, also can be helpful, because paratrabecular lymphoid infiltrates are almost never reactive.

Anaplastic Large Cell Lymphoma

The systemic form of anaplastic large cell lymphoma (ALCL) involves the bone marrow in about 15% of cases.[278,279] In contrast, bone marrow involvement is rare in primary cutaneous ALCL.[280] ALCL can involve the marrow extensively in a diffuse or nodular pattern (see Figure 13-14, *C* and *D*),[281] but many cases show a more subtle, interstitial infiltration pattern. In particular, the small cell variant of ALCL can be difficult to diagnose in the bone marrow and may present as a leukemic form lacking lymphadenopathy.[282] Such leukemic cases manifest as highly atypical lymphoid cells with lobulated nuclei in the blood and bone marrow aspirate; the neoplastic cells in the bone marrow biopsy specimen may be revealed only by staining for CD30 and ALK protein.[282,283] However, in most cases, the diagnosis of ALCL already has been established on an extramedullary biopsy, and the bone marrow examination is performed for staging.

The neoplastic cells of ALCL express CD30 and EMA, as well as ALK protein in ALK+ ALCL.

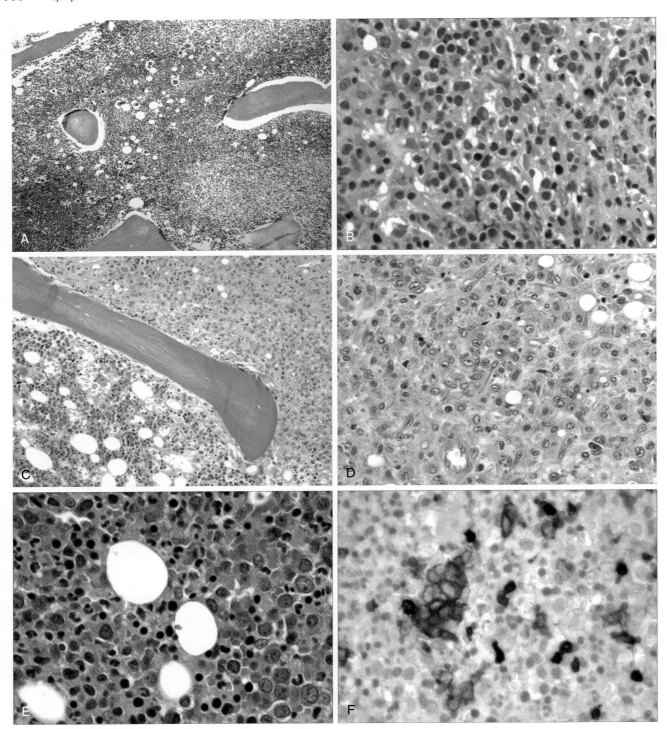

Figure 13-14 Peripheral T-cell lymphomas. **A,** Angioimmunoblastic T-cell lymphoma (AITL) with ill-defined, large nodules in a hypercellular marrow. **B,** The cells in AITL are atypical on high-power view, showing irregular nuclei and a polymorphous appearance. **C,** Anaplastic large cell lymphoma (ALCL) involving the marrow as a large paratrabecular aggregate. **D,** On high-power view, the ALCL cells have pleomorphic nuclei and abundant, pink cytoplasm, including hallmark cells. **E,** Hepatosplenic T-cell lymphoma (HSTCL), with an ill-defined cluster of large cells *(lower right portion of panel)* that is difficult to distinguish from background left-shifted hematopoietic elements. **F,** By immunohistochemistry, the medium-sized to large neoplastic cells in HSTCL often are intravascular and are weakly positive for CD3, in contrast to the benign interstitial small lymphocytes that stain strongly for CD3.

These immunostains can be helpful for disclosing subtle lymphomatous involvement, and most authors recommend immunostaining of all marrow biopsy specimens to stage ALCL.[146] Bone marrow involvement in ALCL, whether histologically

overt or detectable only on immunostains, is associated with an adverse prognosis.[278] In one study on pediatric patients with ALK+ ALCL, reverse transcriptase polymerase chain reaction (RT-PCR) for *NPM-ALK* fusion detected minimal bone marrow involvement in a high proportion of cases that was not seen on routine histologic examination.[279] In this study, patients with molecularly defined minimal involvement had inferior progression-free survival compared to patients with RT-PCR–negative bone marrow. However, no difference in overall survival was seen, and currently, the role of molecular testing for minimal marrow involvement by ALCL remains uncertain. For current staging purposes, a positive marrow should show ALCL cells that are detectable on routine histology or immunohistochemistry or both.

Hepatosplenic T-Cell Lymphoma

Hepatosplenic T-cell lymphoma (HSTCL) is an aggressive T-cell lymphoma that preferentially infiltrates the sinusoids of the liver and spleen, causing hepatomegaly and splenomegaly; the bone marrow is almost invariably involved.[284] Although affected patients often present with anemia and thrombocytopenia, lymphocytosis or circulating neoplastic cells are rare, and the cytopenias usually are due to the concomitant splenomegaly rather than to bone marrow replacement by lymphoma.[285,286] A hemophagocytic syndrome may be present in some cases.[287] HSTCL may also present as a type of post-transplant lymphoproliferative disorder that usually is EBV-negative.[288] Because of the cytopenic presentation and lack of lymphadenopathy, a bone marrow biopsy specimen often is the first diagnostic sample taken in a patient presenting with HSTCL.

The associated systemic symptoms and broad clinical differential of hepatosplenomegaly can distract from consideration of lymphoma in the differential diagnosis. HSTCL usually shows a mixed intrasinusoidal and interstitial infiltration pattern that can be easily overlooked on routine stains.[289,290] The neoplastic cells in both the bone marrow biopsy sample and aspirate vary in size, presenting a spectrum of small, medium-sized, and large forms with round to slightly irregular nuclei, dispersed chromatin, and distinct nucleoli.[146,290] In aspirate smears, the neoplastic cells are large and have basophilic cytoplasm and dispersed chromatin; they usually are infrequent and may be mistaken for blasts.[290]

The characteristic immunophenotype of HSTCL that involves the bone marrow is similar to that seen in extramedullary organs[291] (see Chapter 6). Immunohistochemistry for CD3 is helpful for revealing the neoplastic cells in the bone marrow biopsy (see Figure 13-14, E and F). Similar to angioimmunoblastic T-cell lymphoma, the bone marrow may show hypercellularity, plasmacytosis, and increased vascularity. Hyperlobated megakaryocytes and dyserythropoiesis, presumably reactive in nature, also have been reported.[290]

Cutaneous T-Cell Lymphomas

Mycosis fungoides (MF) and Sézary syndrome (SS) are primary cutaneous T-cell lymphomas that involve the bone marrow in 6% to 22% of cases.[292,293] The International Society for Cutaneous Lymphomas and the European Organization of Research and Treatment of Cancer (ISCL/EORTC) recommend bone marrow staging in patients with cutaneous T-cell lymphomas who have a high blood tumor burden (defined as 1000 Sézary cells/mm^3 or higher) with demonstration of a peripheral blood T-cell clone.[294] However, the utility of this is uncertain, because bone marrow involvement has not been shown to be an independent prognostic variable in multivariate analyses of cases of cutaneous T-cell lymphoma.[295,296]

When present in the peripheral blood or bone marrow, the neoplastic cells of cutaneous T-cell lymphomas (called Sézary cells) are small to medium sized and have markedly convoluted to cerebriform nuclei. Sézary cells also can be detected in the peripheral blood by flow cytometry as an expanded CD4+, CD3+ T-cell population (CD4/CD8 ratio of 10 or higher), with or without an aberrant phenotype in the context of a clonal T-cell population confirmed by PCR.[294] While the presence or absence and degree of peripheral blood involvement are critical determinants in the staging of MF and SS, bone marrow involvement does not factor into the ISCL/EORTC staging system. In fact, there is poor interobserver reproducibility in determining morphologic marrow involvement by cutaneous T-cell lymphomas.[297]

The nuclear abnormalities that characterize peripheral blood Sézary cells may be less pronounced in the bone marrow. Immunohistochemistry often is unhelpful, because the phenotype of cutaneous T-cell lymphomas overlaps with that of the most prevalent bone marrow lymphocytes, CD4+ T cells. In cases with overt marrow involvement, the lymphoid cells appear pleomorphic and have irregular nuclei. They infiltrate the marrow in an interstitial pattern, often forming small clusters with an associated increased reticulin fiber staining.[297] Clonal TCR gene rearrangements frequently can be detected in the bone marrow, irrespective of whether involvement is detected morphologically. The detection of a T-cell clone in the bone marrow does not appear to correlate with patient outcome in patients with MF and SS.[297]

Peripheral T-Cell Lymphoma Not Otherwise Specified and Other T-Cell Lymphomas

Peripheral T-cell lymphoma not otherwise specified (NOS) involves the bone marrow in about one third of cases. A leukemic presentation is rare at diagnosis (fewer than 5% of patients), although it can occur with disease progression associated with development of a massive tumor burden.[298] Enteropathy-associated T-cell lymphoma involves the bone marrow in fewer than 10% of cases.[298] Subcutaneous panniculitis–like T-cell lymphoma is not reported to involve the bone marrow but may be associated with a hemophagocytic syndrome and marked cytopenias in 15% to 20% of cases, findings that are associated with an adverse outcome.[299]

The bone marrow infiltration pattern of peripheral T-cell lymphoma NOS is variable and often mixed; it includes nodular, interstitial, diffuse, and sometimes intrasinusoidal involvement.[146] Ancillary studies such as immunohistochemistry and/or flow cytometry can be helpful for establishing an aberrant immunophenotype, thereby distinguishing the neoplastic T cells from reactive T-cell populations within the bone marrow.[275] Bone marrow involvement in peripheral T-cell lymphomas is an important negative prognostic feature and is included in a proposed prognostic scoring system.[300]

Classical Hodgkin's Lymphoma

Involvement of the bone marrow in classical Hodgkin's lymphoma constitutes Ann Arbor stage IV disease, with possible important therapeutic and prognostic implications if the disease is upstaged beyond the clinical stage. Overall, about 5% to 10% of adult cases of Hodgkin's lymphoma involve the bone marrow; a lower incidence (about 2%) is seen in pediatric patients.[301-303] Bone marrow involvement is least frequent in the lymphocyte-rich and nodular sclerosis subtypes and is most frequent (up to 75%) in the lymphocyte-depleted subtype.[302,304] The likelihood of bone marrow involvement is directly related to the Ann Arbor stage of disease: bone marrow involvement is rare in clinical stage IA and stage IIA disease (fewer than 1% of cases) but common in clinical stage IV disease (32% of cases).[303,305] For these reasons, the NCCN suggests that bone marrow examination may be omitted in stage IA and stage IIA disease.[306] Some investigators have developed a scoring system model to predict bone marrow involvement. Features associated with a greater likelihood of marrow involvement include B-symptoms, anemia, leukopenia, age 35 years or older, and iliac or inguinal nodal involvement. An elevated erythrocyte sedimentation rate, as well as elevated fibrinogen, alkaline phosphatase, and lactate dehydrogenase (LDH), have also been associated with bone marrow involvement. Based on scoring of these clinical parameters, even some patients with stage III or stage IV disease may not require bone marrow examination if the predicted likelihood of involvement is low.[307] It is uncertain whether marrow involvement in patients who are already stage IV represents an additional adverse prognostic feature.[303,305]

In rare cases, Hodgkin's lymphoma may be diagnosed initially in the bone marrow in patients presenting with fever of unknown origin, cytopenias, and/or hepatosplenomegaly. This primary bone marrow presentation is more common in patients with HIV infection; it accounted for 14% of diagnoses of Hodgkin's lymphoma in the HIV setting in one series.[308] In most such cases, extramedullary disease also is present, even if the presenting symptoms reflect bone marrow infiltration,[309] and if possible, biopsy of an involved lymph node is preferable to establish the diagnosis. However, in some cases in HIV-positive patients, Hodgkin's lymphoma appears predominantly to involve the marrow without any identifiable extramedullary sites of disease. Although identification of mononuclear Reed-Sternberg variants is sufficient to confirm involvement in a staging bone marrow specimen, a diagnosis of primary bone marrow Hodgkin's lymphoma requires the presence of diagnostic Reed-Sternberg cells in the appropriate cellular background. The morphologic features of primary bone marrow Hodgkin's lymphoma are similar to those of extramedullary Hodgkin's lymphoma, with CD30+ and CD15+ neoplastic cells that often are EBV+. Marked fibrosis in the involved areas is common, but eosinophils may be sparse.[308] Although such a primary bone marrow presentation of Hodgkin's lymphoma is rare, this lymphoma should be considered in the differential diagnosis of unexplained focal or diffuse marrow fibrosis, particularly in immunosuppressed patients. The outcome for these patients is poor, although administration of chemotherapy results in remission and prolonged survival of some patients.[308]

The criteria for confirming bone marrow involvement in patients with an established diagnosis of Hodgkin's lymphoma were established in 1971.[310] They require identification of typical Reed-Sternberg cells and/or mononuclear Reed-Sternberg variants in an appropriate cellular background in the bone marrow biopsy specimen. The cellular background usually is markedly fibrotic and has a polymorphous admixture of histiocytes, eosinophils, plasma cells, and small lymphocytes (Figure 13-15, *A* and *B*). The associated fibrosis explains why Reed-Sternberg cells are found in only 5% to 10% of bone marrow aspirates from cases with involved biopsy specimens, even after careful examination of the smears.[303,311] Foci of fibrosis, necrosis, or a typical cellular background without identifiable Reed-Sternberg cells or their variants are considered to be suggestive or suspicious of involvement by Hodgkin's lymphoma. In such situations, use of immunohistochemistry for CD30 and CD15 and examination of multiple levels of the bone marrow biopsy may allow identification of the tumor cells and definitive diagnosis of involvement (see Figure 13-15, *C* and *D*). However, because CD30 may be less sensitive in decalcified bone marrow cores, a negative result should be interpreted with caution. A repeat contralateral biopsy also can be helpful for confirming involvement in suspicious cases that cannot be resolved by immunohistochemistry.[253]

Hodgkin's lymphoma usually infiltrates the bone marrow in a diffuse pattern, involving large intertrabecular areas and displacing the normal marrow elements; smaller nodular nonparatrabecular or paratrabecular foci of involvement also may occur.[302] Of note, the Reed-Sternberg cells always occur with an abnormal background and are not admixed within normal marrow elements; putative areas of involvement thus are readily detected on low-power inspection. Bone marrow involvement is more often patchy and focal in Hodgkin's lymphoma than in non-Hodgkin's lymphomas, which

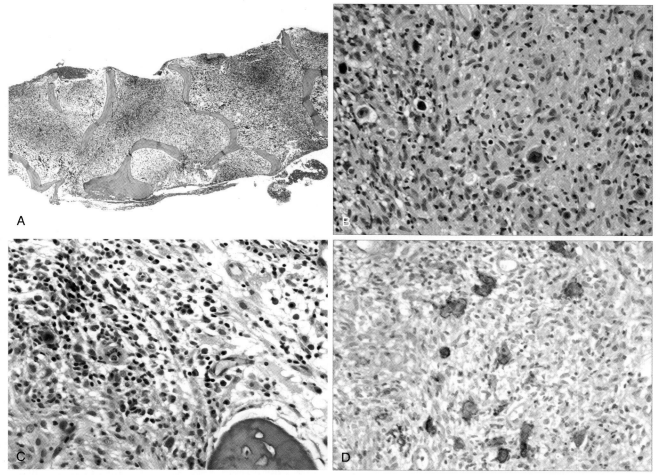

Figure 13-15 Classical Hodgkin's lymphoma. **A,** Bone marrow involvement usually is evident in low-power view as fibrotic areas that often appear hypocellular. **B,** In a high-power view, Reed-Sternberg cells and variants are seen in the typical mixed cellular background with associated fibrosis. **C,** Cases that have a typical background but only occasional atypical cells may require review of additional levels from the paraffin block and immunostaining to reliably demonstrate the Reed-Sternberg variants, highlighted in this case by CD30 **(D).**

has led some investigators to suggest bilateral bone marrow biopsies during staging, particularly when the predicted likelihood of involvement is relatively high.[307,312] The uninvolved hematopoietic areas (either adjacent to foci of Hodgkin's lymphoma or in uninvolved bone marrow from these patients) frequently show nonspecific reactive changes, such as myeloid hyperplasia, eosinophilia, and/or increased megakaryocytes; increased plasma cells, lymphoid aggregates, granulomas, and reticulin fibrosis also may be seen.[313,314] Hemophagocytic syndrome may occur concurrent with bone marrow involved by Hodgkin's lymphoma and may be the presenting manifestation of lymphoma.[315]

The differential diagnosis includes ALCL, T-cell/histiocyte-rich large B-cell lymphoma, primary myelofibrosis, autoimmune myelofibrosis, and metastatic carcinomas or sarcomas. This differential usually can be resolved by using immunohistochemistry to demonstrate CD30 positivity in the large neoplastic cells with lack of strong staining for CD20 and other B-cell markers such as OCT2, BOB1, and CD79a, and negativity for T-cell markers and cytokeratin. Because

of the fibrotic background that surrounds the Reed-Sternberg cells, CD15 often is helpful for diagnosing marrow involvement, because the neoplastic cells are located away from the residual CD15+ normal myeloid elements. Demonstration of weak PAX5 co-expression in the large neoplastic cells also is helpful in excluding other neoplasms, such as CD30+ T-cell lymphomas and ALCL. However, many decalcification procedures may render the characteristically dim PAX5 undetectable in bone marrow Reed-Sternberg cells. CD30+ immunoblasts may be scattered among hematopoietic elements in viral infections such as infectious mononucleosis,[10] but most of the EBV+ cells in infectious mononucleosis do not closely resemble Reed-Sternberg cells and the background is not that of Hodgkin's lymphoma.

Nodular Lymphocyte-Predominant Hodgkin's Lymphoma

Bone marrow involvement in nodular lymphocyte-predominant Hodgkin's lymphoma (NLPHL) is even less common than in classical Hodgkin's lymphoma; it is estimated to occur in only 1% to 2.5% of cases.[304,316] Similar to the bone marrow involvement seen in classical Hodgkin's lymphoma, the involved marrow in NLPHL shows histologic similarities to the primary nodal disease. The pattern of involvement usually is diffuse and less often nodular paratrabecular. Involvement typically is extensive, with tumor occupying a median of 90% of the bone marrow space.[316] The large neoplastic CD20+ "LP cells" resemble those of nodal NLPHL, although nucleoli can be more prominent and centrally located in marrow disease. The LP cells exist as a minority population in a predominant background of CD3+ T cells, histiocytes, and variable numbers of small B cells. Unlike most cases of nodal-based NLPHL, areas of marrow involvement contain relatively few small B cells (typically less prevalent than the T cells) and lack follicular dendritic cells by CD21 staining.[316] CD57+ T cells may be present, but they often are few in number and do not form rosettes around the LP cells. Marrow involvement in NLPHL may be associated with disease that has progressed after therapy or that has adverse features in the extramedullary disease, such as prominent diffuse areas resembling T-cell/histiocyte-rich large B-cell lymphoma or areas of sclerosis. In fact, the features of bone marrow NLPHL closely resemble T-cell/histiocyte-rich large B-cell lymphoma, except that the latter shows a near complete lack of background small B cells.[259,316]

■ OTHER FINDINGS IN BONE MARROW OF LYMPHOMA PATIENTS

The hematopoietic marrow of patients with lymphoma may have abnormal findings apart from merely the presence or absence of lymphoma. The nonneoplastic cells in T-cell lymphomas, hairy cell leukemia, and diffuse large B-cell lymphomas may show dysplastic changes, particularly in the erythroid series.[244,317] These changes, which may be observed even in marrow that is uninvolved by lymphoma, are associated with cytopenias and B-symptoms, which suggests a paraneoplastic phenomenon related to the lymphoma (Figure 13-16, *A*).[248] Increased reticulin fiber deposition often accompanies lymphomatous infiltrates, particularly those in a paratrabecular location; it also may contribute to sampling artifacts such as false-negative results with flow cytometry, and underrepresentation of the lymphoma cells in the bone marrow aspirate smears. Granulomas may be present in marrow involved by Hodgkin's lymphoma[318] or non-Hodgkin's lymphomas, such as hairy cell leukemia.[319]

Hemophagocytic syndromes can be associated with various high-grade lymphomas, including diffuse large B-cell lymphomas, hepatosplenic γδ T-cell lymphoma, aggressive NK-cell leukemia, and peripheral T-cell lymphoma, NOS; many, but not all, such lymphomas are EBV+. Patients with lymphoma-associated hemophagocytic syndrome usually present with systemic symptoms related to splenomegaly, fever, and severe cytopenias.[320] In rare cases hemophagocytic syndrome may precede a diagnosis of lymphoma, but it usually occurs concurrently with the lymphoma, which may or may not involve the bone marrow (see Figure 13-16, *B* to *D*).[320] Hemophagocytosis, in which macrophages in the bone marrow interstitium and/or vascular sinuses contain engulfed red cells and hematopoietic cells, is a hallmark of hemophagocytic syndrome and can be highlighted by CD68 staining of the bone marrow biopsy specimen (see Figure 13-16, *E* and *F*). Reactive cytotoxic CD8+ T cells often are prominent, even in hemophagocytic syndrome cases secondary to B-cell lymphomas. Because the marrow lymphomatous infiltrate may be subtle in such cases, a diagnosis of lymphoma should always be considered for any bone marrow manifesting hemophagocytosis. Immunostains for T-cell and B-cell markers may be helpful for disclosing a subtle infiltrate that may be masked by the prominent reactive histiocytes and small reactive T cells.[320,321] Lymphoma-associated hemophagocytic syndrome has a very poor prognosis.[320]

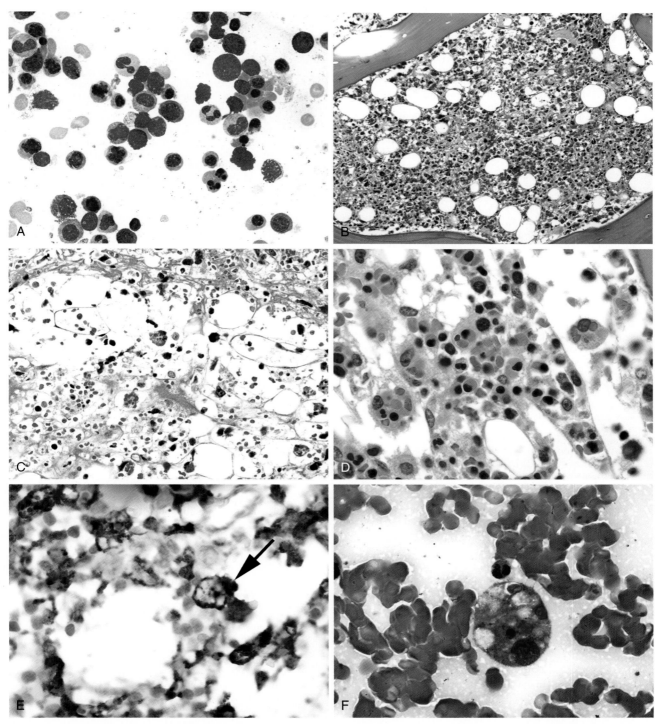

Figure 13-16 Secondary changes observed in the bone marrow of patients with lymphoma. **A,** Morphologic dysplastic changes in the erythroid series in a patient with diffuse large B-cell lymphoma; the bone marrow in this case was negative for lymphoma. **B,** Bone marrow biopsy specimen involved by aggressive NK-cell leukemia and concurrent hemophagocytic syndrome, with a hemorrhagic marrow space containing scattered large, neoplastic lymphoma cells; hemophagocytic syndrome also may occur in marrow uninvolved by lymphoma, such as in subcutaneous panniculitis-like T-cell lymphoma **C. D,** Hemophagocytic histiocytes contain intracytoplasmic erythrocytes and nucleated hematopoietic elements. **E,** CD68 immunohistochemical stain can help highlight the histiocytes that contain ingested cells *(arrow).* **F,** The hemophagocytic histiocytes also may be identifiable on the bone marrow aspirate.

REFERENCES

1. Vega F, Medeiros LJ, Lang WH et al: The stromal composition of malignant lymphoid aggregates in bone marrow: variations in architecture and phenotype in different B-cell tumours, *Br J Haematol* 117:569-576, 2002.

2. Ghia P, Granziero L, Chilosi M, Caligaris-Cappio F: Chronic B cell malignancies and bone marrow microenvironment, *Semin Cancer Biol* 12:149-155, 2002.

3. Cervantes F, Pereira A, Marti JM et al: Bone marrow lymphoid nodules in myeloproliferative disorders: association with the nonmyelosclerotic phases of idiopathic myelofibrosis and immunological significance, *Br J Haematol* 70:279-282, 1988.

4. Thiele J, Zirbes TK, Kvasnicka HM, Fischer R: Focal lymphoid aggregates (nodules) in bone marrow biopsies: differentiation between benign hyperplasia and malignant lymphoma—a practical guideline, *J Clin Pathol* 52:294-300, 1999.

5. Horny HP, Wehrmann M, Griesser H et al: Investigation of bone marrow lymphocyte subsets in normal, reactive, and neoplastic states using paraffin-embedded biopsy specimens, *Am J Clin Pathol* 99:142-149, 1993.

6. Diebold J, Molina T, Camilleri-Broet S et al: Bone marrow manifestations of infections and systemic diseases observed in bone marrow trephine biopsy review, *Histopathology* 37:199-211, 2000.

7. Farhi DC: Germinal centers in the bone marrow, *Hematol Pathol* 3:133-136, 1989.

8. Thiele J, Langohr J, Skorupka M, Fischer R: Reticulin fibre content of bone marrow infiltrates of malignant non-Hodgkin's lymphomas (B-cell type, low malignancy): a morphometric evaluation before and after therapy, *Virchows Arch A Pathol Anat Histopathol* 417:485-492, 1990.

9. Osborne BM, Butler JJ: Hypocellular paratrabecular foci of treated small cleaved cell lymphoma in bone marrow biopsies, *Am J Surg Pathol* 13:382-388, 1989.

10. Anagnostou D: Pitfalls in the pattern of bone marrow infiltration in lymphoproliferative disorders, *Curr Diagn Pathol* 11:170-179, 2005.

11. Rosse C, Kraemer MJ, Dillon TL et al: Bone marrow cell populations of normal infants: the predominance of lymphocytes, *J Lab Clin Med* 89:1225-1240, 1977.

12. Chetty R, Echezarreta G, Comley M, Gatter K: Immunohistochemistry in apparently normal bone marrow trephine specimens from patients with nodal follicular lymphoma, *J Clin Pathol* 48:1035-1038, 1995.

13. Thaler J, Greil R, Dietze O, Huber H: Immunohistology for quantification of normal bone marrow lymphocyte subsets, *Br J Haematol* 73:576-577, 1989.

14. Costes V, Duchayne E, Taib J et al: Intrasinusoidal bone marrow infiltration: a common growth pattern for different lymphoma subtypes, *Br J Haematol* 119:916-922, 2002.

15. Borowitz MJ, Chan JKC: B lymphoblastic leukaemia/lymphoma, not otherwise specified. In Swerdlow S, Campo E, Harris N et al, editors: *WHO classification: tumours of haematopoietic and lymphoid tissues,* ed 4, Lyon, 2008, IARC.

16. Gurney JG, Severson RK, Davis S, Robison LL: Incidence of cancer in children in the United States: sex-, race-, and 1-year age-specific rates by histologic type, *Cancer* 75:2186-2195, 1995.

17. Kahwash SB, Qualman SJ: Cutaneous lymphoblastic lymphoma in children: report of six cases with precursor B-cell lineage, *Pediatr Dev Pathol* 5:45-53, 2002.

18. Maitra A, McKenna RW, Weinberg AG et al: Precursor B-cell lymphoblastic lymphoma: a study of nine cases lacking blood and bone marrow involvement and review of the literature, *Am J Clin Pathol* 115:868-875, 2001.

19. Subira M, Domingo A, Santamaria A et al: Bone marrow involvement in lymphoblastic lymphoma and small noncleaved cell lymphoma: the role of trephine biopsy, *Haematologica* 82:594-595, 1997.

20. Nelson BP, Treaba D, Goolsby C et al: Surface immunoglobulin positive lymphoblastic leukaemia in adults; a genetic spectrum, *Leuk Lymphoma* 47:1352-1359, 2006.

21. Borowitz MJ, Chan JK: B lymphoblastic leukaemia/lymphoma with recurrent genetic abnormalities. In Swerdlow S, Campo E, Harris N et al, editors: *WHO classification: tumours of haematopoietic and lymphoid tissues,* ed 4, Lyon, 2008, IARC.

22. Schultz KR, Pullen DJ, Sather HN et al: Risk- and response-based classification of childhood B-precursor acute lymphoblastic leukemia: a combined analysis of prognostic markers from the Pediatric Oncology Group (POG) and Children's Cancer Group (CCG), *Blood* 109:926-935, 2007.

23. Borowitz MJ, Devidas M, Hunger SP et al: Clinical significance of minimal residual disease in childhood acute lymphoblastic leukemia and its relationship to other prognostic factors: a Children's Oncology Group study, *Blood* 111:5477-5485, 2008.

24. Huh YO, Smith TL, Collins P et al: Terminal deoxynucleotidyl transferase expression in acute myelogenous leukemia and myelodysplasia as determined by flow cytometry, *Leuk Lymphoma* 37:319-331, 2000.

25. Tiacci E, Pileri S, Orleth A et al: PAX5 expression in acute leukemias: higher B-lineage specificity than CD79a and selective association with t(8;21)-acute myelogenous leukemia, *Cancer Res* 64:7399-7404, 2004.

26. van der Velden VH, Bruggemann M, Hoogeveen PG et al: TCRB gene rearrangements in childhood and adult precursor-B-ALL: frequency, applicability as MRD-PCR target, and stability between diagnosis and relapse, *Leukemia* 18:1971-1980, 2004.

27. Komrokji R, Lancet J, Felgar R et al: Burkitt's leukemia with precursor B-cell immunophenotype and atypical morphology (atypical Burkitt's leukemia/lymphoma): case report and review of literature, *Leuk Res* 27:561-566, 2003.

28. Navid F, Mosijczuk AD, Head DR et al: Acute lymphoblastic leukemia with the (8;14)(q24;q32) translocation and FAB L3 morphology associated with a B-precursor immunophenotype: the Pediatric Oncology Group experience, *Leukemia* 13:135-141, 1999.

29. Stamatoullas A, Buchonnet G, Lepretre S et al: De novo acute B cell leukemia/lymphoma with t(14;18), *Leukemia* 14:1960-1966, 2000.

30. Ozdemirli M, Fanburg-Smith JC, Hartmann DP et al: Differentiating lymphoblastic lymphoma and Ewing's sarcoma: lymphocyte markers and gene rearrangement, *Mod Pathol* 14:1175-1182, 2001.

31. McKenna RW, Washington LT, Aquino DB et al: Immunophenotypic analysis of hematogones (B-lymphocyte precursors) in 662 consecutive bone marrow specimens by 4-color flow cytometry, *Blood* 98:2498-2507, 2001.

32. Dworzak MN, Fritsch G, Fleischer C et al: Multiparameter phenotype mapping of normal and post-chemotherapy B lymphopoiesis in pediatric bone marrow, *Leukemia* 11:1266-1273, 1997.

33. Kroft SH: Role of flow cytometry in pediatric hematopathology, *Am J Clin Pathol* 122(suppl):S19-S32, 2004.

34. Borowitz MJ, Chan JK: T lymphoblastic leukaemia/lymphoma. In Swerdlow S, Campo E, Harris N et al, editors: *WHO classification: tumours of haematopoietic and lymphoid tissues,* ed 4, Lyon, 2008, IARC.

35. Goldberg JM, Silverman LB, Levy DE et al: Childhood T-cell acute lymphoblastic leukemia: the Dana-Farber Cancer Institute acute lymphoblastic leukemia consortium experience, *J Clin Oncol* 21:3616-3622, 2003.

36. Borowitz MJ, Bene M-C, Harris NL et al: Acute leukaemias of ambiguous lineage. In Swerdlow S, Campo E, Harris N et al, editors: *WHO classification: tumours of haematopoietic and lymphoid tissues,* ed 4, Lyon, 2008, IARC.

37. Karube K, Aoki R, Nomura Y et al: Usefulness of flow cytometry for differential diagnosis of precursor and peripheral T-cell and NK-cell lymphomas: analysis of 490 cases, *Pathol Int* 58:89-97, 2008.

38. Robertson PB, Neiman RS, Worapongpaiboon S et al: 013 (CD99) positivity in hematologic proliferations correlates with TdT positivity, *Mod Pathol* 10:277-282, 1997.

39. Graux C, Cools J, Michaux L et al: Cytogenetics and molecular genetics of T-cell acute lymphoblastic leukemia: from thymocyte to lymphoblast, *Leukemia* 20:1496-1510, 2006.

40. Weng AP, Ferrando AA, Lee W et al: Activating mutations of NOTCH1 in human T cell acute lymphoblastic leukemia, *Science* 306:269-271, 2004.

41. Lin CW, Liu TY, Chen SU et al: CD94 1A transcripts characterize lymphoblastic lymphoma/leukemia of immature natural killer cell origin with distinct clinical features, *Blood* 106:3567-3574, 2005.

42. Binet JL, Auquier A, Dighiero G et al: A new prognostic classification of chronic lymphocytic leukemia derived from a multivariate survival analysis, *Cancer* 48:198-206, 1981.

43. Muller-Hermelink HK, Montserrat E, Catovsky D et al: Chronic lymphocytic leukaemia/small lymphocytic lymphoma. In Swerdlow S, Campo E, Harris N et al, editors: *WHO classification: tumours of haematopoietic and lymphoid tissues,* ed 4, Lyon, 2008, IARC.

44. National Comprehensive Cancer Network Clinical Practice Guidelines, www.nccn.org/professionals/physician_gls/PDF/nhl.pdf, accessed 4/12/10.

45. Frater JL, McCarron KF, Hammel JP et al: Typical and atypical chronic lymphocytic leukemia differ clinically and immunophenotypically, *Am J Clin Pathol* 116:655-664, 2001.

46. Montserrat E, Villamor N, Reverter JC et al: Bone marrow assessment in B-cell chronic lymphocytic leukaemia: aspirate or biopsy? A comparative study in 258 patients, *Br J Haematol* 93:111-116, 1996.

47. Rozman C, Montserrat E, Rodriguez-Fernandez JM et al: Bone marrow histologic pattern—the best single prognostic parameter in chronic lymphocytic leukemia: a multivariate survival analysis of 329 cases, *Blood* 64:642-648, 1984.

48. Bergmann MA, Eichhorst BF, Busch R et al: Prospective evaluation of prognostic parameters in early stage chronic lymphocytic leukemia (CLL): results of the CLL1-protocol of the German CLL Study Group (GCLLSG), *Blood* 110:165, 2007.

49. Henrique R, Achten R, Maes B et al: Guidelines for subtyping small B-cell lymphomas in bone marrow biopsies, *Virchows Arch* 435:549-558, 1999.

50. Carulli G, Stacchini A, Marini A et al: Aberrant expression of CD8 in B-cell non-Hodgkin lymphoma: a multicenter study of 951 bone marrow samples with lymphomatous infiltration, *Am J Clin Pathol* 132:186-191; quiz, 306; 2009.

51. Delgado J, Matutes E, Morilla AM et al: Diagnostic significance of CD20 and FMC7 expression in B-cell disorders, *Am J Clin Pathol* 120:754-759, 2003.

52. Matutes E, Owusu-Ankomah K, Morilla R et al: The immunological profile of B-cell disorders and proposal of a scoring system for the diagnosis of CLL, *Leukemia* 8:1640-1645, 1994.

53. Morice WG, Kurtin PJ, Hodnefield JM et al: Predictive value of blood and bone marrow flow cytometry in B-cell lymphoma classification: comparative analysis of flow cytometry and tissue biopsy in 252 patients, *Mayo Clin Proc* 83:776-785, 2008.

54. Rai KR, Han T: Prognostic factors and clinical staging in chronic lymphocytic leukemia, *Hematol Oncol Clin North Am* 4:447-456, 1990.

55. Dohner H, Stilgenbauer S, Benner A et al: Genomic aberrations and survival in chronic lymphocytic leukemia, *N Engl J Med* 343:1910-1916, 2000.

56. Shanafelt TD, Witzig TE, Fink SR et al: Prospective evaluation of clonal evolution during long-term follow-up of patients with untreated early-stage chronic lymphocytic leukemia, *J Clin Oncol* 24:4634-4641, 2006.

57. Hamblin TJ, Davis Z, Gardiner A et al: Unmutated Ig V(H) genes are associated with a more aggressive form of chronic lymphocytic leukemia, *Blood* 94:1848-1854, 1999.

58. Tobin G, Soderberg O, Thunberg U, Rosenquist R: V(H)3-21 gene usage in chronic lymphocytic leukemia: characterization of a new subgroup with distinct molecular features and poor survival, *Leuk Lymphoma* 45:221-228, 2004.

59. Rassenti LZ, Huynh L, Toy TL et al: ZAP-70 compared with immunoglobulin heavy-chain gene mutation status as a predictor of disease progression in chronic lymphocytic leukemia, *N Engl J Med* 351:893-901, 2004.

60. Wiestner A, Rosenwald A, Barry TS et al: ZAP-70 expression identifies a chronic lymphocytic leukemia subtype with unmutated immunoglobulin genes, inferior clinical outcome, and distinct gene expression profile, *Blood* 101:4944-4951, 2003.

61. Hamblin TJ, Orchard JA, Ibbotson RE et al: CD38 expression and immunoglobulin variable region mutations are independent prognostic variables in chronic lymphocytic leukemia, but CD38 expression may vary during the course of the disease, *Blood* 99:1023-1029, 2002.

62. Foucar K, Rydell RE: Richter's syndrome in chronic lymphocytic leukemia, *Cancer* 46:118-134, 1980.

63. Tsimberidou AM, Keating MJ: Richter's transformation in chronic lymphocytic leukemia, *Semin Oncol* 33:250-256, 2006.

64. O'Malley DP, Vance GH, Orazi A: Chronic lymphocytic leukemia/small lymphocytic lymphoma with trisomy 12 and focal cyclin D1 expression: a potential diagnostic pitfall, *Arch Pathol Lab Med* 129:92-95, 2005.

65. Matutes E, Morilla R, Owusu-Ankomah K et al: The immunophenotype of splenic lymphoma with villous lymphocytes and its relevance to the differential diagnosis with other B-cell disorders, *Blood* 83:1558-1562, 1994.

66. Rawstron AC, Green MJ, Kuzmicki A et al: Monoclonal B lymphocytes with the characteristics of "indolent" chronic lymphocytic leukemia are present in 3.5% of adults with normal blood counts, *Blood* 100:635-639, 2002.

67. Marti G, Abbasi F, Raveche E et al: Overview of monoclonal B-cell lymphocytosis, *Br J Haematol* 139:701-708, 2007.

68. Rawstron AC, Bennett FL, O'Connor SJ et al: Monoclonal B-cell lymphocytosis and chronic lymphocytic leukemia, *N Engl J Med* 359:575-583, 2008.

69. Hallek M, Cheson BD, Catovsky D et al: Guidelines for the diagnosis and treatment of chronic lymphocytic leukemia: a report from the International Workshop on Chronic Lymphocytic Leukemia updating the National Cancer Institute Working Group 1996 guidelines, *Blood* 111:5446-5456, 2008.

70. Kremer M, Quintanilla-Martinez L, Nahrig J et al: Immunohistochemistry in bone marrow pathology: a useful adjunct for morphologic diagnosis, *Virchows Arch* 447:920-937, 2005.

71. Pezzella F, Munson PJ, Miller KD et al: The diagnosis of low-grade peripheral B-cell neoplasms in bone marrow trephines, *Br J Haematol* 111:369-376, 2000.

72. Campo E, Catovsky D, Montserrat E et al: B-cell prolymphocytic leukaemia. In Swerdlow S, Campo E, Harris N et al, editors: *WHO classification: tumours of haematopoietic and lymphoid tissues,* ed 4, Lyon, 2008, IARC.

73. Krishnan B, Matutes E, Dearden C: Prolymphocytic leukemias, *Semin Oncol* 33:257-263, 2006.

74. Del Giudice I, Davis Z, Matutes E et al: IgVH genes mutation and usage, ZAP-70 and CD38 expression provide new insights on B-cell prolymphocytic leukemia (B-PLL), *Leukemia* 20:1231-1237, 2006.

75. Lens D, De Schouwer PJ, Hamoudi RA et al: p53 abnormalities in B-cell prolymphocytic leukemia, *Blood* 89:2015-2023, 1997.

76. Matutes E: Immunophenotyping and differential diagnosis of hairy cell leukemia, *Hematol Oncol Clin North Am* 20:1051-1063, 2006.

77. Ya-In C, Brandwein J, Pantalony D, Chang H: Hairy cell leukemia variant with features of intrasinusoidal bone marrow involvement, *Arch Pathol Lab Med* 129:395-398, 2005.

78. Morice WG, Chen D, Kurtin PJ et al: Novel immunophenotypic features of marrow lymphoplasmacytic lymphoma and correlation with Waldenström's macroglobulinemia, *Mod Pathol* 22:807-816, 2009.

79. Lin P, Hao S, Handy BC et al: Lymphoid neoplasms associated with IgM paraprotein: a study of 382 patients, *Am J Clin Pathol* 123:200-205, 2005.

80. Remstein ED, Hanson CA, Kyle RA et al: Despite apparent morphologic and immunophenotypic heterogeneity, Waldenström's macroglobulinemia is consistently composed of cells along a morphologic continuum of small lymphocytes, plasmacytoid lymphocytes, and plasma cells, *Semin Oncol* 30:182-186, 2003.

81. Owen RG, Barrans SL, Richards SJ et al: Waldenström macroglobulinemia: development of diagnostic criteria and identification of prognostic factors, *Am J Clin Pathol* 116:420-428, 2001.

82. Vitolo U, Ferreri AJ, Montoto S: Lymphoplasmacytic lymphoma/Waldenström's macroglobulinemia, *Crit Rev Oncol Hematol* 67:172-185, 2008.

83. Dimopoulos MA, Kyle RA, Anagnostopoulos A, Treon SP: Diagnosis and management of Waldenström's macroglobulinemia, *J Clin Oncol* 23:1564-1577, 2005.

84. Arber DA, George TI: Bone marrow biopsy involvement by non-Hodgkin's lymphoma: frequency of lymphoma types, patterns, blood involvement, and discordance with other sites in 450 specimens, *Am J Surg Pathol* 29:1549-1557, 2005.

85. Bartl R, Frisch B, Mahl G et al: Bone marrow histology in Waldenström's macroglobulinaemia: clinical relevance of subtype recognition, *Scand J Haematol* 31:359-375, 1983.

86. Swerdlow SH, Berger F, Pileri SA, Harris NL, Jaffe ES, Stein H. Lymphoplasmacytic lymphoma. In Swerdlow S, Campo E, Harris N et al, editors: *WHO classification: tumours of haematopoietic and lymphoid tissues,* ed 4, Lyon, 2008, IARC.

87. Varghese AM, Rawstron AC, Ashcroft AJ et al: Assessment of bone marrow response in Waldenström's macroglobulinemia, *Clin Lymphoma Myeloma* 9:53-55, 2009.

88. Leleu X, Soumerai J, Roccaro A et al: Increased incidence of transformation and myelodysplasia/acute leukemia in patients with Waldenström macroglobulinemia treated with nucleoside analogs, *J Clin Oncol* 27:250-255, 2009.

89. Lin P, Mansoor A, Bueso-Ramos C et al: Diffuse large B-cell lymphoma occurring in patients with lymphoplasmacytic lymphoma/Waldenström macroglobulinemia: clinicopathologic features of 12 cases, *Am J Clin Pathol* 120:246-253, 2003.

90. Tournilhac O, Santos DD, Xu L et al: Mast cells in Waldenström's macroglobulinemia support lymphoplasmacytic cell growth through CD154/CD40 signaling, *Ann Oncol* 17:1275-1282, 2006.

91. Konoplev S, Medeiros LJ, Bueso-Ramos CE et al: Immunophenotypic profile of lymphoplasmacytic lymphoma/Waldenström macroglobulinemia, *Am J Clin Pathol* 124:414-420, 2005.

92. San Miguel JF, Vidriales MB, Ocio E et al: Immunophenotypic analysis of Waldenström's macroglobulinemia, *Semin Oncol* 30:187-195, 2003.

93. Ocio EM, Schop RF, Gonzalez B et al: 6q deletion in Waldenström macroglobulinemia is associated with features of adverse prognosis, *Br J Haematol* 136:80-86, 2007.

94. Owen RG, Parapia LA, Higginson J et al: Clinicopathological correlates of IgM paraproteinemias, *Clin Lymphoma* 1:39-43; discussion, 44-45; 2000.

95. Valdez R, Finn WG, Ross CW et al: Waldenström macroglobulinemia caused by extranodal marginal zone B-cell lymphoma: a report of six cases, *Am J Clin Pathol* 116:683-690, 2001.

96. Baldini L, Goldaniga M, Guffanti A et al: Immunoglobulin M monoclonal gammopathies of undetermined significance and indolent Waldenström's macroglobulinemia recognize the same determinants of evolution into symptomatic lymphoid disorders: proposal for a common prognostic scoring system, *J Clin Oncol* 23:4662-4668, 2005.

97. Morice WG, Hanson CA, Kumar S et al: Novel multiparameter flow cytometry sensitively detects phenotypically distinct plasma cell subsets in plasma cell proliferative disorders, *Leukemia* 21:2043-2046, 2007.

98. Hoyer JD, Hanson CA, Fonseca R et al: The (11;14)(q13;q32) translocation in multiple myeloma: a morphologic and immunohistochemical study, *Am J Clin Pathol* 113:831-837, 2000.

99. Audouin J, Le Tourneau A, Molina T et al: Patterns of bone marrow involvement in 58 patients presenting primary splenic marginal zone lymphoma with or without circulating villous lymphocytes, *Br J Haematol* 122:404-412, 2003.

100. Grogg KL, Morice WG, Macon WR: Spectrum of bone marrow findings in patients with angioimmunoblastic T-cell lymphoma, *Br J Haematol* 137:416-422, 2007.

101. Bernstein L, Newton P, Ross RK: Epidemiology of hairy cell leukemia in Los Angeles County, *Cancer Res* 50:3605-3609, 1990.

102. Flandrin G, Sigaux F, Sebahoun G, Bouffette P: Hairy cell leukemia: clinical presentation and follow-up of 211 patients, *Semin Oncol* 11:458-471, 1984.

103. Frassoldati A, Lamparelli T, Federico M et al: Hairy cell leukemia: a clinical review based on 725 cases of the Italian Cooperative Group (ICGHCL)—Italian Cooperative Group for Hairy Cell Leukemia, *Leuk Lymphoma* 13:307-316, 1994.

104. Golomb HM: Hairy cell leukemia: an unusual lymphoproliferative disease: a study of 24 patients, *Cancer* 42:946-956, 1978.

105. Humphries JE: Dry tap bone marrow aspiration: clinical significance, *Am J Hematol* 35:247-250, 1990.

106. Polliack A: Hairy cell leukemia: biology, clinical diagnosis, unusual manifestations and associated disorders, *Rev Clin Exp Hematol* 6:366-388; discussion, 449-450, 2002.

107. Bouroncle BA: Thirty-five years in the progress of hairy cell leukemia, *Leuk Lymphoma* 14(suppl 1):1-12, 1994.

108. Burke JS, Byrne GE Jr, Rappaport H: Hairy cell leukemia (leukemic reticuloendotheliosis). I. A clinical pathologic study of 21 patients, *Cancer* 33:1399-1410, 1974.

109. Sharpe RW, Bethel KJ: Hairy cell leukemia: diagnostic pathology, *Hematol Oncol Clin North Am* 20:1023-1049, 2006.

110. Lee WM, Beckstead JH: Hairy cell leukemia with bone marrow hypoplasia, *Cancer* 50:2207-2210, 1982.

111. Burke JS, Rappaport H: The diagnosis and differential diagnosis of hairy cell leukemia in bone marrow and spleen, *Semin Oncol* 11:334-346, 1984.

112. Hasserjian RP, Pinkus GS: DBA.44: an effective marker for detection of hairy cell leukemia in bone marrow biopsies, *Appl Immunohistochem* 2:197-204, 1994.

113. Cessna MH, Hartung L, Tripp S et al: Hairy cell leukemia variant: fact or fiction, *Am J Clin Pathol* 123:132-138, 2005.

114. Kent SA, Variakojis D, Peterson LC: Comparative study of marginal zone lymphoma involving bone marrow, *Am J Clin Pathol* 117:698-708, 2002.

115. Bardawil RG, Groves C, Ratain MJ et al: Changes in peripheral blood and bone marrow specimens following therapy with recombinant alpha 2 interferon for hairy cell leukemia, *Am J Clin Pathol* 85:194-201, 1986.

116. Pittaluga S, Verhoef G, Maes A et al: Bone marrow trephines: findings in patients with hairy cell leukaemia before and after treatment, *Histopathology* 25:129-135, 1994.

117. Zak P, Chrobak L, Podzimek K et al: Dyserythropoietic changes and sideroblastic anemia in patients with hairy cell leukemia before and after therapy with 2-chlorodeoxyadenosine, *Neoplasma* 45:261-265, 1998.

118. Macon WR, Kinney MC, Glick AD, Collins RD: Marrow mast cell hyperplasia in hairy cell leukemia, *Mod Pathol* 6:695-698, 1993.

119. Burthem J, Cawley JC: The bone marrow fibrosis of hairy-cell leukemia is caused by the synthesis and assembly of a fibronectin matrix by the hairy cells, *Blood* 83:497-504, 1994.

120. Carulli G, Cannizzo E, Zucca A et al: CD45 expression in low-grade B-cell non-Hodgkin's lymphomas, *Leuk Res* 32:263-267, 2008.

121. Chen YH, Tallman MS, Goolsby C, Peterson L: Immunophenotypic variations in hairy cell leukemia, *Am J Clin Pathol* 125:251-259, 2006.

122. Foucar K: Chronic lymphoid leukemias and lymphoproliferative disorders, *Mod Pathol* 12:141-150, 1999.

123. Jasionowski TM, Hartung L, Greenwood JH et al: Analysis of CD10+ hairy cell leukemia, *Am J Clin Pathol* 120:228-235, 2003.

124. Robbins BA, Ellison DJ, Spinosa JC et al: Diagnostic application of two-color flow cytometry in 161 cases of hairy cell leukemia, *Blood* 82:1277-1287, 1993.

125. Del Giudice I, Matutes E, Morilla R et al: The diagnostic value of CD123 in B-cell disorders with hairy or villous lymphocytes, *Haematologica* 89:303-308, 2004.

126. Matutes E: Contribution of immunophenotype in the diagnosis and classification of haemopoietic malignancies, *J Clin Pathol* 48:194-197, 1995.

127. Matutes E, Morilla R, Owusu-Ankomah K et al: The immunophenotype of hairy cell leukemia (HCL): proposal for a scoring system to distinguish HCL from B-cell disorders with hairy or villous lymphocytes, *Leuk Lymphoma* 14(suppl 1): 57-61, 1994.

128. Went PT, Zimpfer A, Pehrs AC et al: High specificity of combined TRAP and DBA.44 expression for hairy cell leukemia, *Am J Surg Pathol* 29:474-478, 2005.

129. Hounieu H, Chittal SM, al Saati T et al: Hairy cell leukemia: diagnosis of bone marrow involvement in paraffin-embedded sections with monoclonal antibody DBA.44, *Am J Clin Pathol* 98:26-33, 1992.

130. Miranda RN, Briggs RC, Kinney MC et al: Immunohistochemical detection of cyclin D1 using optimized conditions is highly specific for mantle cell lymphoma and hairy cell leukemia, *Mod Pathol* 13:1308-1314, 2000.

131. Brito-Babapulle V, Ellis J, Matutes E et al: Translocation t(11;14)(q13;q32) in chronic lymphoid disorders, *Genes Chromosomes Cancer* 5:158-165, 1992.

132. Brito-Babapulle V, Matutes E, Oscier D et al: Chromosome abnormalities in hairy cell leukaemia variant, *Genes Chromosomes Cancer* 10:197-202, 1994.

133. Johrens K, Happerfield LC, Brown JP et al: A novel CD11c monoclonal antibody effective in formalin-fixed tissue for the diagnosis of hairy cell leukemia, *Pathobiology* 75:252-256, 2008.

134. Basso K, Liso A, Tiacci E et al: Gene expression profiling of hairy cell leukemia reveals a phenotype related to memory B cells with altered expression of chemokine and adhesion receptors, *J Exp Med* 199:59-68, 2004.

135. Matutes E, Wotherspoon A, Catovsky D: The variant form of hairy-cell leukaemia, *Best Pract Res Clin Haematol* 16:41-56, 2003.

136. Sainati L, Matutes E, Mulligan S et al: A variant form of hairy cell leukemia resistant to alpha-interferon: clinical and phenotypic characteristics of 17 patients, *Blood* 76:157-162, 1990.

137. Zinzani PL, Tani M, Marchi E et al: Long-term follow-up of front-line treatment of hairy cell leukemia with 2-chlorodeoxyadenosine, *Haematologica* 89:309-313, 2004.

138. Melo JV, Hegde U, Parreira A et al: Splenic B cell lymphoma with circulating villous lymphocytes: differential diagnosis of B cell leukaemias with large spleens, *J Clin Pathol* 40:642-651, 1987.

139. Traverse-Glehen A, Baseggio L, Bauchu EC et al: Splenic red pulp lymphoma with numerous basophilic villous lymphocytes: a distinct clinicopathologic and molecular entity? *Blood* 111:2253-2260, 2008.

140. Kanellis G, Mollejo M, Montes-Moreno S et al: Splenic diffuse red pulp small B-cell lymphoma: revision of a series of cases reveals characteristic clinico-pathological features, *Haematologica* 95:1122-1129, 2010.

141. Loughran TP Jr: Clonal diseases of large granular lymphocytes, *Blood* 82:1-14, 1993.

142. Herling M, Khoury JD, Washington LT et al: A systematic approach to diagnosis of mature T-cell leukemias reveals heterogeneity among WHO categories, *Blood* 104:328-335, 2004.

143. Dhodapkar MV, Li CY, Lust JA et al: Clinical spectrum of clonal proliferations of T-large granular lymphocytes: a T-cell clonopathy of undetermined significance? *Blood* 84:1620-1627, 1994.

144. O'Malley DP: T-cell large granular leukemia and related proliferations, *Am J Clin Pathol* 127:850-859, 2007.

145. Morice WG, Kurtin PJ, Tefferi A et al: Distinct bone marrow findings in T-cell granular lymphocytic leukemia revealed by paraffin section immunoperoxidase stains for CD8, TIA-1, and granzyme B, *Blood* 99:268-274, 2002.

146. Dogan A, Morice WG: Bone marrow histopathology in peripheral T-cell lymphomas, *Br J Haematol* 127:140-154, 2004.

147. Lima M, Almeida J, Dos Anjos Teixeira M et al: TCRalphabeta+/CD4+ large granular lymphocytosis: a new clonal T-cell lymphoproliferative disorder, *Am J Pathol* 163:763-771, 2003.

148. Bourgault-Rouxel AS, Loughran TP Jr, Zambello R et al: Clinical spectrum of gammadelta+ T cell LGL leukemia: analysis of 20 cases, *Leuk Res* 32:45-48, 2008.

149. Sandberg Y, Almeida J, Gonzalez M et al: TCRgammadelta+ large granular lymphocyte leukemias reflect the spectrum of normal antigen-selected TCRgammadelta+ T-cells, *Leukemia* 20:505-513, 2006.

150. Langerak AW, van Den Beemd R, Wolvers-Tettero IL et al: Molecular and flow cytometric analysis of the Vbeta repertoire for clonality assessment in mature TCRalphabeta T-cell proliferations, *Blood* 98:165-173, 2001.

151. Lima M, Almeida J, Santos AH et al: Immunophenotypic analysis of the TCR-Vbeta repertoire in 98 persistent expansions of CD3(+)/TCRalphabeta(+) large granular lymphocytes: utility in assessing clonality and insights into the pathogenesis of the disease, *Am J Pathol* 159:1861-1868, 2001.

152. Hoffmann T, De Libero G, Colonna M et al: Natural killer–type receptors for HLA class I antigens are clonally expressed in lymphoproliferative disorders of natural killer and T-cell type, *Br J Haematol* 110:525-536, 2000.

153. Osuji N, Beiske K, Randen U et al: Characteristic appearances of the bone marrow in T-cell large granular lymphocyte leukaemia, *Histopathology* 50:547-554, 2007.

154. Evans HL, Burks E, Viswanatha D, Larson RS: Utility of immunohistochemistry in bone marrow evaluation of T-lineage large granular lymphocyte leukemia, *Hum Pathol* 31:1266-1273, 2000.

155. Huh YO, Medeiros LJ, Ravandi F et al: T-cell large granular lymphocyte leukemia associated with myelodysplastic syndrome: a clinicopathologic study of nine cases, *Am J Clin Pathol* 131:347-356, 2009.

156. Posnett DN, Sinha R, Kabak S, Russo C: Clonal populations of T cells in normal elderly humans: the T cell equivalent to "benign monoclonal gammapathy," *J Exp Med* 179:609-618, 1994.

157. Herling M, Patel KA, Teitell MA et al: High TCL1 expression and intact T-cell receptor signaling define a hyperproliferative subset of T-cell prolymphocytic leukemia, *Blood* 111:328-337, 2008.

158. Matutes E, Brito-Babapulle V, Swansbury J et al: Clinical and laboratory features of 78 cases of T-prolymphocytic leukemia, *Blood* 78:3269-3274, 1991.

159. Matutes E, Garcia Talavera J, O'Brien M, Catovsky D: The morphological spectrum of T-prolymphocytic leukaemia, *Br J Haematol* 64:111-124, 1986.

160. Pawson R, Matutes E, Brito-Babapulle V et al: Sézary cell leukaemia: a distinct T cell disorder or a variant form of T prolymphocytic leukaemia? *Leukemia* 11:1009-1013, 1997.

161. Matutes E, Catovsky D: Similarities between T-cell chronic lymphocytic leukemia and the small-cell variant of T-prolymphocytic leukemia, *Blood* 87:3520-3521, 1996.

162. Matutes E, Coelho E, Aguado MJ et al: Expression of TIA-1 and TIA-2 in T cell malignancies and T cell lymphocytosis, *J Clin Pathol* 49:154-158, 1996.

163. Brito-Babapulle V, Catovsky D: Inversions and tandem translocations involving chromosome 14q11 and 14q32 in T-prolymphocytic leukemia and T-cell leukemias in patients with ataxia telangiectasia, *Cancer Genet Cytogenet* 55:1-9, 1991.

164. Pekarsky Y, Hallas C, Isobe M et al: Abnormalities at 14q32.1 in T cell malignancies involve two oncogenes, *Proc Natl Acad Sci U S A* 96:2949-2951, 1999.

165. Maljaei SH, Brito-Babapulle V, Hiorns LR, Catovsky D: Abnormalities of chromosomes 8, 11, 14, and X in T-prolymphocytic leukemia studied by fluorescence in situ hybridization, *Cancer Genet Cytogenet* 103:110-116, 1998.

166. Stern MH, Soulier J, Rosenzwajg M et al: MTCP-1: a novel gene on the human chromosome Xq28 translocated to the T cell receptor alpha/delta locus in mature T cell proliferations, *Oncogene* 8:2475-2483, 1993.

167. Garand R, Goasguen J, Brizard A et al: Indolent course as a relatively frequent presentation in T-prolymphocytic leukaemia—Groupe Francais d'Hematologie Cellulaire, *Br J Haematol* 103:488-494, 1998.

168. Yamaguchi K: Human T-lymphotropic virus type I in Japan, *Lancet* 343:213-216, 1994.

169. Shimoyama M: Diagnostic criteria and classification of clinical subtypes of adult T-cell leukaemia-lymphoma: a report from the Lymphoma Study Group (1984-87), *Br J Haematol* 79:428-437, 1991.

170. Matutes E: Adult T-cell leukaemia/lymphoma, *J Clin Pathol* 60:1373-1377, 2007.

171. Aouba A, Lambotte O, Vasiliu V et al: Hemophagocytic syndrome as a presenting sign of transformation of smoldering to acute adult T-cell leukemia/lymphoma: efficacy of antiretroviral and interferon therapy, *Am J Hematol* 76:187-189, 2004.

172. Ohshima K, Jaffe E, Kikuchi M: Adult T-cell leukaemia/lymphoma. In Swerdlow S, Campo E, Harris N et al, editors: *WHO classification: tumours of haematopoietic and lymphoid tissues,* ed 4, Lyon, 2008, IARC.

173. Tamura K, Unoki T, Sagawa K et al: Clinical features of OKT4+/OKT8+ adult T-cell leukemia, *Leuk Res* 9:1353-1359, 1985.

174. Takeshita M, Akamatsu M, Ohshima K et al: CD30 (Ki-1) expression in adult T-cell leukaemia/lymphoma is associated with distinctive immunohistological and clinical characteristics, *Histopathology* 26:539-546, 1995.

175. Karube K, Ohshima K, Tsuchiya T et al: Expression of FoxP3, a key molecule in CD4CD25 regulatory T cells, in adult T-cell leukaemia/lymphoma cells, *Br J Haematol* 126:81-84, 2004.

176. Tsukasaki K, Tsushima H, Yamamura M et al: Integration patterns of HTLV-I provirus in relation to the clinical course of ATL: frequent clonal change at crisis from indolent disease, *Blood* 89:948-956, 1997.

177. Ohshima K, Suzumiya J, Sato K et al: Survival of patients with HTLV-I–associated lymph node lesions, *J Pathol* 189:539-545, 1999.

178. Shirono K, Hattori T, Takatsuki K: A new classification of clinical stages of adult T-cell leukemia based on prognosis of the disease, *Leukemia* 8:1834-1837, 1994.

179. Suzuki R, Suzumiya J, Nakamura S et al: Aggressive natural killer–cell leukemia revisited: large granular lymphocyte leukemia of cytotoxic NK cells, *Leukemia* 18:763-770, 2004.

180. Song SY, Kim WS, Ko YH et al: Aggressive natural killer cell leukemia: clinical features and treatment outcome, *Haematologica* 87:1343-1345, 2002.

181. Siu LL, Chan JK, Kwong YL: Natural killer cell malignancies: clinicopathologic and molecular features, *Histol Histopathol* 17:539-554, 2002.

182. Hasserjian RP, Harris NL: NK-cell lymphomas and leukemias: a spectrum of tumors with variable manifestations and immunophenotype, *Am J Clin Pathol* 127:860-868, 2007.

183. Chan JKC, Jaffe E, Ralfkiaer E, Ko YH: Aggressive NK-cell leukaemia. In Swerdlow S, Campo E, Harris N et al, editors: *WHO classification: tumours of haematopoietic and lymphoid tissues,* ed 4, Lyon, 2008, IARC.

184. Ryder J, Wang X, Bao L et al: Aggressive natural killer cell leukemia: report of a Chinese series and review of the literature, *Int J Hematol* 85:18-25, 2007.

185. Morice WG: The immunophenotypic attributes of NK cells and NK-cell lineage lymphoproliferative disorders, *Am J Clin Pathol* 127:881-886, 2007.

186. Chan JK, Sin VC, Wong KF et al: Nonnasal lymphoma expressing the natural killer cell marker CD56: a clinicopathologic study of 49 cases of an uncommon aggressive neoplasm, *Blood* 89:4501-4513, 1997.

187. Oshimi K, Kawa K, Nakamura S et al: NK-cell neoplasms in Japan, *Hematology* 10:237-245, 2005.

188. Nakashima Y, Tagawa H, Suzuki R et al: Genome-wide array-based comparative genomic hybridization of natural killer cell lymphoma/leukemia: different genomic alteration patterns of aggressive NK-cell leukemia and extranodal NK/T-cell lymphoma, nasal type, *Genes Chromosomes Cancer* 44:247-255, 2005.

189. Suzuki R, Murata M, Kami M et al: Prognostic significance of CD7+ CD56+ phenotype and chromosome 5 abnormalities for acute myeloid leukemia M0, *Int J Hematol* 77:482-489, 2003.

190. Dalmazzo LF, Jacomo RH, Marinato AF et al: The presence of CD56/CD16 in T-cell acute lymphoblastic leukaemia correlates with the expression of cytotoxic molecules and is associated with worse response to treatment, *Br J Haematol* 144:223-229, 2009.

191. Lima M, Almeida J, Montero AG et al: Clinicobiological, immunophenotypic, and molecular characteristics of monoclonal CD56-/+dim chronic natural killer cell large granular lymphocytosis, *Am J Pathol* 165:1117-1127, 2004.

192. Rabbani GR, Phyliky RL, Tefferi A: A long-term study of patients with chronic natural killer cell lymphocytosis, *Br J Haematol* 106:960-966, 1999.

193. Morice WG, Leibson PJ, Tefferi A: Natural killer cells and the syndrome of chronic natural killer cell lymphocytosis, *Leuk Lymphoma* 41:277-284, 2001.

194. Oshimi K: Leukemia and lymphoma of natural killer lineage cells, *Int J Hematol* 78:18-23, 2003.

195. Morice WG, Kurtin PJ, Leibson PJ et al: Demonstration of aberrant T-cell and natural killer–cell antigen expression in all cases of granular lymphocytic leukaemia, *Br J Haematol* 120:1026-1036, 2003.

196. Zambello R, Loughran TP Jr, Trentin L et al: Serologic and molecular evidence for a possible pathogenetic role of viral infection in CD3-negative natural killer–type lymphoproliferative disease of granular lymphocytes, *Leukemia* 9:1207-1211, 1995.

197. Villamor N, Morice WG, Chan WC, Foucar K: Chronic lymphoproliferative disorders of NK cells. In Swerdlow S, Campo E, Harris N et al, editors: *WHO classification: tumours of haematopoietic and lymphoid tissues,* ed 4, Lyon, 2008, IARC.

198. Tefferi A, Li CY: Bone marrow granulomas associated with chronic natural killer cell lymphocytosis, *Am J Hematol* 54:258-262, 1997.

199. Cohen PL, Kurtin PJ, Donovan KA, Hanson CA: Bone marrow and peripheral blood involvement in mantle cell lymphoma, *Br J Haematol* 101:302-310, 1998.

200. Wasman J, Rosenthal NS, Farhi DC: Mantle cell lymphoma: morphologic findings in bone marrow involvement, *Am J Clin Pathol* 106:196-200, 1996.

201. Argatoff LH, Connors JM, Klasa RJ et al: Mantle cell lymphoma: a clinicopathologic study of 80 cases, *Blood* 89:2067-2078, 1997.

202. Todorovic M, Pavlovic M, Balint B et al: Immunophenotypic profile and clinical characteristics in patients with advanced stage mantle cell lymphoma, *Med Oncol* 24:413-418, 2007.

203. Viswanatha DS, Foucar K, Berry BR et al: Blastic mantle cell leukemia: an unusual presentation of blastic mantle cell lymphoma, *Mod Pathol* 13:825-833, 2000.

204. Bernard M, Gressin R, Lefrere F et al: Blastic variant of mantle cell lymphoma: a rare but highly aggressive subtype, *Leukemia* 15:1785-1791, 2001.

205. Matutes E, Parry-Jones N, Brito-Babapulle V et al: The leukemic presentation of mantle-cell lymphoma: disease features and prognostic factors in 58 patients, *Leuk Lymphoma* 45:2007-2015, 2004.

206. Schenka AA, Gascoyne RD, Duchayne E et al: Prominent intrasinusoidal infiltration of the bone marrow by mantle cell lymphoma, *Hum Pathol* 34:789-791, 2003.

207. Fernandez V, Salamero O, Espinet B et al: Genomic and gene expression profiling defines indolent forms of mantle cell lymphoma, *Cancer Res* 70:1408-1418, 2010.

208. Wong KF, So CC, Chan JK: Nucleolated variant of mantle cell lymphoma with leukemic manifestations mimicking prolymphocytic leukemia, *Am J Clin Pathol* 117:246-251, 2002.

209. Brito-Babapulle V, Pittman S, Melo JV et al: Cytogenetic studies on prolymphocytic leukemia. I. B-cell prolymphocytic leukemia, *Hematol Pathol* 1:27-33, 1987.

210. Ruchlemer R, Parry-Jones N, Brito-Babapulle V et al: B-prolymphocytic leukaemia with t(11;14) revisited: a splenomegalic form of mantle cell lymphoma evolving with leukaemia, *Br J Haematol* 125:330-336, 2004.

211. National Comprehensive Cancer Network Clinical Practice Guidelines, http://www.nccn.org/professionals/physician_gls/PDF/nhl.pdf, accessed 12/3/09.

212. Senff NJ, Kluin-Nelemans HC, Willemze R: Results of bone marrow examination in 275 patients with histological features that suggest an indolent type of cutaneous B-cell lymphoma, *Br J Haematol* 142:52-56, 2008.

213. Iancu D, Hao S, Lin P et al: Follicular lymphoma in staging bone marrow specimens: correlation of histologic findings with the results of flow cytometry immunophenotypic analysis, *Arch Pathol Lab Med* 131:282-287, 2007.

214. Melo JV, Robinson DS, De Oliveira MP et al: Morphology and immunology of circulating cells in leukaemic phase of follicular lymphoma, *J Clin Pathol* 41:951-959, 1988.

215. Hsieh YC, Lee LP, Chuang SS: Follicular lymphoma with many circulating buttock cells: a leukemic presentation mimicking mantle cell leukemia, *Am J Hematol* 81:294-295, 2006.

216. Canioni D, Brice P, Lepage E et al: Bone marrow histological patterns can predict survival of patients with grade 1 or 2 follicular lymphoma: a study from the Groupe d'Etude des Lymphomes Folliculaires, *Br J Haematol* 126:364-371, 2004.

217. Torlakovic E, Torlakovic G, Brunning RD: Follicular pattern of bone marrow involvement by follicular lymphoma, *Am J Clin Pathol* 118:780-786, 2002.

218. Hanson CA, Kurtin PJ, Katzmann JA et al: Immunophenotypic analysis of peripheral blood and bone marrow in the staging of B-cell malignant lymphoma, *Blood* 94:3889-3896, 1999.

219. Schmidt B, Kremer M, Gotze K et al: Bone marrow involvement in follicular lymphoma: comparison of histology and flow cytometry as staging procedures, *Leuk Lymphoma* 47:1857-1862, 2006.

220. Naughton MJ, Hess JL, Zutter MM, Bartlett NL: Bone marrow staging in patients with non-Hodgkin's lymphoma: is flow cytometry a useful test? *Cancer* 82:1154-1159, 1998.

221. Cheson BD, Horning SJ, Coiffier B et al: Report of an international workshop to standardize response criteria for non-Hodgkin's lymphomas—NCI Sponsored International Working Group, *J Clin Oncol* 17:1244, 1999.

222. Zhang QY, Foucar K: Bone marrow involvement by Hodgkin and non-Hodgkin lymphomas, *Hematol Oncol Clin North Am* 23:873-902, 2009.

223. Paszkiewicz-Kozik E, Kulik J, Fabisiewicz A et al: Presence of t(14;18) positive cells in blood and bone marrow does not predict outcome in follicular lymphoma, *Med Oncol* 26:16-21, 2009.

224. Kurtin PJ: Indolent lymphomas of mature B lymphocytes, *Hematol Oncol Clin North Am* 23:769-790, 2009.

225. Franco V, Florena AM, Campesi G: Intrasinusoidal bone marrow infiltration: a possible hallmark of splenic lymphoma, *Histopathology* 29:571-575, 1996.

226. Matutes E, Oscier D, Montalban C et al: Splenic marginal zone lymphoma proposals for a revision of diagnostic, staging and therapeutic criteria, *Leukemia* 22:487-495, 2008.

227. Isaacson PG, Piris MA, Berger F et al: Splenic B-cell marginal zone lymphoma. In Swerdlow S, Campo E, Harris N et al, editors: *WHO classification: tumours of haematopoietic and lymphoid tissues*, ed 4, Lyon, 2008, IARC.

228. Mollejo M, Camacho FI, Algara P et al: Nodal and splenic marginal zone B cell lymphomas, *Hematol Oncol* 23:108-118, 2005.

229. Berger F, Felman P, Thieblemont C et al: Non-MALT marginal zone B-cell lymphomas: a description of clinical presentation and outcome in 124 patients, *Blood* 95:1950-1956, 2000.

230. Giannouli S, Paterakis G, Ziakas PD et al: Splenic marginal zone lymphomas with peripheral CD5 expression, *Haematologica* 89:113-114, 2004.

231. Catovsky D, Matutes E: Splenic lymphoma with circulating villous lymphocytes/splenic marginal-zone lymphoma, *Semin Hematol* 36:148-154, 1999.

232. Franco V, Florena AM, Stella M et al: Splenectomy influences bone marrow infiltration in patients with splenic marginal zone cell lymphoma with or without villous lymphocytes, *Cancer* 91:294-301, 2001.

233. Thieblemont C, Berger F, Dumontet C et al: Mucosa-associated lymphoid tissue lymphoma is a disseminated disease in one third of 158 patients analyzed, *Blood* 95:802-826, 2000.

234. Raderer M, Streubel B, Woehrer S et al: High relapse rate in patients with MALT lymphoma warrants lifelong follow-up, *Clin Cancer Res* 11:3349-3352, 2005.

235. Arcaini L, Burcheri S, Rossi A et al: Nongastric marginal-zone B-cell MALT lymphoma: prognostic value of disease dissemination, *Oncologist* 11:285-291, 2006.

236. National Comprehensive Cancer Network Clinical Practice Guidelines, www.nccn.org/professionals/physician_gls/PDF/nhl.pdf, accessed 4/12/10.

237. Ferry JA, Yang WI, Zukerberg LR et al: CD5+ extranodal marginal zone B-cell (MALT) lymphoma: a low grade neoplasm with a propensity for bone marrow involvement and relapse, *Am J Clin Pathol* 105:31-37, 1996.

238. Palacio C, Acebedo G, Navarrete M et al: Flow cytometry in the bone marrow evaluation of follicular and diffuse large B-cell lymphomas, *Haematologica* 86:934-940, 2001.

239. Talaulikar D, Dahlstrom JE, Shadbolt B et al: Role of immunohistochemistry in staging diffuse large B-cell lymphoma (DLBCL), *J Histochem Cytochem* 56:893-900, 2008.

240. Campbell J, Seymour JF, Matthews J et al: The prognostic impact of bone marrow involvement in patients with diffuse large cell lymphoma varies according to the degree of infiltration and presence of discordant marrow involvement, *Eur J Haematol* 76:473-480, 2006.

241. Chung R, Lai R, Wei P et al: Concordant but not discordant bone marrow involvement in diffuse large B-cell lymphoma predicts a poor clinical outcome independent of the International Prognostic Index, *Blood* 110:1278-1282, 2007.

242. Lim ST, Tao M, Cheung YB et al: Can patients with early-stage diffuse large B-cell lymphoma be treated without bone marrow biopsy? *Ann Oncol* 16:215-218, 2005.

243. Talaulikar D, Dahlstrom JE: Staging bone marrow in diffuse large B-cell lymphoma: the role of ancillary investigations, *Pathology* 41:214-222, 2009.

244. Ponzoni M, Li CY: Isolated bone marrow non-Hodgkin's lymphoma: a clinicopathologic study, *Mayo Clin Proc* 69:37-43, 1994.

245. Kajiura D, Yamashita Y, Mori N: Diffuse large B-cell lymphoma initially manifesting in the bone marrow, *Am J Clin Pathol* 127:762-769, 2007.

246. Mitterbauer-Hohendanner G, Mannhalter C, Winkler K et al: Prognostic significance of molecular staging by PCR-amplification of immunoglobulin gene rearrangements in diffuse large B-cell lymphoma (DLBCL), *Leukemia* 18:1102-1107, 2004.

247. Baiyee D, Warnke R, Natkunam Y: Lack of utility of CD20 immunohistochemistry in staging bone marrow biopsies for diffuse large B-cell lymphoma, *Appl Immunohistochem Mol Morphol* 17:93-95, 2009.

248. Nardi V, Abramson JS, Hasserjian R: Morphologic dysplasia in staging marrow from high-grade non-Hodgkin's lymphoma patients: a paraneoplastic phenomenon associated with adverse clinical outcome, *Mod Pathol* 23:314A, 2010.

249. Morice WG, Rodriguez FJ, Hoyer JD, Kurtin PJ: Diffuse large B-cell lymphoma with distinctive patterns of splenic and bone marrow involvement: clinicopathologic features of two cases, *Mod Pathol* 18:495-502, 2005.

250. Kremer M, Spitzer M, Mandl-Weber S et al: Discordant bone marrow involvement in diffuse large B-cell lymphoma: comparative molecular analysis reveals a heterogeneous group of disorders, *Lab Invest* 83:107-114, 2003.

251. Campbell JK, Matthews JP, Seymour JF et al: Optimum trephine length in the assessment of bone marrow involvement in patients with diffuse large cell lymphoma, *Ann Oncol* 14:273-276, 2003.

252. Luoni M, Declich P, De Paoli AP et al: Bone marrow biopsy for the staging of non-Hodgkin's lymphoma: bilateral or unilateral trephine biopsy? *Tumori* 81:410-413, 1995.

253. Wang J, Weiss LM, Chang KL et al: Diagnostic utility of bilateral bone marrow examination: significance of morphologic and ancillary technique study in malignancy, *Cancer* 94:1522-1531, 2002.

254. Robertson LE, Redman JR, Butler JJ et al: Discordant bone marrow involvement in diffuse large-cell lymphoma: a distinct clinical-pathologic entity associated with a continuous risk of relapse, *J Clin Oncol* 9:236-242, 1991.

255. Yan Y, Chan WC, Weisenburger DD et al: Clinical and prognostic significance of bone marrow involvement in patients with diffuse aggressive B-cell lymphoma, *J Clin Oncol* 13:1336-1342, 1995.

256. Park S, Lee J, Ko YH et al: The impact of Epstein-Barr virus status on clinical outcome in diffuse large B-cell lymphoma, *Blood* 110:972-978, 2007.

257. Sevilla DW, Weeden EM, Alexander S et al: Nodular pattern of bone marrow infiltration: frequent finding in immunosuppression-related EBV-associated large B-cell lymphomas, *Virchows Arch* 455:323-336, 2009.

258. Cadranel J, Wislez M, Antoine M: Primary pulmonary lymphoma, *Eur Respir J* 20:750-762, 2002.

259. Skinnider BF, Connors JM, Gascoyne RDL: Bone marrow involvement in T-cell-rich B-cell lymphoma, *Am J Clin Pathol* 108:570-578, 1997.

260. Macon WR, Williams ME, Greer JP et al: T-cell-rich B-cell lymphomas: a clinicopathologic study of 19 cases, *Am J Surg Pathol* 16:351-363, 1992.

261. Scarpa A, Bonetti F, Zamboni G et al: T-cell-rich B-cell lymphoma, *Am J Surg Pathol* 13:335-337, 1989.

262. Nakamura S, Ponzoni M, Campo E: Intravascular large B-cell lymphoma. In Swerdlow S, Campo E, Harris N et al, editors: *WHO classification: tumours of haematopoietic and lymphoid tissues*, ed 4, Lyon, 2008, IARC.

263. Ferreri AJ, Campo E, Seymour JF et al: Intravascular lymphoma: clinical presentation, natural history, management and prognostic factors in a series of 38 cases, with special emphasis on the "cutaneous variant," *Br J Haematol* 127:173-183, 2004.

264. Murase T, Yamaguchi M, Suzuki R et al: Intravascular large B-cell lymphoma (IVLBCL): a clinicopathologic study of 96 cases with special reference to the immunophenotypic heterogeneity of CD5, *Blood* 109:478-485, 2007.

265. Dufau JP, Le Tourneau A, Molina T et al: Intravascular large B-cell lymphoma with bone marrow involvement at presentation and haemophagocytic syndrome: two Western cases in favour of a specific variant, *Histopathology* 37:509-512, 2000.

266. DiGiuseppe JA, Nelson WG, Seifter EJ et al: Intravascular lymphomatosis: a clinicopathologic study of 10 cases and assessment of response to chemotherapy, *J Clin Oncol* 12:2573-2579, 1994.

267. Tucker TJ, Bardales RH, Miranda RN: Intravascular lymphomatosis with bone marrow involvement, *Arch Pathol Lab Med* 123:952-956, 1999.

268. Gordon DS, Jones BM, Browning SW et al: Persistent polyclonal lymphocytosis of B lymphocytes, *N Engl J Med* 307:232-236, 1982.

269. Feugier P, De March AK, Lesesve JF et al: Intravascular bone marrow accumulation in persistent polyclonal lymphocytosis: a misleading feature for B-cell neoplasm, *Mod Pathol* 17:1087-1096, 2004.

270. Delage R, Roy J, Jacques L, Darveau A: All patients with persistent polyclonal B cell lymphocytosis present bcl-2/Ig gene rearrangements, *Leuk Lymphoma* 31:567-574, 1998.

271. Soussain C, Patte C, Ostronoff M et al: Small noncleaved cell lymphoma and leukemia in adults: a retrospective study of 65 adults treated with the LMB pediatric protocols, *Blood* 85:664-674, 1995.

272. Cairo MS, Sposto R, Perkins SL et al: Burkitt's and Burkitt-like lymphoma in children and adolescents: a review of the Children's Cancer Group experience, *Br J Haematol* 120:660-670, 2003.

273. Borowitz MJ, Hunger SP, Carroll AJ et al: Predictability of the t(1;19)(q23;p13) from surface antigen phenotype: implications for screening cases of childhood acute lymphoblastic leukemia for molecular analysis: a Pediatric Oncology Group study, *Blood* 82:1086-1091, 1993.

274. Cho YU, Chi HS, Park CJ et al: Distinct features of angioimmunoblastic T-cell lymphoma with bone marrow involvement, *Am J Clin Pathol* 131:640-646, 2009.

275. Gaulard P, Kanavaros P, Farcet JP et al: Bone marrow histologic and immunohistochemical findings in peripheral T-cell lymphoma: a study of 38 cases, *Hum Pathol* 22:331-338, 1991.

276. Attygalle A, Al-Jehani R, Diss TC et al: Neoplastic T cells in angioimmunoblastic T-cell lymphoma express CD10, *Blood* 99:627-633, 2002.

277. Lachenal F, Berger F, Ghesquieres H et al: Angioimmunoblastic T-cell lymphoma: clinical and laboratory features at diagnosis in 77 patients, *Medicine (Baltimore)* 86:282-292, 2007.

278. Fraga M, Brousset P, Schlaifer D et al: Bone marrow involvement in anaplastic large cell lymphoma: immunohistochemical detection of minimal disease and its prognostic significance, *Am J Clin Pathol* 103:82-89, 1995.

279. Mussolin L, Pillon M, d'Amore ES et al: Prevalence and clinical implications of bone marrow involvement in pediatric anaplastic large cell lymphoma, *Leukemia* 19:1643-1647, 2005.

280. Benner MF, Willemze R: Bone marrow examination has limited value in the staging of patients with an anaplastic large cell lymphoma first presenting in the skin: retrospective analysis of 107 patients, *Br J Dermatol* 159:1148-1151, 2008.

281. Weinberg OK, Seo K, Arber DA: Prevalence of bone marrow involvement in systemic anaplastic large cell lymphoma: are immunohistochemical studies necessary? *Hum Pathol* 39:1331-1340, 2008.

282. Bayle C, Charpentier A, Duchayne E et al: Leukaemic presentation of small cell variant anaplastic large cell lymphoma: report of four cases, *Br J Haematol* 104:680-688, 1999.

283. Grewal JS, Smith LB, Winegarden JD III et al: Highly aggressive ALK-positive anaplastic large cell lymphoma with a leukemic phase and multi-organ involvement: a report of three cases and a review of the literature, *Ann Hematol* 86:499-508, 2007.

284. Wong KF, Chan JK, Matutes E et al: Hepatosplenic gamma delta T-cell lymphoma: a distinctive aggressive lymphoma type, *Am J Surg Pathol* 19:718-726, 1995.

285. Belhadj K, Reyes F, Farcet JP et al: Hepatosplenic gammadelta T-cell lymphoma is a rare clinicopathologic entity with poor outcome: report on a series of 21 patients, *Blood* 102:4261-4269, 2003.

286. Cooke CB, Krenacs L, Stetler-Stevenson M et al: Hepatosplenic T-cell lymphoma: a distinct clinicopathologic entity of cytotoxic gamma delta T-cell origin, *Blood* 88:4265-4274, 1996.

287. Kadin ME, Kamoun M, Lamberg J: Erythrophagocytic T gamma lymphoma: a clinicopathologic entity resembling malignant histiocytosis, *N Engl J Med* 304:648-653, 1981.

288. Abramson JS, Kotton CN, Elias N et al: Case records of the Massachusetts General Hospital: case 8-2008—a 33-year-old man with fever, abdominal pain, and pancytopenia after renal transplantation, *N Engl J Med* 358:1176-1187, 2008.

289. Marafioti T, Paterson JC, Ballabio E et al: Novel markers of normal and neoplastic human plasmacytoid dendritic cells, *Blood* 111:3778-3792, 2008.

290. Vega F, Medeiros LJ, Bueso-Ramos C et al: Hepatosplenic gamma/delta T-cell lymphoma in bone marrow: a sinusoidal neoplasm with blastic cytologic features, *Am J Clin Pathol* 116:410-419, 2001.

291. Farcet JP, Gaulard P, Marolleau JP et al: Hepatosplenic T-cell lymphoma: sinusal/sinusoidal localization of malignant cells expressing the T-cell receptor gamma delta, *Blood* 75:2213-2219, 1990.

292. Marti RM, Estrach T, Reverter JC et al: Utility of bone marrow and liver biopsies for staging cutaneous T-cell lymphoma, *Int J Dermatol* 35:450-454, 1996.

293. Salhany KE, Greer JP, Cousar JB, Collins RD: Marrow involvement in cutaneous T-cell lymphoma: a clinicopathologic study of 60 cases, *Am J Clin Pathol* 92:747-754, 1989.

294. Olsen E, Vonderheid E, Pimpinelli N et al: Revisions to the staging and classification of mycosis fungoides and Sézary syndrome: a proposal of the International Society for Cutaneous Lymphomas (ISCL) and the Cutaneous Lymphoma Task Force of the European Organization of Research and Treatment of Cancer (EORTC), *Blood* 110:1713-1722, 2007.

295. Beylot-Barry M, Parrens M, Delaunay M et al: Is bone marrow biopsy necessary in patients with mycosis fungoides and Sézary syndrome? A histological and molecular study at diagnosis and during follow-up, *Br J Dermatol* 152:1378-1379, 2005.

296. Zackheim HS, Amin S, Kashani-Sabet M, McMillan A: Prognosis in cutaneous T-cell lymphoma by skin stage: long-term survival in 489 patients, *J Am Acad Dermatol* 40:418-425, 1999.

297. Sibaud V, Beylot-Barry M, Thiebaut R et al: Bone marrow histopathologic and molecular staging in epidermotropic T-cell lymphomas, *Am J Clin Pathol* 119:414-423, 2003.

298. Lopez-Guillermo A, Cid J, Salar A et al: Peripheral T-cell lymphomas: initial features, natural history, and prognostic factors in a series of 174 patients diagnosed according to the R.E.A.L. classification, *Ann Oncol* 9:849-855, 1998.

299. Willemze R, Jansen PM, Cerroni L et al: Subcutaneous panniculitis–like T-cell lymphoma: definition, classification, and prognostic factors: an EORTC Cutaneous Lymphoma Group study of 83 cases, *Blood* 111:838-845, 2008.

300. Gallamini A, Stelitano C, Calvi R et al: Peripheral T-cell lymphoma unspecified (PTCL-U): a new prognostic model from a retrospective multicentric clinical study, *Blood* 103:2474-2479, 2004.

301. Mahoney DH Jr, Schreuders LC, Gresik MV, McClain KL: Role of staging bone marrow examination in children with Hodgkin disease, *Med Pediatr Oncol* 30:175-177, 1998.

302. Franco V, Tripodo C, Rizzo A et al: Bone marrow biopsy in Hodgkin's lymphoma, *Eur J Haematol* 73:149-155, 2004.

303. Howell SJ, Grey M, Chang J et al: The value of bone marrow examination in the staging of Hodgkin's lymphoma: a review of 955 cases seen in a regional cancer centre, *Br J Haematol* 119:408-411, 2002.

304. Diehl V, Sextro M, Franklin J et al: Clinical presentation, course, and prognostic factors in lymphocyte-predominant Hodgkin's disease and lymphocyte-rich classical Hodgkin's disease: report from the European Task Force on Lymphoma Project on Lymphocyte-Predominant Hodgkin's Disease, *J Clin Oncol* 1999;17:776-783, 1999.

305. Munker R, Hasenclever D, Brosteanu O et al: Bone marrow involvement in Hodgkin's disease: an analysis of 135 consecutive cases—German Hodgkin's Lymphoma Study Group, *J Clin Oncol* 13:403-409, 1995.

306. National Comprehensive Cancer Network Clinical Practice Guidelines, www.nccn.org/professionals/physician_gls/PDF/hodgkins.pdf, accessed 4/15/10.

307. Vassilakopoulos TP, Angelopoulou MK, Constantinou N et al: Development and validation of a clinical prediction rule for bone marrow involvement in patients with Hodgkin lymphoma, *Blood* 105:1875-1880, 2005.

308. Ponzoni M, Fumagalli L, Rossi G et al: Isolated bone marrow manifestation of HIV-associated Hodgkin lymphoma, *Mod Pathol* 2002;15:1273-1278, 2002.

309. Karcher DS: Clinically unsuspected Hodgkin disease presenting initially in the bone marrow of patients infected with the human immunodeficiency virus, *Cancer* 71:1235-1238, 1993.

310. Rappaport H, Berard CW, Butler JJ et al: Report of the Committee on Histopathological Criteria Contributing to Staging of Hodgkin's Disease, *Cancer Res* 31:1864-1865, 1971.

311. Moid F, DePalma L: Comparison of relative value of bone marrow aspirates and bone marrow trephine biopsies in the diagnosis of solid tumor metastasis and Hodgkin lymphoma: institutional experience and literature review, *Arch Pathol Lab Med* 129:497-501, 2005.

312. Brunning RD, Bloomfield CD, McKenna RW, Peterson LA: Bilateral trephine bone marrow biopsies in lymphoma and other neoplastic diseases, *Ann Intern Med* 82:365-366, 1975.

313. Joshi A, Aqel NM: Hodgkin's disease of bone marrow masquerading as a heavy plasma cell infiltration and fibrosis, *Br J Haematol* 122:343, 2003.

314. Te Velde J, Den Ottolander GJ, Spaander PJ et al: The bone marrow in Hodgkin's disease: the non-involved marrow, *Histopathology* 2:31-46, 1978.

315. Kojima H, Takei N, Mukai Y et al: Hemophagocytic syndrome as the primary clinical symptom of Hodgkin's disease, *Ann Hematol* 82:53-56, 2003.

316. Khoury JD, Jones D, Yared MA et al: Bone marrow involvement in patients with nodular lymphocyte predominant Hodgkin lymphoma, *Am J Surg Pathol* 28:489-495, 2004.

317. Auger MJ, Nash JR, Mackie MJ: Marrow involvement with T cell lymphoma initially presenting as abnormal myelopoiesis, *J Clin Pathol* 39:134-137, 1986.

318. Sacks EL, Donaldson SS, Gordon J, Dorfman RF: Epithelioid granulomas associated with Hodgkin's disease: clinical correlations in 55 previously untreated patients, *Cancer* 41:562-567, 1978.

319. Schmidt HH, Hofler G, Beham-Schmid C et al: Bone marrow granulomas in hairy cell leukaemia, *Histopathology* 29:291-292, 1996.

320. Allory Y, Challine D, Haioun C et al: Bone marrow involvement in lymphomas with hemophagocytic syndrome at presentation: a clinicopathologic study of 11 patients in a Western institution, *Am J Surg Pathol* 25:865-874, 2001.

321. Takeshita M, Kikuchi M, Ohshima K et al: Bone marrow findings in malignant histiocytosis and/or malignant lymphoma with concurrent hemophagocytic syndrome, *Leuk Lymphoma* 12:79-89, 1993.

CHAPTER 14

Intravascular Lymphomas

Judith A. Ferry

INTRODUCTION

Intravascular lymphoma was first described in 1959 by Pfleger and Tappeiner,[1] but because of its localization within blood vessels, it initially was thought to be a neoplasm of endothelial origin. Over the following years, it was called "malignant angioendotheliomatosis" and "neoplastic angioendotheliosis," reflecting this concept.[2-4] With the advent of immunohistochemistry, it became clear that the neoplastic cells were actually lymphoid in origin,[5-7] and the neoplasm received new names, including *angiotropic lymphoma*[6] and *intravascular lymphomatosis*.[7]

Most intravascular lymphomas are B-lineage, and intravascular large B-cell lymphoma now is recognized as a distinct entity by the World Health Organization (WHO), which defined it as a rare subtype of extranodal diffuse large B-cell lymphoma characterized by the selective growth of neoplastic cells within the lumens of small blood vessels[8] (some cases with minor extravascular components of lymphoma nonetheless are considered examples of the same disease[9]). Within the entity of intravascular large B-cell lymphoma are the classical, visceral form of the disease (also referred to as the "Western form" of intravascular large B-cell lymphoma), a cutaneous variant, and an Asian variant, each with distinct distribution of disease and different clinical manifestations (Table 14-1).

INTRAVASCULAR LARGE B-CELL LYMPHOMA

Classical Form of Intravascular Large B-Cell Lymphoma

Clinical Features

Intravascular large B-cell lymphoma affects middle-aged and older adults. Patients present with protean symptoms related to vascular obstruction in a wide variety of extranodal sites. Fever also is common.[9-11] The onset of symptoms usually is subacute. Intravascular large B-cell lymphoma usually is disseminated at presentation. Sites commonly involved include the central nervous system (CNS), kidneys, adrenals, lungs, and skin, but many other sites can be involved, including the liver, heart, gastrointestinal tract, and genitourinary tract (Figures 14-1 through 14-3).[9,12-16] Some series report a subset of patients with involvement of the spleen and bone marrow.[17]

The most common findings at presentation are related to CNS involvement; they include confusion; lethargy; dementia; seizures; abnormalities of gait, speech, and vision; and others.[9,11] Renal involvement often manifests as proteinuria and renal insufficiency; some patients have hematuria.[10,12,18-20] Because of the frequency of renal involvement, biopsy of the kidney has been suggested as an effective means of establishing a diagnosis of intravascular large B-cell lymphoma.[18] Rare cases of intravascular large B-cell lymphoma appear to be limited to the kidney; patients with "kidney limited" intravascular large B-cell lymphoma appear to have a good outcome when treated with aggressive combination chemotherapy,[20] but more experience is required to confirm the existence of this possible variant and to delineate its clinicopathologic characteristics. Among adrenal lymphomas, a relatively high proportion (25% in one study) exhibits intravascular growth.[21] Extensive bilateral adrenal involvement by intravascular lymphoma can be associated with adrenal insufficiency.[9,22] Pulmonary involvement leads to dyspnea. Despite the widespread intravascular involvement, neoplastic cells are only rarely identified in peripheral blood.[14,16]

In contrast to many other types of lymphoma, intravascular lymphoma tends to show preferential sparing of lymph nodes. The highly variable and nonspecific nature of the clinical findings often leads to a delay in diagnosis; some cases go undiagnosed until autopsy. Rare patients have a history

TABLE 14-1

Intravascular Large B-Cell Lymphomas			
Type of Lymphoma	**Patients Affected**	**Pathologic Findings**	**Prognosis**
Intravascular large B-cell lymphoma (IVLBCL), classical (or Western) form	Middle-aged and older adults	• *Sites involved:* CNS, kidneys, adrenals, lungs, skin, liver, heart, GI tract, GU tract, others • Lymph node and peripheral blood involvement uncommon	Historically poor, but better with prompt diagnosis and appropriate chemotherapy
IVLBCL, cutaneous variant	Younger patients than in classical form of IVLBCL; females affected more often than males	• *Sites involved:* Dermis, with or without subcutis	Better than for classical form of IVLBCL
IVLBCL, Asian variant	Asians; rare Westerners	• Hemophagocytosis and hepatosplenomegaly are characteristic • *Sites involved:* Bone marrow, liver, lungs, adrenals, others • Involvement of CNS and skin less common than in classical form	Similar to classical form of IVLBCL

CNS, Central nervous system; *GI*, gastrointestinal; *GU*, genitourinary.

of a low-grade B-cell lymphoma[10,14]; in these cases, the intravascular lymphoma may represent large cell transformation of the low-grade lymphoma.

The most common laboratory abnormalities are anemia, elevated lactate dehydrogenase (LDH) levels, and an elevated erythrocyte sedimentation rate. Radiographic studies often do not yield specific information. Neuroimaging studies do not detect abnormalities in all patients with intravascular lymphoma,[14] and when an abnormal result is found, the features often are not specific for lymphoma.[11]

Pathologic Features

On gross examination, tissues involved by intravascular lymphoma may show hemorrhage, necrosis, or vascular thrombosis; however, not all involved tissues show an obvious gross abnormality.[9] Small extravascular foci of lymphoma can be found in some cases, particularly if a complete autopsy is performed.[9,10]

The histologic hallmark of this disorder is blood vessels filled with and distended by large transformed lymphoid cells, usually with the appearance of centroblasts or immunoblasts, often without distortion of the architecture of the involved tissue (see Figures 14-1 through 14-3). The infiltrate may be associated with thrombosis. Rare cases have been described in which tumor cells are located within the blood vessels of other neoplasms, including renal cell carcinoma, hemangioma,[10] and lymphangioma.[23]

Immunophenotyping shows that these cells express the leukocyte common antigen (CD45) and pan–B-cell antigens such as CD20.[9,10] Co-expression of CD5 appears to be more common than in diffuse large B-cell lymphoma without intravascular spread.[23,24] CD5 expression in this setting does not indicate an association with chronic lymphocytic leukemia or mantle cell lymphoma.[23] Neoplastic cells usually are MUM1/IRF4+ and are CD10+ in a small minority of cases.[8,16] In one large Japanese series, 38% of cases were CD5+, and CD5+ cases differed from CD5– cases with respect to some features[25]; however, most of the cases in this series were examples of the Asian variant (see Asian Variant of Intravascular Large B-Cell Lymphoma, later in the chapter),[25] and the results could differ for cases

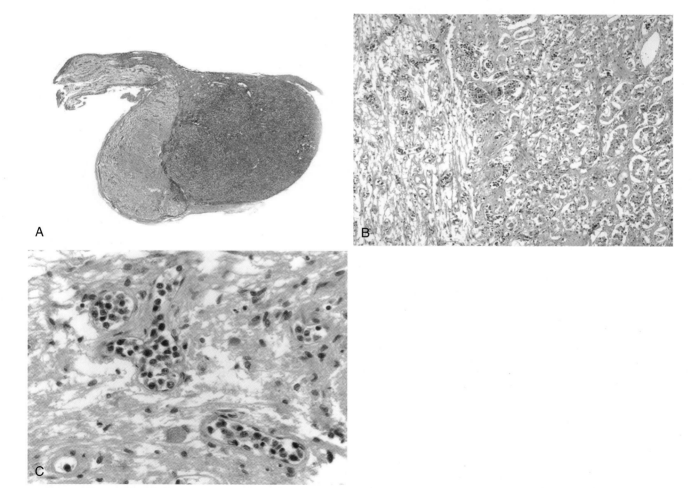

Figure 14-1 Intravascular large B-cell lymphoma involving the pituitary, at autopsy. **A,** Whole mount of the pituitary shows that its architecture is intact. Multiple small blood vessels contain small clusters of lymphoid cells, but they are not readily seen at low power. Higher power view shows involvement of both the anterior pituitary *(right)* and the posterior pituitary *(left)*. **C,** The stem of the pituitary also is involved by intravascular lymphoma. The large, dark neoplastic cells fill small blood vessels and are associated with slight dilatation of those blood vessels.

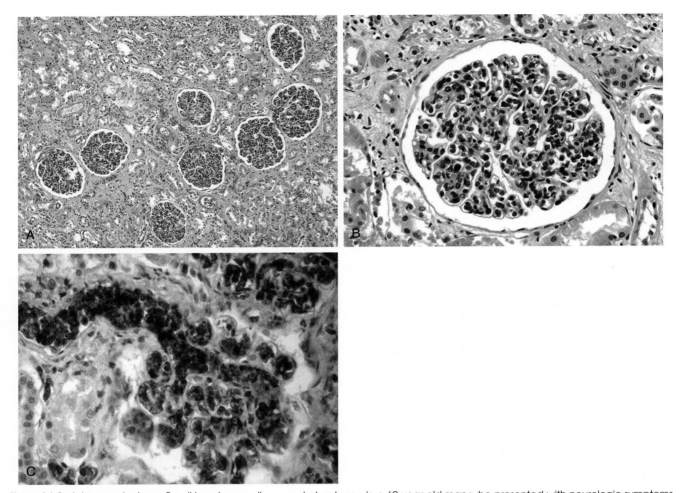

Figure 14-2   Intravascular large B-cell lymphoma, diagnosed at autopsy, in a 69-year-old man who presented with neurologic symptoms and with respiratory and renal failure. Intravascular lymphoma involved multiple sites, including the brain, leptomeninges, heart, lungs, liver, pancreas, thyroid, and kidney. **A,** This section of kidney shows glomeruli that are prominently hypercellular because of the presence of large lymphoid cells in glomerular capillaries. Large lymphoid cells are present in smaller numbers in peritubular capillaries. **B,** High-power view of a glomerulus shows numerous large, dark lymphoid cells filling glomerular capillaries. **C,** Lymphoid cells in vessels within and entering the glomerulus are CD45+. (Immunostain on a paraffin section.)

among Western patients. In a smaller series from the United States, the features of CD5+ cases were similar to those without CD5.[23]

We have seen a case of human herpes virus type 8–positive (HHV8+) intravascular large B-cell lymphoma in an HIV-positive male; intravascular large B-cell lymphoma positive for HHV8 had not been reported previously. As for other HHV8+ lymphomas, this intravascular lymphoma had an immunophenotype that corresponded to a late stage in B-cell differentiation (CD20–, MUM1/IRF4+, CD79a+; Figure 14-4).[26] (See Lymphomas of the Pleura and Pleural Cavity in Chapter 4 for additional information on HHV8+ lymphomas.)

Clonal rearrangement of the immunoglobulin heavy chain gene has been demonstrated in some cases of intravascular large B-cell lymphoma.[23] Although only a small number of cases has been studied, most cases appear to be characterized by the presence of somatic hypermutation, consistent with an origin from post-germinal center B cells, and most cases used the immunoglobulin heavy chain V_H3 gene family.[24] The proportion of replacement and silent mutations found on sequencing suggests that the cell of origin is not typically an antigen-selected B cell.[24]

Adequate tissue for conventional cytogenetics has been obtained in a relatively small number of cases, but intravascular large B-cell lymphoma is characterized by a complex karyotype, and both numeric and structural abnormalities commonly are found.[16] A subset of cases has additional chromosomal material from 11q (extra copies of chromosome 11 or duplications involving 11q) in the area of the mixed lineage leukemia *(MLL)* gene, leading to speculation about a role for this gene, or possibly another gene in the area, in the pathogenesis of a subset of cases of intravascular large B-cell lymphoma.[16]

The pathogenesis of this unusual lymphoma is uncertain; some have postulated that the neoplastic cells harbor a homing receptor defect.[9,27,28] Lack of the adhesion molecule CD54 (ICAM-1), as well as

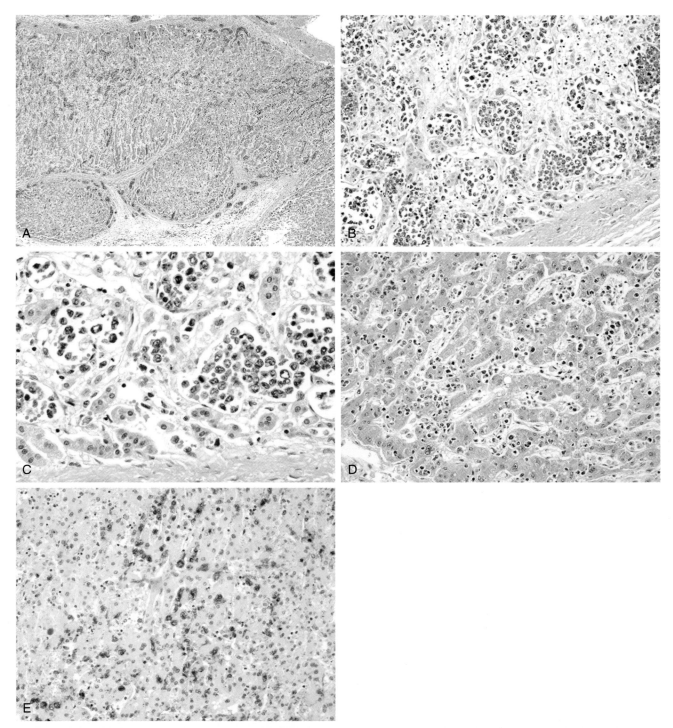

Figure 14-3   Intravascular large B-cell lymphoma, diagnosed at autopsy, in a 64-year-old woman who presented with fever, night sweats, weight loss, metabolic acidosis, and coagulopathy; she was thought to be septic. Postmortem examination revealed intravascular lymphoma involving multiple sites. **A,** Low-power examination of the adrenal shows viable adrenal gland with intact architecture but with many sinusoidal vascular spaces containing atypical lymphoid cells, most numerous in the right side of the image. **B,** Multiple thin-walled blood vessels are filled and distended by large lymphoid cells. **C,** The neoplastic cells are large discohesive cells with vesicular nuclei, distinct nucleoli, and scant cytoplasm. **D,** The hepatic sinusoids also contain large atypical lymphoid cells. **E,** The large cells in the sinusoids are CD20+. (Immunoperoxidase technique on paraffin sections.)

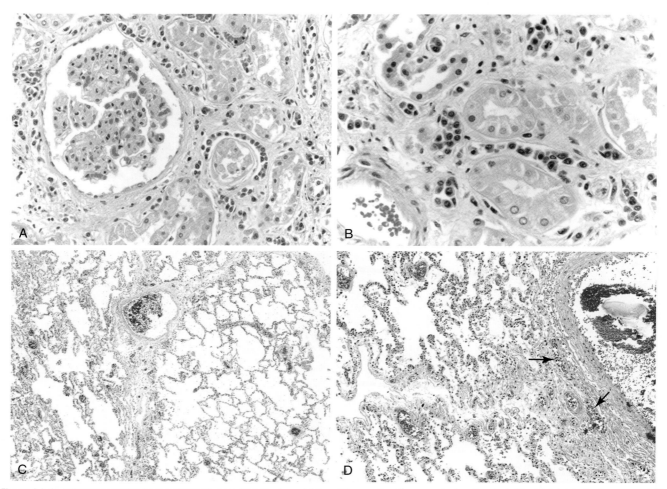

Figure 14-4   Intravascular large B-cell lymphoma, HHV8+, in an HIV-positive male, diagnosed at autopsy. **A,** The histologic features are similar to those of HHV8– intravascular large B-cell lymphomas. In the kidney in this case, lymphoma is more conspicuous in peritubular than in glomerular capillaries. **B,** High-power view shows small clusters and cords of atypical lymphoid cells in peritubular capillaries. Some atypical cells have moderately abundant, eccentrically placed cytoplasm, indicating plasmacytic differentiation. **C,** Low-power examination of the lung shows that the architecture is preserved, and abnormalities are subtle. **D,** On closer inspection, small blood vessels contain many nucleated cells *(arrows)*, and alveolar septae appear hypercellular.

CD29 (beta$_1$ integrin) expression by neoplastic cells, has been described; this is not specific for intravascular lymphoma, but it has been suggested to play a role in the intravascular localization and widespread distribution of intravascular lymphoma.[10]

A case of intravascular large B-cell lymphoma has been described, which presented with cutaneous involvement but likely also had systemic involvement, in which the neoplastic lymphoid cells expressed CXCR3 and the vascular endothelium expressed its ligand, CXCL9.[15] The interaction between CXCR3 and CXCL9 could have contributed to the intravascular localization of tumor cells in this case; whether this is an important factor in other intravascular large B-cell lymphomas remains to be investigated.

Staging, Treatment, and Outcome

The mortality rate for the classical form of intravascular large B-cell lymphoma is high, but the prognosis appears to be better when therapy appropriate for the

lymphoma is given in a timely manner. The high mortality rate is partly due to the unusual symptomatology, because of which diagnosis is delayed in many cases or is established only on postmortem examination. Patients promptly diagnosed and treated with anthracycline-containing chemotherapy have a better prognosis than those who do not receive that therapy. In one series, 52% of patients so treated achieved complete remission, and the 2-year overall survival rate was 46%.[17] Patients who receive chemotherapy in combination with rituximab appear to have a better outcome than those treated with conventional chemotherapy alone, although this has been best studied in Asian series (see Asian Variant of Intravascular Large B-Cell Lymphoma, later in the chapter).[29]

Differential Diagnosis

Once a biopsy of involved tissue has been obtained, establishment of a diagnosis usually is straightforward, provided careful attention is paid to the

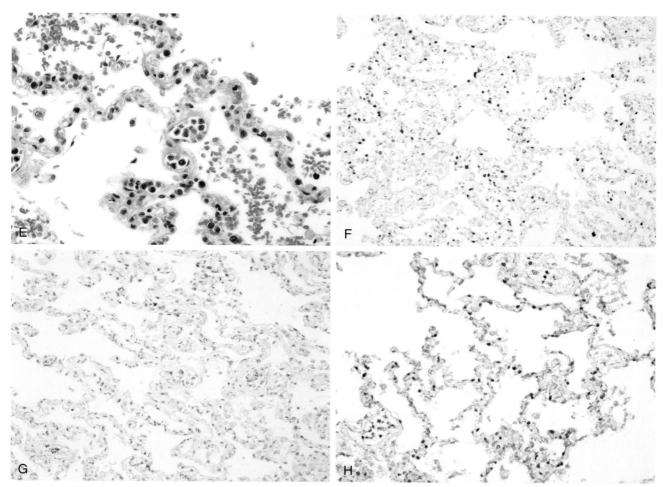

Figure 14-4, cont'd E, High-power view shows large lymphoid cells filling alveolar capillaries. **F,** Staining with antibody to HHV8 highlights neoplastic B cells in alveolar capillaries. **G** and **H,** The HHV8+ cells are negative for CD20 **(G),** in contrast to other intravascular large B-cell lymphomas; however, they express nuclear MUM1/IRF4 **(H),** which is consistent with a late stage in B-cell differentiation. (*F* to *H,* Immunoperoxidase technique on paraffin sections.)

morphology of cells present in blood vessels. The challenging aspect of establishing a diagnosis of intravascular lymphoma is that the clinical manifestations are nonspecific, often raising the question of nonneoplastic processes such as systemic inflammatory disorders, including infection. The neurologic manifestations can mimic cerebrovascular accident, encephalomyelitis, Guillain-Barré syndrome, vasculitis, multiple sclerosis, or some form of dementia.[11]

Cutaneous Variant of Intravascular Large B-Cell Lymphoma

The cutaneous variant of intravascular lymphoma is defined as being confined to the vessels of the skin. This type represents a minority of cases of intravascular lymphoma, accounting for 26% in one series.[14] These cases show a female preponderance, and the disease affects younger patients than are affected by the classical form of intravascular lymphoma.

Skin lesions may be single but more often are multiple; they are located mostly on the trunk and lower extremities. They take the form of erythematous or violaceous macules, plaques, nodules, or large tumors, sometimes with ulceration. The lesions often are painful.[14,30] Microscopic examination reveals large lymphoid cells in the lumens of blood vessels in the superficial and deep dermis and sometimes the subcutaneous tissue.[30]

Patients with the cutaneous variant have a better prognosis than those with the classical form,[14] and patients with single lesions have a better prognosis than those with multiple lesions.[14] Some patients who present with skin involvement also have systemic involvement[27]; these patients do not have the favorable prognosis associated with intravascular lymphoma confined to the skin. In one review, only 10% of patients with intravascular lymphoma confined to the skin died, whereas 85% of those who also had systemic involvement had a fatal outcome.[30] Cases with systemic involvement cannot be distinguished from those without such involvement on the basis of the appearance of the skin lesions[30]; this emphasizes the importance of careful staging.

The differential diagnosis on clinical grounds is broad, because intravascular lymphoma in the skin can mimic a variety of inflammatory disorders, including thrombophlebitis, erythema nodosum, and erysipelas.[30]

Asian Variant of Intravascular Large B-Cell Lymphoma

The Asian variant of intravascular lymphoma is characterized by bone marrow involvement and hemophagocytosis.[17,25,31] This variant affects middle-aged and older adults; the median age is in the late 60s. Men and women are affected roughly equally.[25,31,32] Nearly all cases of this type have been described among Asians; rare cases in Western patients may represent the same entity.[33] A history of some form of extranodal inflammatory disease (pulmonary or renal tuberculosis, tuberculous peritonitis, parasitic infection, hepatitis, and others) is reported in a number of cases[31]; whether this is coincidental is uncertain.

Common findings include fever, cytopenias, hepatosplenomegaly, respiratory insufficiency, and evidence of disseminated intravascular coagulation, usually without conspicuous involvement of the skin or central nervous system.

Pathologic evaluation reveals intravascular or intrasinusoidal large atypical lymphoid cells; the most common sites of involvement are the bone marrow, lungs, kidneys, liver, and adrenal glands. The bone marrow also shows hemophagocytosis.[17,31-34] In one large series, 24% of cases had peripheral blood involvement[25]; this feature thus may be more common in the Asian variant than in the classical form of intravascular large B-cell lymphoma. The neoplastic cells are large B cells that are reported to be CD20+ and CD79a+,[32,34] with CD5 expression in a subset of cases.[31,32,34] In one large Japanese series in which most of the cases were examples of the Asian variant, CD5 was expressed in 38% of cases, CD10 in 13%, bcl6 in 26%, bcl2 in 91%, and MUM1/IRF4 in 95%.[25] Among the CD10− cases, CD5 expression was associated with a higher risk of bone marrow or blood involvement and a lower frequency of neurologic abnormalities.[25] The cases studied have shown no evidence of infection with Epstein-Barr virus (EBV), human T-cell leukemia virus type 1 (HTLV-1), or human herpes virus type 8 (HHV8).[25,31] Cytogenetic analysis typically shows complex abnormalities.[31,34]

The lymphomas have been associated with a poor prognosis. Patients often develop multiorgan failure, and in some series, most patients succumbed to lymphoma.[31-33] However, some patients treated with combination chemotherapy have long-term survival,[31] and the addition of the anti-CD20 monoclonal antibody rituximab to the treatment regimen may improve the prognosis.[34] In one large series, those receiving rituximab achieved complete remission more often than those who did not (82% versus 51%); they also had a superior 2-year overall survival rate (66% versus 46%).[29]

In contrast to the usual type of intravascular lymphoma, in the Asian variant, liver, spleen, and marrow involvement and hemophagocytosis are characteristic, and neurologic and cutaneous manifestations are uncommon. Not all cases of intravascular lymphoma that arise in Asians are the Asian variant. Some Asian patients have intravascular lymphoma without hemophagocytosis and have clinical and pathologic features similar to those of Western patients with classical intravascular lymphoma.[17]

■ INTRAVASCULAR LYMPHOMA, T-LINEAGE

Infrequent cases of intravascular lymphoma are T-lineage. In one series of 38 cases of intravascular lymphoma, only one was T-lineage.[14] Intravascular T-cell lymphoma mainly affects middle-aged and older adults, although a few cases in younger patients have been described. A slight male preponderance is seen.[35] Presentation with cutaneous lesions is common; staging often reveals widespread visceral involvement,[35] although T-cell intravascular lymphoma confined to the skin also has been described.[30] The clinical appearance of the lesions is similar to that of intravascular large B-cell lymphoma.[30]

Microscopic examination shows medium-sized to large atypical lymphoid cells in dilated vascular lumens, sometimes with a sparse perivascular inflammatory cell infiltrate.[35] Detailed immunophenotyping has not been performed consistently, but most cases have been CD3+ and CD45RO+, with variable expression of CD5 and with CD4 or CD8 expression in a minority of cases. A few cases have been positive for CD56 and for cytotoxic granule proteins (TIA-1, perforin, granzyme B), and also for EBV by in situ hybridization; the possibility that some of these cases actually are of natural killer (NK)-cell origin cannot be excluded, because clonal T-cell gene rearrangement has not been demonstrated in some of these cases. A well-documented case of T-lineage, CD8+, EBV+ intravascular lymphoma has been described in an HIV-positive man.[36] T-cell intravascular lymphomas with and without hemophagocytosis have been described,[17] analogous to the Asian and classical types of intravascular large B-cell lymphoma.

Intravascular T-cell lymphoma has a poor prognosis; most patients succumb to the disease in less than 1 year.[35] Currently, the distinction between intravascular lymphoma of T-cell origin and that of NK-cell origin (see the following section) is not clinically significant, because the two appear to have similar behavior.

■ INTRAVASCULAR LYMPHOMA, NK-LINEAGE

Rare cases of intravascular lymphoma of NK lineage have been described in adults 41 to 71 years of age.[35,37,38] These patients presented with cutaneous lesions (erythematous plaques, patches, or nodules) or evidence of widespread disease (fever, neurologic symptoms, pancytopenia). All had large atypical lymphoid cells confined to vascular lumens.

The usual immunophenotype of the affected cells was CD2+, CD3+, and CD7+ or CD7−, CD4−, CD8−, CD5−, and CD56+; the cells also were positive for cytotoxic granule proteins (TIA-1, perforin, and/or granzyme B) and did not express B-cell, myeloid, or histiocytic markers. T-cell receptor *(TCR)* and immunoglobulin heavy chain *(IGH)* genes did not show clonal rearrangements. EBV was detected by in situ hybridization in most cases. Follow-up was limited. Patients with disease apparently confined to the skin at presentation sometimes did well, but most patients developed progressive disease and died.[35,37,38] The disease may have a rapidly fatal course.[38]

REFERENCES

1. Pfleger L, Tappeiner J: Zur Kenntnis der systemisierten Endotheliomatose der cutanen Blutgefässe (Reticuloendotheliose?), *Hautarzt* 10:359-363, 1959.
2. Fulling K, Gersell D: Neoplastic angioendotheliomatosis: histologic, immunohistochemical, and ultrastructural findings in two cases, *Cancer* 51:1107-1118, 1983.
3. Petito CK, Gottlieb GJ, Dougherty JH, Petito FA: Neoplastic angioendotheliosis: ultrastructural study and review of the literature, *Ann Neurol* 3:393-399, 1978.
4. Keahey T, Guerry D, Tuthill R, Bondi E: Malignant angioendotheliomatosis proliferans treated with doxorubicin, *Arch Dermatol* 118:512-514, 1982.
5. Ansell J, Bhawan J, Cohen S et al: Histiocytic lymphoma and malignant angioendotheliomatosis: one disease or two? *Cancer* 50:1506-1512, 1982.
6. Sheibani K, Battifora H, Winberg C et al: Further evidence that "malignant angioendotheliomatosis" is an angiotropic large-cell lymphoma, *N Engl J Med* 314:943-948, 1986.
7. Wick M, Mills S, Scheithauer B et al: Reassessment of malignant "angioendotheliomatosis": evidence in favor of its reclassification as "intravascular lymphoma," *Am J Surg Pathol* 10:112-123, 1986.
8. Nakamura S, Ponzoni M, Campo E: Intravascular large B-cell lymphoma. In Swerdlow S, Campo E, Harris N et al, editors: *WHO classification: tumours of haematopoietic and lymphoid tissues,* ed 4, Lyon, 2008, IARC.
9. Ferry JA, Harris NL, Picker LJ et al: Intravascular lymphomatosis (malignant angioendotheliomatosis): a B-cell neoplasm expressing surface homing receptors, *Mod Pathol* 1:444-452, 1988.
10. Ponzoni M, Arrigoni G, Gould VE et al: Lack of CD 29 (beta1 integrin) and CD 54 (ICAM-1) adhesion molecules in intravascular lymphomatosis, *Hum Pathol* 31:220-226, 2000.
11. Zuckerman D, Seliem R, Hochberg E: Intravascular lymphoma: the oncologist's "great imitator," *Oncologist* 11:496-502, 2006.
12. DiGiuseppe JA, Nelson WG, Seifter EJ et al: Intravascular lymphomatosis: a clinicopathologic study of 10 cases and assessment of response to chemotherapy, *J Clin Oncol* 12:2573-2579, 1994.
13. Stroup RM, Sheibani K, Moncada A et al: Angiotropic (intravascular) large cell lymphoma: a clinicopathologic study of seven cases with unique clinical presentations, *Cancer* 66:1781-1788, 1990.
14. Ferreri AJ, Campo E, Seymour JF et al: Intravascular lymphoma: clinical presentation, natural history, management and prognostic factors in a series of 38 cases, with special emphasis on the "cutaneous variant," *Br J Haematol* 127:173-183, 2004.
15. Kato M, Ohshima K, Mizuno M et al: Analysis of CXCL9 and CXCR3 expression in a case of intravascular large B-cell lymphoma, *J Am Acad Dermatol* 61:888-891, 2009.
16. Deisch J, Fuda FB, Chen W et al: Segmental tandem triplication of the MLL gene in an intravascular large B-cell lymphoma with multisystem involvement: a comprehensive morphologic, immunophenotypic, cytogenetic, and molecular cytogenetic antemortem study, *Arch Pathol Lab Med* 133:1477-1482, 2009.
17. Ferreri AJ, Dognini GP, Campo E et al: Variations in clinical presentation, frequency of hemophagocytosis and clinical behavior of intravascular lymphoma diagnosed in different geographical regions, *Haematologica* 92:486-492, 2007.
18. Agar JWM, Gates PC, Vaughan SL, Machet D: Renal biopsy in angiotropic large cell lymphoma, *Am J Kidney Dis* 24:92-96, 1994.
19. Ferry JA, Harris NL, Papanicolaou N, Young RH: Lymphoma of the kidney: a report of 11 cases, *Am J Surg Pathol* 19:134-144, 1995.
20. Kameoka Y, Takahashi N, Komatsuda A et al: Kidney-limited intravascular large B cell lymphoma: a distinct variant of IVLBCL? *Int J Hematol* 89:533-537, 2009.
21. Ohsawa M, Tomita Y, Hashimoto M et al: Malignant lymphoma of the adrenal gland: its possible correlation with the Epstein-Barr virus, *Mod Pathol* 9:534-543, 1996.
22. Levy N, Young WJ, Habermann T et al: Adrenal insufficiency as a manifestation of disseminated non-Hodgkin's lymphoma, *Mayo Clin Proc* 72:818-822, 1997.
23. Khalidi HS, Brynes RK, Browne P et al: Intravascular large B-cell lymphoma: the CD5 antigen is expressed by a subset of cases, *Mod Pathol* 11:983-988, 1998.
24. Kanda M, Suzumiya J, Ohshima K et al: Analysis of the immunoglobulin heavy chain gene variable region of intravascular large B-cell lymphoma, *Virchows Arch* 439:540-546, 2001.
25. Murase T, Yamaguchi M, Suzuki R et al: Intravascular large B-cell lymphoma (IVLBCL): a clinicopathologic study of 96 cases with special reference to the immunophenotypic heterogeneity of CD5, *Blood* 109:478-485, 2007.
26. Ferry JA, Sohani AR, Longtine JA et al: HHV8-positive, EBV-positive Hodgkin lymphoma-like large B-cell lymphoma and HHV8-positive intravascular large B-cell lymphoma, *Mod Pathol* 22:618-626, 2009.
27. Kutzner H, Jaffe E: Intravascular large B-cell lymphoma. In LeBoit P, Burg G, Weedon D, Sarasin A, editors: *Pathology and genetics: skin tumours,* Lyon, 2006, IARC.
28. Gatter K, Warnke R: Intravascular large B-cell lymphoma. In Jaffe E, Harris N, Stein H, Vardiman J, editors: *Pathology and genetics of tumours of haematopoietic and lymphoid tissues,* Lyon, 2001, IARC.
29. Shimada K, Matsue K, Yamamoto K et al: Retrospective analysis of intravascular large B-cell lymphoma treated with rituximab-containing chemotherapy as reported by the IVL study group in Japan, *J Clin Oncol* 26:3189-3195, 2008.
30. Roglin J, Boer A: Skin manifestations of intravascular lymphoma mimic inflammatory diseases of the skin, *Br J Dermatol* 157:16-25, 2007.
31. Murase T, Nakamura S, Kawauchi K et al: An Asian variant of intravascular large B-cell lymphoma: clinical, pathological and cytogenetic approaches to diffuse large B-cell lymphoma associated with haemophagocytic syndrome, *Br J Haematol* 111:826-834, 2000.
32. Narimatsu H, Morishita Y, Saito S et al: Usefulness of bone marrow aspiration for definite diagnosis of Asian variant of intravascular lymphoma: four autopsied cases, *Leuk Lymphoma* 45:1611-1616, 2004.
33. Dufau JP, Le Tourneau A, Molina T et al: Intravascular large B-cell lymphoma with bone marrow involvement at presentation and haemophagocytic syndrome: two Western cases in favour of a specific variant, *Histopathology* 37:509-512, 2000.
34. Shimizu I, Ichikawa N, Yotsumoto M et al: Asian variant of intravascular lymphoma: aspects of diagnosis and the role of rituximab, *Intern Med* 46:1381-1386, 2007.

35. Cerroni L, Massone C, Kutzner H et al: Intravascular large T-cell or NK-cell lymphoma: a rare variant of intravascular large cell lymphoma with frequent cytotoxic phenotype and association with Epstein-Barr virus infection, *Am J Surg Pathol* 32:891-898, 2008.

36. Merchant SH, Viswanatha DS, Zumwalt RE, Foucar K: Epstein-Barr virus–associated intravascular large T-cell lymphoma presenting as acute renal failure in a patient with acquired immune deficiency syndrome, *Hum Pathol* 34:950-954, 2003.

37. Kuo TT, Chen MJ, Kuo MC: Cutaneous intravascular NK-cell lymphoma: report of a rare variant associated with Epstein-Barr virus, *Am J Surg Pathol* 30:1197-1201, 2006.

38. Wu H, Said JW, Ames ED et al: First reported cases of intravascular large cell lymphoma of the NK cell type: clinical, histologic, immunophenotypic, and molecular features, *Am J Clin Pathol* 123:603-611, 2005.

INDEX

Note: Page numbers followed by "b" indicate boxes, "f" figures; "t" tables.